# Interpersonal Relationships

# Interpersonal Relationships

## Professional Communication Skills for Nurses

*third edition*

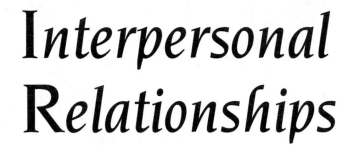

Elizabeth Arnold, PhD, RN, CS-P
Associate Professor
University of Maryland
School of Nursing
Baltimore, Maryland

Kathleen Underman Boggs, PhD, FNP-C
Associate Professor
Family Nurse Practitioner Program
University of North Carolina at Charlotte
Charlotte, North Carolina

**W.B. SAUNDERS COMPANY**
*A Division of Harcourt Brace & Company*
Philadelphia    London    Toronto    Montreal    Sydney    Tokyo

**W.B. SAUNDERS COMPANY**
*A Division of Harcourt Brace & Company*

The Curtis Center
Independence Square West
Philadelphia, Pennsylvania 19106

**Library of Congress Cataloging-in-Publication Data**

Arnold, Elizabeth.
Interpersonal relationships : professional communication skills for nurses / Elizabeth Nolan Arnold, Kathleen Underman Boggs.—3rd ed.

p.     cm.

Includes bibliographical references and index.

ISBN 0–7216–8103–4

1. Nurse and patient.     2. Interpersonal communication.     I. Boggs, Kathleen Underman.     II. Title.

RT86.3.A76 1999     610.73′06′99—dc21                                                                 98-38372

INTERPERSONAL RELATIONSHIPS:
PROFESSIONAL COMMUNICATION SKILLS FOR NURSES                       ISBN 0–7216–8103–4

Last digit is the print number:     9     8     7     6     5     4     3     2     1

To my beloved husband, George B. Arnold

*Elizabeth Arnold*


In memory of
Eileen Kelly Underman and Rita Weiber Boggs

*Kathleen Underman Boggs*

# Contributors

**Kristin Lynn Bussell, MS, RN, CS-P**
Clinical and Classroom Instructor
University of Maryland
School of Nursing
Baltimore
Program Therapist
Developmental School Foundation
Rockville, Maryland

**Verna Benner Carson, PhD, RN, CS-P**
National Director of Restore Behavioral
 Health
Staff Builders Home Health & Hospice
Fallston, Maryland

**Ann O'Mara, PhD, RN, AOCN**
Assistant Professor
University of Maryland
School of Nursing
Baltimore, Maryland

**Judith W. Ryan, PhD, RN, CRNP**
Director of Clinical Support Services
EverCare
Linthicum, Maryland

**Shirley A. Smoyak, RN, PhD, FAAN**
Professor
The Bloustein School of Planning and Public
 Policy
The Institute for Health, Health Care Policy,
 and Aging Research
Rutgers University
New Brunswick

Adjunct Professor
University of Medicine and Dentistry of New
 Jersey
Robert Wood Johnson Medical School
School of Public Health
Family Health Track
New Brunswick, New Jersey

# Reviewers

**Shirley Anderson, MSN, RN**
Department of Health Sciences
Kirkwood Community College
Cedar Rapids, Iowa

**Joyce Begley, PhD, RN**
Baccalaureate and Graduate Nursing
Eastern Kentucky University
Richmond, Kentucky

**Janet Burton, MSN, RN**
Department of Nursing
Bob Jones University
Greenville, South Carolina

**Agnes J. Janoscrat, MSN, RN**
Department of Nursing
Delaware State University
Dover, Delaware

**David R. Langford, DNSc, RN**
Department of Family and Community Nursing
University of North Carolina at Charlotte
Charlotte, North Carolina

**Christine Massey, MSN, RN**
Department of Nursing
Barton College
Wilson, North Carolina

**Deena Nardi, MSN, RN**
Department of Nursing
Indiana University Northwest
Gary, Indiana

**Shirley Newberry, MSN, RN**
Department of Nursing
Winona State University
Winona, Minnesota

**Kathleen O'Connell, MSN, RN, NP**
Department of Nursing
Indiana University–Purdue University
Fort Wayne, Indiana

**Enid Rossi, MSN, RN**
Department of Nursing
Northern Arizona University
Flagstaff, Arizona

**Jo Stejskal, MSN, RN**
Department of Nursing
Winona State University
Winona, Minnesota

**Mary Wilhite, EdD, RN**
College of Nursing
University of North Dakota
Grand Forks, North Dakota

The authentic experience of understanding begins with communication. As nurses we are answerable to our clients, our profession, and ourselves to communicate with clients in a very specific sense, at once physical, psychological, and ethical regardless of what nursing intervention is employed. Despite the technological advances in diagnosis and treatments available to clients and their families, communication remains the single most important, and sometimes under-rated, dimension of nursing practice. We believe that the third edition of *Interpersonal Relationships: Professional Communication Skills for Nurses* will serve as a primary reference source for nurses seeking to improve their communication skills in a variety of health care settings. This text offers a comprehensive and critical analysis of the communication process that occurs with clients of all ages and in a variety of clinical situations.

The third edition strives to spell out the implications of the accountability and the shared reciprocity between nurse, client, and health care system for each client's health and well-being. As the health care system changes, so does the context of our communication with clients and other professionals. This edition has been revised to reflect current trends in health care, specifically shorter encounters, communication technology, and a greater focus on health promotion.

This edition presents new information on critical thinking skills, care of the grieving client, delegation, and incorporation of theoretical concepts related to changes in health care, as well as updated references and revised exercises. A wealth of experiential exercises offers you, as nurse and student, the opportunity to practice, observe, and critically evaluate your own communication skills and those of others. Case examples provide a basis for discussion by helping students to understand and appreciate clients' perspectives and needs. Communication principles assist the student to think through and experiment with alternative approaches to "human encounter with presence" in the daily care of clients and families.

The book is divided into five parts, using a format similar to that in the second edition of presenting the basic concepts of the chapter subject followed by clinical applications. Part I, Conceptual Foundations of Nurse–Client Relationships, provides a theoretical framework and professional guides to practice. Part II, The Nurse–Client Relationship, explores the essential components of this relationship. Two new chapters, one focused on ethical decision making and critical thinking skills and the other on communicating with the grieving client, broaden the therapeutic application of the communication process in contemporary health care. Part III, Therapeutic Communication, examines communication skills related to the needs of population groups. This material has been updated to reflect a greater emphasis on the client as partner in his or her health care. Part IV, Responding to Special Needs, addresses lifespan issues in communication as well as those with clients who require specific adaptations. Finally, Part V, Professional Issues, discusses issues pertaining to communication and documentation with other health care providers on delegation strategies and use of technology. As in previous editions, the third edition of *Interpersonal Relationships: Communication Skills for Nurses* has been designed for use as individual teaching modules or across the curriculum.

Those of us who accept the responsibility of professional nursing as a life commitment are most fortunate because we can constantly learn and grow professionally and personally from our interpersonal encounters with the clients we serve. Ask almost any nurse: These encounters are what make nursing special and replenish our resolve. Some encounters with clients are remembered with joy and satisfaction; others with pain at the missed opportunity to be fully present or to have that "encounter with presence" experienced by a client. But with each interpersonal encounter, the nurse has yet another chance to appreciate the richness of human experience, the magnificence of the human being, and the many different opportunities for fulfilling human potential through the medium of relationship.

The goal of the experiential format is to enable the student to learn, grow, and develop new insights about communication and relationship concepts brought to life through active involvement in the process. The exercises are designed to foster self-awareness and to provide an opportunity for students to practice communication skills in a safe learning environment with constructive feedback to encourage analysis and synthesis of content. Through collegial sharing of experiences with students and faculty, students are better able to integrate theory with practice-applications and to generalize the classroom experience of communication skills to the larger world of professional nursing.

Additional experiential exercises can be found in the accompanying *Instructor's Manual*, along with strategies for teaching and learning and brief chapter summaries with teaching tips. The test bank in the *Instructor's Manual* has been completely revised to reflect the content of this third edition.

Our hope is that *Interpersonal Relationships: Communication Skills for Nurses* will serve as a conceptual "staging area" for reflective communication, offering room to push off from in the refinement of interpersonal relationships in professional practice. We encourage students and faculty to "prepare the passage for the future" via ever renewed interpretations of the type of behavioral responses that calm, educate, and promote the healing process of our client and compel reasoned action through communication in the service of the client, the family, and the profession.

ELIZABETH ARNOLD
KATHLEEN UNDERMAN BOGGS

# Acknowledgments

This third edition carries forward the ideas and efforts of students, valued colleagues, clients, and the editorial staff at WB Saunders. The evolution of this text began with an interpersonal relationship seminar that was part of the curriculum in an upper division baccalaureate nursing program at the University of Maryland. It became clear that using experiential exercises to reinforce communication concepts provided a richer learning experience for students. Faculty and students have deepened the understanding of the materials presented in this text through the caring, creativity, and competence evidenced in professional relationships. Their voices find consistent expression in each chapter.

The material also reflects the perspectives of communication in interpersonal relationships derived from the professional reflections of leaders in the field of communication and nursing. Hildegard Peplau's classic work on interpersonal relationships in professional nursing practice provides the nursing framework for this text. Contributors from outside the realm of nursing provide a broader understanding of the communication process to guide therapeutic conversations with clients and professionals involved with their care.

The editorial staff at WB Saunders deserves special acknowledgment for their commitment to the preparation of this book. We owe a special debt of thanks to Terri Wood, our nursing editor, for her encouragement and consistent support in developing the text. Her quick and ready response to issues that arose during the development of the text kept us on track with a tight publication schedule. We also wish to acknowledge the careful attention to detail and the strong working relationship that Marie Thomas, editorial assistant, provided throughout the process. We also want to acknowledge the useful and supportive suggestions made by our reviewers.

We feel most fortunate to have had the competent services of Rachel Bedard once again as developmental editor for the text. Her clarity of thinking, sensitive understanding of the material, revision of the glossary, and suggestions related to editorial revisions was exceptional and deeply appreciated.

Finally, we need to acknowledge the loving support of our families. We are particularly grateful to our spouses, George B. Arnold and Michael J. Boggs, for their unflagging encouragement and support.

# Contents

## Part V

## Professional Issues

## PART I

# Conceptual Foundations of Nurse–Client Relationships

## 1

# Theory as a Guide to Practice

### Elizabeth Arnold

**OBJECTIVES**

At the end of this chapter, the student will be able to

1. Describe the nature and purpose of nursing theory
2. Identify the historical development of nursing theory
3. Compare and contrast different levels of nursing knowledge
4. Describe the implications of Peplau's nursing theory for the nurse–client relationship
5. Analyze psychological models relevant to nurse–client relationships
6. Specify the use of communication theory in nursing practice

*Nursing theory ought to guide research and practice, generate new ideas, and differentiate the focus of nursing from other professions.*

Chinn & Jacobs, 1987

❖❖ Chapter 1 focuses on the role of theory as a necessary foundation for the nurse–client relationship. Dienemann (1998) suggested that theories "enable a person to critically analyze what otherwise would be too difficult to comprehend" (p. 269). Included in the chapter are the structural components of nursing knowledge and a brief overview of theoretical perspectives found in the nurse–client relationship drawn from nursing and other disciplines.

Having nursing models to describe professional nursing is more important than ever in today's health care environment. As we enter the 21st century, a variety of factors—economics, multidisciplinary approaches to health care delivery, and advances in technology—are changing nursing's professional landscape (Booth, Kenrick, & Woods, 1997). Such changes obviously affect the traditional formats of the nurse–client relationship but not its essence. Basic therapeutic communication principles and theory-based applications of the nurse–client relationship persist as valuable and current. This is because client reactions to illness and health have not changed despite the revolution in health care delivery.

Life for each individual still is a personal tale of comedy and tragedy, joys and sorrows, peak moments and despair, accomplishment and defeat, happiness and pains, an original adventure story. Some people are born with or acquire defects that alter the human story. For others, physical and emotional disturbances, injuries, and personal life situations occur to create a new chapter. When a human story takes a turn requiring health care, people seek help from nursing professionals to reduce their sense of discomfort, to find relevant answers to difficult problems, and to rediscover the meaning of their lives now changed through illness or injury (Paterson & Zderad, 1988).

Nurses see clients at their most vulnerable in health care situations. They share peak moments, both good and bad, with their clients in birth, death, and much of life in between. Feeling centered as a personal self is difficult when clients are confronted with life-altering health conditions. The learning clients experience in the process of redefining their identity while maintaining continuity of self is unique and intensely personal. In each nursing intervention, the nurse–client relationship serves as its foundation for helping clients maintain continuity of self while expand-

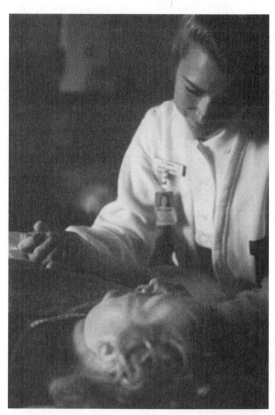

The nurse integrates three fundamental forms of nursing knowledge—theoretical, technical, and creative—in the nurse–client relationship. (Courtesy of the University of Maryland School of Nursing.)

ing their definition to include a distinct change in health status.

Nursing interventions cover the spectrum of care ranging from health promotion to caring for clients in the home, caring for critically ill clients in the hospital, caring for clients in prisons and nontraditional settings, and caring for the dying client in a hospice.

## BASIC CONCEPTS
### Definition of Theory

*Theory* comes from the Greek word *theoria*, meaning "something examined into, a viewing" (Shipley, 1945, p. 333). A theory represents a theorist's thoughtful examination of a phenomenon, defined as a concrete situation, event, circumstance, or condition of interest. Theory takes raw data about phenomena, fashions the data into a meaningful whole, provides a common language to describe the data, and gives a collective shape to the phenomena that people understand. This examination takes place over a long time and leads the theorist to make educated guesses about its nature. The theorist describes the significant elements (concepts) that make up the phenomenon and includes tentative assumptions about the relationships among them. Tentative assumptions become hypotheses that other scientists can test empirically.

A theory is neither reality nor truth. In examining theoretical frameworks or models, nurses need to explore a theory's usefulness in explaining behaviors rather than to question its truthfulness. Theoretical models are subject to change and adaptation as new information develops. A simple illustration: Descartes convinced many people of the full separation of mind and body in medieval times. This theoretical understanding, widely accepted for centuries, we now know to be false. Early nursing theorists viewed health from a disease perspective, as the absence of disease, and focused on body systems or physical interventions as a way of organizing data about an individual in need of nursing care. Their views mirrored popular understandings at the time. Modern nursing theories have broadened the definition of health to focus on well-being as the desired health outcome with a strong emphasis on disease prevention and health promotion.

There can be, and usually is, more than one theory about the same phenomenon. Each theorist focuses on different aspects and consequently draws contrasted conclusions, and this is good. Just as there is no one universal truth applicable in all situations, there is no one universal explanation for a particular phenomenon. Some theories are more useful in certain nursing situations than others. For example, Peplau's (1952, 1997) theory of interpersonal relationships is particularly useful as a framework for nurses working in psychiatric and long-term settings but much less so to nurses working with comatose clients or critically ill newborns. On the other hand, Levine's theory of energy conservation could prove helpful to neonatal intensive care unit (NICU) nurses and would not be as effective in psychiatric settings. Most nurses take elements from different theories to develop a personally relevant theory of nursing to guide their clinical practice.

### Purpose of Nursing Theory

Theory informs nursing practice by (1) furnishing a distinct body of nursing knowledge governing the scope of practice, (2) providing professional values to guide nurses in the decision-making processes, and (3) portraying the expected role of the nurse in a multidisciplinary health care environment. Nursing theories provide practitioners with a systematic way to view client situations and a logical way to organize and interpret health data (Raudonis & Acton, 1997). In all nursing theory frameworks, the client is the central focus, and the goal of nursing is to promote and maintain the health and well-being of individuals, families, and communities (Doheny, Cook, & Stopper, 1997).

Nurses often question the relevance of nursing theory for professional practice (Kim, 1994). Nursing theory seems abstract and so far removed from what nurses do every day. Yet having a body of knowledge that is distinctly nursing, separate from, but related to, what nurses actually do, is critical to the survival of nursing as a profession. Without a body of knowledge to characterize the nature of professional nursing and to describe its distinctive elements, registered nurses have no independent identity as a profession. For example, how is the nursing role different from the medical or the social work role or distinct from the paraprofessional role? Is the nurse an autonomous practitioner? If so, what is the body of knowledge that governs and guides his or her practice?

McKenna (1993) argued that nursing theory provides nurses with a distinct health care identity in collaborating with other members of the interdisciplinary health care team. General theories of nursing lay out the domain of the profession, establish the boundaries of professional nursing, provide a basis for research, and serve as a guide for curriculum development and clinical practice.

Nursing is not applied theory (Allmark, 1995). The effective practice of nursing depends on more than nursing theory. It includes critical thinking and clinical judgment based on integrated applications from scientific, ethical, and personal knowledge. Most theorists describe nursing as both an art and a science.

The artistic aspect includes, but is not limited to, tender care, attentive compassion and concern, advocacy and various hands-on practices to enhance the comfort and well-being of sick people. The developing scientific component of nursing includes knowledge applied for understanding of a broad range of human problems and psychosocial difficulties, as well as for health restoration and maintenance (Peplau, 1997, p. 162).

To sustain critical membership as part of the interdisciplinary health care team, nurses need to view nursing practice as an arena for new theory development as well as for applying nursing knowledge (Reed, 1997). Nursing theory models provide a framework for discussion, research, and the development of new thinking about the profession. They force the reader to challenge what is and to create fresh alternatives.

### Nursing Theory Development

Theory development in nursing began with Florence Nightingale and her classic work *Notes on Nursing* (1940). She described nursing as "the care that puts the patient in the best condition for nature to act." She defined health as "not only to be well, but to use well every power that we have." The validity of her ideas is represented in the timelessness of their applicability.

After Nightingale's work there was a long period of silence about nursing until the 1950s.

Nurses in the early part of the 20th century were trained using an apprenticeship model in hospital-based schools that viewed nurses as ancillary personnel or semiprofessionals rather than as professionals. Their training followed the medical model, and in most settings nurses were regarded as the handmaiden of the physician or angel of mercy rather than as autonomous competent practitioners of professional nursing.

The primary impetus for the development of a body of knowledge distinctively described as professional nursing came in the 1950s from universities where nursing leaders found themselves coping unsuccessfully with confusion and ambiguity about the role of nurses, particularly those with higher degrees. That "a nurse is a nurse is a nurse," regardless of educational preparation, was hard to dispute without a specific body of knowledge labeled professional nursing and descriptive of its nature. At about the same time, nursing education in college settings began to emerge as the preferred educational route for registered nurses, and hospital-based diploma training of nurses was replaced with associate degree and baccalaureate education.

Nursing leaders in higher education began to insist on defining the domain of professional nursing practice. They saw it as critical to the evolution of nursing as a profession to establish a logical academic structure of professional nursing education with a distinctive body of knowledge, clearly linked to what nurses actually do. Since that time, theorists such as Virginia Henderson, Myra Levine, Martha Rogers, Imogene King, Sister Callista Roy, Madeline Leininger, Dorothea Orem, Jean Watson, Dorothy Johnson, Betty Neuman, and Rosemarie Parse have devoted their professional lifetimes to developing theories about the body of knowledge unique to professional nursing.

As we enter the 21st century, nursing education is part of the career ladder that many nurses use to enhance their practice; more and more nurses elect to pursue advanced education at the master's level. Nursing theory continues to be relevant as curricular and practice threads for the associate degree, baccalaureate degree, and advanced practice with a master's degree.

The scholarly thinking of graduate nursing students has helped to further nursing theory development. Graduate nursing students have

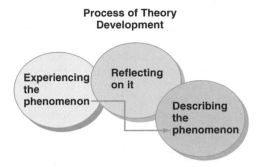

**Process of Theory Development**

Experiencing the phenomenon

Reflecting on it

Describing the phenomenon

Figure 1–1. Process of theory development.

provided ideas, struggled to understand the language and meaning of concepts, critiqued ideas, and developed important research studies to support the validity of nursing theory (Fig. 1–1). Thus, the nursing theories that guide professional practice today have a richness evolving from scholarly inquiry and an integrity springing from the commitment of its primary and contributing authors to explaining the phenomenon of professional nursing.

Nursing theories are classified as grand theory and midrange theory. *Grand theories* encompass thinking about nursing as a whole and are the most abstract of theoretical knowledge. Examples include Martha Rogers's theory of unitary beings and Dorothea Orem's self-care model.

*Midrange theories* cover more discrete aspects of a phenomenon and describe concepts in professional nursing in depth rather than exploring all aspects of phenomena. Hildegard Peplau's theory of interpersonal relationships in nursing is an example of a midrange theory (Armstrong & Kelly, 1995). More recent midrange theories cover topics such as therapeutic touch, pain, resiliency, dignity, and presence. Exercise 1–1 provides an opportunity for students to critique an article using nursing theory in clinical practice.

## Structure of Nursing Knowledge

### Metaparadigm

Nursing knowledge proceeds from general to more specific in a structural hierarchy that begins with the broadest level of nursing knowledge—nursing's metaparadigm—and proceeds to the most discrete level of nursing knowledge—nursing theory. A *paradigm* is a broad worldview. A *metaparadigm* contains the common ideas held across all paradigms. Nursing's metaparadigm reflects the central elements of nursing practice held to be valid regardless of setting: (1) person, (2) environment, (3) health, (4) nursing (Marriner-Tomey, 1994). Early theorists added nursing as a separate component to reinforce its importance, and caring as a fifth essential

---

◆ Exercise 1–1. **Critiquing a Nursing Theory Article**

**Purpose:** To provide the student with an opportunity to understand the connection of nursing theory to clinical practice

**Procedure:**
1. Select an article from a professional journal that describes the use of nursing theory or nursing concepts.
2. Suggestions of journals include *Nursing Science Quarterly, Journal of Advanced Nursing, Journal of Professional Nursing, Advances in Nursing Science.*
3. Read the article carefully and critique the article to include (1) how the author applied the theory or concept, (2) relevance of the concept or theory for nursing practice, (3) how you could use the concept in your own clinical practice, and (4) what you learned from reading the article.

**Discussion:**
In your class group, share some of the insights you obtained from the article and engage in a general discussion about the relevance of nursing theory for the professional nursing role.

element finds advocates in later works. Figure 1–2 provides a diagram of the structural hierarchy of nursing knowledge.

**Concept of a Person.** *Person* is a unitary concept with integrated physiological, psychological, spiritual, and social dimensions. When a person suffers a physical change in health status, he or she also has a psychological response to it. The change will influence social and spiritual meanings about the change.

The holism of person is key to effective nursing practice. The nurse views the client as a whole person, "not as an additive summation, but rather as a gestalt" (Paterson & Zderad, 1988, p. 25). The concept of person helps the nurse understand what makes an individual human and allows for protection of the person within the critically ill newborn, the comatose client, and mentally ill client as with the most contributing member of society. Nurses usually are the health professionals most intimately involved in promoting a person's health and well-being, preventing further injury and providing practical intervention to the client, with educational and emotional support given to their families.

The nurse–client relationship always begins with the understanding of each individual client as a holistic being even before considering the nature of the specific health care problem. Preserving and protecting the client's basic health rights as a person is in the forefront as an ethical responsibility of nurse to client in the nurse–client relationship.

**Concept of Environment.** *Environment* refers to the cultural, developmental, physical, and psychosocial conditions that influence the client's perception and behaviors, growth, and development. Just as plant growth cannot be fully understood without an analysis of its environment (i.e., the soil and the balance between sun and shade required for each plant's development), persons cannot be fully understood without an analysis of the environment that supports or compromises their existence.

Environmental factors do not simply include tangible physical settings. Psychosocial environmental elements, such as family, social norms, culture, and religion, are important factors for the nurse to consider. For example, a new mother may be anxious about her ability to care for her child depending on the amount and type of family assistance that she will receive when she goes home. Cultural or religious beliefs can make it difficult for the client to comply with treatment if they are in conflict with prescribed treatment. What a child sees parents doing at home can reduce the effectiveness of the best health prevention education about drug use or sexually responsible behavior.

**Concept of Health.** Harvey (1998) observed that "Americans are moving away from the idea of *health* as the absence of disease and the result of medical intervention to a broader definition that includes both personal responsibility and quality of life" (p. 187). Prevention, self-care, and optimal well-being are the focus of new conceptualizations of health and healthy behaviors.

In today's health care environment, the client is a consumer and an active partner in determining the focus and in planning and implementing health care measures. The personal meaning of health varies, affected by many factors, including the person's perception of wellness or illness (Frean & Malin, 1998).

Empowering clients to take primary responsibility for their health through education, emo-

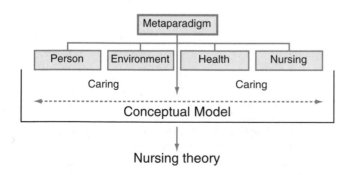

Figure 1–2. Hierarchy of nursing knowledge.

tional support, and early referral becomes increasingly important. Health promotion, emphasizing those factors that influence healthy lifestyle behaviors, is a natural part of nursing intervention regardless of personal clinical diagnosis (Antrobus, 1997; Polk, 1997). Meleis (1990) argued that health is a broader concept than a purely personal one. It should be considered as a social concern, particularly for people who do not have personal control over their health or the necessary resources to enhance their health status.

The concept of health is multidimensional with physical, emotional, social, and spiritual elements. The physical dimensions are self-explanatory. In today's society, more people engage in some health-seeking behaviors (e.g., exercise, diet, rest, leisure activities) that help them feel more healthy and better able to cope.

Emotional concepts of health have to do with positive attitudes and hope (Fryback, 1993). Finding reasons to enjoy the moment and allowing oneself to experience the caring of others enhances health and well-being regardless of physical diagnosis.

The spiritual domain of health emphasizes a personal relationship with a higher power and recognition of a person's mortality. There is "a level of awareness that exceeds ordinary, physical boundaries and limitations" (Reed, 1996, p. 33). The spiritual dimension of health often sustains people when physical or emotional assaults threaten continuity of self in health care. Exercise 1–2 provides an opportunity to explore the meaning of health.

**Concept of Nursing.** *Nursing* has many meanings to people. In 1956, Margaret Mead pointed to the complexity of describing nursing at a National Nursing Conference. A similar dilemma persists almost 50 years later. Mead said

I have tried to identify this thing that everybody who is a nurse does and how the service you give to our society could be phrased. It seems to me that you protect the vulnerable, that you protect all those who are or could be in danger, in any kind of danger—from illness, from strain, from grief; that every spot in this society where there are those who are in danger and who need continuous concern, this is the place where you might function (p. 1001).

Of particular interest in the nurse–client relationship is its root definition as "a process of nourishing, of promoting the development or progress of something" (Reed, 1997, p. 76). The goal of nursing interventions is to empower clients and to provide them with the support they need to achieve health and well-being. Taken in this context, modern nursing moves away from a conceptualization of nursing as an externally applied process to one that is intimately tied to a unique partnership with clients in health care. Pullen et al. (1994) defined nursing in today's

---

◆ **Exercise 1–2. Understanding the Meaning of Health as a Nursing Concept**

**Purpose:** To help students understand the dimensions of health as a nursing concept

**Procedure:**
1. Write a one- to two-page essay on the characteristics of a healthy person that you know.
2. In small groups of three or four, read your stories to each other. As you listen to other students' stories, write down themes that you note.
3. Compare themes, paying attention to similarities and differences and developing a group definition of health derived from the students' stories.
4. In a larger group, share your definitions of health and defining characteristics of a healthy person.

**Discussion:**
1. Is it possible to have a chronic disability and still be healthy?
2. How is health determined?
3. In what ways can the nurse support the health of a client?

health care environment as "the provision of essential health services to promote health, prevent illness, and promote cure of/or adaptation to illness" (p. 202). Nurses are in a strong position to provide a continuum of services ranging from health education to direct care and research evaluation.

Central to professional nursing as defined by many theorists is the core concept of caring. In a reflective study of caring stories, graduate nursing students identified the basic characteristics of caring as involving (1) giving of self, (2) involved presence, (3) intuitive knowing and empathy, and (4) supporting the patient's integrity, with (5) professional competence underscoring caring interventions in professional nursing practice (Arnold, 1997).

### Patterns of Knowing

Another form of nursing knowledge comes from an interconnected body of knowledge that nurses bring to their practice (Berragau, 1998). In her classic work, Carper (1995) described four patterns of **knowing**—empirical, personal, aesthetic, and ethical—embedded in nursing practice (Carr, 1996; Sherman, 1997). *Empirical patterns of knowing* are grounded in the scientific principles a nurse consistently incorporates in all phases of the nursing process. For example, nurses use scientific ways of knowing as the basis for most skilled nursing interventions. *Personal ways of knowing* acknowledge the humanness of another. Carper noted that "personal knowledge is concerned with the knowing, encountering and actualizing of the concrete, individual self. One does not know *about* the self; one strives simply to *know* the self" (Carper, 1995, p. 251). Personal knowledge occurs when the nurse is able to intuitively understand and tailor nursing responses to each person as unique.

*Aesthetic patterns of knowing* allow the nurse to understand the client from a different plane (i.e., to transcend mundane experience of a person into an event of beauty) (Chinn, Maeve, & Bostick, 1997). Aesthetic knowing includes creative applications in the relationship through the use of literature, poetry, art, and music to connect with clients. This pattern of nursing knowledge permits the nurse to capture moments of connection and caring in the nurse–client relationship experienced by both participants (Jacobs-Kramer & Chinn, 1995).

An *ethical pattern of knowing* relates to the choices that nurses have to make in the best interest of their client's well-being. Ethical ways of knowing encompass knowledge of what is right and wrong, attention to standards and codes in making moral choices, and taking responsibility for one's actions as well as professional values in providing health care.

## Nursing in the 21st Century

Nursing is in a state of developmental crisis, and how this crisis is resolved depends as much on the profession coming together as it does on societal and political understandings. Many factors contribute to the state of crisis: managed care, complexity of medical technology, and access to care issues for the elderly, the mentally ill, and the poor. Health care resources are increasingly rationed in a "one size fits all" model of care delivery. Nursing practice is becoming community based in a health care delivery system that is market driven, with no single discipline dominating health care delivery.

Redman (1998) suggests that "perhaps the largest threat to the construction of nursing practice in the new paradigm is the cavalier way in which its basic resources—its knowledge and human resources—are used" (p. 45). Because nurses historically are the only health professionals responsible for 24-hour care and surveillance, they can assume new roles as clinical educators and clinical experts valued by those within and outside the profession. Nurses play a decisive role in the direction the profession takes in the next millennium, but only if they find their collective voice.

Zalumas (1995) noted that "the practicing nurse is almost invisible in the nursing literature" (p. 89). This needs to change. If nurses do not definitively describe their professional knowledge and skills they bring to the health care situation, other disciplines will attempt to define their work.

To maintain their credibility as a professional discipline, nurses need to have a theoretical model of practice that is holistic, inclusive, and relevant to society. They need to communicate effectively to consumers, other health care professionals, and third-party insurers and within their own profession educational requirements, scope of practice, and their role in an interdisciplinary health care approach to care provision. Nurses need to understand the paradigm shift in a health care environment in which the driving force increasingly is to provide cost-effective, time-efficient quality care.

The public needs to hear not only from its nursing leaders but also from the practicing nurse telling the story of professional nursing from the caretaking role. Cash et al. (1997) suggested that nurses need to become more reflective practitioners, engaging in self-awareness and critical analysis of clinical anecdotes and able to synthesize the meaning of nursing experiences. This process enhances the nurse's capacity to share reflective clinical practice stories that tell the story of nursing. Exercise 1–3 provides an opportunity to reflect on the meaning of being a nurse.

## Conceptual Models

The conceptual model is the second level of nursing knowledge. **Conceptual models** are mental images or abstract representations of nursing that operate as a frame of reference for describing the four elements of nursing's metaparadigm: person, environment, health, and nursing. They help organize facts, clarify principles of interest to nursing, and provide scientific rationales for provision of nursing care. A conceptual model provides a logical structure for thinking about

and interpreting the meaning of each element from a nursing perspective, outlining the boundaries of professional knowledge.

*Concepts* are broad, comprehensive ideas that serve as the building blocks of conceptual models by presenting key ideas that make up the model in a logical and focused manner. A theorist uses a word or label to convey the broader meaning of the concept. For example, energy fields, openness, pandimensionality, and pattern are basic concepts in Martha Rogers's conceptual model of unitary beings. These terms describe the idea that person and environment draw energy from each other, that people develop certain patterns of behavior, and that we possess many dimensions of self that are not always seen on first encounter.

Concepts incorporate the theorist's assumptions. *Assumptions* are belief statements that form the basis for development of a concept. For example, the belief statement that "human beings are different from and more than the sum of their parts" is a basic assumption of Martha Rogers's life process model. Conceptual models cannot be empirically tested because they do not display the relationships between concepts; they simply describe them.

## Theory

Nursing theory respresents the third and most discrete level of nursing knowledge. A theory defines the relationships among concepts, as-

---

◆ **Exercise 1–3. What Is Professional Nursing?**

**Purpose:** To help students develop an understanding of professional nursing

**Procedure:**
1. Interview a professional nurse, asking each to describe (1) what he or she considers professional nursing to be today, (2) in what ways he or she thinks nurses make a difference, and (3) what would he or she describe as the most significant achievement in professional nursing.
2. In small groups of three to five students, discuss findings and develop a group definition of professional nursing.

**Discussion:**
1. What does nursing mean to you?
2. Is your understanding of nursing different from those of the nurses you interviewed?
3. As a new nurse, how would you want to present yourself?

sumptions, and propositions in a nursing model. *Propositions* are statements that describe the relationships between concepts. For example, Rogers's model proposes that "the continuous mutual flow of energy of human beings and their environments creates constant changes in the life process" (George, 1995, p. 18). This proposition demonstrates the connection between person and environment by taking the position that human beings continuously affect and are affected by their environment in ways that influence their health and well-being. For example, think of how you are influenced by positive and negative comments from others in your environment. A well-placed compliment on your performance can make your day; criticism can dampen your spirits. A positive approach on your part can affect the response of others.

Nursing theories can be tested empirically. Although it is beyond the scope of this text to detail nursing knowledge other than in the nurse–client relationship, regular reading of professional journals provides nurses with explanations of nursing theory in professional nursing practice, its use, and related clinical research.

## APPLICATIONS
## Nursing Theory in the Nurse–Client Relationship
### Hildegard Peplau

Dr. Peplau (1952) was the first nurse theorist to describe the nurse–client relationship as the foundation of nursing practice. In shifting the focus from what nurses do *to* clients to what nurses do *with* clients, Peplau masterminded a major paradigm shift from a nursing model focused on medical treatments to an interpersonal model of nursing practice. The strength of her work lies in giving nurses a structural basis to guide their interactions with clients, families, and communities (Feely, 1997; Fowler, 1995; Reynolds, 1997). Peplau viewed nursing as a "developmental educational instrument" designed to help individuals, families, and communities achieve changes in health care status and well-being.

Peplau's work continues to make a major contribution to nursing knowledge and clinical practice as we enter the 21st century. Observation,

description, formulation, interpretation, validation, and intervention form the essence of a nurse–client relationship in which the nurse helps the client transform raw data into a meaningful shared experience that both can understand (Thelander, 1997). As nurses observe and listen to their clients, they develop impressions and general ideas about the meaning of the clients' situation. The nurse validates these inferences by checking with the client for accuracy. Peplau (1992) believed illness can be a unique opportunity for experiential learning, personal growth, and improved coping strategies for living.

The dynamic nursing approach Peplau advocated is not that of a passive spectator. As participant-observers, nurses actively engage with their clients, simultaneously observing clients' behavior and their own responses, providing assistance, information, and encouragement as needed. Peplau identified six professional roles the nurse assumes in the nurse–client relationship (see Box 1–1).

### Developmental Phases

In her classic work on the nurse–client relationship, *Interpersonal Relations in Nursing*, Peplau (1952) described four developmental phases of the relationship that overlap and build on one another (Peplau, 1992). She characterized the nurse–client relationship as a dynamic learning experience out of which personal-social growth can occur for both nurse and client. Clarification and continuity are communication threads interwoven through each phase (Forchuk, 1991).

In today's health care environment, nurse–client relationships are of short duration, and nursing interventions have to be brief, concise, and effective. The principles of engaging the client, developing a working partnership, exploiting available resources, and successfully terminating a relationship remain salient but with a stronger emphasis on fortifying the client with information and referrals to be carried out later. Case management strategies, ongoing home health care interventions, and care in long-term and psychiatric settings lend themselves to the phases of relationship development as originally described by Peplau.

Peplau maintained that the **orientation phase**

---

**Box 1-1. Peplau's Six Nursing Roles**

*Stranger role:* receives the client the same way one meets a stranger in other life situations; provides an accepting climate that builds trust

*Resource role:* answers questions, interprets clinical treatment data, gives information

*Teaching role:* gives instructions and provides training; involves analysis and synthesis of the learner experience

*Counseling role:* helps client understand and integrate the meaning of current life circumstances; provides guidance and encouragement to make changes

*Surrogate role:* helps client clarify domains of dependence, interdependence, and independence and acts on client's behalf as advocate

*Active leadership role:* helps client assume maximum responsibility for meeting treatment goals in a mutually satisfying way

---

sets the stage for the rest of the relationship. Nurse and client encounter each other as strangers. They must develop a working partnership before work on health care problems occurs. Nurse and client begin to analyze a problem situation and related client needs. From this analysis, the nurse develops relevant nursing diagnoses. This phase correlates with the assessment phase of the nursing process.

Once nurse and client together define the problem in the orientation phase, they move into the **working phase.** The working phase is subdivided into two aspects: identification and exploitation. The identification component focuses on mutual clarification of ideas and expectations. The nurse also helps the client express feelings of helplessness, dependency, and despair; discover personal strengths; and identify potential resources. The composite data become the basis of an individualized nursing care plan. Nurse and client mutually develop goals related to resolution of identified client health needs and decide on the type of assistance needed to achieve them. In the exploitation phase, the nurse assists the client to seek out and use health care services and personal strengths in resolving the issues for which the client initially sought treatment. Corresponding to the implementation phase of the nursing process, the nurse fosters the client's self-direction in promoting health and well-being. Peplau categorized the client role as dependent, interdependent, or independent, based on the amount of responsibility the client is willing or able to assume for personal care.

Peplau referred to the final phase of the rela-

tionship as the **resolution** (termination) phase, corresponding to the evaluation phase of the nursing process. The nurse assists the client in evaluating the resolution of issues that initially brought the client into treatment. If modifications, including referrals, are necessary, the nurse takes responsibility for making additional plans that extend beyond the relationship with other health care providers.

## Contributions from Other Disciplines

Theory principles from other disciplines can help nurses understand what goes on in the successful nurse–client relationship. Selected theory contributions from psychiatry and psychology reinforce the importance of the nurse–client relationship, providing psychological understanding of behaviors and desired outcomes in helping relationships.

### Sigmund Freud

Sigmund Freud (1937, 1959) is of interest in the study of nurse–client relationships for several reasons. He was the first to insist that talking about situations and the feelings accompanying them with a trained professional has a positive effect on reducing tension and resolving maladaptive behaviors.

Freud's ideas about **transference** (in which the client projects irrational attitudes and feelings from the past onto people in the present) are useful in understanding difficult behaviors in nurse–client relationships. For example, the client who says to the young nurse, "Get a real nurse—you're young enough to be my daughter and I don't want to talk with you about my personal life," has a transference reaction having little to do with the nurse's competence. Recognizing this statement as a transference reaction helps the nurse depersonalize the client's comment, allowing for a more appropriate response. Peplau (1992) suggested that a constructive way of handling this situation would be "(a) to get the patient to specify the similarity between the familiar other and the nurse, and (b) to specify some differences" (p. 15).

**Countertransference** feelings refer to the attitudes or feelings the nurse may develop toward a client. They can emerge in response to a client's provocative transference behaviors, usually sexual or hostile. Alternatively, they can reflect the nurse's biases and past experiences with similar situations or people. For example, feeling anger or frustration, strong attraction, acting on the basis of stereotypes, or feeling like a child with a powerful client can be countertransference feelings stemming either from the client's behavior, the nurse's personal needs, or past encounters with similar behaviors. Unrecognized countertransference feelings sabotage the relationship. Acknowledged countertransference feelings are an important source of information. Usually nurses find it useful to talk about them with a trusted colleague or mentor so that they do not get in the way of successful relating.

Freud also was the first to identify biopsychosocial stages of development as a way of describing personality development. He maintained that each person passes through a series of biologically determined stages of personality development, each with its own set of problems and conflicts. Freud believed that people who do not resolve a specific maturational stage at the appropriate age are destined to retain an immature behavioral response pattern for the rest of their lives. They remain "fixated" at that developmental stage. Behaviors and emotions out of proportion to a situation may indicate a lack of psychosocial maturity in resolving earlier developmental stages. For example, a client who experienced little parental support in early childhood may find it difficult to trust that anyone, including helping professionals, will help.

Freud identified **ego defense mechanisms** as

self-talk a person uses to protect the self from anxiety, for example, denial, rationalization, and projection of anger that occur on a regular basis in stressful clinical situations. Nurses use these concepts as they strive to understand their clients' and their own behaviors in the nurse–client relationship.

## Carl Jung

Jung's work (1963, 1971) helps nurses examine the many dimensions of a person. For example, Jung challenged the idea that men and women are automatically locked into gender-related roles and behaviors from birth. He believed that men have tenderness and sensitivity, commonly thought of as feminine traits, and that women have equally male-associated assertive behavior traits that need recognition if a person is to be whole. Although these ideas were considered radical in Jung's day, today both men and women enjoy the broadened expression of behavior. Men take pleasure from active parenting behaviors, and women enjoy the choice of working outside of the home in previously male-dominated occupations. Men choose nursing as a career and women select medicine, something unheard of in Jung's time. The world is better for the more open-minded perspective.

While respecting the concept of cultural diversity, Jung (1963) reminded nurses of our universal heritage as human beings. He viewed all people, regardless of race, socioeconomic status, religion, or culture, as sharing common human qualities: gentleness, strength, love, and anger. Nurses' recognition of the common human bonds shared with all clients helps promote understanding and acceptance of people as human beings first and foremost. Jung (1969) also introduced spirituality as an integral dimension of self.

Jung's concepts of adult development are useful in understanding changes in values and things of importance to the older adult. He noted that "we cannot live the afternoon of life according to the values of life's morning" (1971) and described an inward turning in which a person begins to question the meaning of his or her life, examines what is really important, and is less concerned with the approval of others.

Jung likened the role of a helping person in a therapeutic relationship to a "midwife, assisting in bringing into the light of day a natural process, the process of coming into one's self" (Von Franz, 1975). The nurse uses a similar metaphor in working with the client. The client does the work and the nurse assists in a natural life process, using his or her expertise.

## Harry Stack Sullivan

Peplau credited Sullivan's work as the foundation for her ideas of the nurse–client relationship. Harry Stack Sullivan (1953), an American psychoanalyst, introduced the idea of the therapeutic relationship as being a human connection that heals. Without this human connectivity recognized by nurse and client as meaningful, Sullivan contended, the relationship fails, no matter how technically correct the interventions.

People learn their humanness from significant others in their environment (see Chapter 3). Sullivan believed that individuals experience anxiety when they do not feel secure within their interpersonal environment. Having a corrective interpersonal experience in adulthood with a helping professional helps individuals find the self-security they missed in childhood.

Working mostly with schizophrenic patients, Sullivan introduced the concept that people cannot always relate to a helping person with personal data. Individuals experiencing shock, panic, serious mental illness, or brain damage are unable to recall past events. They cannot plan effectively for the future because they have trouble connecting the past, present, or future in their minds. Understanding this behavioral construct allows the nurse to act empathetically with clients who simply cannot function in a relationship at a higher level (Peplau, 1992).

## Martin Buber

The I–thou relationship described by Martin Buber (1958) captures the essence of the relationship desired in the nurse–client relationship. In an **I–thou relationship,** each individual responds to the other as a unique person in a mutually respectful manner. Neither is an "object" of study. Instead, there is a process of mutual discovery. Each person in an I–thou relationship feels free to be authentic and to relate compassionately and responsibly with the other. Always there is a focus on confirming the essential dig-

nity of the human being with the potential for becoming more through the relationship. Paterson and Zderad (1988) suggested that "Buber's I–thou relating emphasizes awareness of each being's uniqueness without a superimposing, or a deciding about the other without a knowing" (p. 44).

Buber's work forms the theoretical foundation for using confirming responses. He described this way of responding as follows: "Man wishes to be confirmed in his being by man and wishes to have a presence in the being of the other. Secretly and bashfully, he watches for a yes which allows him to be" (Buber, 1957, p. 104). Nurses confirm the humanity of clients each time they respect their human dignity, even when clients are difficult or unappreciative.

## Carl Rogers

Carl Rogers's person-centered model of therapeutic relationships emphasizes an I–thou relationship as essential to healing and points to the primacy of person as the agent of healing. According to Rogers (1961), "if I can provide a certain type of relationship, the other person will discover within himself the capacity to use that relationship for growth and change, and personal development will occur." Rogers identified helper characteristics essential to the development of client-centered relationships: unconditional positive regard and empathy and genuineness. Many of the characteristics that Rogers described as necessary to a successful therapeutic relationship are similar to the creative compo-

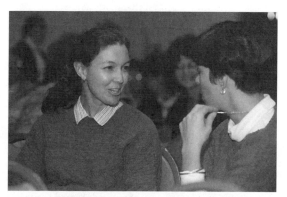

In an I–thou relationship, the client is never treated like an object.

nents of nurse–client relationships. They are discussed as bridges to relationship in Chapter 5. Rogers's concepts of a person-centered relationship are relevant for establishing appropriate learning environments for client teaching.

### Erik Erikson

Erik Erikson (1982, 1994) described human development from birth to death as a series of psychosocial crises, each with associated tasks. The word *development* means "unfolding." Erikson viewed developmental maturation as a linear process from lower to higher development, with each stage representing a more complex formation of identity development and incorporating previous stage development.

Erikson viewed identity as the central life task and self-definition as a lifelong process. He described maturation as occurring according to an epigenetic principle, which states that "anything that grows has a ground plan . . . and out of this ground plan all parts arise, each part having its time of ascendancy, until all parts have arisen to form a functioning whole" (1959). The transition from one developmental stage to another precipitates a psychosocial crisis because previous patterns of psychosocial adaptation no longer work effectively.

Individuals mature by developing more complex social skills and successfully resolving psychosocial developmental crises. Society confirms the process of identity and successful resolution of developmental crises through markers in the life cycle such as confirmations, graduations, weddings, and retirement. Developmental remnants of earlier experiences persist, to be constantly reworked and interwoven into the tapestry of life by each individual (Erikson & Erikson, 1981). To illustrate, a person newly diagnosed with a serious illness may feel much the same need to trust the helping professional felt by the newborn dependent on mother at the beginning to provide direction.

Differences in parenting, death of a parent, divorce, and other life experiences can "fast forward" a child through crisis periods (e.g., into assuming adult responsibilities without going through normal childhood phases). Other children exhibit arrested psychosocial development brought about by drug abuse or overprotection.

Cultural diversity also can influence the exact timetable and behavioral expression of different developmental stages (e.g., some cultures favor early marriages or prolonged childhood).

Erikson considered unexpected life circumstances that affect appropriate mastery of developmental life tasks (e.g., illness, job promotion, marriage, job loss) as horizontal threads in a life tapestry. When they arise in conjunction with normal developmental crises, the developmental crisis is more intense and difficult to resolve (Dowd, 1990). Box 1–2 contrasts psychosocial development constructs. Exercise 1–4 provides students with a personalized understanding of psychosocial development throughout the life span. Exercise 1–5 provides an opportunity to learn about the integration of psychosocial development through the life cycle.

### Abraham Maslow

Abraham Maslow's theory of self-development describes progressive stages of personal growth needs, beginning with physiological survival needs and ending with self-actualization. His theory is useful in helping nurses prioritize nursing interventions. At the lowest level of Maslow's model are basic **physiological needs.** Satisfying hunger, thirst, and sexual and sensory stimulation needs has an emotional component requiring satisfaction as well. The second level of needs, **safety and security needs,** includes physical safety and emotional security. Once a person meets safety and security needs, a person seeks to meet **love and belonging needs,** the need to be part of a family or community. As people feel part of a community, they experience self-esteem. A sense of dignity, respect, and approval by others for the self within is the hallmark of successfully meeting **self-esteem needs.**

Maslow's highest level of need satisfaction, **self-actualization,** represents "the human being at his best," using talents and personality to the best of his or her ability for the betterment of society. To become self-actualized, a person must achieve a sufficient level of need fulfillment at all the lower stages.

Self-actualized individuals are not superhuman. They are subject to the same feelings of insecurity and vulnerability all individuals experience. However, they accept this part of their

◆ Box 1–2. Personality Development

| Age (Years) | Erikson's Psychosocial Stages | Primary Person Orientation | Strengths | Qualities | Freud's Psychosexual Stages | Jung's Psychosocial Orientation |
|---|---|---|---|---|---|---|
| 0–2 | Trust vs. mistrust | Mother | Hope | To receive, to give | Oral | Largely unconscious |
| 2–4 | Autonomy vs. shame-guilt | Father | Willpower | To control, to let go | Anal | |
| 4–6 | Initiative vs. guilt | Basic family | Purpose | To make, to play-act | Oedipal | Beginning ego consciousness |
| 6–12 | Industry vs. inferiority | Neighborhood, school | Competence | To make things, to put things together | Latency | |
| 13–19 | Identity vs. identity diffusion | Peer groups | Fidelity | To be one's self | Puberty | Individual consciousness |
| Young adult | Intimacy vs. self-absorption | Partners in marriage, friendship | Love | To share one's self with another | Genitality | Social adaptation, achievement |
| Adult | Generativity vs. self-absorption | Children, community | Care | To take care of, to create | | Inner reflection, individuation |
| Old age | Integrity vs. despair | Humankind | Wisdom | To accept being, to accept not being | | Self-knowledge of the meaning of one's existence |

Adapted from Erikson E. (1982). The Life Cycle Completed New York, Norton. Used with permission.

◆ Exercise 1–4. **Time Line**

**Purpose:** To give students experience with understanding psychosocial development through the life span

**Procedure:**
1. Draw a time line of your life to date. Include all significant events and the age at which they occurred. Identify horizontal threads.
2. Insert Erikson's stages as markers in your time line.

**Discussion:**
In a large group, discuss the following:

1. In what ways did Erikson's stages provide information about expected tasks in your life?
2. In what ways did they deviate?
3. To what would you attribute the differences?
4. How could you use this exercise in your nursing care of clients?

---

◆ **Exercise 1–5. Completing the Life Cycle**

**Purpose:** To help you understand the integration of psychosocial development through the life cycle

**Procedure:**
1. Interview an older adult who has reached at least the sixth decade of life.
2. Identify Erikson's psychosocial tasks and ask the person to identify what factors in his or her life contributed to or interfered with mastery of the task of each stage.
3. Describe in short summary the factors that you believe contributed or interfered with each stage of the person's adult life.

**Discussion:**
1. In the larger group, share your examples.
2. For each stage compile on the board a list of the factors identified.
3. Discuss the impact certain factors may have on the outcome of development through the life span.

---

humanness and strive to share it with others. Self-actualized people take important personal stands on issues; saying no when it is appropriate and fully committing themselves to personal goals that enrich their sense of self and contribute to the lives of others. Box 1–3 describes characteristics of self-actualized people.

Nurses use Maslow's theory to understand and reflect on where to begin care. Basic needs come before growth needs. For example, attempting to collect any but the most essential information

---

◆ **Box 1–3. Characteristics of Self-Actualization**

Quality of genuineness

Passion for living

Ability to get along well with others

Strong sense of personal worth

View of life situations as opportunities, not threats

Ability to experience each moment fully

Moments of intense emotional meaning, "peak experience"

Full acceptance of self and others

Identification with fellow human beings

High sense of responsibility with a strong desire to serve humanity

Integrity of purpose

---

when the client is in pain or suffering a heart attack is inappropriate. The nurse meets the client's physiological need for pain relief before collecting general information for a nursing data base. Exercise 1–6 provides the student with practice using Maslow's categories of need, and Exercise 1–7 provides practice with a case study. Figure 1–3 presents selected nursing diagnoses related to each stage of Maslow's theory.

## Communication Theory

Communication is the primary means through which the nurse–client relationship occurs. The concept includes nonverbal behaviors as well as verbal communication. Four basic assumptions serve as the foundation for the concept of communication (Box 1–4).

### Linear Theory

Current communication models build on linear concepts of the communication process, originally conceptualized as having three basic elements: sender, message, and receiver. *Communication* is defined as an interpersonal activity involving the transmission of messages by a source to a receiver for the purpose of influencing the receiver's behavior (Miller & Nicholson, 1976). Personal channels of communication are sensory receptors through which a person transmits information through one or more of the five senses: sight, hearing, taste, touch, and smell.

◆ Exercise 1-6. **Maslow's Hierarchy of Needs**

**Purpose:**  To help students apply Maslow's hierarchy of needs theory to care of clients

**Procedure:**
1. Divide the class into small groups with each group taking a step of Maslow's hierarchy. Each group will then brainstorm examples of that need as it might present in clinical practice.
2. Identify potential responses from the nurse related to each need.
3. Each group will share its examples with the larger group and discuss the concept of prioritization of needs using Maslow's hierarchy.

**Discussion:**
1. In what ways is Maslow's hierarchy helpful to the nurse in prioritizing client needs?
2. What limitations do you see with the theory?

The **sender** is the source or initiator of the message. The sender *encodes* the message (i.e., puts the message into verbal or nonverbal symbols that the receiver can understand). To encode a message appropriately requires a clear understanding of the receiver's mental frame of reference (feelings, personal agendas, past experiences) as well as knowledge of the desired objective of the communicated message. The sender organizes the message content to focus on key ideas that the sender wishes to convey. By expressing an internal thought or feeling, the sender assumes responsibility for the accuracy of the content and the emotional tone of the message.

The **message** consists of a verbal or nonverbal

◆ Exercise 1-7. **Case Application of Maslow's Theory**

**Purpose:**  To examine the use of Maslow's theory in a specific case

**Procedure:**  In groups of three or four students, consider the following case study and apply Maslow's hierarchy of needs theory to Mr. Rodgers's case from the time of admission to the coronary care unit until his discharge and follow-up care. Include any considerations for changing priorities because of fluctuations in his condition.

Mr. Rodgers is admitted to the cardiac intensive care unit with an acute myocardial infarction. He is an internationally known middle-aged businessman, a corporate vice president of a major company, and very well liked by his employees. His blood pressure for the past 2 years has never fallen below a diastolic reading of 95, and he is being treated with a mild diuretic. Before this hospitalization, he had never been admitted to a hospital. Mr. Rodgers is anxious and perspiring profusely. He has many of the predisposing factors for heart problems present in his history, family, and lifestyle.

**Discussion:**
1. At what stage of Maslow's hierarchy is this client?
2. With what needs is the client likely to require nursing intervention during his hospitalization and after discharge?
3. In the large group, share your conclusions and recommendations for prioritizing Mr. Rodgers's care with a rationale.

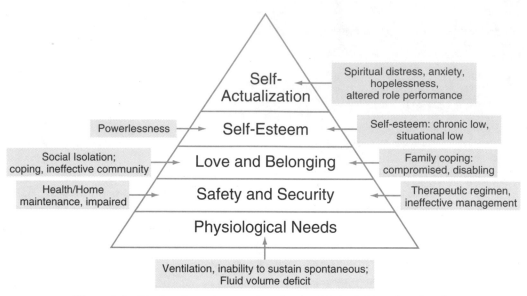

**Figure 1–3.** Nursing diagnosis categories related to Maslow's hierarchy of needs.

expression of thoughts or feelings transmitted from the sender to the receiver. The most effective messages are authentic and expressed in a language the receiver can understand. *Feedback* is the term used to describe the message the receiver sends in response to the sender's message.

The **receiver** is the recipient of the message. Once received, the receiver *decodes* it (i.e., translates the message into word symbols and internally interprets its meaning to make sense of the message). An open attitude and suspension of

judgment strengthens the possibility of decoding the sender's message accurately (Fig. 1–4).

## Circular Transactional Theoretical Models

A circular model is a transactional model that expands linear models to include the context of the communication. With this model, the sender and receiver construct a mental picture of the other that influences the message, including perceptions of the other person's attitude and potential reaction to the message. Two communication characteristics expand linear constructs by adding systems theory concepts: feedback and validation.

Circular models are based on systems concepts that describe how the human system influences and is influenced by the communication it receives. Communication is conceptualized as a continuous, mutually interconnected activity in which sender and receiver influence each other in the transmission and receiving of a message. Accordingly, a human system receives information from the environment (input), internally processes the information and reacts to it based on its own internal functions (throughput), and

---

### ◆ Box 1–4. Basic Assumptions of Communication Theory

It is impossible not to communicate (Bateson, 1979).

We only know about ourselves and others through communication.

Faulty communication results in flawed feeling and acting.

Feedback is the only way we know that our perceptions are valid.

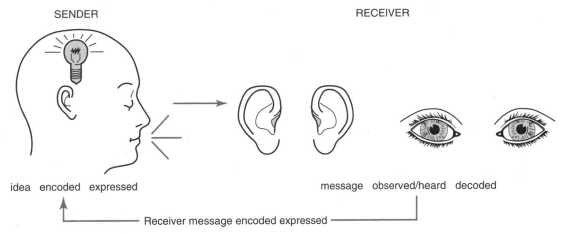

SENDER                                    RECEIVER

idea  encoded  expressed                    message  observed/heard  decoded

Receiver message encoded expressed

**Figure 1–4.** Linear model of communication.

produces new information or behavior (output) as a result of the process. The system provides information about the process and output through the mechanism of feedback. Feedback allows the system to correct or sustain its original input.

A circular transactional model proposes that "every communication has a content and a relationship aspect such that the latter classifies the former and is therefore **metacommunication**" (Waltzlawick, 1967, p. 54). Metacommunication is a nonverbal message about how the receiver should interpret the message. For example, a person may tell someone, "This is important, let's talk about it." If that person then sits down in a relaxed position with good eye contact and actively listens, the verbal and nonverbal messages are congruent. If, however, the sender delivers the same verbal message while looking at the clock or remains in a standing position, the metacommunication that accompanies the verbal message is that the sender is in a hurry and does not have time to listen. Another interpretation the receiver might make is that the topic really is not important.

Circular models also take into account the role relationships between communicators. People take either *symmetrical* or *complementary* roles in communicating. When communicators are equal in status there is a ***symmetrical relationship*** and either can assume responsibility for the direction of the communication. In complementary rela-

tionships, one participant assumes the leadership role and the other follows. Complementary relationships occur when one party has a higher status than the other. Consider, for example, the type of communication a nurse might have with a supervisor or physician versus a peer. The nurse–client relationship has elements of both types of roles. The nurse takes a complementary role in providing education and a symmetrical role in working with the client on developing mutually defined goals and the means to achieve them.

**Feedback** is the verbal or nonverbal response the receiver gives to the sender about the message. Feedback always occurs. Even by not responding, the receiver provides feedback. Feedback can focus on the content, the relationship between people, and events, or the receiver can provide it through behavior. It affects all future communication (Dance, 1967).

**Validation** is a form of feedback providing verbal and nonverbal confirmation that both participants have the same basic understanding of the message and the feedback. Both concepts are discussed in detail in Chapter 10. Figure 1–5 is a diagram of the model. Exercise 1–8 provides an opportunity to experiment with linear versus circular models of communication.

## Therapeutic Communication

Therapeutic communication is a basic tool used in the helping relationship. Ruesch (1961) coined

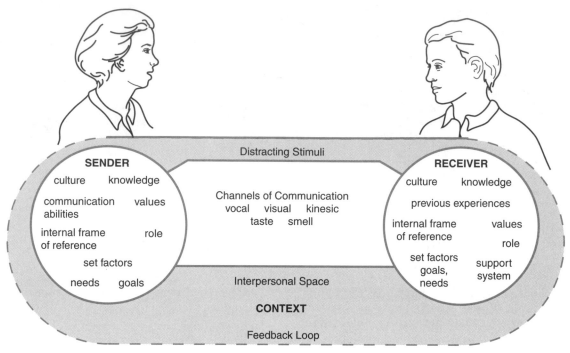

Figure 1–5. Circular transactional model of communication.

the term *therapeutic communication* and proposed that "communication is a universal function of man that is not tied to any particular place, time, or context, and basically communication which produces a therapeutic effect in no way differs from what happens in ordinary exchanges" (pp. 30–31).

The quality of the communication process, to a large extent, determines the caliber of the relationship. Doheny et al. (1997) observed that

---

◆ Exercise 1–8. **Differences Between Linear and Circular Models of Communication**

**Purpose:**   To help you see the difference between linear and circular models of communication

**Procedure:**
1. Role-play a scenario in which one person provides a scene that might occur in the clinical area using a linear model: sender, message, receiver.
2. Role-play the same scenario using a circular model, framing questions that recognize the context of the message and its potential impact on the receiver, and provide feedback.

**Discussion:**
1. Was there a difference in your level of comfort? If so, in what ways?
2. Was there any difference in the amount of information you had as a result of the communication? If so, in what ways?
3. What implications does this exercise have for your future nursing practice?

"when certain skills are used to facilitate communication between nurse and client in a goal directed manner, the therapeutic communication process occurs" (p. 5). Therapeutic communication is not a method but rather a specialized application of basic communication principles designed to promote the client's well-being and self-actualization.

Knowledge of communication theory not only helps the nurse examine client interactions in a more systematic way, but also helps steer the direction of the relationship. This process allows the nurse and the client to become working partners in the client's care. Nurses use therapeutic communication skills to provide new information, correct misinformation, promote understanding of client responses to health problems, explore options for care, assist in decision making, and facilitate client well-being (Sellick, 1991).

## SUMMARY

Chapter 1 introduces theoretical concepts that contribute to the understanding of the nurse–client relationship. The nurse–client relationship consists of three components: theoretical, technical, and creative. Use of theoretical models in the implementation of the nurse–client relationship brings order to nursing practice, provides a cognitive structure for developing a body of knowledge identifiable with the profession, and contributes a basis for nursing research. Four elements critical to an understanding of nursing practice are person, health, nursing, and environment. These elements form the metaparadigm for professional nursing, the basis for professional nursing.

Hildegard Peplau's theory of interpersonal relationships in professional nursing practice forms the basic theory structure for the nurse–client relationship. She described three phases of the relationship: orientation, working, and resolution. Building on the work of Harry Stack Sullivan, Peplau believed that the interpersonal relationship is the crux of effective nursing practice.

Nursing borrows concepts and principles related to the development of interpersonal relationships from other disciplines. Sigmund Freud's contributions include the therapeutic

value of talking about painful experiences, the concepts of transference and countertransference, and ego defense mechanisms. Carl Jung proposed several controversial ideas that today are recognized as valid regarding spirituality, the influence of culture on behavior, adult development, and gender roles. Erikson broadened the scope of earlier thinking on personality development to include humans' interaction with the larger social environment. Buber and Rogers offered basic concepts concerning the characteristics the nurse needs for developing effective interpersonal relationships with clients. Maslow's needs theory provides a basis for determining priorities in all phases of the nursing process.

Communication is the foundation and basic tool of the nurse–client relationship. Circular transactional models broaden linear models within a larger social context. Using the elements outlined in these models in creative applications of therapeutic conversations with clients will increase the depth and meaning of interpersonal interactions.

## REFERENCES

Allmark P. (1995). A classical view of the theory-practice gap in nursing. Journal of Advanced Nursing 22(1):18–23.

Antrobus S. (1997). Developing the nurse as a knowledge worker in health—learning the artistry of practice. Journal of Advanced Nursing 25(4):829–835.

Armstrong M, Kelly A. (1995). More than the sum of their parts: Martha Rogers and Hildegard Peplau. Archives of Psychiatric Nursing 9(1):40–44.

Arnold E. (1997). Caring from the graduate student perspective. International Journal for Human Caring 1(3):32–42.

Bateson G. (1979). Mind and Nature. New York, Dutton.

Berragau L. (1998). Nursing practice draws upon several different ways of knowing. Journal of Clinical Nursing 7(3):209–217.

Booth K, Kenrick M, Woods S. (1997). Nursing knowledge, theory and method revisited. Journal of Advanced Nursing 26(4):804–811.

Buber M. (1957). Distance and relation. Psychiatry 20: 97–104.

Buber M. (1958). I and Thou (2nd ed., Smith R, trans.). New York, Scribner.

Carper B. (1995). Fundamental patterns of knowing. In Nicholl L (ed.), Perspectives on Nursing Theory (3rd ed.). Philadelphia, JB Lippincott.

Carr E. (1996). Reflecting on clinical practice: Hectoring talk or reality? Journal of Clinical Nursing 5(5):289–295.

Cash P, Brooker J, Penney W, Reinbold J, Strangis L. (1997).

Reflective inquiry in nursing practice on revealing images. Nursing Inquiry 4(4):246–256.

Chinn P, Jacobs MK. (1987). Theory and Nursing (2nd ed.). St. Louis, CV Mosby.

Chinn P, Maeve M, Bostick C. (1997). Aesthetic inquiry and the art of nursing. Scholarly Inquiry in Nursing Practice. 11(2):83–96.

Dance FEX. (1967). Human Communication Theory. New York, Holt, Rinehart & Winston.

Dienemann J. (1998). Assessing organization. In Dienemann J (ed.), Nursing Administration: Managing Patient Care (2nd ed.). Stamford, CT, Appleton & Lange.

Doheny M, Cook C, Stopper M. (1997). The Discipline of Nursing. Stamford, CT, Appleton & Lange.

Dowd J. (1990). Ever since Durkheim: The socialization of human development. Human Development 33:138–159.

Erikson E. (1994). Identity and the Life Cycle. New York, WW Norton.

Erikson E. (1993). Childhood and Society. New York, WW Norton.

Erikson E. (1982). Life Cycle Completed. New York, WW Norton.

Erikson E, Erikson J (1981). On generativity and identity: From a conversation with Erik and Joan Erikson. Harvard Educational Review 51:251.

Erikson E. (1959). Youth and Identity. New York, WW Norton.

Feely M. (1997). Using Peplau's theory in nurse-patient relations. International Nursing Review 44(4):115–120.

Forchuk C. (1991). Peplau's theory: Concepts and their relations. Nursing Science Quarterly 4(2):54–60.

Fowler J. (1995). Taking theory into practice: Using Peplau's model in the care of a patient. Professional Nurse 10(4):226–230.

Frean M, Malin S. (1998). Health promotion: Theoretical perspectives and clinical applications. Holistic Nursing Practice 12(2):1–7.

Freud S. (1937). The Basic Writings of Sigmund Freud (Brill AA, trans. and ed.). New York, Modern Library.

Freud S. (1959). Collected Papers (Strachey J, ed.). New York, Basic Books.

Fryback P. (1993). Health for people with a terminal illness. Nursing Science Quarterly 6(3):147–159.

George J. (1995). Nursing Theories: The Base for Professional Nursing Practice (4th ed.). Stamford, CT, Appleton & Lange.

Harvey J. (1998). Marketing in the new health care environment. In Dienemann J (ed.), Nursing Administration: Managing Patient Care (2nd ed.). Stamford, CT, Appleton & Lange.

Hickman J. (1995). An introduction to nursing theory. In George J (ed.), Nursing Theories: The Base for Professional Nursing Practice (4th ed.). Stamford, CT, Appleton & Lange.

Jacobs-Kramer M, Chinn P. (1995). Perspectives on knowledge: A model of nursing knowledge. In Nicholl L (ed.), Perspectives on Nursing Theory (3rd ed.). Philadelphia, JB Lippincott.

Jung CG. (1963). Memories, Dreams and Reflections (Winston R, trans.). New York, Vintage.

Jung CG. (1969). Psychology and religion: West and east. In Collected Works of CG Jung (Hull RFC, trans.). Princeton, NJ, Princeton University Press.

Jung CG. (1971). The stages of life. In Campbell J (ed.), The Portable Jung. New York, Viking.

Kim HS. (1994). Practice theories in nursing and a science of nursing practice. Scholarly Inquiry for Nursing Practice 8(2):145–158.

Marriner-Tomey A. (1994). Nursing Theorists and Their Work (3rd ed.). St. Louis, CV Mosby.

McKenna G. (1993). Unique theory—Is it essential in the development of a science of nursing? Nursing Education Today 13(2):121–127.

Mead M. (1956). Nursing—Primitive and civilized. American Journal of Nursing 56(8):1001–1004.

Meleis A. (1990). Being and becoming healthy: The core of nursing knowledge. Nursing Science Quarterly 3(3):107–114.

Miller GR, Nicholson HE. (1976). Communication Inquiry: A Perspective on Process. Reading, MA, Addison-Wesley.

Nightingale F. (1940). Notes on Nursing. New York: Appleton-Century-Crofts.

Paterson J, Zderad L. (1988). Humanistic Nursing. New York, National League for Nursing.

Peplau H. (1952). Interpersonal Relations in Nursing. New York, Putnam.

Peplau H. (1992). Interpersonal relations: A theoretical framework for application in nursing practice. Nursing Science Quarterly 5(1):13–18.

Peplau H. (1997). Peplau's theory of interpersonal relations. Nursing Science Quarterly 10(4):162–167.

Polk L. (1997). Toward a mid-range theory of resilience. Advances in Nursing Science 19(3):1–13.

Pullen C, Edwards J, Lenz C, Alley N. (1994). A comprehensive primary health care delivery model. Journal of Professional Nursing 10(4):201–208.

Raudonis B, Acton G. (1997). Theory-based nursing practice. Journal of Advanced Nursing 26(1):138–145.

Redman B. (1998). The health policy process and nursing. In Dienemann J (ed.), Nursing Administration: Managing Patient Care (2nd ed.). Stamford, CT, Appleton & Lange.

Reed P. (1996). Transforming practice knowledge into nursing knowledge—A revisionist analysis of Peplau. Image: Journal of Nursing Scholarship 28(1):29–33.

Reed P. (1997). Nursing: The ontology of the discipline. Nursing Science Quarterly 10(2):76–79.

Reynolds W. (1997). Peplau's theory in practice. Nursing Science Quarterly 10(4):168–170.

Rogers C. (1961). On Becoming a Person. Boston, Houghton Mifflin.

Ruesch J. (1961). Therapeutic Communication. New York, Norton.

Sellick KJ. (1991). Nurse's interpersonal behaviors and the development of helping skills. International Journal of Nursing Studies 28(1):3–11.

Sherman D. (1997). Death of a newborn: Healing the

pain through Carper's patterns of knowing in nursing. Journal of the New York State Nurses Association 28(1): 4–6.

Shipley J. (1945). Dictionary of Word Origins (2nd ed.). New York: Philosophical Library.

Sullivan HS. (1953). The Interpersonal Theory of Psychiatry. New York, Norton.

Thelander B. (1997). The psychotherapy of Hildegard Peplau in the treatment of people with serious mental illness. Perspectives in Psychiatric Care 33(3):24–32.

Von Franz M. (1975). CG Jung: His Myth in Our Time. Boston, Little, Brown.

Waltzlawick P. (1967). Pragmatics of Human Communication. New York, Norton.

Zalumas J. (1995). Caring in Crisis. Philadelphia: University of Pennsylvania Press.

# 2

# Professional Guides to Action in Interpersonal Relationships

### Elizabeth Arnold

---

**OBJECTIVES**

At the end of the chapter, the student will be able to

1. Define professional nursing
2. Discuss the implications of nurse practice acts in the nurse–client relationship
3. Identify professional standards of care
4. Discuss legal standards
5. Discuss implications of the code of ethics with interpretive statements for the nurse–client relationship
6. Describe the nursing process as a framework for professional nursing practice and the nurse–client relationship
7. Discuss critical pathways as a method of communication

---

*If a man's actions are not guided by thoughtful considerations, then they are guided by inconsiderate impulse, unbalanced appetite, caprice or the circumstances of the moment.*

John Dewey (1933)

---

❖❖ Chapter 2 introduces the student to the professional, legal, and ethical standards of practice that provide essential parameters for professional therapeutic activities occurring within the nurse–client relationship. Also included in the chapter are brief overviews of the nursing process and critical pathways used to sequence nursing actions in the nurse–client relationship and to chart client progress.

Nursing, like other professional disciplines, has professional, legal, and ethical standards that identify scope of practice and govern its actions. They offer the clinician and the consumer a common way of understanding a professional service relationship. When a client goes to a physician, the client assumes the physician will use a defined body of knowledge and will provide care consistent with discipline-specific practice, legal and ethical standards. The client expects the physician to use an organized, systematic method of data collection and to prescribe an appropriate treatment. Similar expectations are found in the legal system. Clients seek lawyers who have knowledge of specific legal codes and procedures. They expect their lawyer to guide them in legal matters to achieve mutually determined goals. As a professional discipline, nurses require similar professional, legal, and ethical standards to guide their practice.

## BASIC CONCEPTS
### American Nurses Association's Definition of Professional Nursing Practice

The American Nurses Association (ANA) has developed a statement of nursing practice that forms the basis for definitions developed in state Nurse Practice Acts.

The practice of professional nursing means the performance for compensation of professional services requiring substantial specialized knowledge of the biological, physical, behavioral, psychological, and sociological sciences and of nursing theory as a basis for assessment, diagnosis, planning, intervention, and evaluation in the promotion and maintenance of health; the case finding and management of illness, injury, or infirmity; the restoration of optimum function; and the achievement of a dignified death. Nursing practice includes, but is not limited to, administration, counseling, supervision, delegation,

and evaluation of practice and execution of the medical regimen, including administration of medications and treatments prescribed by any person authorized by the state to prescribe. Each registered nurse is directly accountable and responsible to the consumer for the quality of nursing care provided (ANA, 1981).

### Professional Licensure

The registered nurse's professional license ensures that each individual nurse has successfully completed nursing program requirements and can demonstrate the knowledge, skills, and competencies to function as a health provider of safe, effective nursing care. All persons practicing nursing are required by law to have a current license in the state in which they practice and to update their licensure yearly. This license requires anyone practicing nursing to comply with all state laws governing practice. The ANA tests core nursing knowledge before granting a nurse a professional license. Nursing licensure helps maintain standards for nursing. Each state currently has the right to determine who does and who does not practice in that state.

### Nurse Practice Acts

*Nurse Practice Acts* are legal documents developed at the state level that define professional nursing's scope of practice and outline the nurse's rights, responsibilities, and licensing requirements in providing care to individual clients, families, and communities. *Scope of practice* refers to the legal boundaries of practice for professional nurses established by each state and defined in written state statutes. Nurse Practice Acts are the single most important statutory laws governing the provision of professional nursing care through the nurse–client relationship (Betts & Waddle, 1993).

Within the Nurse Practice Act, each state or territory identifies specific nursing actions and functions defined as nursing practice, including providing direct care, effectively managing emergency and crisis situations, administering medications, monitoring changes in client conditions, teaching and coaching, prioritizing and coordinating care, supervising unlicensed personnel, and delegating.

Each state legislature approves its Nurse Practice Act and charges state nursing boards, composed of nurses appointed by the governor, to interpret and enforce their mandates through licensing requirements and disciplinary actions if needed. Because the Nurse Practice Act so directly affects professional nursing functions, nurses should pay close attention to legislation and state statutory definitions of nursing practice affecting their practice.

Nurse Practice Acts are written by representative nurses who are appointed by the governor to act as a state board of nursing. Nurse Practice Acts authorize state boards of nursing to interpret the legal boundaries of safe nursing practice and give them the authority to punish violations (ANA, 1995). Violations of the Nurse Practice Act are serious, and professional nurses can lose their licensure to practice or have it suspended for a period of time.

Each state develops and executes its own Nurse Practice Act. Consequently, if a nurse practices in one state and then moves to another, the nurse has to apply for licensure in that state. Scope of practice and the rules governing them may differ as well. Because all Nurse Practice Acts reflect standards of nursing care developed by the ANA (1991), they usually do not differ significantly, but the nurse is advised to have a working knowledge of the Nurse Practice Act in each state of planned employment.

## Professional Standards of Care

Professional Standards of Care, developed by the ANA and revised in 1991, provide guidelines for the provision and evaluation of professional nursing care (ANA, 1991). They are important criteria by which the nurse's actions will be evaluated should legal questions arise about adequate provision of care (Craven & Heinle, 1992). Professional standards help nurses articulate the core of professional nursing to consumers and provide a benchmark for holding practitioners accountable regardless of clinical setting. Specialty groups within the profession have developed additional standards of practice for specific areas such as oncological, geronto-

logical, and psychiatric nursing. Box 2–1 presents Professional Standards of Nursing Care, and Box 2–2 provides descriptors of actions the nurse can take in the nurse–client relationship to implement those standards.

## Legal Standards

In addition to providing nursing care according to professional nursing standards and in accord with Nurse Practice Acts, other important legal tenets have particular relevance for the nurse–client relationship. The nurse is bound legally by the principles of tort law to provide a *reasonable standard of care*, defined as a level of care that a reasonably prudent nurse would provide in a similar situation (Cournoyer, 1991). If taken to court, this statement will be the benchmark against which the nurse's actions will be judged. Criteria for judging negligence in professional nursing practice are found in Box 2–3.

In the nurse–client relationship, the nurse is responsible for maintaining the professional conduct of the relationship. Any form of conduct that could compromise the client's health or welfare is considered unprofessional. Examples of unprofessional conduct in the nurse–client relationship include

- Breaching client confidentiality
- Verbally or physically abusing a client
- Assuming nursing responsibility for actions without having sufficient preparation
- Delegating care to unlicensed personnel that could result in client injury
- Following a doctor's order that would result in client harm
- Failing to report or document changes in client health status
- Falsifying records

### Confidentiality

**Confidentiality,** defined as providing only that information needed to provide care for the client with other health professionals directly involved in the care of the client, is essential to the development of trust. The nurse is bound legally to respect the client's privacy. This means that the nurse must have the client's permission to share information provided in the nurse–client rela-

---

**◆ Box 2–1. Professional Standards Guiding the Nurse–Client Relationship**

**Standards of Care**

I. Assessment
   The nurse collects client health data.

II. Diagnosis
   The nurse analyzes the assessment data in determining diagnoses.

III. Outcome Identification
   The nurse identifies expected outcomes individualized to the client.

IV. Planning
   The nurse develops a plan of care that prescribes interventions to attain expected outcomes.

V. Implementation
   The nurse implements the interventions identified in the plan of care.

VI. Evaluation
   The nurse evaluates the client's progress toward attainment of outcomes.

**Standards of Professional Performance**

I. Quality of Care
   The nurse systematically evaluates the quality and effectiveness of nursing practice.

II. Performance Appraisal
   The nurse evaluates his/her own nursing practice in relation to professional practice standards and relevant statutes and regulations.

III. Education
   The nurse acquires and maintains current knowledge in nursing practice.

IV. Collegiality
   The nurse contributes to the professional development of peers, colleagues, and others.

V. Ethics
   The nurse's decisions and actions on behalf of clients are determined in an ethical manner.

VI. Collaboration
   The nurse collaborates with the client, significant others, and health care providers in providing client care.

VII. Research
   The nurse uses research findings in practice.

VIII. Resource Utilization
   The nurse considers factors related to safety, effectiveness, and cost in planning and delivering client care.

Reprinted with permission from Standards of Clinical Nursing Practice, © 1991, American Nurses Association, Washington, DC.

---

tionship, even with involved family members. Exceptions to this legal mandate include cases involving children in certain circumstances or situations in which withholding of information might cause harm to the client or innocent others. Other exceptions include the required reporting of certain communicable diseases, gunshot wounds, and child abuse. An increasing number of states have introduced legislation to protect privileged communication between nurse and patient statutorily. Chapter 5 provides further information on confidentiality.

In addition to protecting the client's privacy in terms of what is actually discussed in the relationship, the nurse has a legal responsibility to ensure against invasion of privacy related to the following:

- Releasing information about the client to unauthorized parties
- Unwanted visitations in the hospital
- Discussing client problems in public places or with people not directly involved in the client's care
- Taking pictures of the client without consent or using the photographs without the client's permission

---

◆ Box 2-2. Relationship of the Nursing Process to Patient Care Standards in the Nurse–Client Relationship

I. Assess

Collects data

The nurse collects data throughout the nursing process related to client strengths, limitations, available resources, and changes in the client's condition.

Analyzes data

The nurse organizes cluster behaviors and makes inferences based on subjective and objective client data and personal and scientific nursing knowledge.

The nurse verifies data and inferences with the client to ensure validity.

II. Diagnosis

Formulates biopsychosocial statements

The nurse develops a comprehensive biopsychosocial statement that captures the essence of the client's health care needs/problems and validates the accuracy of the statement with the client; the statement becomes the basis for the nursing diagnoses.

Establishes nursing diagnosis

The nurse develops relevant nursing diagnoses and prioritizes them based on the client's most immediate needs in the current health care situation.

III. Plan

Identifies expected outcomes

The nurse and client mutually develop expected outcomes realistically, based on client needs, strengths, and resources.

Specifies short-term goals

The nurse and client mutually develop realistic short-term goals and choose actions to support achievement of expected outcomes.

IV. Implement

Takes agreed-on action

The nurse encourages, supports, and validates the client in taking agreed-on actions to achieve goals and expected outcomes through integrated, therapeutic nursing interventions and communication strategies.

V. Evaluation

Evaluates goal achievement

The nurse and client mutually evaluate attainment of expected outcomes and survey each step of the nursing process for appropriateness, effectiveness, adequacy, and time efficiency, modifying the plan as indicated by evaluation.

---

- Performing procedures such as acquired immunodeficiency testing without the client's permission
- Publishing data about a client in any way that makes the client identifiable without the client's permission (Cournoyer, 1991)

## Informed Consent

*Informed consent,* defined as giving the client enough information on which to base a knowledgeable decision, is another aspect of legal considerations needed in the nurse–client relation-

---

### ◆ Box 2–3. Definition and Examples of Negligent Actions

| Definition of Negligent Action | Example |
|---|---|
| Performing a nursing action that a reasonably prudent nurse would *not* perform | Carrying out a physician's order that would have been questioned by other reasonably prudent nurses in similar circumstances |
| Failing to perform a nursing action that a reasonably prudent nurse would perform | Failing to report child or sexual abuse |
| Failure to provide routine or customary care | Failing to check vital signs pre- and post-surgery; failing to perform post partum checks on a client |
| Conduct that a reasonably prudent nurse would recognize as posing an unreasonable risk to a client | Failing to give accurate information in a manner that the client can understand regarding choice of treatment and known side effects; sharing confidential information with a client's family or work without the client's permission |
| Failing to protect a client from unnecessary harm | Not putting up the guardrails on a bed with a newly diagnosed client suffering from a stroke; allowing unlicensed personnel to do a nursing procedure without appropriate experience or supervision |

---

ship. This is most commonly associated with research studies, treatment decisions, and permission for invasive procedures. Although it typically is the physician's responsibility to supply the information needed for informed consent, nurses play an important role in making sure the conditions for informed consent are met within the nurse–client relationship. Unless there is a life-threatening emergency, all clients have the right to give informed consent. For legal consent to be valid, it must contain three elements (Northrop & Kelly, 1987):

- Consent must be voluntary.
- The client must have full disclosure about the risks, benefits, cost, potential side effects or adverse reactions, and other alternatives to treatment.
- The client must have the capacity and competency to understand the information and to make an informed choice.

### *Protecting Client Rights*

The nurse can take several actions to legally safeguard the rights of clients in professional relationships and to protect the nurse's practice. Important protective strategies are knowledge of and adherence to professional nursing standards. Nurses also are responsible for careful documen-

tation of nursing assessments, care given, and behavioral responses of the client. In the eyes of the law, failure to document in written form any of these elements means the actions were not taken (Betts & Waddle, 1993). In addition, the nurse is accountable for informing other members of the health care team of changes in the client's condition, for appropriately supervising ancillary personnel, and for questioning unclear or controversial orders made by the physician.

## Ethical Code for Nurses

In addition to their legal responsibility to uphold professional standards of nursing practice, nurses have a moral accountability to the clients they serve (Fry, 1991). The purpose of having Codes of Ethics is to promote ethical behaviors by providing guidelines designed to protect the client's rights, provide a mechanism for professional accountability, and educate professionals about sound ethical conduct (Creasia & Parker, 1991). Guidelines for the nurses are found in the ANA Code of Ethics. Nurses need to interpret ethical guidelines not only in the context of each nursing situation but also with an understanding of cultural meanings attached to client behaviors. Chapter 7 describes ethical decision-making processes in more detail.

Ethical principles are guides to actions in the nurse–client relationship and should be a basic consideration in a nurse's choice of words and actions. Erlen (1997) suggested that nurses confront ethical situations every day as they interact with clients, families, and other health care providers. The code of ethics developed by the ANA (Box 2–4) does not contain explicit definitions of right and wrong. Rather, it forms a broad conceptual framework for identifying the moral dimensions of nursing practice that the nurse can incorporate in choosing ethical ways of meeting client needs. Personal moral principles combined with critical thinking and ethical decision-making frameworks become increasingly important in a health care environment driven by cost containment (Moss, 1995). We hope that the reader will see applications of the code threaded throughout the boxes and exercises presented in this text (see Exercise 2–1).

Of particular importance to the nurse–client relationship are ethical directives related to the nurse's primary commitment to the client's welfare, respect for client autonomy, recognition of each individual as unique and worthy of respect, accountability, and collaboration with other health professionals.

In 1991, the U.S. Congress passed the Patient Self Determination Act. This legislation gives clients the autonomy to choose whether or not to have life-prolonging treatment should they become mentally unable to make this decision. Individual preferences regarding treatment options can be put in writing and are recognized by state law. Advance directives provide a new dimension of care and respect for the autonomy of adult clients that formerly was not an explicit issue in nurse–client relationships. Unfortunately, even with an advance directive in place, family members sometimes override the wishes of the client. This can create an ethical conflict for the nurse who frequently is called on to play a significant role in helping families make difficult decisions when the client is unable to do so.

## APPLICATIONS
### Nursing Process

The nursing process was originally developed from general systems theory by the North

---

### ◆ Box 2–4. American Nurses Association Code for Nurses

1. The nurse provides services with respect for human dignity and the uniqueness of the client unrestricted by considerations of social or economic status, personal attributes, or the nature of health problems.

2. The nurse safeguards the client's right to privacy by judiciously protecting information of a confidential nature.

3. The nurse acts to safeguard the client and the public when health care and safety are affected by the incompetent, unethical, or illegal practice of any person.

4. The nurse assumes responsibility and accountability for individual nursing judgments and actions.

5. The nurse maintains competence in nursing.

6. The nurse exercises informed judgment and uses individual competence and qualifications as criteria in seeking consultation, accepting responsibilities, and delegating nursing activities to others.

7. The nurse participates in activities that contribute to the ongoing development of the profession's body of knowledge.

8. The nurse participates in the profession's efforts to implement and improve standards of nursing.

9. The nurse participates in the profession's effort to establish and maintain conditions of employment conducive to high-quality nursing care.

10. The nurse participates in the profession's effort to protect the public from misinformation and misrepresentation and to maintain the integrity of nursing.

11. The nurse collaborates with members of the health professions and other citizens in promoting community and national efforts to meet the health needs of the public.

◆ **Exercise 2-1. Applying the Nurses' Code of Ethics to Professional and Clinical Situations**

**Purpose:** To help you identify applications of the nursing code of ethics

**Procedure:**
1. In small groups of four to five students, each student is to think of a potential ethical dilemma in the clinical care of clients or an actual situation in which he or she has been involved as a caregiver, client, or family member. The dilemma is written as a short summary.
2. Each person shares his or her ethical dilemma and the group problem-solves collaboratively on how the nurse's code of ethics can be used to work through the situation.

**Discussion:**
1. What types of difficulty did your group encounter in resolving different scenarios?
2. What type of situation offers the most challenge ethically?
3. Were there any problems in which the code of ethics was not helpful?
4. How can you use what you learned in this exercise in your nursing practice?

American nursing profession to serve as an organizing framework for ordering and evaluating nursing care (Mason & Attree, 1997). Its use provides a consistent, comprehensive, and coordinated approach to the delivery of nursing care to clients. This systematic process represents a clinical management framework, recognized by all nursing theorists as an organizing structure for clinical nursing practice. It provides a structure for nurses in planning and providing individualized care by identifying and treating responses to potential and actual alterations in health (Alfaro-Lefevre, 1994). In 1991, the ANA expanded the nursing process to include outcome identification as a specific component of the planning phase. The nursing process consists of five progressive phases: (1) assessment, (2) diagnosis, (3) outcome identification and planning, (4) implementation, and (5) evaluation.

The ANA uses the progressive steps of the nursing process as a structural format for identifying measurement criteria related to the professional standards of care described in Box 2-2. The nursing process offers the nurse guidelines to identify the type of nursing a client requires, the scope of nursing activities needed to meet health goals, and the means to evaluate whether the individual's nursing care needs were met.

## Nursing Process and Professional Relations

The nurse–client relationship, as shown in Figure 2–1, affects every aspect of the nursing process, which in turn provides the basic format for all activities carried out in the relationship. The relationship acts as a continuous feedback system for nursing interventions and incorporates a thoughtful process of analysis, synthesis, and critical thinking when working with clients to decide what needs to be done and how best to meet the individualized needs of clients (Taylor, 1997). Within the relationship, the nurse uses the nursing process to analyze client information.

The assessment and nursing diagnosis phases of the nursing process correspond with the orientation phase of the relationship. Here the nurse gathers data from the client (primary source) and other secondary sources such as family, laboratory tests, physical examination, and so on. In the orientation phase, the nurse tries to understand the client as a person responding to an alteration in health status. Data collection includes a description of the health problem or need from the client's perspective, the client's expectations for treatment, strengths and resources available to the client, and a working diagnosis that will serve as the basis for planning and therapeutic intervention.

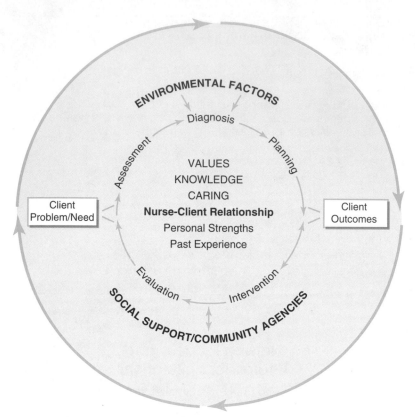

Figure 2–1. The nursing process and the nurse–client relationship feedback loop.

The outcome identification and planning phase of the nursing process bridges the orientation and working phases of the relationship. Here nurse and client develop goals that will direct further work together. Implementation strategies are part of the working phase and consist of client activities toward goal achievement and nursing interventions needed to support them. Evaluation strategies are a significant focus in the resolution phase of the nurse–client relationship as nurse and client review progress, determine necessary modifications, and terminate the relationship. The goals of communication as they relate to the nursing process are directed toward

- Helping clients to promote, maintain, or restore health or to achieve a peaceful death
- Facilitating client management of difficult health care issues
- Providing quality nursing care in an efficient manner

## Assessment

Assessment begins with the first contact between client and nurse. The nurse asks the client to tell his or her story as it relates to the current request for nursing services. A simple statement such as "Can you tell me what prompted you to seek treatment at this time?" usually is sufficient to start the conversation. The initial assessment, usually completed on admission to the health care agency, is very comprehensive. The nurse will collect data not only of the current problem for which the client seeks treatment but also of the client's perception of his or her health, presence of other health risk and protective factors, and the client's coping patterns and support system. In addition to collecting data from all possible sources, the assessment phase includes

1. Organizing the data into a coherent whole
2. Validating the data with the client and others involved in the client's care

3. Identifying patterns and clustering related data
4. Making initial inferences and validating them with the client
5. Reporting data

The nurse uses a structured format for collecting both subjective and objective data from a client and the client's family. *Subjective data* refers to the client's perception of data and what the client says about the data: "I have a severe pain in my chest." *Objective data* refers to data that are directly observable or verifiable through physical examination or tests (e.g., an abnormal electrocardiogram). Combined, these data will present a complete picture of the client's health problem. One without the other is insufficient. In addition, the nurse uses *data cues*, defined as small pieces of data that taken by themselves would not reveal much, but when considered within the total assessment picture can lead the nurse to ask further questions and often turn out to be extremely important (Avant, 1991). For example, hesitancy about a certain topic, complaints of hunger or thirst, dry skin, or agitation should raise questions in the nurse's mind to look beyond the symptom for a fuller explanation. Throughout the data collection, the nurse should consistently validate information with the client to make sure that the information and the nurse's interpretation of it are complete and accurate.

The nurse also collects data related to relevant history (e.g., previous hospitalizations, family history, past medical and psychiatric treatment, and medications). Christensen and Kenney (1990) cautioned that the data should reflect information from as many sources as needed for complete accuracy. Sources of data would include interview, history, physical assessment, and review of records. The nurse identifies potential as well as actual problems and asks the client for confirmation that the nurse's perceptions and problem analysis are correct. It cannot be stressed too often that until the client or significant other (if the client is unable to validate data) validates the data, the assessment is incomplete and in some instances can be invalid. This is an important intersection between the nurse–client relationship and the nursing process.

The nurse identifies health deviations specific to the client and does not make global assumptions about a patient's situation without evidence to support the assumptions. In each clinical situation, the client's behavioral response might be assessed differently. For example, maintaining a sufficient intake of food would need to be assessed in terms of what is sufficient for this particular individual on the basis of age, activity, height-weight ratio, and present health status. Nutritional needs for an active teenager are greater than those for an older, sedentary adult. Having knowledge of their relevance, the nurse would ask different questions of a diabetic, anorexic, or obese client regarding nutritional intake and food choices than of those without these deviations.

Special situations also warrant individualized assessments. For example, the mother of a newborn with Down syndrome might know how to care for a normal infant but will need help adapting care strategies for her handicapped infant. The first time a person relapses with cancer can be different from multiple relapse. Active listening skills allow the nurse to obtain relevant data.

Observations of the client's nonverbal behaviors lead the nurse to make inferences. An **inference** is an educated guess about the meaning of a behavior or statement. To be sure the inference is factual, the nurse validates the data with the client. For example, because a client is withdrawn and distractible, the nurse infers that the client is struggling with an internal emotional issue. To validate this inference, the nurse might comment, "You seem withdrawn as though something is troubling you. Can you tell me about how you are feeling?"

Assessment data will serve as baseline information throughout the nursing process, alerting the nurse to resolution of nursing problems or the need for a different strategy if client needs and problems are not being addressed. As new information becomes available, the nurse refines and updates nursing diagnoses.

After data collection and identification of the health deviation, problem, or need, the nurse analyzes the data and identifies gaps in the data collection. The nurse compares individual client data with normal health standards, behavior patterns, and developmental norms to identify not only client problems but also client strengths. Identifying client strengths on which to build in seeking solutions to difficult health care problems is particularly important in today's health care environment, when clients have to assume much more responsibility for their health care than previously. Those health care concerns judged potentially responsive to nursing intervention form the basis for the selection of nursing diagnoses.

## Diagnosis

The second step in the nursing process is development of relevant nursing diagnoses. Nursing diagnoses provide a common language for discussing client problems. Written as client-centered statements, an actual diagnosis consists of three parts (North American Nursing Diagnosis Association, 1996). The stem of the diagnosis labels the problem requiring nursing intervention. The second part of the statement identifies the cause or risk factors associated with the health care problem. For example, "Impaired communication related to cerebral vascular accident" or "Alteration in body image related to partial mastectomy" are clear, simple connecting statements about client health care concerns requiring nursing intervention. The third part of the statement identifies the clinical evidence that supports the diagnosis, for example, "Impaired communication related to a cerebral vascular accident, as evidenced by incomplete sentences and slurred words."

Nurses need to express a nursing diagnosis in clear, precise language so that any member of the health care team can look at the statement and be able to identify relevant issues for the client. Levine (1989) suggested that "the nursing diagnosis should be as informative and useful to the physician as the medical diagnosis is to the nurse" (p. 5). Exercise 2–2 gives practice in writing nursing diagnoses. Chapter 23 elaborates on the use of the nursing process with a focus on appropriate, accurate documentation.

## Planning and Outcome Identification

Once a nursing diagnosis is in place, the nurse develops a comprehensive treatment plan in collaboration with other members of the health care team that addresses immediate and potential client-specific problems. The Joint Commission on Accreditation of Health Care Organizations (1991) requires that a carefully formulated written plan of care with clearly identified and individualized goals addressing the short- and long-term needs of the client be initiated on admission and reassessed periodically according to agency policy. The plan is sequential, with priority attention focused on the most immediate life-threatening problems and dynamic, meaning that it needs to be continuously updated as the client's condition and needs change.

The care plan contains short- and long-term goals, stated as outcome criteria that direct nursing interventions to meet the desired outcomes. The planning phase requires critical thinking skills developed in Chapter 7 and the development of realistic desired outcome criteria. Outcome criteria are the actions and behaviors that the client will demonstrate once the health problem is resolved, stated in behavioral terms. Corresponding nursing interventions as actions the nurse will take to help the client meet identified goals relate specifically to identified outcome criteria. The ANA (1991) specified that outcomes should be

- Based on diagnoses
- Documented in measurable terms
- Developed collaboratively with the client and other health providers
- Realistic and achievable

For example, an outcome criterion (short-term goal) for a socially isolated client might be written as, "The client will develop a support system within 1 month." The associated nursing intervention might be, "The nurse will encourage the client to call at least one person every 2 days."

Outcome criteria take into account the client's life situation, history and present status, intellectual and emotional capabilities, and strengths and limitations as well as the professional resources available. Care needs to be taken that the client participates to the fullest extent possible in arriving at nursing diagnoses and setting goals (Mitchell, 1991). Important client values and preferences should be factored into the development of relevant outcome criteria. Time limits need to be realistic so that the client does not become discouraged with lack of goal achievement.

Establishing nursing need priorities based on practical considerations and the wishes of the

---

◆ **Exercise 2–2. Writing Nursing Diagnoses**

**Purpose:** To help you develop skill in writing nursing diagnoses

**Procedure:**
1. In small groups of two or three students, develop as many nursing diagnoses as possible for each of the following clinical situations based on the information you have. Indicate what other types of information you would need to make a complete assessment.

   a. Michael Sterns was in a skiing accident. He is suffering from multiple internal injuries, including head injury. His parents have been notified and are flying in to be with him.

   b. Lo Sun Chen is a young Chinese woman admitted for abdominal surgery. She has been in this country for only 8 weeks and speaks very little English.

   c. Marisa LaFonte is a 17-year-old unmarried woman admitted for the delivery of her first child. She has had no prenatal care.

   d. Stella Watkings is an 85-year-old woman admitted to a nursing home after suffering a broken hip.

**Discussion:**
1. What common diagnoses emerged in each group?
2. In what ways were the diagnoses different, and how would you account for the differences?
3. Were there any common themes in the types of information each group decided it needed to make a complete assessment?
4. How could you use what you learned from this exercise in your clinical practice?

---

client help ensure success. The nurse ranks the client's nursing diagnoses in order of physiological and psychological importance, with basic physical imperatives emerging first and inclusive of input from the client, family, and significant others. Maslow's hierarchy of needs, described in Chapter 1, provides a rationale for prioritizing nursing actions, beginning with the most acute and basic needs. Once basic physiological needs (respiration, cardiac status, nutrition, and renal function) are satisfied, the nurse begins to consider the client's safety and self-esteem needs and so on to higher levels on the hierarchy of needs. Nurses may address more than one nursing diagnosis at a time; in fact, often attention to several nursing diagnoses can serve the same outcome. By communicating the results of this decision-making process to other health care providers involved in the treatment of the client, the nurse ensures continuity and an ordered approach to meeting the individualized needs of the client (Carpenito, 1995). The care plan is a dynamic document that the nurse continually updates as the client's condition changes.

Goal achievement forms the rationale for the nurse and client to engage in a therapeutic relationship. The nurse and client mutually develop treatment goals related to the nursing diagnosis that are stated as measurable behavioral objectives to be achieved within a specific time frame. Short-term goals represent the progressive steps needed to achieve a broader and more general long-term goal. For example, "The client will achieve dietary control of his diabetes" might be a long-term goal for a diabetic client, and "The client will identify a sample American Dietetic Association (ADA) diet plan for 1 week" might be a short-term goal.

## Implementation

During the implementation phase, the client and nurse carry out the care plan. Interventions appropriate to the purposes of the nurse–client relationship include giving physical, psychological, social, and spiritual support; health teaching; collaborating with other health professionals on behalf of the client; continuing to make ongoing assessments; documenting client responses; and updating or revising the care plan as needed. ***Independent nursing interventions*** are interventions that nurses can provide without a physician's order or direction from another health professional. Independent nursing interventions are permitted under Nurse Practice Acts and are protected through professional licensure and law. Many forms of direct care assistance, health education, health promotion strategies, and counseling fall into this category, and nurses are particularly well equipped to provide these functions. ***Dependent nursing interventions*** are those that require an oral or a written order from a physician. A prime example is medication administration. In most states, staff nurses cannot administer a medication without having a physician order. The nurse, however, is held accountable for using appropriate knowledge, judgment, and competence in administering the medication a physician orders. Thus, a nurse would not automatically carry out a physician's order without considering first the appropriateness of the medication or without knowing appropriate dosage, mode of action, side effects, and potential adverse reactions.

## Evaluation

The nurse uses the evaluation phase of the nursing process to compare projected behavioral responses and outcomes with what actually occurred. Nurse and client assess the client's progress or lack of progress toward identified goals. They mutually appraise the benefits and limitations of choices made for problem resolution. When there is a lack of progress, the nurse needs to ask the following questions:

- Was the assessment data collected appropriate and complete?
- Was the nursing diagnosis appropriate?
- Were the goals realistic and achievable in the time frame allotted?
- Were the nursing interventions chosen appropriate to the needs of the situation and the capabilities of the client?

The nurse needs to critically think through the meaning of each question. For example, the nursing diagnosis may be appropriate, but the intervention required may be too complex or not achievable in a limited time frame. The nurse needs to analyze the effectiveness, time efficiency, appropriateness, and adequacy of the nursing actions selected for implementation. Paying attention to the reality of the situation, the motivation of the client, and the setting in which the interventions need to be accomplished can prevent unnecessary frustration on the part of both nurse and client. The client gives input regarding actions perceived as helpful or not useful. Mutually agreed-on modification follows in any area of the nursing process requiring it. Figure 2–2 diagrams the steps of the nursing process.

## Critical Pathways

Current changes in the health care delivery system with an emphasis on maximizing resource use and multidisciplinary accountability have fostered the development of new, broader clinical management tools that extend beyond the nursing process (Walsh, 1997). One such strategy is the emergence of critical pathways, sometimes referred to as a clinical pathway or integrated care plan. *Critical pathways* function as interdisciplinary health care guidelines. They begin with a desired client outcome, based on clinical diagnosis rather than with individualized client needs. A critical pathway document is a comprehensive client-centered plan of care that

- Defines desired client outcomes and goals
- Directs collaborative practice
- Provides for coordination and continuity of care involving clients and families
- Focuses on reducing resource requirements (Westra, 1997, p. 1)

Critical pathways usually address a specific diagnosis or procedure such as surgery. Criteria for the development of a critical pathway include high volume, high cost, or difficulty in treatment. They provide a diagram of the expected treatment resources needed to achieve designated outcomes within specified time frames and lessen documentation by using a check-off care plan sheet. Shaughnessy (1997) defines a *health care outcome* as "the change in health status between a baseline time point and a final time point" (p. 1225).

Critical pathways integrate the medical with corresponding nursing plans and predetermined

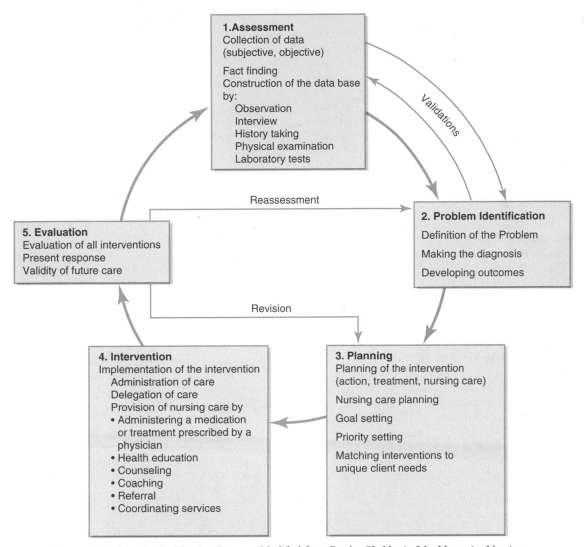

**1.Assessment**
Collection of data
(subjective, objective)

Fact finding
Construction of the data base
by:
    Observation
    Interview
    History taking
    Physical examination
    Laboratory tests

Validations

Reassessment

**2. Problem Identification**
Definition of the Problem

Making the diagnosis

Developing outcomes

**5. Evaluation**
Evaluation of all interventions
Present response
Validity of future care

Revision

**4. Intervention**
Implementation of the intervention
    Administration of care
    Delegation of care
    Provision of nursing care by
    • Administering a medication
      or treatment prescribed by a
      physician
    • Health education
    • Counseling
    • Coaching
    • Referral
    • Coordinating services

**3. Planning**
Planning of the intervention
(action, treatment, nursing care)

Nursing care planning

Goal setting

Priority setting

Matching interventions to
unique client needs

Figure 2–2. Steps in the Nursing Process. (Modified from Reeder SJ, Martin LL: Maternity Nursing, 16th ed. [1987]. Lippincott-Raven Publishers. In McCaffery M, Beebe A. [1989]. Pain: Clinical Manual for Nursing Practice. St. Louis, CV Mosby.)

standards of care. The pathway can include other health care services provided by physical therapy, nutritionists, occupational therapy, social work, and referrals to external health care agencies. In the hospital, critical pathways use days as time frames, and in home care, the time frames are developed around visits. The pathway focuses on critical clinical elements and events necessary to achieve predetermined treatment outcomes. A

critical pathway record is used at any given time as a composite guide to treatment and account of outcome achievement.

Critical pathways have implications for the nurse–client relationship. The nurse frequently is in charge of coordinating the critical pathway and of explaining treatment expectations and the client's role in the process of goal achievement. Critical pathways should be client focused. The role of the client is active and centered on the treatment process. From the start of treatment, the client knows the anticipated short- and long-term outcomes and just what is expected of him or her as a partner in the critical pathway to a successful outcome.

The nursing process can still help the nurse organize nursing care within the critical pathway. Critical pathways spell out desired nursing interventions related to specific medical and nursing diagnoses. Despite the standardized format of critical pathways on paper, the nurse still individualizes nursing care to meet the unique needs of each client through the medium of the nurse–client relationship. Here, as in all other aspects of nursing practice, the nurse uses nursing theory to inform practice and integrates technical knowledge with creative applications of the nursing process to achieve mutually decided-on health care goals.

Often the nurse is accountable for ensuring continuity of care related to the critical pathway. Nurses will assume primary responsibility for coordinating the care given by a number of health care team members as well as for evaluating the client's progress toward expected outcomes and documenting variances.

As documentation becomes increasingly computerized with client data entered at the time of service into an ongoing electronic medical record, critical pathways become essential as a way of organizing and directing health care interventions.

## SUMMARY

Chapter 2 focuses on the nurse's need to have a basic knowledge of the externally imposed legal and ethical variables that influence the nurse's choice of actions in the nurse–client relationship. The chapter provides a brief overview of the nursing process as a framework for the actions taken in the relationship. Knowledge of practice guidelines and ethical principles is necessary for implementing an effective nurse–client relationship.

The nurse–client relationship is contained within the scope of nursing practice as defined by the Nurse Practice Acts. Standards of professional practice provide a measurement standard that should form the foundation of professional nursing. The nurse–client relationship is bound legally by the principles of tort law to provide a reasonable standard of care. This means that the nurse is obligated to provide a level of care that a reasonably prudent nurse would provide in a similar situation. The ANA code of ethics provides a broad conceptual framework for identifying the moral dimensions of nursing practice and is an important guide to choices of actions in nurse–client relationships.

The nursing process serves as a clinical management framework, recognized by all nursing theorists as an organizing structure for clinical nursing practice. It involves five phases: assessment, diagnosis, outcome criteria and planning, implementation, and evaluation. The nursing diagnosis is established at the end of the assessment phase and forms the basis for the remaining phases of the nursing process.

Critical pathways have emerged as an interdisciplinary clinical management framework as a result of radical changes in the health care system and the introduction of managed care. Critical pathways merge medical and nursing care plans, offering a standardized format for ordering and evaluating treatment from admission to discharge.

## REFERENCES

Alfaro-Lefevre R. (1994). Applying Nursing Diagnoses and Nursing Process (3rd ed.). Philadelphia, JB Lippincott.

American Nurses Association. (1981). Definition of the Practice of Professional Nursing. Kansas City, MO, Author.

American Nurses Association. (1985). Code for Nurses with Interpretative Statements. Kansas City, MO, Author.

American Nurses Association. (1991). Standards of Clinical Nursing Practice. Washington, DC, Author.

American Nurses Association. (1995). Nursing: A Social Policy Statement. Washington, DC, Author.

Avant K. (1991). Paths to concept development in nursing diagnosis. Nursing Diagnosis 2(3):105–110.

Betts V, Waddle F. (1993). Legal aspects of nursing. In Chitty K (ed.), Professional Nursing: Concepts and Challenges. Philadelphia, WB Saunders.

Carpenito L. (1995). Nursing Care Plans and Documentation: Nursing Diagnosis and Collaborative Problems (2nd ed.). Philadelphia, JB Lippincott.

Christensen P, Kenney J. (1990). Nursing Process: Application of Conceptual Models (3rd ed.). St. Louis, Mosby-Year Book.

Cournoyer C. (1991). Legal relationships in nursing practice. In Creasia J, Parker B (eds.), Conceptual Foundations of

Professional Nursing Practice. St. Louis, Mosby-Year Book.

Craven R, Heinle C. (1992). Fundamentals of Nursing. Philadelphia, JB Lippincott.

Creasia J, Parker B. (1991). Conceptual Foundations of Professional Nursing Practice. St. Louis, Mosby-Year Book.

Erlen J. (1997). Everyday ethics. Orthopedic Nursing 16(4):60–63.

Fry S. (1991). Ethics in health care delivery. In Creasia J, Parker B (eds.), Conceptual Foundations of Professional Nursing Practice. St. Louis, Mosby-Year Book.

Joint Commission on Accreditation of Health Care Organizations. (1991). Accreditation Manual for Hospitals. Chicago, Author.

Levine M. (1989). The ethics of nursing rhetoric. Image 21(1):4–6.

Mason G, Attree M. (1997). The relationship between research and the nursing process in clinical practice. Journal of Advanced Nursing 26(5):1045–1049.

Mitchell GJ. (1991). Nursing diagnosis: An ethical analysis. Image 23(2):99–103.

Moss M. (1995). Principles, values, and ethics set the stage for managed care nursing. Nursing Economics 13(5):276–284.

North American Nursing Diagnosis Association. (1996). Nursing Diagnoses: Definitions and Classification 1997–1998. Philadelphia, Author.

Northrop C, Kelly M. (1987). Legal Issues in Nursing. St. Louis, CV Mosby.

Shaughnessy P. (1997). Outcomes across the care continuum: Home health care. Medical Care 35(12):1225–1226.

Taylor C. (1997). Problem solving in clinical nursing practice. Journal of Advanced Nursing 26(2):329–336.

Walsh M. (1997). Will critical pathways replace the nursing process? Nursing Standard 11(52):39–42.

Westra B. (1997). Critical pathways in home care. Available: http.//carefacts.com/art2.html.

# 3

# Self-Concept in the Nurse–Client Relationship

Shirley A. Smoyak

---

## OBJECTIVES

At the end of the chapter, the student will be able to

1. Define self-concept
2. Describe the characteristics and functions of self-concept
3. Identify the psychosocial stages of self-development
4. Describe behaviors related to self-concept: body image, personal identity, self-esteem, and spiritual distress
5. Identify nursing interventions relevant to nursing diagnoses of alteration of self-concept
6. Describe the role of self-awareness in the nurse–client relationship

*The greatest gift I can conceive of having from anyone is to be seen by them, heard by them, to be understood and touched by them. The greatest gift I can give is to see, hear, understand and to touch another person. When this is done, I feel contact has been made.*

Virginia Satir, 1976

## BASIC CONCEPTS

At birth, infants do not have a "self." They are simply a biological bundle of drives, predispositions, and tendencies to develop in ways determined by their heritage. These essentially biological beings, interacting with their human socializing agents known as parents, evolve into psychosocial beings, complete with selves and self-esteem. Nurses need to address not only the biological components of patients for whom they provide nursing care but the psychosocial components as well. Culture is the prime determinant of how parents rear and develop their children and is discussed within this chapter, although the main focus is on concepts and dynamics associated with the self or self-concept.

Chapter 3 provides an overview of self-concept as a way of understanding the uniqueness of nurse and client, the basic units of a nurse–client relationship. The chapter defines self-concept, considers its complex nature, and provides applications related to self-concept within nurse–client relationships.

## Definitions

Self, self-concept, and self-system are used interchangeably in the human developmental and psychological literature. Harry Stack Sullivan (1892–1949) is considered the father of the interpersonal theory of psychiatry, and wrote widely about how self develops and what processes mediate its development. Hildegard E. Peplau, considered the mother of psychiatric nursing, studied Sullivan's work and extended it in her many written works and workshops for nurses in the United States and many foreign countries.

The self, **self-concept,** or self-system is an organized network of ideas, feelings, and actions, which every person has as a consequence of experiences and interactions with other people, with parents being the most important in the development process. **Self-esteem** reflects the degree to which one feels valued, important, or satisfied with the concept of self.

### How Self Develops

Peplau described four steps that clearly spell out how the self develops. Over the years, she incorporated these steps into lectures about the self delivered to students in basic education programs, master's programs, and continuing education workshops.

1. Appraisals are made by significant others about the *self.*

In this first step, self is emphasized to show that it does not yet exist but is developing. Mothers and other significant others, such as fathers, grandparents, and older siblings, make appraisals or evaluative statements about the newborn or very young infant. Generally, these appraisals are very warm, positive, or complimentary (e.g., "good girl," "good boy," "beautiful baby," "how wonderful") and said in pleasant tones, accompanied by cuddling or holding gently but securely. The infant cannot comprehend the words, of course, but does absorb the affect and general meaning.

The important idea in this first step is that the appraisal is not based on anything that the infant does or is but rather is based on the expectational set of the evaluator or appraiser. In fact, often the appraisal is really about something that the significant other has done. For instance, when an infant is burped properly and expels air, keeping the milk down, the evaluator (mother or caretaker) says, "good boy!" or "good girl!" When the evaluator burps the infant incorrectly, and he or she spits up milk along with the air, what's said is "Oh, messy baby." In the first instance, the statement really should be "good burper!" or "good Mother" and in the latter "bad burper!" or "bad Mother." If the burper does not get the air up after a feeding and the infant later has gas pains, the statement made is "Oh, what a colicky baby!" or "how irritable" or "how fussy." Again, the infant did not act by itself; the outcome was largely the competence or incompetence of the mother or other caretaker.

Thus, appraisals being made by significant others about the developing self need to be understood as part of the self-system of the developers, not the newborn.

2. Appraisals are repeated, become a pattern, and become incorporated into self.

As time goes on and the infant grows, appraisals being made take on regularity and become patterns. Mothers who feel competent and good about being mothers generally feel positively toward their infants. Mothers who are ill or stressed or having many problems of their own will tend to see their infants in a less positive light. Their appraisals will be more negative.

Expectations held (even if not in full awareness) by significant others are very critical to this process. If the infant's feeding clock is set at 2 hours and the mother thinks infants should eat every 4 hours, negative appraisals will be made about the infant's signal for hunger, crying. If the infant takes 20-minute naps in a random manner, and the mother thinks newborns should sleep several hours at a time during the day, the two are on a collision course, with the outcome being that the infant is appraised negatively.

3. Behavior emerges to match the appraisals.

Even before speech emerges, it is possible to see how infants react to the appraisals. Infants can be observed, and what can be seen are images of generally satisfied, pleasant, or happy little beings or, on the other hand, unhappy, unpleasant beings. These outcomes emerge from the powerful impact of the significant others or caretakers on the developing selves.

When speech emerges, validation of this appraisal is evident by the child's language. Generally, children begin referring to self in the third person, such as "Johnny good," or by pointing to self and smiling, after doing something positive. Later, the first person is used, and we hear "I ate it all up!" or "I did potty right!"

4. With each new era of development, the self is open for reappraisal.

An era of development can be a biophysical maturation, such as sphincter control (so toilet training can be successful) or brain development (so speech is possible), or a change of environment. Going to school, or preschool, presents opportunities for new appraisers and new experiences. Each situational change opens the self-system for a new look at expectations, accomplishments, and possibilities.

In essence, the self joins the process of appraisal by becoming a vital part of the appraisal work. For instance, the self might not agree with a negative appraisal and might correct it. "I'm not naughty; I'm trying to discover things" or "I am not sleepy, or hungry" or "I am."

The development of self is an ongoing process. One is never completely finished with refining one's sense of self, or self-concept. Similarly, one's self-esteem can be damaged at times but then repaired and enhanced.

Throughout life, the self-concept continues to act as an interpreter of life's meaning. It represents "a self-knowledge of one's coherence and authenticity" (Hoare, 1991, p. 47). Self-concept biases what a person focuses on in communication, what a person expects from others, and what a person remembers of a conversation. How open and honest a person is able to be in a relationship with another person is correlated with the self-concept. Differences in people's definition of personally meaningful behavior and those life events that affect them very little can be understood from the perspective of what constitutes the self.

Self-concept affects treatment outcomes. Unanticipated negative outcomes in an illness or during a crisis can reflect self-concept disturbances rather than a lack of motivation or knowledge (Koehler, 1989). People can unconsciously "will" themselves to die or fail to progress because to do otherwise does not fit with their self-concept.

A narrow self-concept tends to thwart adaptation. When dysfunctional thoughts challenge the self-concept, energy becomes bound by those thoughts and feelings. Defense of self-concept restricts thinking about alternatives, resulting in self-defeating behaviors.

Caring human connections often are as healing as medication and specific treatments in influencing human responses to an illness, because they touch and confirm the self-concept. Even when the nurse is unable to promote healing through physical measures, the interpersonal process of understanding the meaning of the illness in the person's life provides a different type of healing. Through the nurse–client relationship, the nurse helps clients lessen the impact of confusion, social alienation, emptiness, or illness.

## Characteristics

The self-concept is a dynamic, holistic, unique mental construct reflecting a person's interaction with the larger social community as well as intrapersonal characteristics. More than the sum of its parts, the self-concept acts as an inner snapshot of a person, helping people experience who they are and what they are capable of becoming physically, emotionally, intellectually, socially, and spiritually in community with others.

### Dynamic Process

The self-concept is a dynamic process, increasing in both diversity and complexity (Markus & Wurf, 1987). Throughout life a person develops and defines self-concepts as generalizations about the self: "I am outgoing," "I have excellent analytical skills," "I am a loser." As the person develops from child to adult, the self-concept becomes increasingly complex, reflecting responses of the self to new challenges in the life cycle. Attitudes about the self are modified by life experience (Cairns & Cairns, 1988).

Self-concepts allow roles to change and enlarge as a person matures. The self-concept of a child broadens through social interactions as the emerging person develops close associations with others to include that of adult, marriage partner, or parent. James (1891) noted that a person "has as many different social selves as there are distinct groups of persons about whose opinion he cares." Appropriate psychosocial development requires the emerging adult to incorporate the self-identity of worker, contributor to the community, spouse, and parent in an evolving spectrum of self-identifying concepts.

### Holistic Construct

Self-concept is a **holistic construct.** It represents the unified whole of a person with each functional aspect of self-concept fitting together and each single element affecting all other parts. Because self-concept functions as an organized whole, disorganization in any one dimension of self affects the functioning of the entire self. Alterations in body image influence personal identity and vice versa. Depression and loss of meaning affect a person's attitudes toward the body and toward role relationships.

In health care the sensitive interconnections among mind, body, and spirit illustrate the close interdependence of self-concepts. Physical illness always creates some type of psychological tension. Current research demonstrates that it is possible to reduce the physical need for pain medication and to diminish the impact of physiological disorders by altering typical patterns of behavior and feelings (Heinrich & Schag, 1985). Irreversible physical ailments in the patient can create emotional exhaustion and moral dilemmas for the caregiver, including the professional nurse (Arnold, 1989). In 1986, the North American Nursing Diagnosis Association (NANDA) developed a Unitary Person Framework for developing a nursing data base, further emphasizing the belief in the whole person as the fundamental concern of professional nursing care.

### Unique Construct

The self-concept is unique to each person (Travelbee, 1971). Individual physiological features and inborn personality traits differ, as do ethnic and cultural heritage. Life experiences are both qualitatively and quantitatively different, even for two individuals living together within the same family environment. Position in the family, encounters with neighbors, physical make-up, basic temperament preferences, and amount of social support are variables that account for differences in experience. One can think of the self-concept basically as being the response to the question, "Who am I?" For each person, the answer is different (Exercise 3–1).

### Social and Cultural Norms

Self-concepts reflect social and cultural norms. **Context** represents a person's environment, defined as all of the intrapersonal and interpersonal circumstances influencing client behaviors. Self-concept is linked emotionally with context through culture and experience but also serves

◆ Exercise 3–1. **Who Am I?**

**Purpose:** To help you understand some of the self-concepts you hold about yourself. May be done as a homework exercise and discussed in class. The class should sit face to face in a circle.

**Procedure:**
Fill in the blanks to complete the following sentences. There are no right or wrong answers.

The thing I like best about myself is _____.

The thing I like least about myself is _____.

My favorite activity is _____.

When I am in a group, I _____.It would surprise most people if they knew I _____.

The most important value to me is _____.

I like _____.

I most dislike _____.

I am happy when _____.

I feel sad when _____.

I feel most self-confident when I _____.

I am _____.

I feel committed to _____.

Five years from now I see myself as _____.

**Discussion:**
1. What were the hardest items to answer? The easiest?
2. Were you surprised by some of your answers? If so, in what ways?
3. Did anybody's answers surprise you? If so, in what ways?
4. Did anyone's answers particularly impress you? If so, in what ways?
5. What did you learn about yourself from doing this exercise?
6. How would you see yourself using this self-awareness in professional interpersonal relationships with clients?

to interpret the meaning of the context. Family, friends, and others in the community are part of a person's interpersonal context (Fig. 3–1). They serve to confirm, support, or negate the self-concept. For example, an American woman might be respected for strong self-expression; the same behaviors would be frowned upon in a traditional Chinese woman.

The capacity of an individual to maintain a stable, adaptive identity depends in part on the nature, timing, and number of the biological, environmental, or psychological assaults to the integrity of the self. For example, any job loss is difficult for a person to absorb emotionally. However, a job loss for someone whose job has been a principal part of his or her identity can have the psychological impact of a significant death.

Threats to the self-concept occurring in rapid succession can have an additive effect, as can

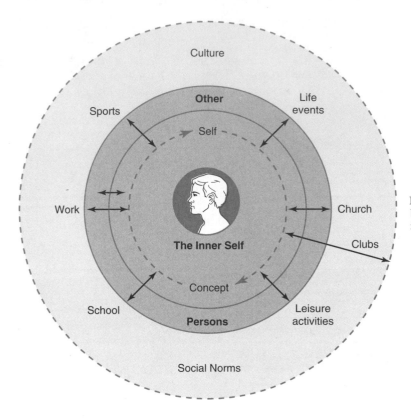

**Figure 3–1.** Reciprocal connections between self-concepts and social influences.

those occurring coincident with normal maturational crises. Consider the cumulative effects of losing both parents and undergoing emergency surgery within a 3-month period. Cumulative tragedies result in significant assaults to self-concept.

## Psychological Centrality

Clinically, certain aspects of the self-concept may be favored or valued more than others, thus achieving a "psychological centrality" (Adler et al., 1986). Psychological centrality refers to the level of emphasis a person places on different aspects of self-concept. For example, the health care team might emphasize body image or personal identity with a trauma victim having disfiguring injuries. Being attached to multiple pieces of equipment and restrained from moving will affect perception, with a related loss of orientation and confusion about self. Body image alterations are very obvious. However, the same injury also may create significant spiritual distress

and questions about the quality of life. Limited socialization and physical disability usually result in redefinition of roles.

Circumstances determine which aspects of self-concept become psychologically central. Psychological centrality is temporary and changes as circumstances convert the focus from one element to another. When students study for a test, they usually focus on how well prepared they feel and on their cognitive ability. They mentally review past performance as an indicator of whether they will pass or fail the test. Even if they know the content, the positive or negative evaluation of their performance ability will affect their test achievement.

After the test, psychological centrality shifts from cognitive aspects of identity to other parts of the self. At the party after the test, social and physical aspects of self will be more primary. The self-concept remains the same, but psychological centrality shifts, much as designs do when seen through a kaleidoscope.

In health care, the impact of being in a hospital assumes psychological centrality for most clients. Differences in client experiences affect the level of shock. Previous experiences and the client's perception of successful outcome are important, as are cultural values about hospitalization and helping professionals. The client who has never been hospitalized has more limited coping skills than one who has had the experience. Simple interventions such as providing anticipatory guidance about procedures, letting children manipulate equipment, and orienting the client and family to the unit help reduce the impact of being in a new and unfamiliar setting.

## Functions of Self-Concept

Self-concepts

- Help explain behavior
- Provide a conceptual framework for decision making
- Shape expectations for the future
- Provide bridges to meaning

Self-concept acts as a decision-making framework within which the individual can evaluate current behaviors and weigh the legitimacy of feelings. Decisions congruent with self-concept affirm the sense of self-identity. Those that conflict with understandings of self diminish self-worth and affect the quality of a person's relationships with others.

Self-concept serves to shape future expectations through the concept of "possible selves" (Cross & Markus, 1991). Possible selves unfold in the form of thoughts about goals, dreams, and fears about events still to come. Future thoughts provide either positive or negative input to the self-concept. For example, the nursing student might think, "I am a nursing student, but I can see myself, one day, as a nurse practitioner." Such thoughts help the novice nurse work harder to achieve professional goals. Possible selves have the capacity to prompt behaviors and aspirations, bringing about a self-fulfilling prophecy (Markus & Nurius, 1986).

Crises and illnesses provide the stage for considering possible selves that would not occur without these life interruptions. This concept is particularly important in health care because possible selves offer clients the hope that the current self-concept can be enlarged to include more positive possibilities. At the same time, negative possible selves (failure, incompetence, powerlessness) can work against the person, providing a negative context for evaluating the current self-concept. The nurse–client relationship provides support for positive possibilities of self and helps clients reframe the negative possible selves.

Self-concept provides interpersonal bridges to meaning. The journey to becoming completely one's own unique self is an intensely personal experience. At different points, the terrain appears dark, lonely, and unfamiliar. The nurse offers the client an interpersonal bridge between external events and internal perceptions, aiding the client in search of the deeper meaning of life. That interpersonal bridge can be simply one's presence and valuing of the client. For example, a nursing student wrote in her journal of a client encounter in which the client felt very depressed about her recent diagnosis of cancer. The student spent a long time with the client, answering her questions not only about her condition but also about why the student had chosen nursing. At the end of the encounter, the client thanked the student for listening and kissed her on the cheek, with tears in her eyes. For both participants, the interaction had meaning. The client felt hope and caring. For the student, it was a peak experience, reaffirming her self-concept as a professional nurse, as her statement reveals: "I know I made her feel much better and I comforted her a great deal; I was truly happy being there and this is what I think of when I picture myself as a future nurse" (Turnes, 1993). There was no one statement that made this meeting memorable; it was the genuine presence of the participants that gave this conversation its I–thou qualities. Exercise 3–2 helps the nurse identify personality variations that contribute to self-concept.

## Erikson's Model of Psychosocial Development

Erik Erikson's (1963, 1982) seminal work on personality development is a primary developmental construct used by nurses in the nurse–client relationship. Concepts related to Erikson's model are described in Table 3–1. What follows is a description of each stage as the nurse might encounter it in the nurse–client relationship.

---

◆ **Exercise 3-2. Contribution of Life Experiences to Self-Concept**

**Purpose:**  To help you identify some of the many personality variations contributing to self-concept. There are no right or wrong responses.

**Procedure:**
1. Pair off with another student, preferably one with whom you are not well acquainted.
2. Student A spends 5 minutes questioning Student B to collect a biography of facts, collecting such information as ethnic background, number of siblings, place of birth, job or volunteer experiences, unusual life experiences, types of responsibilities, favorite leisure activities. The process is then reversed, and Student B interviews Student A.
3. Each student introduces the other to the class, using the information gained from the interview.

**Discussion:**
1. What types of information were chosen for sharing and why?
2. Were you surprised by any of the information you found out?
3. How did your perception of other students change in light of the information shared?
4. In what ways were your perceptions different from your initial impression of your partner after the interview portion of the exercise?
5. To what would you attribute these differences?
6. What types of information were fairly similar and which ones were different among your classmates?
7. How did sharing information about self impact on the life of the group?
8. What did you learn about yourself from doing this exercise?
9. How do you think what you learned might apply to nursing practice?

---

## Trust Versus Mistrust

Erikson labeled the first stage of personality development trust versus mistrust. Infants are completely dependent on their caregivers for all of their needs. The infant needs to trust that the caregiver will respond appropriately. Trust is always a major issue for an infant.

As an adult, trust is a basic feeling that someone important to one's well-being will be there emotionally and physically when needed. Without trust, it is difficult to cooperate, to listen to instructions, or to share one's inner feelings. That is why it is such a basic and initial component in any meaningful relationship.

Whenever a person (because of age, illness, or temporary circumstances) becomes dependent on others for his or her existence, trust resurfaces as an issue. Any new experience will create this phenomenon, but an undesired experience in which one feels a lack of coping skills makes it even worse. There is a sense of insecurity and dependence; one feels a need to rely on others for direction and support. In the hospital, these feelings are quickly activated. The client feels like an outsider in an unfamiliar environment and looks to the nurse for assistance in reconstituting a meaningful self-identity. As a client develops confidence in the nurse's caring, the trust issue recedes into the background. Consistency and reliability foster trust.

## Autonomy Versus Shame and Doubt

Once an infant becomes physically mobile, its interpersonal world looks quite different. Erikson's second developmental crisis involves developing motor autonomy. Coinciding with physical autonomy, the child learns the magic of the word "no" in choosing between alternatives. If denied an opportunity to practice independent behavior or family support to express legitimate feelings freely without fear of reprisal, the child may develop a sense of vulnerability and shame. Self-doubt replaces autonomy in situations call-

Table 3-1. **Erikson's Stages of Psychosocial Development, Clinical Behavior Guidelines, and Stressors**

| STAGE OF PERSONALITY DEVELOPMENT | EGO STRENGTH OR VIRTUE | CLINICAL BEHAVIOR GUIDELINES | STRESSORS |
|---|---|---|---|
| Trust versus mistrust | Hope | Appropriate attachment behaviors<br>Ability to:<br>• ask for assistance with an expectation of receiving it<br>• give and receive information related to self and health<br>• share opinions and experiences easily<br>• differentiate between how much one can trust and how much one must distrust | Unfamiliar environment or routines<br>Inconsistency in care<br>Pain<br>Lack of information<br>Unmet needs, such as having to wait 20 minutes for a bedpan or pain injection<br>Losses at critical times or accumulated loss<br>Significant or sudden loss of physical function, such as a client with a broken hip being afraid to walk |
| Autonomy versus shame and doubt | Will power | Ability to:<br>• express opinions freely and to disagree tactfully<br>• delay gratification<br>• accept reasonable treatment plans and hospital regulations<br>• regulate one's behaviors (overcompliance, noncompliance, suggest disruption)<br>• make age-appropriate decisions | Overemphasis on unfair or rigid regulations, for instance, putting clients in nursing homes to bed at 7 P.M.<br>Cultural emphasis on guilt and shaming as a way of controlling behavior<br>Limited opportunity to make choices in a hospital setting<br>Limited allowance made for individuality |
| Initiative versus guilt | Purpose | Ability to:<br>• develop realistic goals and to initiate actions to meet them<br>• make mistakes without undue embarrassment<br>• have curiosity about health care<br>• work for goals<br>• develop constructive fantasies and plans | Significant or sudden change in life pattern that interferes with role<br>Loss of a mentor, particularly in adolescence or with a new job<br>Lack of opportunity to participate in planning of care<br>Overinvolved parenting that doesn't allow for experimentation<br>Hypercritical authority figures<br>No opportunity for play |
| Industry versus inferiority | Competence | Work is perceived as meaningful and satisfying<br>Appropriate satisfaction with balance in lifestyle pattern, including leisure activities<br>Ability to work with others, including staff<br>Ability to complete tasks and self-care activities in line with capabilities<br>Ability to express personal strengths and limitations realistically | Limited opportunity to learn and master tasks<br>Illness, circumstance, or condition that compromises or obliterates one's usual activities<br>Lack of cultural support or opportunity or training |

*Table continued on following page*

Table 3–1. **Erikson's Stages of Psychosocial Development, Clinical Behavior Guidelines, and Stressors** *Continued*

| STAGE OF PERSONALITY DEVELOPMENT | EGO STRENGTH OR VIRTUE | CLINICAL BEHAVIOR GUIDELINES | STRESSORS |
|---|---|---|---|
| Identity versus identity diffusion | Fidelity | Ability to establish friendships with peers<br>Realistic assertion of independence and dependence needs<br>Demonstration of overall satisfaction with self-image, including physical characteristics, personality, and role in life<br>Ability to express and act on personal values<br>Congruence of self-perception with nurse's observation and perception of significant others | Lack of opportunity<br>Overprotective, neglectful, or inconsistent parenting<br>Sudden or significant change in appearance, health, or status<br>Lack of same-sex role models |
| Intimacy versus isolation | Love | Ability to:<br>• enter into strong reciprocal interpersonal relationships<br>• identify a readily available support system<br>• feel the caring of others<br>• act harmoniously with family and friends | Competition<br>Communication that includes a hidden agenda<br>Projection of images and expectations onto another person<br>Lack of privacy<br>Loss of significant others at critical points of development |
| Generativity versus stagnation and self-absorption | Caring | Demonstration of age-appropriate activities<br>Development of a realistic assessment of personal contributions to society<br>Development of ways to maximize productivity<br>Appropriate care of whatever one has created<br>Demonstration of a concern for others and a willingness to share ideas and knowledge<br>Evidence of a healthy balance among work, family, and self demands | Aging parents, separate or concurrently with adolescent children<br>Obsolescence or layoff in career<br>"Me"-generation attitude<br>Inability or lack of opportunity to function in a previous manner<br>Children leaving home<br>Forced retirement |
| Integrity versus despair | Wisdom | Expression of satisfaction with personal lifestyle<br>Acceptance of growing limitations while maintaining maximum productivity<br>Expression of acceptance of certitude of death as well as satisfaction with one's contributions to life<br>Lack of opportunity | Rigid lifestyle<br>Loss of significant other<br>Loss of physical, intellectual, and emotional faculties<br>Loss of previously satisfying work and family roles |

ing for self-reliant action. An abnormal dependence or obstinacy can develop as the child learns that it is unsafe to choose any action autonomously.

On the other hand, failure to impose limits when they should be applied is equally destructive to self-concepts. The toddler is ill equipped physically and emotionally to be completely independent in making choices or decisions. Lacking judgment, many of the toddler's choices can lead to shame and self-doubt without parental direction. Providing direction and safeguards helps the child learn the limits of freedom in relationships. The child learns to express the self so that legitimate personal needs are met without significantly antagonizing others. Developing a sense of autonomy includes behaviors related to self-control, order, and reliability.

## Initiative Versus Guilt

Initiative broadens the development of autonomy to include the skills involved in deliberately planning and undertaking activities. Independent actions become purposeful and goal directed. As the child discovers pleasure in manipulating tools and experimenting with different roles in play activities, thinking and behaviors become more complex.

## Industry Versus

InferiorityCompetency is important in this stage of psychosocial development. The child begins to experience the pleasures associated with task completion and pride in producing something. Children begin to see themselves as workers and to experience themselves in relation to others, both competitively and cooperatively, in mastering skills and tools.

Emotional mastery becomes more of a focus. Before adolescence, parental relationships were the child's primary guide to developing life strategies. In preadolescence, there is a shift in emotional energy from parents to peers. Group play becomes team play. Industry is a forerunner of the more integrated task of ego identity. The strategies learned in this developmental stage ideally lead to career and personal principled commitment.

## Identity Versus Identity

DiffusionErikson considered resolution of the psychosocial crisis of identity as the central life task. Establishing a clear, firm sense of identity promotes resilience in coping with the various assaults to the self-concept life invariably delivers in unfavorable life circumstances.

Erikson characterized identity as representing

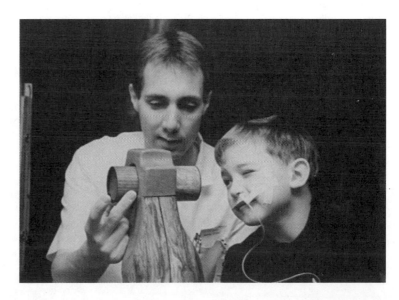

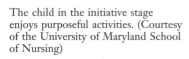
The child in the initiative stage enjoys purposeful activities. (Courtesy of the University of Maryland School of Nursing)

a continuity of self in which personal identity becomes clearer. Truths about self learned from others, self-motivations developed through competencies and values, and the expectations of significant persons in one's life contribute to self-identity. Adolescence marks the transition from child to adult and a new sense of identity. The separation of self from parental figures, which began at birth, becomes more pronounced. A certain amount of identity diffusion or emotional upheaval in the process is considered healthy and normal. There is a loss associated with the necessary change in role to that of the adult. Much of the teenager's emotional turmoil and ambivalence relates to a search for identity, separate from yet very much built on what has gone before.

For many parents, watching teenagers experiment as they attempt to develop "an autonomous definition of self, apart from the nuclear family" (Hoare, 1991) is a painful time. However, adolescents must establish an authentic sense of who they are, repudiating those elements they are not.

Because identity requires that each person become his or her own self-agent, Erikson spoke of commitment to ideals, career identity, and sex role identity as its benchmark. As a core construct of personality, people who choose a commitment corresponding with their talents, skills, and interests generally express self-satisfaction.

Culture and economic conditions play a role in development and expression of identity. Western cultures foster an individualistic approach to identity, but group identity is the preference in many Asian cultures. For many people in today's society, building a solid career identity is threatened by economic uncertainty. Young adults are postponing major life commitments, including marriage, children, and home ownership, because of declining job opportunities and rising costs of housing and education. For economic reasons, many adults in their 20s are still living at home with their parents. Midlife layoffs in previously stable work situations create serious assaults to self-identity. Some people emerge stronger; others are irreparably scarred. Marriage, parenting, and changes in responsibilities, lifestyle, or economic status are capable of re-creating a crisis of identity.

## Intimacy Versus Isolation

Once a person has chosen a vocation, the next life task extends self-concept to a broader shared purpose with another human being. Intimacy is the ability to join with another human being, to connect emotionally as well as physically in mutually satisfying ways. It involves trust of another's good will, a sense of personal identity, and confidence in one's ability to relate effectively with another human being. If a person does not have a clear sense of personal identity, intimacy is difficult to achieve. Other people can enrich, complement, and offer feedback about the self, but they should never be allowed to define it.

## Generativity Versus Stagnation and Self-Absorption

Generativity, the developmental stage associated with midlife, encompasses "procreativity, productivity and creativity" (Erikson, 1982). This time an individual reaffirms the sense of identity by investing the self in the interest of the larger society. Caring becomes central to one's self-definition.

Caring is expressed through commitment. Sharing one's talents with others becomes important. The benchmark associated with this stage of ego maturation does not necessarily relate to the number of family or community obligations a person has. It is possible to fill one's life with activity without being generative or to make many commitments without satisfying any of them. Instead, generativity reflects the quality of investment a person makes to his or her commitments. A person who commits to the betterment of humankind leaves a legacy of experience, knowledge, and caring that affects and inspires future generations. Work, community service, and creative projects, as well as child care, are avenues for generativity. A life in which one has no regrets generally is one that has been generative.

On the other hand, self-absorption or stagnation evolves when an individual makes choices that compromise personal commitments to one's fellow human beings. In hospital settings, where one has little else to think about, it is easy to become self-absorbed. Taking time with a client to explore all aspects of the person, rather than focusing only on the part of the person that is ill, helps refocus clients caught up in self-absorption. The person's contribution to society or his or her sense of self may have to change, but life still can be fulfilling.

## *Integrity Versus Despair*

Erikson's final stage of ego development, integrity versus despair, focuses on the assessment of the meaning and worth of one's life. The crisis of ego integrity is not always age related. Young people facing death as well as old people need to assess their life during the last stage of ego development. They need to understand the meaning of their life as they prepare to exit it. All previous stages are incorporated into this stage of human development, so "a wise Indian, a true gentleman, and a mature peasant share and recognize in one another the final stage of integrity" (Erikson, 1968).

Life review is an important strategy in helping to resolve this stage. A sense of despair develops when an individual realizes that life is almost over and that the opportunity to act differently no longer exists. The nurse can help a client enhance the time left by making attitude changes that permit a different self-appraisal and accepting more fully the positive elements. Exercise 3–3 promotes an understanding of possible selves.

Nurses use Erikson's model as an important part of client assessment. Exercise 3–4 can help apply Erikson's concepts to client situations. Analysis of behavior patterns, using this framework, can identify age-appropriate or arrested development of interpersonal skills (see Table 3–1).

## APPLICATIONS

Figure 3–2 identifies the characteristics of a healthy self-concept. NANDA (1986) separated the nursing diagnosis "Alteration in self-concept" into four discrete elements: body image, personal identity, self-esteem, and role performance. The first three elements are described here. Role relationships are described in Chapter 6 because they have a dual function as an interpersonal bridge between the inner and the outer world of health care.

Although body image, personal identity, self-esteem, and role performance are described as separate processes, the separation is artificial. Sutherland (1993) noted that separation of different elements of self-concept "fails to do justice to the uniqueness of the self as a functioning whole" (p. 4). Throughout the chapter, the student must keep in mind that the simulated division of self-concepts into detached dimensions is for discussion purposes only.

### Body Image

*Body image* represents the physical dimension of self-concept and a person's first awareness of self. Perceptions of the body and its associated elements, not its reality, make up body image. Physical structures associated with body image include not only the actual material body but all

---

### ◆ Exercise 3–3. **A Life of Integrity Through Imaging Possible Selves**

**Purpose:** To promote understanding of the concept of possible selves. Written parts may be done as a homework exercise and the results shared in class

**Procedure:**
Image yourself at a gathering to celebrate your life when you are 60 years old. Write down what you would like the main speaker to highlight about your life. Be as imaginative as possible, but include all of the things you would most like remembered about you if you had full control over how you would live your life.
Share the speech you developed with your class group.

**Discussion:**
1. How did it feel to do this exercise? Were you surprised by any of the feelings you had or by the content of the speech? If so, in what ways?
2. In what ways do you feel the speech you developed reflects your values and life goals?
3. How did it feel to share your speech with your classmates?
4. What new information does the group have that could prove useful in understanding the power of possible selves in nursing practice?

---

◆ Exercise 3–4. **Erikson's Stages of Psychosocial Development**

**Purpose:** To help you apply Erikson's stages of psychosocial development to client situations. May be done as a homework exercise and the results shared in class

**Procedure:**
To set your knowledge of Erikson's stages of psychosocial development, identify the psychosocial crisis(es) each of the following clients might be experiencing:

1. A 16-year-old unwed mother having her first child
2. A 50-year-old executive "let go" from his job after 18 years of employment
3. A stroke victim paralyzed on the left side
4. A middle-aged woman caring for her mother who has Alzheimer's disease
5. A 49-year-old woman dying of pancreatic cancer
6. A 63-year-old woman whose husband announces he has fallen in love with a younger woman and wants a divorce
7. A 17-year-old high school athlete suddenly paralyzed from the neck down

**Discussion:**
1. What criteria did you use to determine the most relevant psychosocial stage for each client situation?
2. In what ways were your answers similar or different from those of your peers?
3. What conclusions can you draw from doing this exercise that would influence how you would respond to each of these clients?

---

somatic sensations of pain, fatigue, pleasure, heat, and cold. The physical self-concepts include the senses as well as the physical presentations of movement expressed through dancing, running, and gestures (Grassi, 1986).

### Functions of Body Image

Schontz (1974) described four functions of body image: (1) a sensory image, (2) an instrument for action and source of drives, (3) a stimulus to self and others, and (4) an expressive instrument. As a sensory register, the body recognizes important information through one or more of its sensory receptors. Touch, for example, provides information about temperature, pressure, and texture (Ackerman, 1990).

The physical self functions as a major instrument for action. Through a remarkable network of muscle, nerve, and cellular interactions, the human body can perform an infinite variety of independent actions. No other physical structure can autonomously decide to move on its own, be able to complete the action, reflect on the meaning of it, and discuss the meaning of it with another.

As a stimulus to self, the mental picture of a person's body and associated feelings (e.g., body weight, shape, and size) affect the value we place on ourselves. Consider how you feel about yourself when you have not showered, shaved, brushed your teeth, or combed your hair; then think how you feel when you know you look your best. Some mental disorders such as major depression, schizophrenia, and eating disorders reflect disturbed body images as part of their symptomatology.

Finally, body image serves as an expressive instrument giving interpersonal signals and information about the self to others. People who dress well and are well groomed generally command more respect than those who do not.

### Types of Alterations

Most people think of body image as describing visible changes in physical characteristics. However, the concept includes more subtle variations related to loss of body function, loss of control, and deviations from the norm.

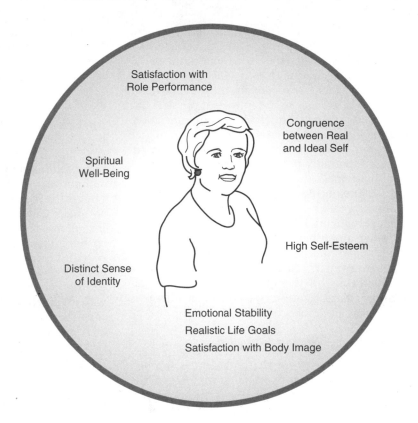

**Figure 3–2.** Characteristics of a healthy self-concept.

Satisfaction with Role Performance

Congruence between Real and Ideal Self

Spiritual Well-Being

High Self-Esteem

Distinct Sense of Identity

Emotional Stability
Realistic Life Goals
Satisfaction with Body Image

**Loss of Body Function.** Loss of body function is an aspect of body image that can be very obvious or well hidden by the client. Inability to move freely, infertility, impotence, and loss of bladder or bowel function are examples of functional loss. The loss is only part of the problem. Many people experience shame about their condition and avoid social situations because of their embarrassment. The mind and body interface so tightly that real or perceived inability to function biologically both affects and is affected by psychological factors. Worrying about it can further compromise functioning. Talking about loss of function with a sympathetic listener makes it more acceptable and more manageable to the client.

**Loss of Control.** Similar in impact to loss of function are alterations in control and loss of sensation. Clients in pain and those subject to seizures, alcoholism, cardiac arrhythmias, or periodic depressions may exhibit few obvious changes in body image. However, the repeated loss of control over the body leaves the client with similar feelings of insecurity and uncertainty. Being able to talk about these realities that dominate some people's feelings about themselves can be enormously reassuring.

**Deviations in Physical Characteristics.** Body image is affected by subtle reactions of others. Those who are too thin or too fat or who look considerably older or younger than they are often are judged on the basis of their looks. Physical attractiveness and conformity to the norm unfortunately result in special treatment, and those who are different or unattractive are not treated so well. People who are different speak of feeling invisible, receiving subtle discrimination, and being misunderstood.

Significant deviations in physical, intellectual, or emotional characteristics have a profound effect on self-concept and self-esteem (Felker, 1974). Understanding differences and working with clients to develop effective coping strategies enhance self-esteem and self-efficacy.

A frequent response to people with long-standing physical deviations is to ignore them or to assume they have gotten used to being different. Lifelong experience with significant deviations in body image does not necessarily make the person unaware of it or any more comfortable with it. Sensitivity to the impact of physical differences is essential to effective communication. Otherwise, nurses can overlook or minimize chronic alterations in body image that are of great importance in assessing the meaning of client behaviors.

**Culture and Body Image.** Culture plays a significant role in our perception of body image by emphasizing some physical characteristics as positive and others as negative. For example, in the United States a slim, trim figure is admired. The overweight individual is thought of as sloppy or unhealthy whether or not this is true. In other cultures, Africa and India, for example, obesity is viewed as a sign of prosperity (Ackerman, 1990).

## How Body Image Develops

Self-knowledge about the body comes through the primary caregiver's human stimulation of the infant. When the infant nurses at the breast or is held, the physical and psychological stimulation enhances the infant's sense of well-being. Deprived of this pleasurable activity, the infant protests by crying and tightening its muscles. Children who never experience the physical and psychological satisfactions of being touched affectionately, kissed, or held often have difficulty expressing and receiving affection in adult relationships. In life, Ackerman (1990) suggested, "touch seems to be as essential as sunlight" (p. 80).

Normal developmental stages affect body image. In adolescence, the rapid surge of physical growth and development, acne, the advent of secondary sex characteristics in puberty, and changes in the endocrine system make the adolescent more vulnerable to concerns about body image (Dempsey, 1972). For the adolescent cancer victim, the hair loss frequently accompanying chemotherapy may be a more difficult side effect with which to cope than a more objectively disabling symptom of pervasive fatigue or nausea.

In later maturity, the body again undergoes major changes; looks fade, the skin becomes wrinkled, muscles sag, the eyes become dim, hearing diminishes, and physical movements slow. The perception of body image is no longer one of youth. To a lesser degree, pregnancy may have a temporary effect on body image.

## Assessment Strategies

Alterations in body image always require some type of adaptation. The extent of adjustment is determined partially by the nature and magnitude of the alteration and the degree to which the alterations interfere with functioning or lifestyle. Highly visible changes usually require more of an adjustment. Likewise, sudden changes in body image may be more difficult to absorb than changes in appearance that occur over time. Important in the human response to alterations in body image are the feelings and attitudes of others, the potential capacity of the client to cope with change, and the availability of sources of support.

Beginning with the first encounter, the nurse seeks to understand the meaning behind the symptoms. The value placed on body image differs from person to person. Some individuals, like Helen Keller and Ray Charles, adapt an objectively negative physical feature of self in ways that benefit not only themselves but all whom they encounter. Others let a physical deviation so dominate self-image that it becomes their only defining characteristic.

The same medical treatment or surgical procedure stimulates different body images. For some women, the prospect of a hysterectomy is viewed with relief; for others, it has serious psychological implications related to attractiveness and physical enjoyment of sex. Understanding these variations in the meaning of physical changes enables the nurse to respond effectively. Instead of simply accepting a single behavioral response as a given, the nurse takes into consideration the personalized meaning of the change for each client in planning care. Assessment data for a nursing diagnosis of self-concept disturbance in body image might include one or more of the following behaviors:

Verbal expression of negative feelings about the body
No mention of changes in body structure and function or preoccupation with changed body image

Reluctance to look at or touch a changed body structure

Expression of worthlessness or hopelessness related to changes in body structure or appearance

Social isolation and loss of interest in friends

The nurse can seek supporting data through open-ended questions or circular questioning related to the client's perception of altered body structure or function. For example, "What has it been like for you since you had your operation?" or "Who do you think could be most helpful to you in making the transition back to work?" Often the concerns of clients relate not only to their perception of the changed appearance or function but also to perceptions of possible reactions of significant others. For example, a client with a speech impediment resulting from surgery or a stroke does not talk because she is anxious about the way her speech sounds to others. A cancer victim fears how she looks to others without her wig.

Other data should include the client's identified strengths and limitations, expressed needs and goals, the nature and accessibility of the client's support system, and the impact of body image change on lifestyle.

## Planning and Intervention

Sensitivity to the client's need to absorb the implications of a change in body image is a critical component of support. Most clients need time to absorb physical changes. Interventions to modify alterations in body image might include

Providing information and support

Modeling acceptance

Introducing adaptive and compensatory functioning

Encouraging the client to share experiences with others

Enhancing social support

*Providing relevant information* and creating opportunities for the client to ask questions make it acceptable for the client to explore an anticipated or actual change in body image. In the case of a new diagnosis, it is important for the nurse to go over information more than once, even if it appears that the client understands it initially. Validation checks, asking whether the client has any questions, and suggesting realistic responses can facilitate communication when the client seems very anxious.

*Modeling acceptance* starts with the nurse. Showing the client that a physical change does not frighten the nurse reduces the fear and panic that a significant change in appearance often presents. Nurses see clients with serious body image changes on a regular basis. For the client it is a unique and potentially horrifying experience. Finding that a significant physical change does not cause the nurse to recoil in disgust allows the client to reframe the situation and to see that the person within remains intact. For example, one client with extensive head and neck surgery would deliberately unwrap his wound to see how each new nurse would react. He needed to know that his nurse would not turn away from him because of his appearance.

As the client demonstrates beginning acceptance through inquiry or a willingness to talk about the physical change, the nurse can slowly introduce the idea of resuming normal functions appropriate to the client's age and developmental level. A warm, supportive, yet tactfully objective interpersonal approach encourages expressions of feelings. For example, the nurse can help a client anticipate and respond with dignity to the reactions of others. *Sharing the experience* with others with a similar ordeal recognizes the legitimacy of having feelings that otherwise might go unexpressed. For example, having a "Reach for Recovery" volunteer visit a mastectomy client to share feelings, hopes, alternative options, and practical suggestions for adapting to changes is a very simple intervention that helps increase the client's adjustment and acceptance of the change. With children, the nurse can act as an advocate in explaining alterations in body image to peers who otherwise might ridicule or avoid a child with a significant physical, cognitive, or emotional deficit.

Finally, the importance of *social support* from family and friends cannot be overestimated. Social support does as much or more for a person than medication and technical skill in alterations in self-concept related to body image. The client needs to know that his or her altered appearance will not disturb relationships. The nurse can suggest that the client call family or friends. Sometimes just a suggestion is enough to put the client in contact with others. At other times the nurse needs to provide encouragement and support to help the client take this step. Anticipatory guidance with visitors to prepare them for dramatic changes in their family member or friend's appearance helps promote acceptance.

### Evaluation

Throughout the relationship, the nurse and client mutually evaluate the effectiveness of the rehabilitation process. Confirming statements about client effort and small steps taken, as well as goals attained, encourage the client to acknowledge short-term goals and point out areas of development that require further modification of the nursing care plan. Appropriate adjustments, if needed, are mutually determined and implemented.

## Personal Identity

*Personal identity* consists of all the psychological beliefs and attitudes people have about themselves: the perceptual, cognitive, emotional, and spiritual elements of self-concept. Personal identity is more difficult to characterize than the physical aspects of self-concept because the nurse cannot actually see it, and it fluctuates with situations. Personal identity is seen in behavior (Rawlinson, 1990).

### Perception

**Perception** is a personal identity construct by which a person transforms external sensory data into personalized images of reality. As an intrapersonal process, perceptions allow a person to choose among sensory images and to cluster sensory images into a meaningful design. Perception is the first gatekeeper of self-concept.

Perception is a function of the mind and not of the senses. Consider the two pictures in Figure 3–3. Depending on how one's eyes focus on the figures in each picture, it is possible to draw quite different conclusions about the images. The same phenomenon is true in life. Reality lies in the eyes of the beholder. Perceptions differ because people develop mindsets that automatically alter sensory data in specific personal ways. Validation of perceptual data is needed because the nurse and the client may not be looking at the same phenomenon.

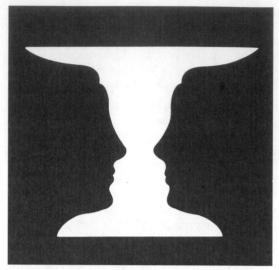

**Figure 3–3.** The figure-ground phenomenon. Are the figures presented in white against a black background or in black against a white background? Does it make a difference in your perception of the figures? (From the Westinghouse Learning Corporation Self-Instructional Unit 12. Perception, 1970. Used with permission.)

### Types of Perceptual Alterations in Self-Concept

**Distorted Reality.** Perceptual processes contribute significantly to the self-concept in the way individuals think about themselves and others. When perceptions are colored by unresolved past conflicts, cultural values, or simple misunderstandings, they contribute to a false sense of self (Snyder, 1984). For example, a young boy with artistic abilities and little interest in sports might think of himself as odd or as not fitting in with his more aggressive, sports-minded schoolmates if there is no support from the environment for his more aesthetic inclinations. A sympathetic teacher or school art club, however, can dramatically reshape his self-concept in much the same manner as occurred in the story of the ugly duckling (Swann, 1982).

Perceptual distortions of reality are found in many mental and neurological disorders. People can create their own little world, which has little to do with reality. Usually if the perceptual distortions are significant, the client is unable to maintain independent living.

**Selective Attention.** This is a less serious interpersonal perceptual process by which a person hears selected parts of a message and fails to absorb other parts because of defensive self needs. A person who has heard only part of the message is unlikely to respond appropriately. For example, people who are depressed hear only the 1 negative comment a person makes and fail to register the 10 positive comments made in the same conversation (Segal, 1988). Some common perceptual filters associated with selective attention include culture, sex, age, physical condition, mood, past experience, similarity of problem, stereotyping, expectations, and interpersonal differences (Table 3–2).

Selective attention focuses on behavior extremes. People pay more attention to stimuli that are attention grabbing and remember them longer. Often it is difficult to erase the perceptual image created by a particularly intense or painful stimulus even if new information contradicts it or the image was only a peripheral aspect of a larger situation. Interestingly, negative impressions are retained longer than favorable impressions (Adler & Rodman, 1988).

## Table 3-2 Perceptual Filters Affecting Attention

| PERCEPTUAL FILTER | IMPLICATIONS |
| --- | --- |
| Culture | Is the object acceptable or alienating? |
| Sex | Is the object of specific gender interest? |
| Age | Does the object have relevance to the observer's group? |
| Physical condition | Is a long period of attentiveness involved, requiring endurance for concentration? |
| Mood | What mood does the observer bring—receptive and focused or antagonistic and distracted? |
| Past experience | Is the observer distracted by early impressions or similar prior experiences? |
| Interpersonal differences | Is "chemistry," tolerance, or understanding lacking for focused attention? |

First impressions contribute to a subtle form of selective attention by blocking subsequent information that would contradict the initial assessment. For example, a coworker tells you that Mrs. Jones in room 300 is difficult and cantankerous, and as you enter her room, she glares at you. Mrs. Jones may be having a bad day, and her behavior may not really reflect her normal behavioral responses. However, the next time you work with her you may approach her as a "difficult" client. Reframing Mrs. Jones's angry symptoms as a cry for help could prevent this stereotyping action on your part.

**Self-Fulfilling Prophecy.** When a person's perceptions of a certain outcome actually influence the person's present and future behaviors, the process is referred to as a self-fulfilling prophecy. For example, Martha receives an evaluation indicating a need for improved confidence. Martha interprets the instructor's comments as meaning she is awkward. Instead of seeing the instructor's comment as about a behavior simple to correct, Martha perceives it as a personal commentary on her self. This perception colors Martha's behavior, and from that point on she performs awkwardly and freezes when asked questions in the clinical area.

**How Perception Develops.** Perceptual development of a recognizable self-identity begins at birth when the infant first encounters his or her parents. The infant acquires perceptual attitudes about the self by observing the reactions of caregivers to his or her behavior. Over time, self-perceptions become more complex and flexible. Children who have multiple opportunities to experiment with different options and situations demonstrate greater perceptual flexibility, provided the experimentation is supported and guided.

Individuals who show evidence of healthy perceptual abilities characteristically are open minded. They develop realistic frames of reference for analyzing data and orienting self to time, place, and person. Problems and complex situations are viewed realistically, without significant distortions. When new information forces the conclusion that previous perceptions are no longer valid, the person can discard them with relative ease. Relationships with others reflect a healthy balance between dependent and independent behaviors.

## Assessment Strategies

A nursing assessment of perceptual difficulty is based on knowledge of the expected developmental level of a particular client and observation of unsatisfactory behavioral responses to stress. Disturbances in perception can be inferred when the client seems to block out parts of his or her experience, projects the blame for personal frustration onto the environment, or is hypercritical of self or others. Hopelessness expressed as an inability to see alternative options also indicates limited perceptual functioning.

Health status, intelligence, life experience, and age are important considerations in assessing the client's perceptual capacity. For example, anxiety, brain trauma or dysfunction, disease, reaction to medication, certain abnormal blood values, sheltered living experiences, and the age-related evolution of thinking in childhood all have a significant impact on perceptual ability.

Assessment of perceptual patterns should take into account the environmental context in which the interaction takes place. People "edit" their behavior to meet their perceived expectations of the other person and the appropriateness of their communication to the current situation. They tend to be more guarded in unfamiliar and exposed settings. If the interview takes place in a less than ideal setting, this should be noted as an environmental variable.

Assessment data should incorporate the cultural diversity of the client. Major and minor language differences between client and nurse can affect the perception of the intent of the message sender or receiver. People are sometimes insulted by comments, gestures, and emblems they perceive as intrusive or degrading when this was not the intent of the message sender. Different cultures have culture-specific norms about the use of eye contact and deference to others. Without an understanding of cultural diversity, the nurse may unintentionally misinterpret a client's response or offend a client. Asking clients about their cultural world helps prevent insensitivity.

Perceptions of both nurse and client may be colored by interests, emotions, or needs that either party carries into the conversation. For example, if the nurse is worried about something happening that morning in her own family, it is likely that some of the client's data may go unnoticed or may be distorted because of the nurse's distraction.

Hospitalization by its very nature narrows perceptual ability. Adjusting to a major physical impairment and a radically different living situation simultaneously may prove overwhelming to a "normal" client and significantly affect that client's perceptual acuity (Swann, 1982).

### ◆ Case Example

Mrs. Segal, a fiercely independent elderly woman, has suddenly been immobilized with a broken hip. After a short hospital stay, she is sent to a nursing home because she can no longer take care of herself. She is bewildered and acts slightly confused.

To reorient herself to the meaning of her new situation, Mrs. Segal might have some of the following concerns: "In what ways am I like or unlike the other nursing home residents? Will I fit in? Is this a temporary or permanent arrangement?" For Mrs. Segal, it is a whole new social milieu. Furthermore, physically helpless, elderly clients who have all of their mental faculties are sometimes treated as though they are mentally incompetent because of stereotypes about aging. The nursing staff needs to understand that just because Mrs. Segal is 90 does not mean she has significant memory problems. She has the same needs as they do: to be valued and treated with dignity. How can Mrs. Segal be helped to communicate her needs without being seen as demanding or out of line?

The art of nursing involves protecting the integrity of her self-concept while giving Mrs. Segal the emotional support and compensatory assistance she needs. Providing information and cues for action are structural interventions the nurse can use. The nurse can also encourage the client to take advantage of activities with gentle verbal support.

## Planning and Intervention

When perceptions are clouded, the nurse may intentionally provide a calm, unhurried interpersonal situation for therapeutic conversations. Timing and interpersonal space are critical in planning interventions. For example, the suspicious client needs shorter and more objective verbal interactions until trust is established. Sometimes the undemanding presence of a nurse allows the client to move closer without fear of reprisal. In the general hospital, taking time to make sure the newly admitted client or family is comfortable, offering a beverage, and introducing yourself are simple actions that reduce the anxiety most clients feel in unfamiliar settings. An uncomplicated game or small talk about a neutral topic can be a useful bridge in working with psychotic clients, for whom perceptions and the relationship are intertwined.

Tone of voice, choice of words, and nonverbal gestures create perceptual barriers if the person experiencing them feels devalued. The person receiving the message may not know the reason for being devalued, but the underlying communication is likely to affect every aspect of the nurse–client relationship and of goal accomplishment.

## Perceptual Checks: A Useful Nursing Strategy

The interpersonal relationship offers an excellent means of reformulating false perceptions through perception checks. Adler and Rodman (1988) offered a three-step process for checking the validity of perceptual inferences.

The first step involves describing precisely the behavior of concern. All aspects of the problem, including the reasons the problem is of major concern at this time, as well as possible causes are considered.

The second step involves offering two alternative explanations for the problem. In most situations, the nurse asks only one question at a time to avoid confusing the client; however, the client with perceptual problems may need alternative suggestions. Adler and Rodman advocated using two possible cause-effect explanations rather than one interpretation as a way of broadening their perspective. Most situations are multidetermined. Offering alternate explanations models the idea that most situations in life carry more than one possible explanation and more than one solution, or perhaps none.

The third step involves requesting feedback. Feedback forces the client to interact with the helping person in checking reality. It reduces the chances of misinterpretations and false assumptions. This three-step process helps a person maintain an accurate picture of reality. In the process of developing shared meanings, people draw closer together. The knowledge that another individual cares enough to find out what is going on within the person affirms the value of the interpersonal relationship for both participants.

---

◆ **Case Example**

**Nurse:** Mr. Jones, I notice that you didn't use the Ames glucose monitor this morning to test your blood for sugar. (Focused description of behavior)

Is that because you didn't understand fully what we went over yesterday, or is it difficult for you to consider using it for more personal reasons? (Two alternative logical explanations of behavior)

**Client:** The idea of pricking myself all the time isn't appealing.

**Nurse:** So it is the needlestick that disturbs you. Can you tell me more about your reluctance to test your blood? (Asking for feedback)

From the client's response, the nurse now knows that use of the glucose monitor, rather than a misunderstanding of instructions, is the major concern for the client. This perceptual check means that further instruction, support, and feedback will center on those parts of the problem of greatest import to the client. Equally important, the client feels heard.

---

Perceptual checks, combined with well-thought-out inferences about the meaning of client behaviors, enhance the quality of decision making in the nurse–client relationship. They allow the nurse to use perceptual data in a conscious, deliberate way to facilitate the relationship process. Because the client feels heard and communication focuses on matters of interest and concern to the client, mutuality occurs with greater frequency. Nursing interventions are more likely to fit the client's needs, resulting in deeper satisfaction and a more successful outcome.

The nurse–client relationship is not the only source of perceptual checks. Referent groups, defined as groups of persons having common interests and concerns, are a form of social support. These informal support groups allow people who perceive that they are alone to find others who have similar physical, emotional, and spiritual situations.

## Evaluation

Behaviors indicating broader perceptual flexibility include the ability to develop different perspectives on the same subject. Willingness to enter a support group and to try different options also suggests perceptual adaptability.

## Cognition

Thinking is a complex, creative cognitive process stimulated by conscious data, internal as well as external. Cognitive processes take perceptual images and categorize them into new informational sets through the process of reflective thinking. Through cognitive thinking processes, a person determines the accuracy of perceptual data and assesses the possible outcomes of alternate options. Without the ability to process the meaning of perceptual images cognitively, people would be unable to develop realistic goals, implement coherent patterns of behavior, and evaluate their efforts.

The cognitive aspects of self-concept are best characterized by the level, clarity, and logic of thinking. New cognitive images are stored in long- or short-term memory, capable of retrieval when needed. When illness, genetic factors, pain, accident, or injury affects cognition, they also have a profound effect on a person's overall sense of personal identity. Although images may enter the psyche, the normal cognitive processes directing behavior can no longer make sense of them.

### How Cognition Develops

Most of what we know about cognitive development of thinking processes emanates from the work of Jean Piaget, who described sensorimotor, preoperational, concrete operational, and formal operational stages of cognitive development. Stages of cognitive development are described in Chapter 18, Communicating with Children.

Cognitive development proceeds from simple to complex. It is important to realize that a child thinks with images as well as with words. For example, a 2-year-old child sees all four-legged animals as the same. As the child progresses in cognitive complexity, distinctions are made between horses and dogs. By the time the child grows up, subtle differences in breeds are also noted. Distinctions regarding the temperament, function, and so on of different breeds are readily stored in and retrieved from memory. The adolescent is capable of making abstract inferences about the data and drawing conclusions about the relationships among them. Because imaging is so important with children, incorporating pictures and allowing children to handle equipment is a necessary part of their learning process.

### Assessment Strategies

The information-processing characteristics of each client are different. Because people think differently about the same issues, it is logical to assume that individuals' cognitive approaches to problem solving differ. Time spent accurately assessing and responding appropriately to the individual learning characteristics of the client saves time for the nurse and minimizes frustration for the client.

Assessment data that might lead the nurse to suspect a disturbance in cognition start with the client's knowledge about his or her illness, treatment protocols, and expectations of therapy. Other information includes the client's knowledge of risk factors; previous illnesses; motivation; orientation to time, place, and person; and memory assessment.

Cognition can be compromised at any time by alterations in an individual's physiological and emotional state. For example, low blood sugar affects cognition in a very direct and immediate way. Pain, hunger, hormones, and chemical imbalances in the body influence cognitive functioning adversely. Strong emotions and intense psychological states can temporarily reduce the level of cognitive function and awareness. To lose one's cognitive functioning is one of the most horrifying circumstances affecting a human being, as Lear (1980) wrote: "The most painful thing was what happened to my mind. Nothing in my life was ever worse than that, or ever will be" (p. 222). His wife observed: "It was not, of course, no memory. It was damaged memory. Of all his disabilities, this was the most devastating. He had always taken memory so far for granted. Who does not when it works? He had no awareness how paralyzed one might be without it. Now he understood the obvious as philosophers do, profoundly. He understood that without memory, life was not human life but vegetation. Without memory, one could not tie a shoe" (Lear, 1980, p. 217).

It is not unusual to see an Alzheimer's disease victim clutching his head as if to make sense out of a meaningless world. Taking into account the agony that loss of cognition creates in its victims enhances the development of appropriate nursing strategies.

When assessing cognition, it is important to differentiate transient memory loss from more permanent loss in the elderly. Elderly clients can appear acutely confused when confronted with the unfamiliar context of a hospitalization, yet the disorientation may completely disappear when they return home.

### Planning and Intervention

Reflective thinking and the ability to express thoughts clearly contribute to effective functioning. Not all thinking processes are clear. Cognitive distortions occur as a result of thoughts about the meaning of a situation that have little to do with reality (Box 3–1). Faulty perceptions lead to cognitive distortions, but it is the thinking about them that leads to disordered behavior. When this occurs, the nurse looks for the cause of the distortion and links the intervention to the nursing diagnosis.

Special modifications of the nurse–client relationship allow for individual differences in cognitive capacities. Clients with dementia have limited functioning because their ability to use knowledge constructively and to put facts together in a systematic way is no longer available to them. Mentally ill clients often are unable to use cognitive problem-solving skills.

Keeping communication simple, breaking instructions down into smaller, sequential steps, presenting ideas one at a time, and using touch to emphasize directions or guide the client help compensate for cognitive deficits. Unless there is a pronounced cognitive deficit, knowledge of the client's educational level influences the type of language the nurse uses. Clients with flexible thinking styles may need less direct structural support from the nurse to assimilate new ideas than clients with more rigid thinking patterns. Older and chronically mentally ill individuals may need more time to process information. Sensory overload can compromise the assimilation of unfamiliar information in clients of all ages.

### Self-Talk

It is difficult to separate thoughts from feelings, and much of the reason that people feel badly about themselves has to do with negative self-talk. **Self-talk** is a cognitive process that produces a thought or thoughts, which then lead to a feeling about a situation. Feelings attach a value to a person's thoughts, characterizing them as good or bad testimony about the self. When the thought carries a negative value connotation, it can affect the individual as though the thought represented the whole truth about the person. The thought "I stuttered in the interview" becomes emotionally translated into "I had a terrible interview and I know I probably won't get the job." If the person thinks about it long enough, negative thoughts and associated feelings escalate to "I'm never going to get a job," "I don't ever interview well," "I'm no good." One part of one interview suddenly becomes a major defining

---

◆ **Box 3–1. Examples of Cognitive Distortions**

"All or nothing" thinking (the situation is all good or all bad; a person is trustworthy or untrustworthy)

Overgeneralizing (one incident is treated as if it happens all the time; picking out a single detail and dwelling on it)

Mind reading and fortune telling (deciding a person does not like you without checking it out; assuming a bad outcome with no evidence to support it)

Personalizing (seeing yourself as flawed instead of separating the situation as something you played a role in but did not cause)

Acting on "should" and "ought to" (deciding in your mind what is someone else's responsibility without perceptual checks; trying to meet another's expectations without regard for whether or not it makes sense to do so)

"Awfulizing" (assuming the worst; every situation has a catastrophic interpretation and anticipated outcome)

statement of self. The pervading thoughts create a decrease in self-esteem. Changing the self-talk resets the thinking process. With positive self-talk as a therapeutic strategy, the person chooses the feeling he or she will have about a situation or person.

Through self-talk, a person can question the legitimacy of cognitive distortions, and often their irrationality becomes apparent. The nurse's comments can support the client's questioning. This can be done with direct challenge when appropriate, such as "Is that really true you have never been successful at anything?," or it can be done with humor, as in the following.

### ◆ Case Example

Grace Ann Hummer is a 65-year-old widow with arthritis, a weight problem, and failing eyesight. She looks older than she is. Admitted for a minor surgical procedure, Ms. Hummer tells the nurse she does not know why she came. Nothing can be done for her because she is too old and decrepit.

**Nurse:** As I understand it, you came in today for removal of your bunions. Can you tell me more about the problem as you see it? (Asking for this information separates the current situation from an overall assessment of ill health.)

**Client:** Well I've been having trouble walking, and I can't do some of the things I like to do that require extensive walking. I also have to buy "clunky" shoes that make me look like an old woman.

**Nurse:** So you are not willing to be an old woman yet? (Taking the client's statement and challenging the cognitive distortion presented in her initial comments with humor allows the client to view her statement differently.)

**Client:** (Laughing) Right, there are a lot of things I want to do before I'm ready for a nursing home.

**Nurse:** What are some of the things you would like to do that will be possible after the surgery? (Questions relating the shared experience of the surgery to shared possible outcomes of the surgery stimulate the client to think about possible options and subtly diminish the validity of the client's overgeneralized negative thinking about life being over for her.)

Exercise 3–5 gives practice in recognizing and responding to cognitive distortions.

### Developing a Prevention Plan

A therapeutic intervention that combines self-talk strategies with social support forms the basis for a prevention plan designed to correct cognitive distortions. First, it is important to separate the person from the problem. This thinking process allows the client to step back and view the situation as an objective observer might, before beginning to resolve it. A certain amount of emotional distance is required to resolve difficult issues. When this condition is met, the client is able to develop and evaluate concrete strategies to cope with the issues. Even when the solutions chosen are appropriate and effective, however, the client may need to have ongoing support to implement them. Enlisting the help of others for support and advice gives rise to more effective problem solving.

Feedback and social support are powerful antidotes to cognitive distortions about responsibility. Although a plan to correct cognitive distortions is easier to articulate than to implement, these guidelines have proved useful in helping people to relinquish crooked thinking patterns and to take constructive action instead.

### Emotions

Emotions are an important part of personal identity. They clarify the nature of relationships as, for example, happy, sad, fearful, or angry. The person who is feeling angry and despondent because he has just lost a job and the person who is ecstatic because he has had a promotion are each expressing their self-consistent reactions to the relationship between self and the job. To the extent that a person, object, or situation has positive or negative value, there always is emotional involvement. Emotions color a person's perceptions and thinking processes through an additional filter of value-laden feelings.

Feeling awareness of self profoundly affects how we experience another person's humanity. Feelings allow people to experience compassion and sensitivity for another's experience even if they do not fully understand it. Feelings may also contribute to negative actions. Much of the brutality and inhumanity that occur in society relate to a suppression of feeling or strong negative feelings about the value of others.

Emotions are an inseparable part of all human

◆ **Exercise 3-5. Correcting Cognitive Distortions**

**Purpose:** To provide you with practice in recognizing and responding to cognitive distortions. May be done in small groups of four to five students

**Procedure:**
1. Using the definitions of cognitive distortions presented in the text, identify the type of cognitive distortion and the response you might make in each of the following situations:

a. I shouldn't feel anxious about making this presentation in class.
b. My wife never listens to me. If she really loved me, she would listen.
c. I am boring and people don't like to talk to me.
d. I shouldn't get upset when people don't approve of me.
e. If I hadn't been raised in a dysfunctional family, I would be a different person.
f. People should hire you because you can do the job, not because they like you or not.
g. If I don't expect a situation to turn out well, it means that I won't be disappointed if it doesn't turn out the way I would like.
h. If people really knew what I was like, they would never want to be my friend.
i. Self-actualized people never make mistakes.
j. If I don't get high grades, my family will think less of me.
k. I can't experience true satisfaction unless I do things perfectly.

**Discussion:**
1. Which situations were hardest to develop answers for?
2. What were your thoughts and feelings in doing this exercise?
3. How do cognitive distortions affect behavior?
4. In what ways can you use this exercise to enhance your nursing practice and personal relationships?

experience. In nursing, emotions are an important part of the commitment to caring. Nursing actions performed with genuine feeling for a client are qualitatively different from those executed without feeling. A touch that communicates empathy for the client's situation differs from one that occurs without compassion. Conversations that value and respect the uniqueness of the client contrast markedly with half-hearted communications. The difference lies in the presence or absence of feeling for the client or one's work.

Almost without exception, feelings are significant pieces of information in the nurse–client relationship. Frequently, it is the emotional sharing in the therapeutic relationship that stands out as most meaningful to both nurse and client. The emotional encounters are remembered with intensity, positively or negatively, long after the

tangible nurse–client relationship has terminated.

### Emotions as Social Responses

Expressions of feeling are influenced by culture as well as by the personal characteristics of the individual. They do not occur in a vacuum but in the form of a social response to a situation. To understand happiness, sadness, and anger, one must also understand the situations and symbols that stimulate them (Kippax et al., 1988). How people handle emotions depends on the intensity of the experience stimulating the emotion, cultural norms, genetic temperament, and family constellation. Cultures express sadness, shame, guilt, and other feelings in many different ways. In our culture, men until recently were socialized to repress feelings of emotional fragility. Exposing vulnerable feelings by crying or showing pain was not considered manly. Some cultures, such as Latin and Mediterranean cultures, permit free expression of emotions. Others, such as Oriental and British Isles cultures, restrict the use of spontaneous, openly expressed emotion.

Family rules in dysfunctional families often prevent members from understanding and accepting legitimate emotions. Unacceptable feelings are automatically replaced with an emotional void or more socially acceptable emotions. Rules about emotional expression are very difficult to understand without knowing the "script" of the family.

### Interplay with Physical and Cognitive Processes

Although expression of emotion can occur verbally, it is more often and more truly communicated nonverbally through facial expression and behaviors such as smiling, laughing, frowning, striking out, and crying. Specific physiological changes in the body such as a quickening of the heartbeat, blushing, headache, muscle tension, or relaxation accompany the experience and expression of strong emotion. Thus, there is a close connection between physical and emotional expressions of personal identity.

### Complexity of Emotions

Emotions can occur as simple expressions of a momentary feeling. They can also be so complicated that even the person experiencing the emotions is not fully aware of their existence or able to describe them. Persons may know what they feel but not why. A person may feel conflicting emotions about someone or something simultaneously: outrage, fear, love all at once. Nurses are an important resource in helping clients clarify their emotions and develop productive ways of expressing them.

### Balanced Emotions

Healthy expression of feelings allows people to express who they are. In emotional maturity, emotions inform but do not dominate relationships. The person is able to feel the emotion, step back from it, and use it as a form of data without getting caught up in it. Likewise, a person may find it necessary to make a decision that

causes painful emotions; the emotionally healthy person is able to make that decision and cope with the resulting emotions: for example, a decision to leave a destructive relationship. The emotionally healthy person does not deny the existence of emotions, even when they are irrational, but uses them as signals about life experiences in need of attention.

Properly harnessed, emotions provide energy to direct, motivate, and enrich life experiences. Careful expression of feelings can draw people closer as they strive to resolve difficult issues. Feelings energize relationships, inviting people to enter more deeply into a relationship or cautioning them to be wary of it. Emotionally healthy people generally have high self-esteem.

### Unhealthy Emotional Expression

Feelings are dangerous only when they get out of control and serve to diminish the self or another person. Unresolved feelings tend to distance partners in a relationship. Behavior usually is an indicator that something is wrong, but if the reason for the behavior is not apparent, feelings have no chance of being clarified. "Unacceptable" feelings can be camouflaged by a calm, exterior demeanor or hidden behind a mask of superrationality. Feelings that have been strongly repressed are sometimes expressed with an intensity that is significantly out of proportion to the situation. When the receiver of a communication feels angry about a neutral message and there is no personal reason for having such a response, the receiver may be picking up strong hostile feelings about which the sender has little awareness.

### How Emotions Develop

People first learn about emotions from their families. They learn which emotions can be expressed in what interpersonal contexts and under what conditions. Emotional memories of subjectively significant events play an important role in self-esteem and in how people continue to express themselves emotionally as adults.

In dysfunctional families, children learn to internalize and mask legitimate feelings. Unacceptable feelings are unconsciously replaced with feelings of shame, unworthiness, or anger, which erupt unexpectedly whenever the person encounters a situation with similar elements. Unless the person is able to correct the emotionally distorted information about a situation and to accept, resolve, or discard that information as irrelevant, the feeling tones will continue to dominate human responses (Carr, 1984).

## Assessment Strategies

The emotions the nurse is most likely to encounter in health care settings include helplessness, frustration, hopelessness, powerlessness, anger, inadequacy, joy, anxiety, peacefulness, fearfulness, and apathy. In assessing the health of emotional self-concepts, the nurse considers several factors. Does the emotion fit the nature of the stimulus? Does it reflect a correct understanding of a situation or circumstances? When feelings do not match the nature of the behavioral stimulus (e.g., too much, too little, contradictory, or unrelated), there may be an emotional block.

Does communication get blurred, or are tasks left unfinished for no known reason? For example, a client who refuses to take medication as instructed may be experiencing emotional barriers of anger or anxiety rather than a cognitive lack of understanding.

Do the emotions support the communicated message and match the body language of the participants? Emotions are important message carriers. Besides the actual verbal message, the sender and receiver steadily exchange emotionally laden nonverbal communication signals through facial expression, tone of voice, choice of words and gestures, emphasis, omissions, and timing of the communication.

The receiver of the message may hear only part of the message through an additional emotional filter that has little to do with the ongoing conversation. Feelings about the sender as well as about the content of the message influence how the message is received and interpreted. If the receiver feels threatened by the sender of the message or by the message itself, the receiver may read into the situation things that are not meant. The margin of distortion hides the true meaning of an experience to the client; factors contributing to this are presented in Figure 3–4. Exercise 3–6 helps develop skill in clarifying feelings.

## Planning and Intervention

Feelings do not obey the rules of logic, so arguing the legitimacy of a feeling wastes time and energy. The presence of emotions needs no justification; feelings simply exist, in all people. However, acting on emotions is not always in the best interest of the person experiencing the emotions. For example, it may be inappropriate to express anger to one's boss in the same way one might express anger to a friend.

Understanding that the language of emotion is telling you how the client is experiencing a life event or relationship is the key to giving a sensitive response. In highly charged emotional situations, for instance, the nurse frequently encounters angry, belligerent, out-of-control clients and families, and much of the emotion is projected onto the nurse or innocent family members. Armed with an understanding of the underlying feelings, such as intense fear, anguish about an anticipated loss, and lack of power in an unfamiliar situation, the nurse provides the opening for the client to tell his or her story. The nurse might identify a legitimate feeling: "It

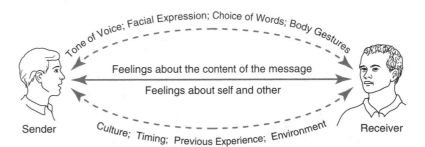

**Figure 3–4.** Affective margin of distortion in communication.

---

### ◆ Exercise 3-6. **Clarifying Feelings**

**Purpose:** To provide an opportunity to develop skill in recognizing underlying emotions and responding effectively to them. Break into small groups of three to five

**Procedure:**
A class has been assigned a group project for which all participants will receive a common group grade. Each group consists of six students.

1. Identify two possible underlying feelings for each participant.
2. Develop a group understanding of the feelings and a response to each of the following situations. Consider the possible consequences of your intervention in each case.

   a. Don tells the group that he is working full time and will be unable to make any group meetings. There are so many class requirements that he also is not sure he can put much effort into the project, although he would like to help and the project interests him.

   b. Martha is very outspoken in group. She expresses her opinion about choice of the group project and is willing to make the necessary contacts. No one challenges her or suggests another project. At the next meeting, she informs the group that the project is all set up and she had made all the arrangements.

   c. Jackie is very quiet. She rarely says anything in group, and when she does it doesn't seem to get much response. Martha says, ``Jackie, you are so quiet. Don't you have anything to say?'' to which Jackie replies, ``Not at this time.''

   d. Joan promises she will have her part of the project completed by a certain date. The date comes, and Joan does not have her part completed.

   e. Mary agrees to edit the group project. She spends an entire weekend editing. When she presents her completed work to the group, they do not like how she has ``altered their work.'' They don't feel it represents what they wanted to say.

   f. John feels like an outsider in the group. Every contribution he makes is challenged by Martha, or someone abruptly changes the subject. John is considered one of the weaker students in the class because English is his second language and he doesn't do well on objective written tests.

**Discussion:**
1. Identify common themes and difficulties in responding to emotional elements in a situation.
2. What would be the most appropriate response to each of these participants?
3. What are some actions the participants can take to move the group forward?
4. How can you use this exercise as a way of understanding and clarifying feelings in clinical work situations?

---

must be frustrating to feel that your questions go unanswered" and then say, "How can I help you?" From a nonreactive position, the nurse can demonstrate caring about the client as a person by helping the client obtain the needed information and seeking validation of legitimate client concerns.

Clients caught up in the emotion of an event may need the nurse's permission to take a break.

A simple comment from the nurse, such as "Why don't you go down to the cafeteria and get something to eat? We'll contact you immediately if your mother's condition changes," gives the family needed respite from an overly intense emotional involvement. Recognizing escalating emotions before they get out of control and acknowledging their legitimacy help relieve tension.

When setting limits on out-of-control behaviors, how the limit is presented is as important as the content of the message. In highly charged emotional situations, communication about limits can be expressed as clear, definite expectations (Lowe, 1992): "Mr. Smith, I can see that you are really upset about the doctor not being here. But your anger isn't helping your wife. Would you come with me, please, so that we can straighten this out?" Expectations should be clear and not open to interpretation. In a qualitative research study, the categories that emerged as most important in defusing intense emotion included a calm, dispassionate approach, honesty, assessment of prodromal signs of escalating tension, the giving of opportunities for face-saving alternatives, positive reinforcement of appropriate emotional display, and use of touch (Gertz, 1980).

## Spiritual Aspects of Personal Identity

Spiritual aspects of personal identity are sometimes spoken of as spiritual perspectives. Like other aspects of personal identity, they are intangible and are inferred from behaviors (Fig. 3–5).

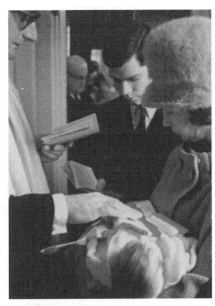

**Figure 3–5.** Spirituality plays a large part in personal identity.

Hasse et al. (1992) defined a spiritual perspective as "an integrating and creative energy based on belief in, and a feeling of interconnectedness with, a power greater than self" (p. 143). This inner energy allows a person to consider possibilities one would not ordinarily ponder. Even if one feels worthless, connections with a higher power can restore hope. Spirituality is also described as the "soul," or the core, of a person's humanness and basic self-integrity (Kinerk, 1985).

Fowler (1985) viewed spiritual perspectives as faith, "a patterned process or structure underlying and giving form to the contents of believing, valuing, knowing and committing" (p. 135). For other authors, spiritual self-concepts represent a world view or self-transcendence (Hoshinko, 1993; Labun, 1988; Reed, 1991). Spiritual self-concepts help us answer vital questions about what is human, which human events have depth and value, and what are imaginative possibilities of being. Spiritual dimensions of self make significance possible and sustain a person's belief that he or she is worthy of respect as a human being. Although spiritual perspectives can occur within the framework of an organized religion, many deeply spiritual people do not embrace any organized religious group.

Having the courage and determination to do and say what one believes to be right rather than what is easy or currently fashionable is a benchmark for determining spiritual health. For the person with integrity, the goals or outcomes are important. The means by which the goals are achieved are equally significant. A person with integrity is motivated by a desire to create and to do things that matter to others as well as to self. The language of the soul is found not only in words and actions but also in music, poetry, and art, mediums that stir our inner depths and create new and broader meanings in life.

### Spirituality in Health Care

Suffering is a personal experience that summons a person to look more closely at unsettled questions of faith. The crisis of illness can be a time of spiritual renewal, when one discovers new inner resources, strengths, and capacities never before tested. In contrast, it can be a time of spiritual desolation, leaving the individual feeling powerless to control or change important life circumstances.

Dugan (1987) described spiritual pain as "a loss of one's sense of personal integrity, a fragmenting of one's sense of internal togetherness" (p. 27). The realization that there are some things beyond our control, some realities and circumstances that can leave us temporarily immobilized, perhaps never to be settled to our satisfaction, can be overwhelming. Because human spiritual nature touches on the innermost core of an individual, the depth of a spiritual need is not always readily observable either to the nurse or to the client.

Unlike physical pain, spiritual pain can only be inferred from the client's behavior and what the client is willing to share verbally. Spiritual well-being and being able to see the purpose and meaning of one's life are particularly important concepts when one is ready to leave this life. If the nurse can assist a client to find a connectedness with the meaning of his or her life in a larger cosmic process, the client can find healing and acceptance (Levine, 1987). From the nurse's perspective, self-integrity through action embodies "the ultimate virtues of life in the form of hope, courage, faith, honor, love, acceptance, and meaningful encounter with death" (Arnold, 1989). Centering nursing practice on the development of these qualities strengthens the caring in the nurse–client relationship through commitment to personal integrity and high ethical standards.

## How Faith Develops

Fowler's (1985) stages of faith development parallel those of Piaget, Erikson, and Kohlberg in that they emerge from a simple, global understanding to increasingly more complex self-understandings of faith. Described in progressive stages of development, people experience a growing self-awareness of faith beginning with the uncritical acceptance of the parent-family values (intuitive-projective faith). As the child develops a stronger sense of self, moral rules and attitudes are assigned to behaviors (mythical-literal faith). Rules are taken literally at first. However, as the child's world and sense of self begin to expand, faith becomes increasingly more complex (synthetic-conventional faith). The next stage of faith development, the individuating-reflective stage, takes place in late adolescence. There is a qualitative shift in belief; the individual realizes that he or she must take personal responsibility for choosing commitments to a certain lifestyle and set of beliefs. In the adult stages of spiritual development (paradoxical-consolidative faith), the person is able to recognize the integrity and truth of others as well as of self, although this may be a threatening prospect. Fowler's highest stage of faith development is reached by relatively few people. Fowler suggested that people who achieve this stage are able to "instinctively know how to relate to us affirmingly, never condescendingly, yet with pricks to our pretense and with genuine bread of life" (p. 141).

Like other aspects of personal development, people are an important source of learning: teachers, role models, and even momentary encounters with people who spark meanings for us. Life events also provide a stimulus to spiritual growth (Newman, 1989).

In concluding that a person is a part of a larger scheme, disturbing questions of faith arise. Is there something or someone beyond ourselves that represents a deeper truth? Is it understandable? How then does one account for all of the evil that occurs, the misfortunes that beset innocent victims, or the randomness with which catastrophe seems to strike some people and not others? There are no easy answers to these questions. Perhaps the mystery of life is that one can only live it successfully with faith. As people grow in faith, the presence of a higher power generally becomes a matter of knowledge and experience as well as of feeling.

## Assessment Strategies

Spiritual distress can occur in the form of pain experienced through loss; separation from a faith community; or treatments that create spiritual anxiety, guilt, anger, or despair. Carson (1989) referred to four areas of spiritual concern as a framework for assessment:

A person's personal concept of God
Personal sources of energy and hope
Relevance of specific religious practices to the individual
Areas of spiritual concern activated by the illness

## Assessing a Person's Personal Concept of God

The client's personal concept of God and spiritual needs may be quite obvious and initially responsive to clergy and pastoral counselors and to readings. The nurse notes the client's comments about God, a higher power, or "the man upstairs." Often, however, the spiritual needs of the client are ambivalent, cloaked in feelings of anger and disappointment toward a God who let this happen. For example, a lack of faith in the value of humanity may represent a need to find a spiritual meaning for life. Other clients may express the need in the form of anger. C. S. Lewis (1976), the noted author of traditionally spiritual books, calls his God "the cosmic sadist" as he experiences his personal grief following the death of his wife. Yet few would doubt the depth of his spirituality.

## Personal Sources of Hope

Spirituality manifests itself in the form of hope. Hope energizes a person to take steps that increase competency, peace, and self-transcendence (Hasse et al., 1992). Hope enables people to seek new alternatives for achieving positive future goals. Quite distinct from the optimism surrounding magical thinking, which may or may not be based in truth, hope as a spiritual resource is grounded in reality (Progoff, 1985).

It is well known that hope is critical in maintaining the spirit of a person in health care settings (Miller, 1989). How else can one explain the will to live or the complete serenity of some individuals in the face of life's most adverse circumstances? Jourard (1964) suggested that "it is probably the spirit-response which is mobilized by any event that signifies hope or confidence in self or in the future; it is probably the spirit-response which, when weakened, permits illness to flourish." Societal sources of hope may be found in organized religions, in self-help books, in support groups, and in poetry and music. The nurse might ask the client, "What do you see as your primary sources of strength at the present time?," and "In the past, what have been sources of strength for you in difficult times?" as ways of focusing attention on sources of hope and energy in the current situation.

## Current Spiritual Practices

When assessing the current spiritual preferences of the client, the nurse also needs to consider past religious affiliations. It is not unusual for the religion listed on the client's chart to be quite different from the religious practices the client actually follows. Cultural orientation and practices influence not only beliefs but the way they are expressed. Questions the nurse might ask during the nursing assessment interview are as follows:

Are there special spiritual practices that are particularly important to you now?
Would it be helpful for me to arrange a visit from the hospital chaplain or your pastor? (There should be client data to warrant this question.)

The nurse also explores areas of special concern the client has expressed. Inquiring about religious rituals important to the client can be very helpful. Baptisms, last rites, and ethnic practices in preparing the body can occur within the hospital setting and can provide peace for a client experiencing spiritual and emotional pain.

## Planning and Intervention

Carson (1989) suggested that the compassionate presence of the nurse in the nurse–client relationship is the most important tool the nurse uses in helping the client reinforce and confirm spiritual self-concepts. From the moment the client enters the hospital, orientation to available religious services should be an essential component of the relationship. It is important, however, for the nurse to be aware of his or her own spiritual beliefs and not impose them on the client. This can be particularly tempting in times of crisis or when death seems imminent. Client autonomy requires that the client give the nurse permission for the pastoral counselor or clergy to visit.

Praying with a client, even when the client is of a different faith, can be soothing. If the client professes no faith, the nurse can help the client identify actions that bring peace and meaning in times of stress. Exercise 3–7 helps in understanding spiritual responses to distress.

## Developing the Next Step

Long-term goals are not always the primary focus in promoting, maintaining, or restoring spiritual health. Only the "next step" is important. Break-

◆ Exercise 3–7. **Responding to Issues of Spiritual Distress**

**Purpose:** To help you understand responses in times of spiritual distress.

**Procedure:**
Review the following case situations and develop an appropriate response to each.

1. Mary Trachter is unmarried and has just found out she is pregnant. She belongs to a fundamentalist church in which sex before marriage is not permitted. Mary feels guilty about her current status and sees it as ''God is punishing me for fooling around.''

2. Bert Smith, who is 18 years old, has been admitted to a psychiatric unit for conduct disorder. He tells you he is an atheist. His parents are strongly religious and believe he should be exorcised to get rid of the demons responsible for his delinquent behavior.

3. Linda Carter is married to an abusive, alcoholic husband. Linda reads the Bible daily and prays for her husband's redemption. She feels that God will turn the marriage around if she continues to pray for changes in her husband's attitude. ''My trust is in the Lord,'' she says.

4. Bill Compton tells the nurse, ''I feel that God has let me down. I was taught that if I was faithful to God, He would be there for me. Now the doctors tell me I'm going to die. That doesn't seem fair to me.''

**Discussion:**
1. Share your answers with others in your group.
2. Give and get feedback on the usefulness of your responses.
3. Identify common themes.
4. In what ways can you use this new knowledge in your nursing care?

ing down potentially overwhelming problems into manageable steps makes the problem seem workable and stimulates hope. The hopeful person also trusts in a transcendent source to show itself in the form of suggestion and direction about the next step.

### Social Support

Social support can have a spiritual as well as an emotional and a social effect on a client. Usually other people in the immediate situation play a critical role in the stimulation of hope through their encouragement and practical suggestions and sometimes simply through their presence during a stressful time. Carson (1989) offered the following example of a caring intervention with a 16-year-old athlete with a bilateral amputation. Exercise 3–8 may increase your appreciation of the role of social support.

◆ **Case Example**

One morning after shift report, Mrs. Johnson walked into Robert's room and found him crying. Her first response was to leave the room as she thought, "I can't handle this today." However, she was able to stop herself and she went over to Robert and touched his shoulder. He continued to sob and said, "What am I going to do? I wish I were dead. My whole life is sports. I would have qualified for an athletic scholarship if this hadn't happened. I feel like my life is over at 16."

Mrs. Johnson recognized the feelings of despair that Robert was expressing and said to him, "It doesn't seem like life has any meaning at all. You are feeling that this is such an unfair thing to have happened to you. I agree with you, it is. But let's talk about it. We can't change what has happened, but maybe we can start to look at where to go from here." (Carson, 1989, p. 167)

### Evaluation

Client outcomes suggestive of resolution of spiritual distress include reconnection with a higher power, decreased guilt, forgiveness of others, expressions of hope, and evidence that the client finds meaning in his or her current situation.

---

◆ **Exercise 3–8. Social Support**

**Purpose:** To help you understand the role of social support in significant encounters.

**Procedure:**
1. Describe a "special" situation that had deep meaning for you.
2. Identify the person or people who helped make the situation meaningful for you.
3. Describe the actions taken by the people or person identified in Procedure Step 2 that made the situation memorable.

**Discussion:**
1. What common themes emerged from student descriptions of special situations?
2. What did you learn about yourself from doing this exercise?
3. What do you see as the role of social support in making memories?
4. How might you use this information in your practice?

---

### Self-Esteem

**Self-esteem** is not the same as self-concept, but it is intimately related to it (Hamachek, 1985). It refers to the value and significance people place on their self-concepts. It is an emotional process of self-judgment, an orientation to the self, ranging on a continuum from feelings of self-efficacy and respect to a feeling of being fatally flawed as a person (Branden, 1983).

Self-esteem is subjective. It develops from individuals' perceptions of their personal being and achievements, particularly in interpersonal relations. It is possible to have many objective achievements and to have low self-esteem. People with few achievements but with the knowledge that they have conducted themselves as well as possible can have high self-esteem. Although self-esteem can be reinforced by confirming relationships, the inner worth of a person can be experienced only by that person.

Self-esteem reflects a delicate balance between fitting into a larger social community and retaining the support and affirmation of others for being unique. Wanting the approval of others at the expense of personal integrity decreases self-respect, which in turn affects the admiration of others and leads to social alienation.

A relationship exists between self-esteem and the level of psychological adaptation. People who value themselves become freer to know and to cherish the intrinsic value of others. Energy is not wasted on self-defensive behavior. People with high self-esteem have a strong emotional as well as intellectual conviction that they are worthy of respect and recognition, with something unique and useful to offer to society. When individuals do not feel as though there is much value to who they are as human beings or what they are able to contribute to others, they experience low self-esteem. Box 3–2 identifies characteristic behaviors related to self-esteem.

Self-esteem is not a fixed concept. It fluctuates whenever the self-concept is challenged by life transitions or crises, illnesses, or changes in status or role. Turning points of self-meaning related to developmental, situational, relational, and spiritual circumstances affect self-esteem. Sources of low self-esteem include loss of a job; loss of an important relationship; change in appearance, role, or status; and criticism by significant others.

Perceptions of the opinions and feelings of significant others have a profound effect on self-esteem. Contrast, for example, a social situation in which you are considered an authority or a prized guest with one in which you clearly are on a different social level and have less life experience or fewer credentials than most of the other people present. Most probably there was a significant difference in the value you felt you had in each of these situations. If people feel valued by others, they begin to experience themselves as being worthy. Criticism, disconfirming comments, and devaluing by others through insensitive actions usually have the opposite effect.

---

### ◆ Box 3–2. Self-Esteem Characteristics

People with high self-esteem

- Expect people to value them
- Are active self-agents
- Have positive perceptions of their skills, appearance, sexuality, and behaviors
- Perform equally well when being observed as when not
- Are nondefensive and assertive in response to criticism
- Can accept compliments easily
- Evaluate their performance realistically
- Are relatively comfortable relating to authority figures
- Express general satisfaction with life
- Have a strong social support system
- Have a primary internal locus of control

People with low self-esteem

- Expect people to be critical of them
- Are passive or obstructive self-agents
- Have negative perceptions of their skills, appearance, sexuality, and behaviors
- Perform less well when being observed
- Are defensive and passive in response to criticism
- Have difficulty accepting compliments
- Have unrealistic expectations about their performance
- Are uncomfortable relating to authority figures
- Are dissatisfied with their lot in life
- Have a weak social support system
- Rely on an external locus of control

---

### Self-Esteem in Health Care

Epstein (1973) suggested that a sudden decrease in self-esteem is experienced as a greater loss than a more gradual decline. In most chronic or major illnesses, there is a lowering of self-esteem because the individual is no longer able to function as before in ways that inspired higher levels of self-esteem. In many cases, neither is there any real reason to believe there will be a return to normal activities or a positive change in functioning. Yet high levels of self-esteem can accompany even the most debilitating illness if the client is given enough social support.

When illness occurs, at least two outcomes are possible. The client may become emotionally immobilized by the threat to self-identity that a symptom imposes, and loss of self-esteem results. Alternatively, the client may feel challenged by the illness to develop new coping skills, and there is an increase in self-esteem. The nurse, in providing support and confirmation of the client's efforts, plays an important role in a client's decisions and subsequent actions.

### Assessment Strategies

Assessment of self-esteem tends to be observational. The nurse notes what the client says about him- or herself. Does the client devalue accomplishments, project blame for problems on others, minimize personal failures, or make self-deprecating remarks? Does the client express shame or guilt? Does the client seem hesitant to try new things or situations or express concern about ability to cope with events? Lack of culturally appropriate eye contact, poor hygiene, self-destructive behaviors, hypersensitivity to criticism, need for constant reassurance, and an inability to accept compliments are behaviors associated with low self-esteem.

### Planning an Intervention

When people have low self-esteem, they feel they have little worth and that no one really cares enough to bother with them. The nurse helps clients increase self-esteem by being psychologically present as a sounding board. Just the process of engaging with another human being who offers a different perspective can have an effect of enhancing self-esteem. The implicit message the nurse conveys with personal presence and interest, information, and a guided exploration of the problem is twofold. First is confirmation of the client: "You are important and I will stay with you through this uncomfortable period." Second is the introduction of the possibility of hope: "There may be some alternatives you haven't thought of that can help you cope with this problem in a meaningful way." Once a person starts to take charge of his or her life, a higher level of well-being can result.

Self-esteem affects the ability to weather stress without major changes in self-perception. With a positive attitude about self, an individual is more likely to view life as a glass half full rather than half empty.

The nurse can use several strategies to help a client experience deeper levels of self-esteem. Modeling is very effective. The nurse can convey a positive self-image, which is contagious.

The nurse's questions can be deliberately designed to assist clients in reflecting on their strengths and accomplishments. The nurse can say, "Tell me the achievement you are most proud of" or "Tell me some things you like about yourself." The nurse can give the client positive feedback: "The thing that impresses me about you is . . ." or "What I notice is that although your body is so much weaker, it seems as if your spirit is stronger. Is that your perception as well?" Such questions help the client focus on positive strengths. Exercise 3–9 strengthens the nurse's skill in this area.

When the nurse helps the client make independent judgments about health care, the process strengthens the client's self-esteem. The act of taking charge and choosing among alternatives indirectly suggests that the client can cope with difficult problems. Communication, combined with compassionate health care information and actions, confirms the value of a person as worthwhile.

### Evaluation

Self-esteem behaviors are evaluated by comparing the number of positive self statements with those originally observed. Behaviors suggestive of enhanced self-esteem include

Taking an active role in planning and implementing self-care
Verbalizing personal psychosocial strengths
Expressing feelings of satisfaction with self and ways of handling life

### Self-Awareness

**Self-awareness** is the means by which a person gains knowledge and understanding of all aspects of self-concept. An interpersonal approach focusing on human responses in the client and nurse is quite different from one approaching self-understanding from a behavioristic or psychoanalytic perspective. In professional relationships with clients and colleagues, the nurse engages with other human beings from a position in which all that a person is capable of being becomes stretched to the utmost.

The nurse's self-concept in the nurse–client relationship is as important as that of clients (Box 3–3). Nurses who are comfortable with themselves can help clients use a similar process of self-reflection in understanding themselves. Creating an interpersonal environment that heals—one that permeates the human senses as well as meets daily needs—is possible only if self-awareness skills are built into the communication process (Rawlinson, 1990).

Self-awareness provides an inner frame of reference for connecting emotionally with the experience of another. Self-awareness occurs through the mechanism of intrapersonal communication, defined as communication taking place within the self, in contrast to interpersonal communication, which takes place between people. The two concepts are very much interwoven in most interpersonal relationships.

Self-awareness provides an external structure for inquiring into and interpreting important behavioral inferences related to illness. Throughout the therapeutic relationship the questions, "How is this illness affecting the client?" and "What is the meaning of the treatment process for this client?" frame the interpersonal experience. Describing the meaning of an illness and one's human responses to it is an interpersonal process that relies heavily on the client as a self-interpreting being.

### Self-Reflection

Nurses learn about themselves through self-reflection and the feedback of others. Self-reflection is a mental process by which we are able consciously to examine the meaning of our motives and actions. It is a mental faculty available only to humans. Leary and Miller (1986) argued that "without the ability to think consciously about ourselves, we could not contemplate alternative courses of action, or consider

◆ Exercise 3–9. **Positive Affirmations: Contributions to Self-Esteem**

**Purpose:**   To help you experience the effects of interpersonal comments on self-esteem.

**Procedure:**

1. This exercise may be done in a group or used as a homework assignment and later discussed in class.
2. List a positive affirming comment you received recently, something someone did or said that made you feel good about yourself.

_____

_____

_____

3. List a disconfirming comment you received recently, something someone did or said that made you feel bad about yourself.

_____

_____

_____

4. What have you done recently that you feel helped enhance someone else's self-esteem?

_____

_____

_____

5. In class, write phrases on a chalkboard that capture the essence of the positive affirming comment.
6. Do the same for the negative disconfirming comment.

**Discussion:**

1. In general, what kinds of actions help enhance self-esteem?
2. What are some things people do or fail to do that diminish self-esteem?
3. What are some specific things you might be able to do in a clinical setting that might help a client develop a sense of self-worth?
4. What did you learn about yourself from doing this exercise?

the impact of our behaviors on other people. We would be unable to ponder the meaning of our actions and lives, systematically plan for the future, or purposefully attempt to better our lives." Taking time alone to explore and to discover what is happening or has happened in human relationships puts the pain and human suffering a nurse encounters on a daily basis into better perspective.

Self-reflection increases the nurse's capacity to be genuine. Knowing personal motivations, prejudices, strengths, and limitations helps nurses connect with clients in a straightforward manner. Self-awareness helps the nurse avoid using the therapeutic interpersonal relationship with clients to meet personal rather than client needs. Consider, for example, the nurse who strongly believes that breast-feeding is more beneficial than bottle-feeding. Without self-awareness, the nurse may unconsciously project her personal values about breast-feeding on a teenage mother who has no desire to breast-feed her infant.

---

**◆ Box 3-3. Questions to Encourage Self-Awareness in the Nurse–Client Relationship**

1. Can I behave in some way which will be perceived by the other person as trustworthy, dependable, or consistent in some deep sense?
2. Can I be expressive enough as a person that what I am will be communicated unambiguously?
3. Can I let myself experience positive attitudes toward this other person: attitudes of warmth, caring, liking, interest, respect?
4. Can I be strong enough as a person to be separate from the other?
5. Am I secure enough within myself to permit the client separateness?
6. Can I let myself enter fully into the world of the client's feelings and personal meanings and see these as the client does?
7. Can I receive the client as he or she is? Can I communicate this attitude?
8. Can I act with sufficient sensitivity in the relationship that my behavior will not be perceived as a threat?
9. Can I free the client from the threat of external evaluation?
10. Can I meet this other individual as a person who is in the process of becoming, or will I be bound by his or her past and by my past?

Adapted from Rogers CR. (1958). The characteristics of the helping relationship. Personnel and Guidance Journal 37(1). Used with permission.

---

### Role Modeling

To be a role model for clients in a professional relationship, nurses need first to recognize their own needs and find ways to meet them in their personal lives. It is difficult for nurses to be considerate and sensitive to the needs of others if they are unable to be gentle and understanding of similar needs within themselves. If nurses cannot see themselves as worthy of being cared for, it is difficult to convince others of their worth. It is difficult to role model self-respect or to give to others from a barren stockpile.

### Becoming Centered

The basic goal of any constructive relationship is to help the participants enlarge self-knowledge and enhance their potential by integrating disowned, neglected, unrecognized, or unrealized parts of the self into the personality. This process is referred to as being centered. Expected outcomes include

Enhanced self-respect
Increased resourcefulness and sense of what the person can do
Greater productivity
Increased personal satisfaction

Attainment of these goals is impossible without a personal experiential knowledge of the self-concept and its effect on the development and maintenance of relationships.

## SUMMARY

At birth, infants are biological bundles, with no psychosocial component, referred to as "self." Self emerges from the appraisals of significant others and is reappraised with each new era of development.

Self-concept is a major nursing diagnosis that involves four components: body image, personal identity, self-esteem, and role performance. Body image alterations encompass loss of function and control as well as physical changes. Included in personal identity are the psychospiritual, cognitive, emotional, and perceptual dimensions of self-concept. Erikson's model of psychosocial development is the framework used to assess client attainment of normal psychosocial tasks.

Self-concept influences communication through perceptual and cognitive processes such as selective attention and self-fulfilling prophecies. Emotional tagging of images affects how a person interacts with others in social situations. Spiritual self-concepts add meaning.

Self-esteem, described as the emotional valuing of the self-concept, stems from perceptual images viewed by the person as good or bad assessments of self. A healthy self-concept results in behaviors reflective of satisfaction with body image, a realistic relationship between actual and ideal self, high self-esteem, general satisfaction with role performance, and a distinct sense of identity and spiritual well-being. Strategies to enhance the development of a positive self-concept and psychospiritual well-being result in higher self-esteem.

## REFERENCES

Ackerman D. (1990). A Natural History of the Senses. New York, Random House.

Adler R, Rodman L. (1988). Understanding Human Communication (3rd ed.). New York, Holt, Rinehart & Winston.

Adler R, Rosenfal L, Towne N. (1986). Interplay: The Process of Interpersonal Communication (3rd ed.). New York, Holt, Rinehart & Winston.

Arnold E. (1989). Burnout as a spiritual issue. In Carson V (ed.), Spiritual Dimensions of Nursing Practice. Philadelphia, WB Saunders.

Branden N. (1983). Honoring the Self. New York, Bantam Books.

Cairns RB, Cairns BD. (1988). The sociogenesis of self-concepts. In Bolger N, Caspi A, Downey G, Moorehouse M (eds.), Persons in Context: Developmental Processes. Cambridge, England, Cambridge University Press.

Carr J. (1984). Communicating and Relating. Dubuque, IA, William C. Brown.

Carson V. (1989). Spiritual Dimensions in Nursing Practice. Philadelphia, WB Saunders.

Cross S, Markus H. (1991). Possible selves across the life span. Human Development 34:230–255.

Dempsey M. (1972). Development of body image in the adolescent. Nursing Clinics of North America 7:609.

Dugan D. (1987). Death and dying: Emotional, spiritual and ethical support for patients and families. Journal of Psychosocial Nursing 25(7):21–29.

Epstein S. (1973). The self-concept revisited: Or a theory of a theory. American Psychologist 5:414.

Erikson E. (1963). Childhood and Society (2nd ed.). New York, Norton.

Erikson E. (1968). Identity: Youth and Crisis. New York, Norton.

Erikson E. (1982). The Life Cycle Completed: A Review. New York, Norton.

Felker D. (1974). Building Positive Self-Concepts. Minneapolis, Burgess.

Fowler J. (1985). Stages of faith development. In Gorman M (ed.), Psychology and Religion. New York, Paulist Press.

Gertz B. (1980). Training for prevention of assaultive behavior in a psychiatric setting. Hospital and Community Psychiatry 31:628–630.

Grassi J. (1986). Changing the World Within. Mahwah, NJ, Paulist Press.

Hamachek D. (1985). The self's development and ego growth: Conceptual analysis and implications for counselors. Journal of Counseling and Development 64:136–142.

Hasse J, Britt T, Coward D, et al. (1992). Simultaneous concept analysis of spiritual perspective, hope, acceptance and self-transcendence. Image 24(2):140–147.

Heinrich RL, Schag CC. (1985). Stress and activity management: Group treatment for cancer patients and spouses. Journal of Consulting and Counseling Psychology 53:439–446.

Hoare C. (1991). Psychosocial identity development and cultural others. Journal of Counseling and Development 70(1):45–53.

Hoshinko B. (1993). Worldview as a model of spirituality. Presented at the First Annual Conference on Spirituality, University of Maryland School of Nursing, Baltimore, May 7, 1993.

James W. (1891). The Principles of Psychology. New York, Henry Holt.

Jourard S. (1964). The Transparent Self. New York, Van Nostrand Reinhold.

Kinerk E. (1985). Toward a method for the study of spirituality. In Gorman M (ed.), Psychology and Religion. New York, Paulist Press.

Kippax S, Crawford J, Benton P, et al. (1988). Constructing emotions: Weaving meaning from memories. British Journal of Social Psychology 27:19–33.

Koehler D. (1989). The relationship between self concept and successful rehabilitation. Rehabilitation Nursing 14(1):9–12.

Labun E. (1988). Spiritual care: An element in nursing care planning. Journal of Advanced Nursing 13:314–320.

Lear M. (1980). Heartsounds. New York: Simon & Schuster.

Leary M, Miller K. (1986). Social Psychology and Dysfunctional Behavior. New York, Springer.

Levine S. (1987). Healing into Life and Death. Garden City, NY, Anchor Press.

Lewis CS. (1976). A Grief Observed. New York, Bantam Books.

Lowe T. (1992). Characteristics of effective nursing interventions in the management of challenging behavior. Journal of Advanced Nursing 17:1226–1232.

Markus H, Nurius P. (1986). Possible selves. American Psychologist, pp. 954–969.

Markus H, Wurf E. (1987). The dynamic self-concept: A social psychological perspective. Annual Review of Psychology 38:299–337.

Miller J. (1989). Hope-inspiring strategies of the critically ill. Applied Nursing Research 2:23–29.

Newman M. (1989). The spirit of nursing. Holistic Nursing Practice 3:1–6.

North American Nursing Diagnosis Association. (1986). Classification of Nursing Diagnoses: Proceedings of the Sixth Conference. St. Louis, CV Mosby.

Progoff I. (1985). The Dynamics of Hope. New York, Dialogue House Library.

Rawlinson J. (1990). Self-awareness: Conceptual influences,

contributions to nursing, and approaches to attainment. Nurse Education Today 10:111–117.

Reed P. (1991). Spirituality and mental health in older adults: Extant knowledge in nursing. Family and Community Health 14(2):14–25.

Schontz F. (1974). Body image and its disorders. International Journal of Psychiatric Medicine 5:464.

Segal Z. (1988). Appraisal of self-schema construct in cognitive models of depression. Psychological Bulletin 103(2):147–162.

Snyder M. (1984). When belief creates reality. In Berkowitz L (ed.), Advances in Experimental Social Psychology. San Diego, Academic Press.

Sutherland J. (1993). The autonomous self. Bulletin of the Menninger Clinic 57(1):4–23.

Swann WB. (1982). When our identities are mistaken: Reaffirming self-conceptions through social interaction. Journal of Social Psychology 43:59.

Travelbee J. (1971). Interpersonal Aspects of Nursing. Philadelphia, FA Davis.

Turnes A. (1993). Unpublished student journal, University of Maryland School of Nursing.

## PART II

# The Nurse–Client Relationship

## 4

# Structuring the Relationship

Elizabeth Arnold

**OBJECTIVES**

At the end of the chapter, the student will be able to

1. Discuss key concepts in the nurse–client relationship
2. Identify the four phases of the therapeutic relationship
3. Contrast tasks in each of the four phases of the relationship
4. Specify effective nursing interventions in each phase of the relationship

_Something, however imperceptible, happens between the two, no matter whether it is marked at the time by any feeling or not. The only thing that matters is that for each . . . the other happens as the particular other, that each becomes aware of the other and is thus related to him in such a way that he does not regard and use him as his object, but as his partner in a living event._

Martin Buber (1965)

❖❖ Chapter 4 focuses on the structure of a therapeutic nurse–client relationship. Peplau (1997) defined this relationship as a primary human connection and "central in a fundamental way to providing nursing care" (p. 163). Therapeutic relationships form the basis for providing total physical care to a client at one extreme of the illness–wellness continuum, emotional support throughout the relationship, and health education at the other extreme. Certain guiding principles—purpose, mutuality, authenticity, empathy, active listening, confidentiality, and respect for the dignity of the client—strengthen the entire process and flow through the three identifiable phases of a relationship. Whereas some therapeutic relationships extend over weeks or months, most will take place within hours or days. Some will be a single session. Although all relationships involve human connections, a therapeutic relationship is different in that it has a health-related purpose, defined boundaries, a one-way focus on the client, and identifiable stages of development.

Healing requires more than medicine and treatment applications. Because illness affects the whole person, it is as important to discover the particular personal meanings woven into the fabric of an illness as it is to address the physical and psychological origins of the disorder. In health care, human connections are essential to the healing process and effective health care delivery. The nurse becomes a "skilled companion" on the illness journey, encouraging, supporting, and challenging the client as needed (Pearson et al., 1997).

Peplau (1997) suggested that "at their best, relationships confirm self-worth, provide a sense of connectedness with others and support self-esteem" (p. 166). The goals of therapeutic nurse–client relationships are threefold: (1) to enhance client well-being, (2) to promote recovery, and (3) to support the self-care functioning of the client. The desired outcome of the nurse–client relationship is to find meaning in the illness experience related to the specific health needs or problems for which a client is seeking health care intervention. Health care needs can include health promotion and preventive care needs as well as actual physiological and emotional needs requiring nursing intervention. Several authors pointed to nurses helping clients achieve a sense of meaning from their illness and suffering as one of the most important and rewarding aspects of relationship in nursing practice (Frankl, 1955; Travelbee, 1971).

## BASIC CONCEPTS
## Characteristics of a Therapeutic Relationship

Therapeutic relationships represent a "modified social relationship" and share many of the same characteristics (Ramos, 1992). All effective relationships involve personal contact and a discovery of the other person: his or her needs, feelings, and ideas in an I–thou relationship (Buber, 1958). Box 4–1 presents the distinctions between a therapeutic helping relationship and a social relationship.

### *Client-Centered Approach*

A client-centered communication involves an individualized focus on the client such that clients feel comfortable sharing intimate personal experiences and the meanings these experiences have for them. Entering the client's world with empathetic objectivity, the nurse is in a unique position to provide the client with another perspective on a potentially overwhelming situation.

Client-centered approaches start where the client is and are designed to meet the distinctive needs of each client. There is no one way to approach a client and no single interpersonal technique that works equally well with every client. Some clients clearly are more emotionally accessible and attractive to work with than others. When a client seems unapproachable or uninterested in human contact, it can be quite disheartening for the nurse. It is not uncommon for the nurse to report the following kind of initial contact with a client:

---
◆ **Case Example**

"I tried, but he just wasn't interested in talking to me. I asked him some questions, but he didn't really answer me. So I tried to ask him about his hobbies and interests. It didn't matter what I asked him. He just turned away. Finally, I gave up because it was obvious that he just didn't want to talk to me."

---

Although from the nurse's perspective, this cli-

---

◆ **Box 4-1. Development of Interpersonal Relationship: Comparison of a Helping Relationship with a Social Relationship**

Both involve at least two persons.
There is a connection between the involved persons for an "established or discoverable reason."

### Helping

One person is taking the *responsibility* of helping while the other is seeking help. There is a specific *purpose* to the relationship. The relationship is *goal* directed. The *focus* of the relationship is the needs of the helpee. *Behaviors* are based on persons taking roles of professional and client, respectively. The relationship is entered into through necessity. The *choice of whom* to enter the relationship with is usually not available to helper or helpee. *Behavior* on the part of the helper is purposefully planned, implemented, and evaluated. It is not necessary that persons involved *like* each other. The helping person seeks to be *nonjudgmental*. Sharing of personal or intimate *set factors* (self-disclosure) is usually a one-way process: helpee to helper. *Empathetic* feelings for the helpee are translated into helpful action. The helper is in control of the situation: the helper is influencing behavior in a positive way. There is usually a definite and anticipated ending to the relationship, ideally when the goals of the relationship have been accomplished. The helper possesses self-knowledge.

### Social

Persons are not in a position of having responsibility for helping the other. Specific purpose is not necessary. The relationship is not necessarily goal directed. A person seeks to have own needs met as well as meet the needs of the other. Certain social behavior is expected of persons in social roles. The relationship is entered into by choice. Persons can choose whom they care to become involved with. Behavior on the part of participants is spontaneous. Feelings of liking, fondness, or love for the other are usually involved. Persons may be judgmental in attitude. There is mutual sharing of intimacies. Feelings for the other may enhance or prevent helpful action. Control is more evenly shared. The relationship may continue indefinitely, and the ending is usually not anticipated.

---

ent's behavior may represent a lack of desire for a relationship, in most cases the rejection is not personal. The stress of hospitalization can heighten emotional responses, and coldness toward the nurse may be the only way a client can cope constructively with his or her predicament. Rarely does it have much to do with the personal approach used by the nurse in the early stages of a relationship, unless the nurse is truly insensitive to the client's feelings or the needs of the situation. Sometimes a simple statement such as "I can see that you don't want to talk right now, but I want you to know that I am here for you and I will stop back later to check on you" prompts a different response at a later time.

For novice nurses, it is important to recognize that all nurses have experienced some form of client rejection at one time or another. More often than not, rejection means that the client is bored, frightened, insecure, upset, or physically uncomfortable. The nurse needs to explore whether the timing was right, whether the client was in pain, and what other circumstances might have contributed to the client's attitude. Behaviors that initially seem maladaptive may appear quite adaptive when the full circumstances of the client's situation are understood.

### ◆ Case Example

A third-year student nurse, Joan Thoms, stops at the hospital to pick up her next day's assignment. Mrs. Groot, her client, is scheduled for a radical mastectomy. Joan enters Mrs. Groot's room to introduce herself but finds her client in tears and unable to talk. Joan gives her a tissue and sits with her, holding her hand. After about 5 minutes, Joan asks, "Would you like to talk for a while? You seem really upset." Mrs. Groot replies, "I'd rather be alone." Joan states, "There are times when we all need to have some time alone. I'll pull your curtains around your bed to give you some privacy, and I will be back to see you later, before I leave the unit."

In this anecdote, the nurse acknowledges the client's immediate need to be alone while at the same time setting the stage for further contact. Meeting the client's needs nonverbally when the client is reluctant to communicate verbally demonstrates respectful interest without pressure. You may have to use this technique several times before you see any results, but it is a highly effective therapeutic maneuver.

Checking with the staff before entering a client's room and reviewing the chart before seeing a client in the community can provide the nurse with important data about the client that can influence initial approaches to a client. Exercise 4–1 examines nonverbal cues in relationships.

### Empowerment

Integral to all interventions in the nurse–client relationship is the concept of *empowerment*. *Webster's Dictionary* defines empower as "to endow with an ability or to enable." The current focus in health care on self-care and a partner relationship emphasizes the importance of using an empowerment model in the nurse–client relationship. This model focuses on helping people develop the knowledge skills and other resources they need to set their own health agendas and to take a primary role in their health care. Rodwell (1996) described the process of empowerment as "enabling people to choose to take control over and make decisions about their lives. It is also a process which values all those involved" (p. 309).

Nurses "empower" clients every time they foster their client's self-direction in choosing treatment options, goal setting, and problem solving the best way to achieve them as partners in care. Providing relevant information, validating the client's personal strengths, and helping clients and families recognize opportunities for choice are other strategies that help empower clients. For example, giving the client information about what to expect after surgery, who to contact if experiencing side effects, and what to look for with medications empowers clients. Allowing clients to do as much for themselves as possible while providing enough support neces-

---

### ◆ Exercise 4–1. **Nonverbal Messages**

**Purpose:** To provide practice in validation skills in a nonthreatening environment

**Directions:**
1. Each student in turn tries to communicate the following feelings to other members of the group without words. They may be written on a piece of paper, or the student may develop one directly from the following list.
2. The other students must guess what behaviors the student is trying to enact.

| | |
|---|---|
| Pain | Anger |
| Sadness | Confidence |
| Anxiety | Disapproval |
| Relief | Uncertainty |
| Shock | Disbelief |
| Disgust | Acceptance |
| Disinterest | Rejection |
| Despair | "Uptightness" |

**Discussion:**
1. Which emotions were harder to guess from their nonverbal cues? Which ones were easier?
2. Was there more than one interpretation of the emotion?
3. How would you use the information you developed today in your future care of clients?

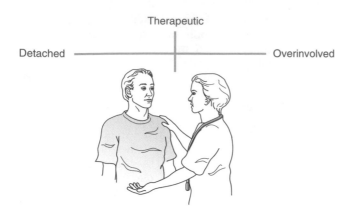

Detached ———————————————————— Overinvolved

Therapeutic

Figure 4–1. Therapeutic relationships require a combination of full presence and emotional objectivity.

sary for them to feel successful empowers clients and enhances self-esteem.

## Role of the Nurse

A therapeutic relationship represents a conscious commitment on the part of the professional nurse to understand how an individual client and his or her family perceive, feel, and respond to their world. From beginning to end, listening closely to verbal and nonverbal messages, focusing on the client's concerns, and attempting to understand the client as a unique person reinforce the client's value as a human being. The underlying

theme in all nursing actions is a respect for the human dignity of the client.

Therapeutic relationships require thoughtful attention. The relationship can be a well-intentioned but ineffectual process if it lacks a planned direction to guide the participants. The purposeful thinking behind the actions taken in the relationship best distinguishes the nurse's role from other types of relationships. Activities to establish and maintain healing relationships are threaded through all stages of therapeutic relationships. The care of the client takes precedence, requiring the full attention and participation of the nurse (Fig. 4–1).

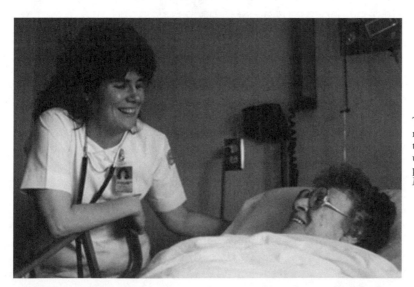

The underlying theme in all nursing interactions is respect for the client and a desire to understand the client as a unique person. (Courtesy University of Maryland School of Nursing)

## Self-Awareness

From the very first encounter, self-awareness is important. The psychological mindset of the nurse influences emotional availability for developing the relationship. Preoccupation with other matters or biases about behaviors or classes of people can get in the way of therapeutic conversations. For example, if the nurse resents being on night duty or is preoccupied with personal matters, interpersonal availability will be affected. Stereotypes about the client's behavior, appearance, or illness make it easier or harder to relate empathetically.

By accepting primary responsibility for the development of the relationship, the nurse consciously sets aside all personal prejudices, interests, and anxieties. Peplau (1997) noted that nurses must observe their own behavior as well as the client's with "unflinching self-scrutiny and total honesty in assessment of their behavior in interactions with patients" (p. 162). By critically and simultaneously examining the behaviors of the client and the nurse and what is going on in the relationship, nurses can create a safe, trustworthy, and caring relational structure. This structure supports and empowers clients as they try to understand and respond productively to difficult circumstances in their lives.

Self-awareness allows nurses to treat each client with respect, as a person having value, even if the nurse cannot understand or approve of certain behaviors. In working closely with clients, nurses will have all sorts of feelings about their clients because they are human. Our humanity is what makes us good nurses, but it also makes nurses more vulnerable to caring too much or too little. Nurses need to acknowledge overinvolvement, avoidance, anger, frustration, or detachment from a client when it occurs and begin to work on developing a deeper understanding of the underlying interpersonal issues. The ethical principle "First, do no harm" should be foremost in the nurse's mind throughout the relationship.

### ◆ Case Example

Kelly, age 20, has been admitted with a tentative medical diagnosis: "Rule out AIDS." John is a 21-year-old student nurse assigned to care for Kelly. He expresses concern to his instructor about the client's sexual orientation. The instructor notes that John spends the majority of his time with his only other assigned client, who is in for treatment of a minor heart irregularity.

---

What conclusions might be drawn regarding the reason John spends so little time caring for Kelly? If you were John, what would be important to you in understanding and resolving your feeling?

## Professional Boundaries

***Professional boundaries*** in a therapeutic relationship are invisible structures imposed by legal, moral, and professional standards of nursing that respect nurse and patient rights. They include defining the time and length of contact, maintaining confidentiality regarding what the client says, and providing an appropriate setting for the relationship, including which people may be involved in various interactions. Most important is the professional conduct of the nurse in relating to the client as a helping person, not as a friend, not as a judge, but as a skilled professional companion committed to helping the client achieve mutually defined health care goals (Briaut & Freshwater, 1998).

The boundaries of a professional relationship make it safe for the client. Just as guardrails protect the public from falling into danger when observing a tourist attraction, professional boundaries protect the client from becoming injured in self-observation. The client must be able to trust that all kinds of feelings are possible without fear of misunderstanding or retaliation (Gallop, 1998).

The nurse is ethically bound to observe the boundaries needed to make a relationship therapeutic. Clients seek health care in good faith from licensed professionals from a vulnerable position as persons in need of help. They have every right to expect that the professionals who care for them will be active, responsive participants and guides in the clients' progress toward optimal health and well-being. Closely related to the concept of boundaries is the nurse's level of involvement.

## Level of Involvement

The nurse–client relationship is an interdependent relationship. Each partner in the relationship has an impact on the other, and each relationship represents a special opportunity for personal growth on the part of both participants (Yuen, 1986). The nurse enters each nurse–client relationship with a certain body of knowledge, a genuine desire to help others, and an openness to experiencing the client as a special and unique person who is worthy of personalized as well as professional attention and respect (Henson, 1997). The client enters the relationship with a health care need potentially responsive to nursing intervention. To be effective, nurses must maintain emotional objectivity.

Heinrich (1992) noted that nurses consistently walk a fine line between having compassion for a client and developing a relationship that is too close, resulting in a friendship with potential serious complications for the client as well as the nurse. Overinvolvement can occur when there are shared positive feelings about the relationship, the client is needy and effusively grateful, or the client reminds the nurse of a similar previously unresolved care situation.

Whenever overinvolvement occurs, the nurse loses the necessary detachment and objectivity needed to support the client in meeting health goals. Lost is the needed balance between compassion and professionalism, a primary ingredient in successful nurse–client relationships. Ethical commitments made to the client to serve as protector and facilitator of the client's personal growth are placed in serious jeopardy. Boundaries meant to safeguard the purposes of the relationship become obscured.

Overinvolvement has effects that extend beyond the individual client. It also can compromise the nurse's obligation to the institution, professional commitment to the treatment regimen, collegial relationships with other health team members, and professional responsibilities to other clients (Morse, 1991).

Warning signs that the nurse is becoming overinvolved include

- Giving extra time and attention to certain clients
- Visiting the client in off hours
- Doing things for clients they could do for themselves
- Discounting the actions of other professionals
- Feeling resentment about the ways other health team members care for the client
- Persistently thinking about the client off duty

Carmack (1997) suggested the following actions that the nurse can take to regain perspective:

- Assume responsibility for care while acknowledging that the outcome may not be within your control.
- Focus on the things that you can change while acknowledging that there are things over which you have no control.
- Be aware and accepting of your personal and professional limits and boundaries.
- Self-monitor your reactions.
- Balance client care with self-care without feeling guilty.

At the other end of the engagement process, nurses sometimes find themselves withdrawing from clients because of their behavior or because they cannot bear their suffering. Dugan (1996) suggested that "to be with a person who is anguished is to risk experiencing the cry that is way down deep inside of us" (p. 40). Clients who fail to progress, who suffer intensely or have a lingering death, or who have significant changes in appearance or condition drain the nurse emotionally. Sometimes nurses will detach from relationship with the client because they cannot bear to watch. When this occurs, the client is left to suffer alone. Morse et al. (1992) note that "sufferers watch for any signs of rejection, dismay or horror in their caregivers' faces. If the caregiver does reveal these feelings, and if the patient recognizes these feelings, he/she may become alarmed and lose hope" (p. 818). Support groups for nurses working in high-stress situations and mentoring of new nurses help to offset lack of balance in the nurse–client relationship.

Nurses also tend to detach from clients who are sexually provocative, complaining, hostile, or extremely anxious or depressed. Patients who smell or who are unkempt or have marked physical disabilities or altered appearance are also vulnerable. It is much harder to stay present with such clients because they trigger feelings in the nurse. Signs of disengagement include withdrawal, limited perfunctory contacts, minimizing the client's suffering, and defensive or judgmental communication. Rogers and Cowles (1997) note that these withdrawal behaviors further intensify the loss or perceived loss of self-integrity so often found with clients in profound emotional pain.

## Presence

The most striking quality of an effective nurse–client relationship is the nurse's ability to be fully present with another human being. Being fully present with another is not always comfortable or pleasant. Presence involves the capacity to know when to provide help and when to stand back, when to speak frankly, and when to withhold comments because the client is not ready to hear them (Taylor, 1992). Sometimes staying present is one of the hardest caring acts a nurse can perform for another human being. Yet the relationship may be the only stable element in the client's life, so that the nurse's presence becomes an extremely significant component of the healing process. For the nurse willing to engage in such a relationship, it can be like none that one has ever experienced before, filling the nurse with awe and respect for the humanness of suffering and the magnificence of humanity.

## Therapeutic Use of Self

Bonnivier (1996) suggested that "nurses are 'safe' but real people on whom to try out new social skills, modify dysfunctional relationship patterns, and reveal emotional vulnerabilities" (p. 38). Therapeutic use of self requires nurses to be authentic and clear about their personal values, feelings, and thoughts in responding to a client. For example, a homeless client tells the nurse, "I know you want to help me, but you can't understand my situation because you have money and a husband to support you. You don't know what it is like out on the streets." Instead of feeling defensive, a more appropriate response is to agree with the client that the nurse does not know what it is like to be homeless and to ask the client to tell her more about it. After this discussion, the nurse might address the loneliness, fear, and helplessness the client is experiencing. These are universal feelings and not foreign feelings for most people, including the nurse, from time to time.

Even mistakes can be a forum for genuine communication. For example, a nurse promises the client to return immediately with a pain medication and then forgets to do so because of other pressing demands. When the nurse brings the medication, the client accuses her of being uncaring and incompetent. It would be appropriate for the nurse to apologize for forgetting the medication and for any extra discomfort suffered by the client. To be truly effective, the nurse must have a keen sense of self-awareness that provides direction and acts as a barometer of the relationship process.

## Self-Disclosure

Nurses do not share intimate details of their life with their clients. The nurse, not the client, is responsible for regulating the amount of disclosure needed to facilitate the relationship. If the

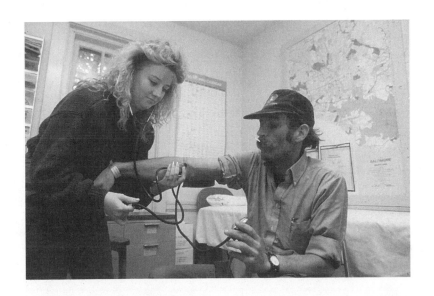

Concepts of the therapeutic relationship are present even in brief encounters.

client asks a nonoffensive superficial question, the nurse may answer briefly with a minimum of information and return to a client focus. For example, questions such as "Are you from around here?", "Where did you go to nursing school?", and "Do you have any children?" may represent the client's effort to establish common ground for conversation (Morse, 1991). Answering them briefly with a return to focus on the client is appropriate. If the client persists with questions, the nurse can say simply, "I'd really like to talk about you, can you tell me about . . . ?"

Requests for intimate information about the nurse do not need to be answered. The nurse may need to redirect the client by saying, "You know, John, I'm not sure my answering your question is relevant and I think we should talk about you," or simply indicate that the question is off limits and return to a client focus. Exercise 4–2 examines appropriate and inappropriate use of self-disclosure.

## APPLICATIONS
### Phases of the Relationship

In 1952, Peplau described four sequential phases of a nurse–client relationship, each characterized by specific tasks and interpersonal skills: preinteraction, orientation, working (active intervention), and termination. Each phase serves to broaden as well as deepen the scope of emotional connection with clients. The therapeutic relationship is a potentially fragile alliance if not handled with care. In any phase of the developing

---

◆ **Exercise 4-2. Recognizing Role Limitations in Self-Disclosure**

**Purpose:** To help you differentiate between a therapeutic use of self-disclosure and spontaneous self-revelation

**Procedure:**
1. Make a list of phrases that describe your own personality, such as

   I am shy.
   I get angry when criticized.
   I'm nice.
   I'm sexy.
   I find it hard to handle conflicts.
   I'm interested in helping people.

2. Mark each descriptive phase with one of the following:

   A = Too embarrassing or intimate to discuss in a group.
   B = Could discuss with a group of peers.
   C = This behavior characteristic might affect my ability to function in a therapeutic manner if disclosed.

3. Share your responses with the group.

**Discussion:**
1. What criteria were used to determine the appropriateness of self-disclosure?
2. How much variation is there in what each student would share with others in a group or clinical setting?
3. Were there any behaviors commonly agreed on that would never be shared with a client?
4. What interpersonal factors about the client would facilitate or impede self-disclosure by the nurse in the clinical setting?
5. What did you learn from doing this exercise that could be used in future encounters with clients?

relationship, the process can break down. Remaining at the superficial, social level of the orientation phase hampers the active, problem-solving process needed for successful resolution of health care issues identified in the working phase. Having developed a strong rapport with a client in the orientation and working phases and then failing to terminate adequately with a client calls into question much of the effectiveness of the nurse's efforts during the earlier phases. The chances of the client trusting in the value of future relationships diminish when termination is treated casually.

Flexibility in returning to more superficial levels may be necessary when the client is not ready to discuss sensitive issues. For example, a difficult diagnosis or beginning awareness of a terminal condition may cause the client to become silent. The client may need more time to absorb disturbing changes internally before using the therapeutic relationship to work through potentially overwhelming feelings about a situation.

## Preinteraction Phase

**Creating the Psychological Environment.** Careful preparation usually makes the first encounter with a client go more smoothly. Having a clear knowledge of the theoretical principles and role responsibilities associated with the relationship does not guarantee a successful outcome, but it does, however, prevent the "lost" feeling that comes from not knowing what one is doing or what one hopes to accomplish through one's efforts. Developing professional goals helps the nurse select concrete, specific nursing actions that are purposeful and aligned with individualized client needs.

The goals of a professional relationship dictate that the client is always the architect of the content; the nurse supplies the coaching framework necessary for understanding the nature of the problem-solving process. Having professional goals communicates to the client that the nurse is knowledgeable, in control of nursing role responsibilities, and ready to focus on the needs of the client. Professional goals rarely are communicated directly to the client, but they are implicit in all that the nurse does and says with a client.

Making the interpersonal environment a safe place in which to explore feelings and to work through painful issues is of critical importance in the beginning stages of the relationship. For example, the nurse on a maternity floor should have a different perspective in approaching a client whose infant is in the neonatal intensive care unit because of respiratory distress than in approaching a client who is rooming in with a healthy infant. The few minutes it takes to obtain a quick overview of client status before the initial meeting can make quite a difference in the choice of interpersonal approaches and in the success of the initial encounter.

Obstacles are easier to handle when they have been anticipated. Thinking seriously about potential difficulties gives the nurse more leverage in responding appropriately in the relationship. For example, two clients might have a similar diagnosis of breast cancer. However, the client who has just received the diagnosis and the client who has known about her diagnosis for the past 4 months are likely to respond quite differently to the nurse. Two young women in the hospital to deliver a first child may have quite different needs in the relationship if one is happily married and the pregnancy was planned and the other is single and does not want the infant. Their personal demographic characteristics and antepartal history may be similar, but their interpersonal needs are likely to be different. Knowledge of the differences in their circumstances affords the nurse greater sensitivity in approaching the clients for the first time. This is what is meant by individualized nursing care. Treating critical yet sometimes subtle differences in individual circumstances as important information in the initial encounter respects the uniqueness of the person experiencing them.

Nurses need to schedule interviews with clients in the hospital at times when the client is physically comfortable and free of pain. In the home, the client should select an appropriate time that does not conflict with the nurse's other responsibilities. Offering the client several different times helps with this process. Nurses should set times with the client when they can give the client undivided attention for the full duration of the visit. The client needs to feel comfortable and unhurried. If the relationship is to be ongoing, the nurse should share initial plans related to time, purpose, and other details with staff. Failure to involve staff in the initial planning stages can sabotage the most careful and creative plan.

**Creating the Physical Environment.** The place where the interview takes place should provide the privacy needed to promote communication. A comfortable setting where nurse and client can sit facing each other with comfortable distance between is essential to the objectives of the relationship whether it is a one-time interview or an ongoing relationship. The room should be well lighted, well ventilated, and in a location where others cannot overhear the conversation. Validating that a space is available at the times needed for the relationship prevents spending more time looking for a room than talking to the client.

When the interview takes place at the client's bed in a hospital setting, the curtain should be drawn and the nurse can sit at an angle facing the client. One-to-one relationships with psychiatric clients frequently take place in a designated, noiseless room, apart from the client's bedroom. In the client's home, the nurse is always the client's guest, and the client plays a stronger role in selecting the most appropriate place for the relationship.

Specific client needs can dictate the most appropriate interpersonal setting. For example, the rape victim in a busy emergency room should be accorded privacy in a private room with a staff member even before the interview begins. Although rape may not represent the most physically urgent triage situation, it is one of the most profound psychological emergency situations a woman can experience. The client needs privacy and someone to stay with her. An adolescent or elderly client may appreciate a "walking interview" on the grounds rather than in his or her room. Each time a nurse considers such factors in a nurse–client relationship, the nurse models thoughtfulness, respect, and empathy.

## Orientation Phase

The nurse–client relationship formally begins with the *orientation phase* and ends with the evaluation phase. Tasks for each phase are presented in Table 4–1. All beginnings are important because they set the tone for the relationship. The nurse enters the relationship in the stranger role and begins the process of developing trust by providing the client with basic information about the nurse (name, professional status) and essential information about the purpose, nature, and time available for the relationship (Peplau, 1997). This can be a simple introduction: "I am Susan Smith, a registered nurse, and I am going to be your nurse on this shift." Nonverbal supporting behaviors of a handshake, eye contact, and a smile reinforce the spoken words.

Introductions are important even with clients who are confused, aphasic, or unable to make an objective response because of mental illness or coma. The vocal tone, smile, and warmth accompanying the words connect with the humanity of the client. The nurse can continue with an invitation to the client to share similar information, "How would you prefer to be addressed?", and follow with some basic questions to put the client at ease. From the very first encounter, the nurse conveys to the client an expectation that the relationship will be a partnership (Kasch, 1986). That understanding, in and of itself, sometimes stimulates an atmosphere of hope. The implicit assumption is that the client has something valuable to offer the relationship, and that the nurse will use this information to help the client achieve his or her goals.

**Clarifying the Purpose of the Relationship.** Nurse and client must develop a working partnership before the work on health care problems takes place. In the orientation phase, the nurse provides basic information about the purpose and nature of the interview or relationship, including what information is needed, how the client can participate in the process, what the client can expect from the encounter, and how the information will be used. The nurse can use statements such as, "I'd like to talk with you about how I can help you in the hospital and to do that, I will need to ask you for some information about your health and what you expect here in the hospital." Asking clients whether they have any questions and what they would like to get out of the relationship helps the nurse have an idea of client expectations and potential roadblocks in the relationship.

The goals of the relationship dictate the depth of the orientation to the purposes of the relationship. A basic orientation given to a client by a nurse assigned for a day would be different from that given to a client when the nurse assumes

Table 4–1. **Phases of the Nurse–Client Relationship***

| ORIENTATION PHASE | WORKING PHASE | | TERMINATION PHASE |
| | IDENTIFICATION | EXPLOITATION | |
| --- | --- | --- | --- |
| *Client:* | | | |
| Seeks assistance | Participates in identifying problems | Makes full use of services | Abandons old needs |
| Conveys educative needs | Begins to be aware of time | Identifies new goals | Aspires to new goals |
| Asks questions | Responds to help | Attempts to attain new goals | Becomes independent of helping person |
| Tests parameters | Identifies with nurse | Rapid shifts in behavior; dependent-independent | Applies new problem-solving skills |
| Shares preconceptions and expectations of nurse resulting from past experience | Recognizes nurse as a person | Exploitative behavior | Maintains changes in style of communi-cation and interaction |
| | Explores feelings | Realistic exploitation | Positive changes in view of self |
| | Fluctuates among dependence, independence, and interdependence in relationship with nurse | Self-directing | Integrates illness |
| | | Develops skills in interpersonal relationships and problem solving | Exhibits ability to stand alone |
| | Increases focal attention | Displays changes in manner of communication (more open, flexible) | |
| | Changes appearance (for better or worse) | | |
| | Understands purpose of meeting | | |
| | Maintains continuity between sessions (process and content) | | |
| *Nurse:* | | | |
| Responds to emergency | Maintains separate identity | Continues assessment | Sustains relationship as long as client feels necessary |
| Gives parameters of meetings | Exhibits ability to edit speech or control focal attention | Meets needs as they emerge | Promotes family interaction |
| Explains roles | Testing maneuvers decrease | Understands reason for shifts in behavior | Assists with goal setting |
| Gathers data | Unconditional acceptance | Initiates rehabilitative plans | Teaches preventive measures |
| Helps client identify problem | Helps express needs, feelings | Reduces anxiety | Uses community agencies |
| Helps client plan use of community resources and services | Assesses and adjusts to needs | Identifies positive factors | Teaches self-care |
| Reduces anxiety and tension | Provides information | Helps plan for total needs | Terminates nurse–client relationship |
| Practices nondirective listening | Provides experiences that diminish feelings of helplessness | Facilitates forward movement of personality | |
| Focuses client's energies | Does not allow anxiety to overwhelm client | Deals with therapeutic impasse | |
| Clarifies preconceptions and expectations of nurse | Helps client to focus on cues | | |
| | Helps client develop responses to cues | | |
| | Uses word stimuli | | |

Date Completed: _____ Signatures: _____

*Phases are overlapping.

Adapted from Forchuk C, Brown B. (1989). Establishing a nurse-client relationship. Journal of Psychosocial Nursing and Mental Health Services 27(2):32. Used with permission.

the role of primary care nurse. When the relationship is to be of longer duration, the nurse should be prepared to discuss the parameters of the relationship (e.g., length of sessions, frequency of meetings, role of the nurse).

Initial meetings should have two outcomes. First, the client should emerge from the encounter with a better idea of some of the beginning health issues and possible goals. Second, the client should feel that the nurse is interested in him or her as a person. At the end of the contact, the nurse should thank the client for his or her participation and indicate what will happen next. For example, the nurse might say, "Our time for today (this interview) is up. But I enjoyed talking with you, and I will share this information with the staff so that we can plan your care. I'd like to go over it with you later to make sure that it is a good fit."

When you initially use this introductory strategy, the words may feel mechanical, and you might prefer to be more informal and spontaneous in your communication. Obviously, you can vary the words, but the verbal message needs to contain this combination of data. It may help to remember that clients do not know who you are or what your purpose is in interacting with them. It is frightening for many people to be asked questions without having any idea what is needed or why the person needs the information. By giving clients an opportunity to understand who you are, what you hope to accomplish by interacting with them, and what the boundaries of the relationship are, you will be more likely to gain their cooperation. Having an idea of what you will say initially to a client also should decrease your anxiety. Exercise 4–3 is designed to give you practice in making introductory statements.

Spontaneity can be expressed in the way you present yourself. Are you smiling and relaxed in manner? Do your posture and gestures support your genuine desire to get to know this client? Are you truly receptive to hearing what the client has to share with you? Your accompanying actions are no less important than the words you use. Both your actions and your words are data the client needs to begin trusting you.

**Assessing Client Needs.** The nurse and the client can have different perceptions of reality, and the nurse needs to begin the assessment process with an open mind. How the client perceives his or her health status, reasons for seeking treat-

ment at this time, and expectations for health care are critical data that will form the basis for all nursing interventions. Depending on the client's ability to enter into a productive relationship, the nurse may need to emphasize the importance of providing accurate information to obtain appropriate help and explore reasons for reluctance to share information. Sometimes more time is needed to develop trust, particularly with psychiatric clients. Acknowledging how hard it is to trust health professionals in a new and unfamiliar situation helps, taking the time to hear the client, and asking for a chance to help sometimes alleviate undue anxiety.

Initially, the nurse focuses on the immediate crisis of the hospitalization or clinic visit and begins to identify factors with the client and the client's family that will facilitate or hinder the treatment process. Asking the client to tell you what brought him or her to the hospital (clinic) or to seek treatment elicits the client's perspective on the illness. Once the reason for seeking health care is established, a second question, "What kind of help can we provide for you?", yields information about client expectations. Asking the second question helps prevent client disappointment stemming from unrealistic expectations and provides the nurse with the opportunity to correct misinformation.

Once the nurse establishes rapport and orients the client to the purposes of the interview or relationship, the nurse listens attentively to the client, incorporating sensory data with spoken information. Planning questions to follow a logical sequence and asking only one question at a time help orient the client and provide more complete data. The nurse's nonverbal behavior should convey respect, interest, and acceptance for the dignity of the person as a fellow human being. When information is not clear, the nurse should use communication strategies found in Chapter 10 to clarify meaning.

**Participant Observation.** Nurses mentally form impressions about the client's behavior, mental status, and anxiety level from the moment that they enter the client's room. These impressions, when validated with the client, serve as guides for subsequent actions in the relationship. For the nurse to obtain the full picture, learning as much as possible about a client through data related to the illness experience is crucial.

◆ **Exercise 4-3. Introductions in the Nurse-Client Relationship**

The introductory statement forms the basis for the rest of the relationship. Effective contact with a client helps build an atmosphere of trust and connectedness with the nurse. The following statement is a good example of how one might engage the client in the first encounter:

Hello, Mr. Smith. I am Sally Parks, a nursing student. I will be taking care of you on this shift. During the day I may be asking you some questions about yourself that will help me to understand how I can best help you.

**Directions:**
After reading this introductory statement, identify the who, what, when, and why in the statement. The prior statement is used as an illustration.

Who: Sally Parks, student nurse

What: taking care of you and asking you some questions

When: on this shift

Why: to help me to understand how I can best help you

Think of a recent interaction you have had with a client. Write the statement and identify the who, what, when, and why in the statement.

_____

_____

_____

_____

_____

Who: _____

What: _____

When: _____

Why: _____

**Discussion:**
1. What was the client's response to the introductory statement?
2. If different students experienced a variation in client responses, what variables might have contributed to this finding?
3. What did you learn from doing this exercise?

Adapted from Carkhuff RR. (1983). The Art of Helping V. Student Workbook. Amherst, MA, Human Resource Development Press. Copyright © 1983. Reprinted by permission of HRD Press, Inc., 22 Amherst Rd., Amherst, MA 01002.

◆ **Case Example**

**Dying Client** (*to the nurse*):  It's not the dying that bothers me as much as not knowing what is going to happen to me in the process.

**Nurse:**  It sounds as though you can accept the fact that you are going to die, but you are concerned about what you will have to experience. Tell me more about what worries you.

By asking for more information about the emotional context, before commenting on the content of the client's message, the nurse shows a desire to understand the situation from the client's perspective. Sometimes the full picture looks quite different from the initial presentation of the problem. Furthermore, the nurse is not relying on intuition or assuming the meaning of data without obtaining all applicable information from the client.

A comment on the client's flowers or an observation about the client, "You look as though you would like to be alone" or "Are those pictures of your family?", shows the client that he or she is seen as a person with recognizable individual characteristics.

Nurses need to be aware of the different physical cues clients give with their verbal messages. Noting the factors that seem to be preventing the establishment of the relationship, "You look exhausted" or "You look worried," acknowledges the presence of these factors. Exercise 4–4 is designed to help you pick up another person's nonverbal cues.

As the nurse interacts with the client, there are opportunities to observe client strengths. Every client has healthy aspects of his or her personality and personal strengths that can be used to facilitate individual coping responses. Think about a client you have had or a person you know who has a serious illness. What personal strengths does this person have that could have a healing impact on the illness?

Relying exclusively on client information without soliciting the perceptions of significant others can distort and limit history taking. If there is any reason to suspect the reliability of the client as a historian, significant others can supply information. Nursing judgment is also needed when family and client disagree about diagnosis, treatment goals, or ways to provide care. Comparing client and family data for congruence and differences is an important source of client data. The differences can be just as important as the agreement in developing the most appropriate nursing interventions. For example, if the client has one perception about self-care abilities or other competencies and family members have a completely different perception, these differences become a nursing concern. Specific nursing diagnoses need to address the discrepancies in perceptions.

It is important to strike a balance between communicating with the client and with significant others accompanying the client. Sometimes health professionals treat clients who are elderly, adolescent, or physically handicapped as though they are mentally incapacitated in assessment interviews. Talking only with the adult members of a family instead of including the client in the dialogue, or assuming the elderly or adolescent client has a limited understanding or interest, devalues the person. This subtle and usually unintentional devaluing of the individual increases a sense of dehumanization and loneliness, a frequent occurrence in health care settings.

The last part of the assessment process in the orientation phase relates to determining the kind of help needed as well as who can best provide it. Assessment of the most appropriate source of help is an important but often overlooked part of the evaluation needed in the orientation phase.

**Communication Strategies.** Initial contacts should be exploratory and somewhat tentative. Both the conversation and behaviors in the orientation phase are usually of a superficial nature.

---

◆ **Exercise 4–4. Interpreting Nonverbal Cues**

**Purpose:**  To identify and understand the role of nonverbal cues of the introductory, working, and termination phases of the therapeutic relationship

**Process:**
A variety of photographs of nurse-client interactions will be provided, and each student will choose one. The student will examine the picture and creatively identify a phase it depicts, the tasks being accomplished by the nurse, and the response of the client.

**Discussion:**
Each student will share his or her picture and interpretation. Descriptions of each phase will be compiled on the board.

Neutral topics rather than emotionally loaded subjects usually seem less invasive to the client in the beginning stages of the relationship. Initially, a client feels vulnerable in examining sensitive subjects before a trusting bond is established. Discussion of deep feelings and core issues will come later.

Talking about the client's interests and noncontroversial topics provides the nurse with important information about the client's choices, knowledge base, interests, and characteristic ways of thinking about life. At the same time, the nurse is accumulating information that can be used to assist the client in establishing workable, meaningful goals. Conversations about hobbies, the geographical area the client is from, and the type of work the client does are ones most clients will respond to with ease. Sometimes an article in the client's room, such as a family picture or religious item, serves the same purpose.

### ◆ Case Example

Mrs. Gayle T., age 24, has been admitted to the hospital in the early stages of labor. She is alone in the labor room, knitting a sweater, but she appears somewhat nervous. Karen K., a student nurse, is assigned to care for Mrs. T. Because Karen loves to knit, she begins a conversation with Mrs. T. by focusing the discussion on the art of knitting and of knitting layettes in particular.

Knowledge of the client's developmental stage and current health situation may suggest possible topics for conversation. For example, one of the best ways to engage an adolescent is to demonstrate an awareness of teenagers, their interests, and pastimes. If the client is on the maternity floor, asking about the labor and delivery is relevant, whereas most elderly clients are eager to share anecdotes about their earlier lives. Such topics usually feel familiar, yet they are perceived an nonintrusive to most clients.

During the initial encounters with the nurse, the client begins to assess the nurse's trustworthiness (Forchuk & Brown, 1989). Communication is a two-way process. Kindness, competence, and a willingness to become involved get communicated through the nurse's words and actions. Does the nurse seem to know what she is doing? Is the nurse tactful and respectful of cultural differences? Data regarding the level of the nurse's interest and knowledge base are factored into the client's decision to engage actively in a therapeutic relationship.

Honesty and commitment are critical elements in trust. Consistency, dependability, and honoring commitments to the client foster the development of trust. When it is impossible to honor a commitment, the client receives a full explanation.

### ◆ Case Example

A Mexican client on a psychiatric ward had an excellent working relationship with a young Spanish-speaking student nurse. Because most of the other staff members did not speak Spanish, they looked to the student nurse to serve as translator. One morning the client told the student nurse she had concealed a knife in her room to commit suicide the night before, but now had decided against it. The student nurse told the client she would have to tell the nursing staff. At this point, the client became very angry. She reminded the student of pledged confidentiality and told her if she communicated with the staff, she, the client, would feel betrayed and would sever the relationship with the nurse because it would mean a loss of privileges.

Despite the client's threat, the student felt she needed to communicate the information about the knife to the appropriate nursing and medical staff. She explained her reasons for doing so and emphasized that the safety of the client was her most important concern. Later, the client was able to renew her sense of trust in the student nurse and the relationship became stronger because the student acted in a manner consistent with her role and dealt with the human aspects of the relationship conflict in a firm but compassionate manner.

Trusting the nurse is particularly difficult for the seriously mentally ill, for whom the idea of having a caring relationship is incomprehensible. Having this awareness helps the nurse depersonalize the experience of momentarily feeling overwhelmed by intense human emotions that he or she does not always easily understand. Most mentally ill clients respond better to shorter, frequent contacts until trust is established. Schizophrenic clients often enter and leave the space occupied by the student, almost circling around a space that is within visual distance of the nurse. With patience and tact, the nurse engages the client slowly, respecting the client's anxiety. Brief meetings gradually held over time that involve an invitation and a statement as to when the nurse will return help reduce the client's anxiety (Morath, 1987), as indicated in the following dialogue.

### ◆ Case Example

**Nurse:** (said with eye contact with the client and enough interpersonal space for comfort): Good morning, Mrs. O'Connell, my name is Karen Quakenbush. I will be your nurse today. (Patient looks briefly at the nurse and looks away, gets up and moves away.)

**Nurse:** This may not be a good time to talk with you. Would you mind if I checked back later with you? (The introduction coupled with an invitation for later communication respects the client's need for interpersonal space and allows the client to set the pace of the relationship.)

---

Later, the nurse notices that Mrs. O'Connell is circling around the area the nurse is occupying but does not approach the nurse. The nurse can smile encouragingly and repeat short encounters with the client until the client is more willing to trust. Creating an interpersonal environment that places little demand on either party initially allows the needed trust to develop in the relationship.

**Defining Goals.** Often a client needs assistance in developing relevant health goals, but the level of assistance always should coincide with the client's capacity for self-help. Unless clients are physically or emotionally unable to participate in their own care, they should be treated as active partners in developing meaningful personal goals.

Goals should have meaning to the client. Finding out the client's interests can influence the selection of environmental motivators and the development of specific nursing strategies. For example, modifying the diabetic adolescent exchange lists to include fast foods and substitutions that mimic normal adolescent eating habits may facilitate acceptance of unwelcome dietary restrictions imposed by the illness. The nurse conveys confidence in the client's capacity to solve his or her own problems by expecting the client to provide data, to make constructive suggestions, and to follow through with the agreed-

on plan. Exercise 4–5 gives practice in establishing mutual goals with a client.

**Developing a Therapeutic Contract.** The final step in the orientation phase of the relationship is a therapeutic contract that supports the aims of the relationship and spells out role expectations and goals. This contract can be renegotiated as the original circumstances in the health care situation change. The contract should contain information about the following:

- The frequency and nature of interpersonal contacts
- Mutually agreed-on goals
- Expected role behaviors of both participants

### Working (Active Intervention) Phase

Once nurse and client together define the problem in the orientation phase, they move into the working phase. The working phase is subdivided into two: identification and exploitation. The identification component focuses on mutual clarification of ideas and expectations. Nurses also help clients express feelings of helplessness, dependency, and despair; discover personal strengths; and identify potential resources. The composite data become the basis of an individualized nursing care plan. Nurse and client mutually develop goals related to resolution of identified client health needs and decide on the type of assistance needed to achieve them.

In the *exploitation phase*, nurses assist their clients to seek out and use health care services and personal strengths in resolving the issues for which the client initially sought treatment. Corresponding to the implementation phase of the nursing process, the nurse fosters clients' self-direction in promoting their health and well-being. Peplau categorized the client role as dependent, interdependent, or independent, based on the amount of responsibility the client is willing or able to assume for his or her care.

Characteristic of this stage is an atmosphere of trust and candor that makes it easier for the client to discuss deeper, more difficult issues and to experiment with new roles and actions. By contrast with the orientation phase, in which roles are more individualistic, the working phase is characterized by interdependent role relationships; the client assumes more of a partnership

◆ **Exercise 4–5. Establishing Mutual Goals**

**Purpose:**  To develop awareness of mutuality in treatment planning

**Procedure:**
1. Read the following clinical situation and subsequent nursing goals.
2. Identify each goal as nurse centered (N), client centered (C), or mutual (M).
3. After completion, discuss correct answers. How could nurse or client goals be modified to become mutual treatment goals?

**Nursing Situation:**
Mr. S., age 48, a white, middle-class professional, is recovering from his second myocardial infarction. After his initial heart attack, Mr. S. resumed his 10-hour workday, high-stress lifestyle, and usual high-calorie, high-cholesterol diet of favorite fast foods, alcohol, and coffee. He smokes two packs of cigarettes a day and exercises once a week by playing golf.

Mr. S. is to be discharged in 2 days. He expresses impatience to return to work but also indicates that he would like to ``get his blood pressure down and maybe drop 10 pounds.'' The student nurse caring for Mr. S. establishes the following treatment goals:

1. After three dietary teaching sessions, Mr. S. will be able to identify five foods high in sodium content.
2. After discharge, Mr. S. will nap for 2 hours each day.
3. During the dietary teaching session, Mr. S. will list five foods high in calories and five foods low in calories.
4. Mr S. will exercise moderately for 10 minutes a day and will limit his weekly golf game to three holes.
5. Mr. S.'s diastolic blood pressure will be below 90 mm Hg at his 1-month postdischarge examination.
6. Immediately after discharge, Mr. S. will resume his executive work schedule.
7. Mr. S. will remain symptom free until discharge.

with the nurse in problem solving and implementation.

The working phase integrates mutuality with the client's autonomy. The sorting-out process occurs more easily when nurses are relaxed and willing to understand views different from their own. Peplau (1997) suggested that a general rule of thumb in working with clients is to "struggle with the problem, not with the patient" (p. 164).

Clients need to feel they have played a major role in developing a plan and implementing it in ways that make sense to them. The role of the nurse is to provide enough structure and guidelines for the client to explore problem issues and develop realistic solutions but no more than is needed (Ballou, 1998). The nurse may sometimes take more responsibility for an outcome than the client needs. Such an approach may be easier in the immediate situation, but important learning

is lost. For example, a seemingly more efficient use of the nurse's time may be to give a bath to a stroke victim rather than to watch the client struggle through the bathing process with coaching when the client falters. However, what happens when the client goes home if she has not learned to bathe herself?

The client's right to make important decisions, provided they do not violate self or others, is accepted by the nurse, even when it runs contrary to the nurse's thinking. This is not always easy when the nurse feels that the client is not acting in his or her own best interest. Consider what you would do as the community health nurse in the following situation.

◇ **Case Example**

Mr. McEntee, 54 years old, is admitted for chest pain. His tests show increased occlusion of the cardiac vessels. All of the male members of his family died of coronary disease in their 50s. Three years ago he had coronary bypass surgery. Since the surgery Mr. McEntee has conformed to a proper diet and exercised prudently. Although he was referred to the cardiac rehabilitation unit for after care, he has refused to go. A home visit shows that he is not adhering to his diet but that he goes to the gym daily to work out. The nurse questions his noncompliance and urges him to consider the implications.

---

Listening with heart as well as head, how would you try to understand Mr. McEntee's predicament? Why do you think he is acting in such a self-destructive way? What suggestions can you offer to the home care nurse to increase compliance?

**Defining the Problem.** The success of the working phase lies in properly identifying all elements that have the potential to interfere with goal achievement. Defining the problem itself increases the probability of a satisfactory solution. The nurse acts as a sounding board, asking questions about parts of the communication that are not understood and helping the client describe the problem in specific and concrete terms.

The problem statement should be precise and concrete. "Mrs. K. started to cry when talking about her son's accident" is much more helpful than stating, "Mrs. K. is sad that her son was hurt in a motorcycle accident." The latter statement includes an inference about cause and effect that could be erroneous. In this case, the client's tears could relate to anger, disappointment, or hurt. Without validation from the client, the second statement about the cause of Mrs. K.'s tears could be incorrect, so that an intervention predicated on that information might be inappropriate.

Initially, it might appear that developing the problem definition in more depth repeats the initial assessment data, but good problem definitions are evolving statements that direct planning and implementation. Full participation by the client in defining the problem reinforces the client's feelings of being in control and free to communicate without being criticized. Clients vary in their ability to do this. For some clients, there seems to be a genuine unawareness of a problem or of the connection between their behavior and the problem itself. Start where the client is in

the process. If the client wishes to be active, use an action-oriented approach. With a more passive client, forcing action-oriented solutions may prove counterproductive. Instead, gentle suggestions and a slower pace are more effective.

It is usually easier for the client to talk about factual data related to a problem rather than to express the feelings associated with the issue, or to talk about the feelings as though there were no factual data associated with the problem. Using open-ended questions and compound sentences to link situational facts and emotional effects allows for the most complete understanding. "It sounds as if you feel _____ because of _____" helps the nurse and client look at the strong interrelationship between the situational data and the emotional reactions to it. For many clients, events and feelings represent two separate and unconnected happenings. To experience the connections comes as a revelation.

Another way of helping clients recognize the significant details of critical issues is to describe the problem situation and the response in terms of who, what, where, when, and how, just as you did in your introduction and clarification of the nurse–client contract in the engagement phase. The difference is that now the communication focus is on a real or potential problem in need of nursing intervention instead of on the roles, purpose, and rules of the relationship. This strategy allows the client to perceive the problem in more complete form, and it gives the nurse an opportunity to observe the client's characteristic ways of handling difficult situations.

Whenever the nurse fails to understand a part of the client's problem or expectations, it is appropriate to ask for clarification or for more specific information. The nurse might ask for concrete data to bring the client's needs into sharper focus. For example, "Can you describe for me what happened next?" "Can you tell me something about your reaction to (your problem)?" Time should be allowed between questions for the client to respond fully. Not infrequently, the questions are asked, but not enough time is allowed for the client to respond.

In asking what, who, and why about problem situations, there must be careful observation of the impact of these questions on the client. "Why" questions are the hardest for clients to answer because motivational factors usually are the most difficult to understand and own. Most of the time behavior is multidetermined. Motivations are too complex and too sensitive to describe in answer to a simple "why" question. Often clients are not totally aware of what made them choose one behavioral response over another. The nurse needs to proceed slowly and carefully with such questions. It is important to challenge the client's thinking but not the client's integrity.

**Pacing.** The nurse needs to recognize the legitimacy of the client's need to proceed at a personally comfortable momentum. Throughout the working phase, the nurse needs to be sensitive as to whether the client is still responding at a useful level. Looking at difficult problems and developing strategies to resolve those problems is not an easy process, especially when resolution will require significant behavioral changes. If the nurse is perceived as inquisitive rather than facilitative, communication breaks down.

Pacing the interview in ways that offer support as well as challenge is the responsibility of the nurse, not the client. The client's behavioral responses will serve as a guide for structuring deeper exploration and for understanding client needs. Changes in client behaviors often are the best indicators of data collection that is proceeding beyond the client's tolerance level. Examples of warning signs indicating increased anxiety include loss of eye contact, fidgeting, abrupt changes in subject, crying, inappropriate laughter, or asking to be left alone.

Although the nurse needs to be aware that heightened anxiety precludes discussion of difficult material, strong emotion should not necessarily be interpreted as reflecting a level of interaction stretching beyond the client's tolerance. Tears or an emotional outburst, even a more prolonged negative exchange, may reflect honestly felt emotion. A well-placed comment such as "It seems to make you sad when we talk about your daughter" acknowledges the feeling and may stimulate further discussion. The deciding factor as to whether to drop a subject or to support the client in exploring it is a clinical judgment about whether or not the feelings are appropriate in intensity to the behavioral stimulus, as well as about the capacity of the client to continue with the discussion. Forcing a client to continue with a painful discussion when it is clear that there is too much emotion fails to respect the client's need for self-determination in the relationship.

Sometimes just sitting with calm interest and an open posture is enough to help a client reduce the internal anxiety of expressing strong emotion. A simple statement such as, "It's all right to cry" or "It's okay to feel angry; nobody would want this to happen to him" acknowledges the feeling component, gives the client permission to express it, and implicitly offers assistance in coping with difficult emotions.

**Developing Realistic Goals.** Goals develop from the nursing diagnosis. The nurse assists the client in developing realistic short-term objectives to meet long-term treatment goals. Breaking a seemingly insoluble problem down into simpler chunks makes it more manageable. Deciding on a course of action for even a small part of the problem helps the client gain some control in the situation and usually reduces anxiety to a tolerable level. For example, a goal of eating three meals a day may seem overwhelming to a person suffering from nausea and loss of appetite associated with gastric cancer. A goal of having Jell-O or chicken soup and a glass of milk three times a day may sound more achievable. Packaging goals in terminology the client understands and accepts is more important than having a goal the client considers beyond his or her capabilities. To be effective, goals should be achievable, behavioral, and realistic.

**Planning Alternative Solutions.** All life situations have some element of choice. In even the most difficult nursing situations, there are some options, even if the choice is to die with dignity or to change one's attitude toward an illness or a family member. Here the nurse and client brainstorm all possible options and strategies to meet agreed-on health objectives. They can discuss the implications of each possible choice and the anticipated reactions of others. Anticipating reactions of others is an important step in the process because even well-thought-out strategies can have unforeseen consequences for self and others. For example, if a client wishes to go home rather than to a nursing home, how is this decision likely to affect other family members who will have to provide the necessary care? How does the client feel about his or her ability to provide self-care, and are these assumptions valid? Each of these questions will have a direct impact on the option chosen. Thinking about them and planning how to handle them strengthens the client's resolve.

During this phase of the relationship, nursing interventions should have a broader focus than simply correcting problem areas. For clients to experience lasting change, there also needs to be an emphasis on strengthening their inner resources. Vocational skills, talents, community resources, and supportive family are advantages clients sometimes take for granted. They fail to appreciate the transferable skills that can be used in the current situation. Exercise 4–6 gives practice in developing alternative strategies.

**Implementing the Plan.** Both nurse and client monitor progress. As the client begins to implement certain actions for coping more successfully with anxiety-provoking situations, the nurse can offer anticipatory guidance and role rehearsal for the more difficult aspects of this process. Sometimes simply anticipating "the worst-case scenario for a given action" allows the client to see that the worst possibility is manageable. Feed-back for the client regarding possible modifications when the situation warrants it is an equally important element of the process.

Implementation does not always mean the course will be smooth and uneventful, even when the plan is appropriate. Mistakes are to be expected. Although mistakes will happen, they will not destroy the work of this phase. The reality is that something can go wrong even with the most perfectly developed plan. Constructive coping mechanisms are as important to support as the actual plan. A useful comment might be, "It is important to keep in mind that you did a good job with this, and no one could have predicted the outcome." This statement removes the blame that so frequently accompanies failed efforts. Coping with unexpected responses can strengthen the client's problem-solving abilities by compelling the person to consider alternative options (Plan B) when the original plan does not bring about the desired results.

Most problems and health care needs have to be worked through slowly, with the client taking two steps forward and one step back. This slow

---

◆ Exercise 4–6. **Selecting Alternative Strategies**

**Purpose:**   To help you develop a process for considering alternative options

**Procedure:**
You have two exams within the next 2 weeks. Your car needs servicing badly. Because of all the work you have been doing, you have not had time to call your mother, and she is not happy. Your laundry is overflowing the hamper. Several of your friends are going to the beach for the weekend and have invited you to go along. How can you handle it all?

1. Give yourself 5 minutes to write down all the ideas that come to mind for handling these multiple responsibilities. Use single words or phrases to express your ideas. Do not eliminate any possibilities, even if they seem far-fetched.
2. In groups of three or four students, choose a scribe, and share the ideas you have written down.
3. Select the three most promising ideas.
4. Develop several small, concrete, achievable actions to implement these ideas.
5. Share the small-group findings with the class group.

**Discussion:**
1. In what ways were the solutions you chose similar or dissimilar to those of your peers?
2. Were any of your ideas or ways of achieving alternative solutions surprising to you or to others in your group?
3. What did you learn from doing this exercise that could help you and a client generate possible solutions to seemingly impossible situations?

progress sometimes is cause for discouragement, and yet, like small children taking their first steps, the process is usually not a straight linear progression. Offering the client reassurance based on the fact that the two small steps were taken and that those steps cannot be erased, even if the client is unable to achieve a short-term goal to complete satisfaction, is a source of valuable support. The more critical question is, "What is it about either the goal, the strategies used to meet the goal, or the appraisal of the need or problem that needs reworking?"

Sometimes the problem with implementation lies with the nurse's availability, but even here there are ways to handle the situation that make a difference in how the client perceives the nurse's interest. Therapeutic responses are clear and focused on the client's need. However, they also respect the nurse's integrity. The two responses to the client's need in the following example take the same amount of time. Which is potentially more satisfying?

### ◆ Case Example

Jenny Johnson, RN, is on her way to the staff lounge to take a much-needed break when Mr. Clemson stops her to discuss his concerns about the cardiac catheterization his son was scheduled for an hour ago. Jenny sighs, glances impatiently at her watch, and comments in a flat voice, "I'd be happy to talk with you about the procedure if you have any questions."

An alternative response, one that recognizes the legitimate needs of both client and nurse, might be as follows:

Nurse (in a warm voice and making direct eye contact): It's natural to be concerned, but this procedure usually takes at least 2 hours. I'll call the recovery room and find out if your son has arrived there yet. If he hasn't arrived, I'll leave a message for them to call me when he does arrive. I'll be off the unit for a short time now, but when I get back, I'd be happy to talk with you about the procedure if you have any questions.

In the second response, the nurse recognizes the legitimacy of the client's need as well as her own and responds accordingly. Because the message is clear and congruent with her expression and action, it is more likely to comfort the client.

**Challenging Resistant Behaviors.** Sometimes in the working phase it is necessary to challenge factors that may get in the way of goal achievement. Challenging resistant behaviors requires a special type of feedback because often the client is only partially aware of what is happening and of his or her role in the process (Garant, 1980). Because of a lack of awareness, these behaviors remain unavailable for direct exploration and negotiation. Before confronting a client, the nurse should determine carefully whether it is warranted and anticipate possible outcomes. It is not necessary to confront a client about a resistant behavior as soon as it occurs, nor is it always useful. Sometimes asking open-ended questions may elicit self-awareness, and the client may come to the same conclusion as the nurse about the existence of a problem in implementing certain actions.

If this strategy does not work and you must challenge the meaning of the client's message, it is important to proceed with interpersonal precision, sensitivity, and accuracy. The nurse needs to appreciate the impact of the confrontation on the client's self-esteem.

Calling a client's attention to a contradiction in behavioral response is usually threatening. It should be accomplished in a tactful manner that welcomes, but does not necessarily demand, an immediate resolution. Constructive feedback involves drawing the client's attention to the existence of unacceptable behaviors or contradictory messages while respecting the fragility of the therapeutic alliance and the client's need to protect the integrity of the self-concept. To be effective, constructive confrontations should be attempted only when the following criteria have been met:

- The nurse has established a firm, trusting bond with the client.
- The timing and environmental circumstances are appropriate.
- The confrontation is delivered in a nonjudgmental and empathetic manner.
- Only those resistances capable of being changed by the client are addressed.
- The nurse is willing to abide by the client's right to self-determination.

Timing is everything. Enough time and interpersonal space should be given to allow the client an opportunity to reflect on the feelings surrounding the behaviors as well as on the thoughts and feelings aroused by the nurse's comments. Discrepancies should never be challenged in a roomful of people unless there is no alternative and the client's behavior represents a danger to self or others. More specific guidelines regarding constructive feedback are presented in subsequent chapters.

### ◆ Case Example

Mary Kiernan is 5 feet 2 inches tall and weighs 260 pounds. She has attended weekly weight management sessions for the past 6 weeks. Although she lost 8 pounds the first week, 4 pounds in Week 2, and another 4 pounds in Week 3, her weight loss seems to have plateaued. Jane Tompkins, her primary nurse, notices that she seems to be able to stick to the diet until she gets to dessert and then she cannot resist temptation. Mary is very discouraged about her lack of further progress.

Consider the effect of each response on the client.

Nurse: You're supposed to be on a 1200-calorie a day diet, but instead you're sneaking dessert. I think you need to face up to the fact that eating dessert while dieting is hypocritical.

Nurse: I can understand your discouragement, but you have done quite well in losing 16 pounds. It seems as though you can stick to the diet until you get to dessert. Do you think we need to talk a little more about what hooks you when you get to dessert? Maybe we need to find alternatives that would help you get over this hump.

The first statement is direct, valid, and concise, but it is likely to be disregarded or experienced as unfeeling by the client. In the second response, the nurse reframes a behavioral inconsistency as a temporary setback, a problem in need of a solution instead of a human failing. By bringing in the observed strength of the progress achieved so far, the nurse confirms her faith in the client's resourcefulness. Both responses would probably require similar amounts of time and energy on the part of the nurse. However, the second response fits the goal of motivating the client to use inner resources. The external rein-

forcement of the nurse allows the client to continue progress toward her goal of losing 50 pounds over a 6-month period.

**Referral.** There are times in the active intervention phase when it becomes obvious that the client needs a different approach to achieve treatment goals. Sometimes it is painful for the nurse to admit that the client's need surpasses the nurse's level of expertise, especially when genuine feelings and the nurse's ego are involved. Referral is an appropriate intervention whenever a client's needs exceed the level of care provided in the interpersonal relationship.

The nurse can play an important role in the referral process by thoroughly discussing with the client the reasons for the referral. Telling the client that you will pave the way or passing along some information about the person who has been referred is a good bridging technique that often alleviates unnecessary anxiety. The nurse should have the client's permission to transmit information to the referred resource. Often the nurse's summary of the relationship is helpful to the referral professional in planning future strategies. Summarizing goal achievement with the client and providing a copy of the summary information reinforces the client's sense of control and continuity of treatment. Peplau (1997) also suggested that nurses can contribute to the advancement of the profession by sharing their experiences with client reactions to the illness experience.

### Termination Phase

Unlike social relationships, therapeutic relationships have a predetermined ending, when the outcome criteria are achieved, the client is discharged, or the number of visits permitted by insurance is reached. Termination refers to the cessation of the relationship and is a time to summarize the major achievements in the relationship. The date of termination should be mentioned well in advance of the actual ending of the relationship. The client needs to be allowed to express feelings related to termination and to discuss the effects of the anticipated loss. Encouraging the client to deal with reactivated feelings from former losses and the nurse's constructive sharing of relevant personal feelings about the relationship and the termination facilitate the process. Together, the nurse and client examine the meaning and value of the relationship, including negative as well as positive elements. Finally, there is a mutual evaluation of goal achievement. Follow-up interventions are identified if needed.

The threads of termination are interwoven throughout the nursing process. Preparation for termination actually begins with the orientation phase, when the nurse explains to the client the times, duration, and focus of the relationship. Just as the orientation phase is linked with the assessment phase, the termination phase of the nurse–client relationship shares characteristics with the evaluation phase. The nurse and client mutually evaluate goal achievement and discuss needed modifications. Feelings surrounding the termination are discussed, and plans for follow-up are initiated, if indicated. With significant and long-term relationships, the nurse and client also evaluate the effectiveness of their communication in the relationship.

Endings are rarely comfortable, but the importance of the termination phase should not be underestimated. Sometimes there is a tendency to shortchange the termination phase because for both the nurse and the client it is more uncomfortable than some of the other stages. This is particularly true when the relationship has meaning. When the participants have invested a lot of themselves in the relational process, it is hard to give it up.

The process of termination will not be the same for every client. Different aspects of the relationship should be emphasized and, ideally, correlated with each client's individualized needs, temperament, and behavioral response. Not every relationship can tolerate a lengthy discussion of termination feelings. The nurse's behavioral response should match the level of other phases in depth and intensity. For very short-term relationships or for a superficial contact, a simple statement of the meaning of the relationship, factual reassurance based on client behaviors observed in the relational experience, and discussion of follow-up plans suffice.

The importance of the relationship, no matter how brief, should not be underestimated. The client may be one of several persons the nurse has taken care of during that shift, but the relationship may represent the only interpersonal

or professional contact available to a lonely and frightened person. In personal relationships, it is customary for the person who is leaving to acknowledge the fact to the people in the immediate surroundings. This custom should carry over into the clinical situation. Even if contact has been minimal, the nurse should endeavor to stop by the client's room to say good-by. The dialogue in such cases can be simple and short: "Mr. Jones, I will be going off duty in a few minutes. I enjoyed working with [meeting] you. Miss Smith, the evening nurse, will be taking care of you this evening." Anticipatory guidance in the form of simple instructions or reiteration of important skills may be appropriate, depending on the circumstances.

Care should be taken to recognize the wide variety of behaviors accompanying termination, including regression and a temporary return of maladaptive ways of coping. Clients react in a variety of ways to separation. Some are grateful but very ready to move on with all they have gained in the relationship. Some become angry; others deny it is happening. Some clients appear to have lost all that was gained personally in the relationship. Behaviors the nurse may encounter with termination include avoidance; minimizing of the importance of the relationship; temporary return of symptoms precipitating the need for nursing care; anger; demands; or additional reliance on the nurse. Sometimes this phase is perplexing for both nurse and client. For the nurse, there is a sense of pride in watching someone grow and develop as a person. It is difficult to give this up or to experience loss of gains during the termination phase. For the client there can be a fear of relapsing and losing ground with the new attitudes and competencies. All of these feelings are normal in the termination phase and are usually temporary. When the client is unable to express feelings about endings, the nurse may recognize them in the client's nonverbal behavior.

◆ **Case Example**

A teenager who had spent many months on a bone marrow transplant unit had developed a real attachment to her primary nurse, who had stood by her during the frightening physical assaults to her body and appearance occasioned by the treatment. The client was unable verbally to acknowledge the meaning of the relationship with the nurse directly, despite having been given many opportunities to do so by the nurse. The client said she couldn't wait to leave this awful hospital and that she was glad she didn't have to see the nurses anymore. Yet this same client was found sobbing in her room the day she left, and she asked the nurse whether she could write to her. The relationship obviously had meaning for the client, but she was unable to express it verbally.

In another clinical situation, a hospitalized formerly psychotic client, who had made remarkable progress in a one-to-one weekly relationship, failed to show up for the last appointment. On questioning the nursing staff, the primary care nurse found that the client had scheduled a clinic appointment off the ward at precisely the time of the nurse–client appointment. The nurse went to the clinic and found the client lying on a bench, waiting to be seen. The nurse told the client that she was disappointed when the client did not come for the appointment and wondered if it had to do with termination. For the first time, the client was able to cry and to address her feelings of abandonment, asking if she could go home with the nurse and become her maid. Although her initial resolution of the termination phase was unrealistic, exploring the meaning behind the request with the nurse allowed this client to express the depth of her feelings about the impending separation.

The nurse was able to appreciate the significance of the relationship to the client and to help her work through some very strong feelings. The meaning and commitment the relationship held for the nurse were effectively demonstrated in her searching out the client, reinforcing the reality that the relationship had significance.

If the relationship has been rewarding, real work has been accomplished. Strong feelings were shared, and often there is a genuine sadness and sense of loss at parting. Nurses need to be sufficiently aware of their own feelings so that they may use them constructively without imposing them on the client. It is appropriate for nurses to share some of the meaning the relationship held for them, as long as such sharing fits the needs of the interpersonal situation and is not excessive or too emotionally intense.

Appropriate self-disclosure in the termination phase might include thanking the client for sharing his or her life with the nurse. Exploration of knowledge gained from the relationship and of attitudes and feelings of client and nurse during the relationship and as they relate to the specific health care concerns of the client adds value to goal achievement. Shared meanings enhance the human outcomes of the therapeutic relationship (Marck, 1990).

In a successful relationship, the client demonstrates the following outcomes:

- Adaptive progression toward health or well-being
- Adequacy of role performance according to developmental level and constraints of the illness
- A self-reported or enacted value shift, indicating a deeper sense of personal integrity

Evaluation of outcomes should take into consideration all phases of the nursing process. Was the problem definition adequate and appropriate for the client? Were the interventions chosen adequate and appropriate to resolve the client's problem? Could the interventions be implemented effectively and efficiently to both the client's and nurse's satisfaction? Negative answers to any of these questions require adjustments in any or all phases of the nursing process.

There are occasions or circumstances in which, because of individual limitations, the policy of the agency, or the nature of the relationship dynamics, it is in the best interest of the client to terminate the relationship. If the relationship needs to be terminated for transfer, therapeutic, or policy reasons, the helping person should be honest, direct, and compassionate as he or she provides a full explanation of the circumstances surrounding the termination. Usually, if the nurse is tactful and considerate in explaining the unplanned end of the relationship, the client has a better chance of working through the termination than if the departure is precipitous and no attention is paid to its impact on the client. Follow-up planning should be initiated and resources identified for continued support.

## SUMMARY

The nurse–client relationship represents a purposeful use of self in all professional relations with clients and other people involved with the client. Respect for the dignity of the client and self, mutuality, person-centered communication, and authenticity in conversation are process threads underlying all communication responses.

By contrast with social relationships, therapeutic relationships have specific boundaries, purposes, and behaviors. They are client focused and are mutually defined by client and nurse. Effective relationships enhance the well-being of the client and the professional growth of the nurse.

The professional relationship is a developmental process characterized by four overlapping yet distinct stages: preinteraction, orientation, working (active intervention), and termination. The preinteraction phase is the only phase of the relationship the client is not part of. During the preinteraction phase, the nurse develops the appropriate physical and interpersonal environment for an optimal relationship, in collaboration with other health professionals and significant others in the client's life.

The orientation phase of the relationship defines the purpose, roles, and rules of the process and provides a framework for assessing client needs. The nurse builds a sense of trust through consistency of actions. Data collection forms the basis for developing relevant nursing diagnoses. The orientation phase ends with a therapeutic contract mutually defined by nurse and client.

Once the nursing diagnosis is established, the working or active intervention phase begins. Essentially, this is the problem-solving phase of the relationship, paralleling the planning and implementation phases of the nursing process. As the client begins to explore difficult problems and feelings, the nurse uses a variety of interpersonal strategies to help the client develop new insights and methods of coping and problem solving.

The final phase of the nurse–client relationship occurs when the essential work of the active intervention phase is finished. Termination involves the deliberate separation of two or more persons from an intimate and meaningful relationship. Each relationship has its own character, strengths, and limitations, and what may be appropriate in one nursing situation may be totally inappropriate in another. Nevertheless, terminations are the final step in the nurse–client relationship, and the ending of it should be thoroughly and compassionately defined. Primary tasks associated with the termination phase of the relationship include summarization and evaluation of completed activities and, when indicated, the making of concrete plans for follow-up.

## REFERENCES

Ballou K. (1998). A concept analysis of autonomy. Journal of Professional Nursing 14(2):102–110.

Benner P. (1984). From Novice to Expert: Excellence and Power in Clinical Nursing Practice. Menlo Park, CA, Addison-Wesley.

Bonnivier M. (1996). Management of self-destructive behaviors in an open outpatient setting. Journal of Psychosocial Nursing 34(2):37–43.

Briant S, Freshwater D. (1998). Exploring mutuality within the nurse-patient relationship. British Journal of Nursing. 7(4):204–206.

Buber M. (1958). I and Thou (2nd ed., RG Smith, trans.). New York, Scribner.

Buber M. (1965). Between Man and Man (RG Smith, trans.). New York, Macmillan.

Carkhuff RR. (1983). The Art of Helping V, Student Workbook. Amherst, MA, Human Resource Development Press.

Carmack B. (1997). Balancing engagement and disengagement in caregiving. Image 29(2):139–144.

Clarke J, Wheeler S. (1992). A view of the phenomenon of caring in nursing practice. Journal of Advanced Nursing 17:1283–1290.

Curtin L. (1983). Trust: An idealistic or realistic goal? In Minckley B, Walters M (eds.), Building Trust Relationships in Nursing. Indianapolis, IN, Midwest Alliance in Nursing.

Dinkmeyer DC, Dinkmeyer DC Jr, Sperry L. (1987). Adlerian Counseling and Psychotherapy (2nd ed.). Columbus, OH, Merrill.

Dugan P. (1996). Excerpts from "Recovering our sense of value after being labeled mentally ill." Journal of Psychosocial Nursing vol 34.

Ersek M. (1992). Examining the process and dilemmas of reality negotiation. Image 24(1):19–25.

Forchuk C, Brown B. (1989). Establishing a nurse-client relationship. Journal of Psychosocial Nursing 27(2):30–34.

Frankl V. (1955). The Doctor and the Soul. New York, Knopf.

Gallop R. (1998). Abuse of power in the nurse-client relationship. Nursing Standard 12(37):43–47.

Garant C. (1980). Stalls in the therapeutic process. American Journal of Nursing 80:2166–2169.

Heinrich K. (1992). When a patient becomes too special. American Journal of Nursing 22(11):62–64.

Henson RH. (1997). Analysis of the concept of mutuality. Image: Journal of Nursing Scholarship. 29(1):77–81.

Kasch C. (1986). Establishing a collaborative nurse-patient relationship: A distinct focus of nursing action in primary care. Image 18(2):44–47.

Kasch C, Dine J. (1988). Person-centered communication and social perspective taking. Western Journal of Nursing Research 10(3):317–326.

Lamb HR. (1988). One-to-one relationships with the long-term mentally ill: Issues in training professionals. Community Mental Health Journal 24(4):328–337.

Marck P. (1990). Therapeutic reciprocity: A caring phenomenon. Advances in Nursing Science 13(1):49–59.

Meize-Grochowski R. (1984). An analysis of the concept of trust. Journal of Advanced Nursing 9:563–572.

Morath J. (1987). Theory-based intervention: A case study using Sullivan's interpersonal theory of psychiatry. Perspectives in Psychiatric Care 24(1):12–19.

Morse J. (1991). Negotiating commitment and involvement in the nurse-patient relationship. Journal of Advanced Nursing 16:455–468.

Morse J, Bottorf J, Anderson G, et al. (1992). Beyond empathy: Expanding expressions of caring. Journal of Advanced Nursing 17:809–821.

Paterson J, Zderad L. (1988). Humanistic Nursing. New York, National League for Nursing.

Pearson A, Borbasi S, Walsh K. (1997). Practicing nursing therapeutically through acting as a skilled companion on the illness journey. Advanced Practice Nursing Quarterly 3(1):46–52.

Peplau HE. (1952). Interpersonal Relations in Nursing. New York, Putnam.

Peplau HE. (1997). Peplau's theory of interpersonal relations. Nursing Science Quarterly 10(4):162–167.

Ramos M. (1992). The nurse-patient relationship: Theme and variations. Journal of Advanced Nursing 17:495–506.

Reynolds W. (1997). Peplau's theory in practice. Nursing Science Quarterly 10(4):168–170.

Roberts S, Krouse J. (1988). Enhancing self-care through active negotiation. Nurse Practitioner 13(8):44–52.

Rodwell C. (1996). An analysis of the concept of empowerment. Journal of Advanced Nursing. 23(2):305–313.

Rogers BL, Cowles KD. (1997). A conceptual framework for human suffering in nursing care and research. Journal of Advanced Nursing 25:1048–1053.

Rogers C. (1973). My philosophy of interpersonal relationships and how it grew. Journal of Humanistic Psychology 13:3.

Seyster K. (1987). A lesson in therapeutic relationship. Imprint 9:56–57.

Taylor B. (1992). Relieving pain through ordinariness in nursing: A phenomenologic account of a comforting nurse-patient encounter. Advances in Nursing Science 15(1):33–43.

Travelbee J. (1971). Interpersonal Aspects of Nursing. Philadelphia, FA Davis.

Yuen FK. (1986). The nurse-client relationship: A mutual learning experience. Journal of Advanced Nursing 11:529–533.

# 5

# Bridges and Barriers in the Therapeutic Relationship

## Kathleen Underman Boggs

**OBJECTIVES**

At the end of this chapter, the student will be able to

1. Identify concepts that enhance development of therapeutic relationships: caring, empowerment, trust, empathy, mutuality, and confidentiality
2. Describe nursing actions designed to promote trust, empowerment, empathy, mutuality, and confidentiality
3. Describe barriers to the development of therapeutic relationships: anxiety, stereotyping, and lack of personal space
4. Identify nursing actions that can be used to reduce anxiety and respect personal space and confidentiality

*We must take our [clients] where we find them and lead them where they are willing to go.*

B. Koesch, cited in Platt (1995)

Chapter 5 focuses on the conceptual components of the nurse–client relationship. The concepts and applications are integrated because they cannot logically be understood apart from one another. To establish a therapeutic relationship, the nurse must understand and apply the concepts of caring, empowerment, trust, empathy, and mutuality. Appreciation of other concepts such as anxiety, stereotyping, personal space, and confidentiality adds to the quality of relationship strategies. Although these concepts are understood as abstract elements of the nurse–client relationship, implementing actions that convey feelings of caring, warmth, acceptance, and understanding to the client is an interpersonal skill that requires careful development. Caring for others in a meaningful way requires patience and practice. Novice students may experience interpersonal situations that leave them feeling helpless and inadequate. Feelings of sadness, anger, or embarrassment, although overwhelming, are common. Discussion of these feelings in peer groups, experiential learning, and theoretical applications help students to grow and learn from prior mistakes. The self-awareness strategies identified in Chapter 3 and the use of educational groups described in Chapter 12 provide useful guidelines for working through these feelings.

## BASIC CONCEPTS
## Bridges to the Relationship
**(Fig. 5–1)**
### Caring

***Caring*** is an intentional human action characterized by commitment and a sufficient level of knowledge and skill to allow the nurse to support the basic integrity of the person being cared for (Clarke, 1992). One person (the nurse) offers caring to another (the client) by means of the therapeutic relationship. The nurse's ability to care develops from a natural response to help those in need, the knowledge that caring is a part of nursing ethics, and respect for self and others. The caring nurse involves clients in their struggle for health and well-being rather than simply doing for clients those actions they cannot perform for themselves.

The focus of the caring relationship is the client and his or her needs. The nurse recognizes the client's need for help and basic vulnerability. Caring represents a selected and informed response to the client's need, the act of giving freely and willingly of oneself to another through warmth, compassion, and concern, and interest. Nurses care for others during times of physical discomfort, emotional stress, and need for health

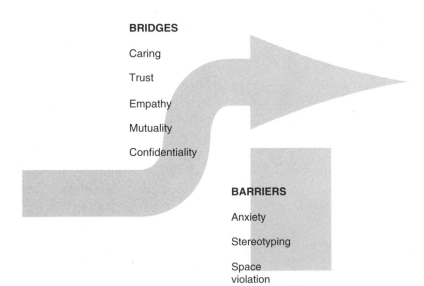

**BRIDGES**

Caring

Trust

Empathy

Mutuality

Confidentiality

**BARRIERS**

Anxiety

Stereotyping

Space violation

Figure 5–1. Relationships can move in a positive or negative direction. Nursing actions can be bridges or barriers to a good nurse–client interaction.

maintenance. Caring has been identified as an ethical responsibility (Harrison, 1990).

Clients want us to understand why they are suffering. Platt (1995) noted that we tend to speak in a language of medicine that values facts, measurable intervals, sizes, sequences, and events. On the other hand clients value associations and causes. To bridge this potential gap, health providers need to convey to clients a sense that they truly care about the clients' perspective. Caring has a positive influence on health status and healing. Caring individuals recognize others as separate and unique persons with varying needs. Clients are treated with kindness and consideration. Through caring, nurses identify client needs, implement appropriate nursing actions, make knowledgeable decisions, and bring about positive changes in their clients (Gault, 1983). In a caring relationship, clients can focus on accomplishing the goals of health care instead of worrying about whether care is forthcoming. The nurse gains from the caring relationship by experiencing the satisfaction of meeting clients' needs accurately and skillfully.

Families also need to experience a sense of caring from the nurse. Many families do not believe that the care provider has a clear understanding of the problems they are encountering while caring for their ill family member. This is especially true if the illness is not an easily observable defect or is a mental illness (Accordino, 1997).

Some people criticize the use of caring as one basis of the nurse–client relationship on the grounds that it is not scientific and is perhaps "feminine" in its origins. However, if competence is defined as having a strong theoretical base from which to make judgments about nursing care, then caring is an important element of the science as well as the art of nursing. Exercise 5–1 will help students focus on the concept of caring.

### Empowerment

*Empowerment* is defined as the "interpersonal process of providing the proper tools, resources and environment to build, develop, and increase the ability of others to set and reach goal" (Hawks, 1992, p. 609). Empowerment is an important underlying thread in every nurse–client relationship. It prepares clients to cope with difficult life situations created by alterations in their health and well-being. Empowerment has to do with people power. This concept encourages us to help clients take maximum control of their lives. Empowerment builds on strengths. Empowerment is purposeful. It encourages clients to assume responsibility for their own health. Personal responsibility, provision of appropriate resources, and ongoing support are given to help them feel empowered.

### Trust

Development of a sense of interpersonal trust has long been considered as an essential skill in humans' development. According to Erik Erikson (1963), *trust* is the reliance on the consistency, sameness, and continuity of experiences that are provided by an organized combination

---

◆ **Exercise 5–1. Application of Caring**

**Purpose:**  To help students apply caring concepts to nursing.

**Procedure:**
Have each student identify some aspect of caring that might be applied to nursing practice. Write each on the chalkboard or a transparency on the overhead projector so the entire group can see.

**Discussion:**
In a large group, discuss examples of how this form of caring could be implemented in a nurse–client situation.

of familiar and predictable things and people. Trust is based on past experiences and begins in infancy through consistent and continual care by the same caregiver. Through trust, one learns how to cope with problems and resolve frustrations.

Trust within a nurse–client relationship appears as attitudes, beliefs, and behaviors (Johns, 1996). These can be characterized as demonstrating respect, honesty, consistency, faith, caring, and hope. Trust impacts not only on communication but in a fundamental way on the healing process. For a client, trust implies a willingness to place oneself in a position of vulnerability, relying on health providers to perform as expected. A therapeutic relationship always begins with trust. Certain interpersonal strategies (Box 5–1) help promote a trusting relationship.

Trust can be replaced with mistrust between nurse and client. Just as some agency managers treat employees as though they are not trustwor-

thy (Johns, 1996), some nurses treat some clients as though they are misbehaving children. Such would be the case if a client fails to follow the treatment regimen and is labeled with the nursing diagnosis of "noncompliant." In another example, the community health nurse who is inconsistent about keeping client appointments or the pediatric nurse who indicates falsely that an injection will not hurt is jeopardizing client trust. It is hard to maintain trust when one person cannot depend on another. Energy that should be directed toward coping with health problems is rechanneled into assessing the nurse's commitment and trustworthiness. Having confidence in the nurse's skills, commitment, and caring allows the client to place full attention on the situation requiring resolution.

Clients can also jeopardize the trust a nurse has in them. In a review of research in the health professions, Thompson (1984) noted that many studies blamed the professional for problematic interactions with clients, ignoring the barriers contributed by clients. Sometimes clients "test" a nurse's trustworthiness by sending the nurse on unnecessary errands or talking endlessly on superficial topics. As long as nurses recognize testing behaviors and set clear limits on their roles and the client's role, it is possible to develop trust. Exercise 5–2 is designed to help students become more familiar with the concept of trust.

### Empathy

**Empathy** is the ability of a person to perceive and understand another person's emotions accurately. Empathetic nurses are able to recognize or communicate the meanings of feelings through verbal and nonverbal behaviors. Empathy is the ability to put oneself into the client's position. According to Feil (1996), an important component of the communication process is conveying respect and empathy, especially if the client is somewhat confused. Objective and nonjudgmental nurses feel the emotions a client feels but at the same time maintain their own separate identities. You should not overidentify with or internalize the feelings of the client. If internalization occurs, objectivity is lost, along with the ability to help the client move through his or her feelings. It is important to recognize that the client's feelings belong to the client, not to you.

---

◆ **Box 5-1. Techniques Designed to Promote Trust**

Convey respect.
Consider the client's uniqueness.
Show warmth and caring.
Use the client's proper name.
Use active listening.
Give sufficient time to answer questions.
Maintain confidentiality.
Show congruence between verbal and nonverbal behaviors.
Use a warm, friendly voice.
Use appropriate eye contact.
Smile.
Be flexible.
Provide for allowed preferences.
Be honest and open.
Give complete information.
Provide consistency.
Plan schedules.
Follow through on commitments.
Set limits.
Control distractions.
Use an attending posture: arms, legs, and body relaxed; leaning slightly forward.

---

◆ **Exercise 5–2. Techniques That Promote Trust**

**Purpose:** To identify techniques that promote the establishment of trust and to provide practice in using these skills.

**Procedure:**
1. Read the list of interpersonal techniques designed to promote trust.
2. Describe the relationship with your most recent client. Was there a trusting relationship? How do you know? Which techniques did you use? Which ones could you have used?

or

3. In triads, one learner interviews a second to obtain a health history, while the third observes and records trusting behaviors. Rotate so that everyone is an interviewer. Interviews should last 5 minutes each. At the end of 15 minutes, each observer shares findings with the corresponding interviewer.

**Discussion:**
Compare techniques.

---

## Levels of Empathy

Attaining high levels of empathy is rewarding to both nurse and client. Carkhuff (1969) identified five levels of empathy. Use information listed in Box 5–2 to understand the following case. Levels of empathy are described from least to most empathetic.

**Level 1.** *Unawareness of the client's message of feelings* is the lowest level of empathy. Because there is no evidence of active listening or understanding of the client's feelings, the nurse's response communicates significantly less than the client's.

### ◆ Case Example

**Client** (frantic):   Jamal (10 months old) has had a terrible cold for more than a week.

**Nurse** (hurriedly, not looking at client):   Is he up to date on his immunizations?

---

In this example, the nurse ignores the feeling tone of the client and changes the subject to obtain the desired information. The nurse's insensitivity may arise from boredom, lack of interest, bias, or differing reasons for the interaction.

**Level 2.** *Superficial acknowledgment of the client's message* minimizes the client's feelings. The nurse shows awareness of superficial feelings but responds in a way that noticeably ignores the client's emotions.

| Box 5–2. Levels of Nursing Actions | | |
|---|---|---|
| Level | Category | Nursing Behavior |
| 1 | Accepting | Uses client's correct name |
| | | Maintains eye contact |
| | | Adopts open posture |
| | | Responds to cues |
| 2 | Listening | Nods head |
| | | Smiles |
| | | Encourages responses |
| | | Uses therapeutic silence |
| 3 | Clarifying | Asks open-ended questions |
| | | Restates the problem |
| | | Validates perceptions |
| | | Acknowledges confusion |
| | Informing | Provides honest, complete answers |
| | | Assesses client's knowledge level |
| | | Summarizes |
| 4–5 | Analyzing | Identifies unknown emotions |
| | | Interprets underlying meanings |
| | | Confronts conflict |

### ◆ Case Example

**Client** (frantic): Jamal (10 months old) has had a terrible cold for more than a week.

**Nurse** (with a casual glance): This is the time of year for colds. Everyone has one. He'll get over it.

In this example, the nurse responds to the content of the statement but not to the feeling tone of the client. The nurse minimizes the client's feelings.

**Level 3.** *Recognition of the client's message and some of the client's feelings* is somewhat helpful. In Level 3, the nurse responds to the meaning of the client's emotions. Verbal and nonverbal behaviors are congruent. The nurse's words reflect the client's concerns and feelings.

### ◆ Case Example

**Client** (frantic): Jamal (10 months old) has had a terrible cold for more than a week.

**Nurse** (tone the same as the client's, making eye contact, leaning forward in chair): You're upset that Jamal has had this cold for more than a week.

**Client** (crying): Yeah. He's so little, and I want him to get better.

**Nurse** (breaking eye contact): He'll get better. The physician will be in soon to examine him.

The nurse's first response shows a Level 3 empathy. The nurse accurately interprets the superficial feeling tone of client. Because the nurse seems to understand, the client feels free to provide more information. The nurse then reverts to a Level 2 response, however, and essentially ignores the client's tears. Level 3 responses are often a prelude to higher level responses, which reflect the client's hidden emotions. Nurses who are unable to cope with deep feelings are unable to develop empathy beyond Levels 2 and 3.

**Level 4.** *Acknowledgment of the message and obvious feelings* demonstrates the nurse's willingness to understand and care about the client's concerns. Although there are still deep, hidden meanings of which the nurse is unaware, there is a forum for discussion. The nurse probes for information

to expand the client's awareness and the nurse's understanding of the situation.

### ◆ Case Example

**Client** (frantic): Jamal (10 months old) has had a terrible cold for more than a week.

**Nurse** (same voice tone as client, making eye contact, with attending, open posture): You are quite upset about this, aren't you?

**Client** (softly, spoken with tears): Yes. He's so little, and he just has to get better.

**Nurse:** You're afraid it might develop into something worse? (Level 4)

**Client:** Could he have pneumonia?

**Nurse:** I don't know. The physician will examine him soon. How would you feel if he had pneumonia? (Gathering data)

**Client:** Oh, I couldn't stand to have him in the hospital away from me.

**Nurse:** You feel anxious about the possibility of hospitalization, in which the two of you would be separated, and what it might do to your close relationship. (Level 4)

**Client:** Yes, being separated would be awful.

In this example, the nurse begins responding on Level 3 and then moves to Level 4 responses. The nurse has not accurately perceived deeper feelings, but gathers more data, which increases knowledge about the client and thus increases the probability of an accurate assessment of emotions.

**Level 5.** *Full therapeutic acknowledgment of the client's hidden message and meaning* adds significantly to the meanings behind the feelings. Because the nurse has a clearer, more objective view than the client, the nurse is able to state deep, hidden feelings unknown to the client.

### ◆ Case Example

Review the example from Level 4 and begin with the client's response.

**Client:** Oh, I couldn't stand to have him in the hospital away from me.

**Nurse:** What is it about the hospital separation from Jamal that makes you so anxious? (Reflects hidden feelings, asks for more information)

**Client:** It's just his being in the hospital.

**Nurse** (questions, still same feeling tone): Have you or anyone close to you been in the hospital?

**Client:** My brother, when he was young.

**Nurse** (seeking more information): And what was he there for?

**Client:** Pneumonia. He died there of complications!

**Nurse:** So now you're frightened that if Jamal has pneumonia and is hospitalized, he will die too, like your brother. (Reflects deep feelings)

Now that the nurse has full information, the interventions are more likely to address the client's individualized needs directly. The nurse then goes on to give information about pneumonia and provide reassurance that it is treatable. Armed with accurate data, the nurse can communicate the client's feelings to the physician so that the physician can discuss Jamal's diagnosis and treatment with the client to lessen the client's anxiety.

Exercise 5–3 will help clarify information about empathetic responses.

### Mutuality

*Mutuality* basically means that the nurse and the client agree on the client's health problems and the means for resolving them, and that both parties are committed to enhancing the client's well-being. This is characterized by respect for the autonomy and value system of the other. In developing mutuality, the nurse maximizes the client's involvement in all phases of the nursing process. Mutuality is collaboration in problem solving.

Mutuality encompasses all phases of the nurs-

---

◆ **Exercise 5–3. Identifying Empathetic Responses**

**Purpose:** To correctly identify levels of empathy for clinical situations.

**Procedure:**
Read the client statement, and then identify the nurse's response as to the correct empathy level (1, 2, 3, 4, or 5); place the number on the line to the left of the response.

1. Client (on the verge of tears): That doctor confused me so. He was in here for 10 minutes and I still don't know what's wrong with me.

Nurse:

_____a. Doctors like that ought to give up medicine.

_____b. You feel the doctor was confusing and didn't explain your medical problem.

_____c. What time is it now?

_____d. You're angry that the doctor was unable to adequately explain your medical condition.

_____e. You feel exasperated about not knowing your current medical problem and helpless in knowing what you should do to take care of yourself.

2. Client (in a hostile voice): I'm sick of being poked at and stuck with needles. Go away and leave me alone.

Nurse:

_____a. You're fed up with needles and wish to be left alone.

_____b. Getting needles is part of being in the hospital.

_____c. You're angry about having all these intrusive procedures and wish you didn't need them.

_____d. Just remember to fill out your menu for tomorrow.

_____e. With all these intrusive procedures, you feel vulnerable and defenseless, ready to go hide to get away from it all.

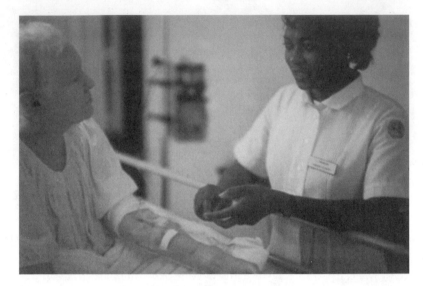

(Courtesy of the University of Maryland School of Nursing)

ing process and enriches nurse–client relationships. Evidence of mutuality is seen in the development of individualized client goals and nursing actions that meet a client's unique health needs. Exercise 5–4 gives practice in evaluating mutuality.

Nurses who are truly sensitive to others' feelings and accept differences between their own lifestyles and those of others have the capacity to develop and attain mutuality in relationships. Such caring nurses show respect by involving clients in the decision-making process. They do not belittle decisions made by clients, nor do clients ever become a "thing" in the nurse's eyes.

Effective use of values clarification assists clients in decision making. As is discussed in Chapter 7, clients who clearly identify their own personal values are better able to solve problems effectively. Decisions then have meaning to the client, who thus has a higher probability of taking steps to achieve success. A mutual relationship is terminated with both parties experiencing a sense of shared accomplishment and satisfaction.

## Confidentiality

*Confidentiality* protects the client's right to decide who can have access to information about any aspect of health care or lifestyle. It refers to the idea that one person feels reassured that the other person will not divulge private information. Within the context of the nurse–client rela-

tionship, the client entrusts the nurse with intimate information and expects it to be held in confidence. The nurse has an ethical responsibility to protect the client's right to privacy.

Chapter 2 presented a discussion of legal issues, including the client's legal right to confidentiality of records and communications with health care professionals.

Information obtained through professional interviewing and history taking is used by the nurse and other health team members to arrive at an individualized client care plan. This information pertains to the client's health status. Relevant data become a part of the client's permanent health record. Emphasis is placed on *pertinent* information. Recorded client data should be neither too sketchy nor too detailed. Information, especially confidential data, that does not contribute to the management of the client's care should not be included in the record. Data about the client or client's condition are not shared with the client's family or health professionals who are not directly involved in the client's care without the competent client's consent.

Discussing private information casually with others is an abuse of confidentiality. Nursing reports and interdisciplinary team case conferences are examples of acceptable forums for the discussion of privileged communication. An explicit norm of such conferences is that the information and feelings shared about a client are not discussed

◆ Exercise 5–4. **Evaluating Mutuality**

**Purpose:** To identify behaviors and feelings on the part of the nurse and the client that indicate mutuality.

**Procedure:**
Complete the following questions by answering yes or no after terminating with a client; then bring it to class. Discuss the answers. How were you able to attain mutuality or why were you unable to attain it?

1. Was I satisfied with the relationship?
2. Did the client express satisfaction with the relationship?
3. Did I share feelings with the client?
4. Did the client share feelings with me?
5. Did I feel or communicate bias toward the client?
6. Did I make decisions for the client?
7. Did I persuade the client to act in a way the client did not want?
8. Did the client feel accepted or understood by me?
9. Did the client feel allowed to make his or her own decisions?
10. Did the client accomplish his or her goals?
11. Did I accomplish my goals?

**Discussion:**
In large group, discuss mutuality.

outside the conference except in the direct application of nursing care (Greve, 1990). To protect privacy, discussion of client care should preferably take place in a conference room with the door closed. This information includes change-of-shift reports, multidisciplinary conferences, one-to-one conversations with other health professionals about specific client care issues, and consultations with clients and their families.

The legal and ethical limitations to confidentiality are discussed in Chapter 2. The nurse can explain that the client's record is kept where only members of the health team have access to it and after discharge is filed in medical records to help ensure the client's privacy. However, in this era of managed care, both nurses and their clients need to be aware that a number of agencies routinely audit records for both quality control and for financial payment requisites. Exercise 5–5 gives more information on confidentiality.

## Barriers to the Relationship

There are barriers in the nurse, the client, and the health care system that can affect the development of the nurse–client relationship. Barriers

affecting the nurse include conflicting values, conflicting professional commitments, lack of a strong sense of self, and lack of value placed on caring. Anxiety, stereotyping, and lack of personal space create barriers within the client. In these days of managed care, barriers within the health care system often reflect cost-containment measures. Such barriers include lack of consistent assignment of nurse to client, increased use of temporary staff such as agency nurses or "floats," lack of time resulting from low staff-client ratios, early discharge, or same-day surgery. In the last 5 years, there has been a marked increase in same-day procedures in which the client is not actually admitted but is treated on an outpatient basis (Naish, 1996). The literature describes agency demand for minimal appointment time with clients. Primary care providers such as nurse practitioners are often constrained to focus just on the chief complaint. Thus, primary care clients are now experiencing "the 15-minute visit."

Other system barriers include communication conflicts with other health professionals, conflicting values, poor physical arrangements, and lack of value placed on caring. These system bar-

◆ Exercise 5–5. **Confidentiality and Setting**

**Purpose:** To identify situations that are a breach of confidentiality and then to correct them.

**Procedure:**
Have students each take one of the following situations, all of which depict a breach of confidentiality. In a group

1. State how confidentiality has been broken.
2. Given the situation, what might be an appropriate response?
3. Change the situation or setting so that confidentiality is maintained.

**Situations:**
1. You are eating lunch in the cafeteria with two fellow pediatric nurses who are discussing the behaviors of an abusive parent.
2. A nurse yells down the hall to you, ``Your patient in 504 is ready to get off the bedpan.''
3. On the postpartum unit, a nurse allows a husband to see his wife's chart.
4. You are riding in the elevator when two operating room nurses step on and comment, ``It took four of us to tie him down for that IV.''
5. You are on rounds. One physician, leaning over Client X, suddenly remembers an order on another client, ``Don't forget Mrs. Smith's enema. Give her a Fleet's enema this morning.''
6. You are at your best friend's house for a dinner party. She is a nurse in the emergency room and begins to discuss a ``terrible accident victim.''

riers limit the nurse's ability to develop substantial rapport with clients. Adequate time is essential to develop therapeutic communication to achieve effective care responsive to client needs (Naish, 1996).

### Anxiety

*Anxiety* is a vague, persistent feeling of impending doom. It is a universal feeling; no one fully escapes it. The impact on the self is always uncomfortable. It occurs when a threat (real or imagined) to one's self-concept is perceived. Anxiety is usually observed through the physical and behavioral manifestations of the attempt to relieve the anxious feelings. Although individuals experiencing anxiety may not know they are anxious, specific behaviors provide clues that anxiety is present. Similarly, although individuals may not be consciously aware of the factors that contribute to the anxiety-producing situation, others may be able to help them identify those factors, thus alleviating the anxiety. Exercise 5–6 identifies behaviors associated with anxiety. Four levels of anxiety are identified by Kreigh and Perko

(1983). Expanding on this information, Box 5–3 shows how an individual's sensory perceptions, cognitive abilities, coping skills, and behaviors relate to the intensity and level of anxiety experienced.

A mild level of anxiety heightens one's awareness of the surrounding environment and fosters learning and decision making. Therefore, it may be desirable to allow a mild degree of anxiety when health teaching is needed or when problem solving is necessary. It is not prudent, however, to prolong even a mild state of anxiety.

Anxiety, other than mild levels, decreases perceptual ability. The anxious state is accompanied by verbal and nonverbal behaviors that inhibit effective individual functioning. Moderate to severe anxiety on the part of either nurse or client hinders the development of the therapeutic relationship. To accomplish goals and attain mutuality, higher levels of anxiety must be reduced. Once the presence of anxiety has been identified, the nurse needs to take appropriate action. Strategies to reduce anxiety are listed in Box 5–4.

Severe anxiety requires medical and psychiat-

---

◆ **Exercise 5–6. Identifying Verbal and Nonverbal Behaviors Associated with Anxiety**

**Purpose:** To broaden the learner's awareness of behavioral responses that indicate anxiety.

**Procedure:**
List as many anxious behaviors as you can think of. Each column has a few examples to start. Discuss the lists in a group, and add new behaviors to your list.

*Verbal*
Quavering voice
Rapid speech
Mumbling
Defensive words

*Nonverbal*
Nail biting
Foot tapping
Sweating
Pacing

_____         _____

_____         _____

_____         _____

_____         _____

---

ric intervention to alleviate the crisis-producing stress. A prolonged panic state is incompatible with life. It is such an extreme level of anxiety that, without immediate medical and psychiatric assistance, suicide or homicide may ensue. Some of these interpersonal strategies used to reduce moderate anxiety also are used during severe anxiety and panic attacks as part of a team approach to client care.

Choosing from various strategies to reduce client anxiety can be difficult because not all methods are appropriate or work equally well with all clients. Although nurses may accurately identify their client's level of anxiety, they should also identify and reduce their own anxiety to help the client fully. Because anxiety can cloud one's perceptions, it can also interfere with relationships.

## Stereotyping and Bias

**Stereotyping** is the process of attributing characteristics to a group of people as though all persons in the identified group possessed them. People may be stereotyped according to ethnic origin, culture, religion, social class, occupation, age, and so on. Even health issues can be the stimulus for stereotyping individuals. For example, alcoholism, sexually transmitted diseases, and acquired immunodeficiency syndrome are fertile grounds for the development of stereotypes.

Stereotypes are learned during childhood and reinforced by life experiences. They may carry positive or negative connotations, as in these examples: all Jewish people are successful in business; Hispanics are basically dishonest—or honest. Nurses may have personal biases based on conscious or often unconscious past learning. They may act on these unknowingly. Stereotypes negate empathy and erode the nurse–client relationship. Nurses must work to develop insight into their own expectations and prejudgments about people. Exercise 5–7 gives practice in identifying stereotypes.

Stereotypes are never completely accurate. There usually are more variations within a group than between groups. All of us like to think that our way is the correct way and that everyone else thinks about life experiences just as we do. The reality is that there are many roads in life, and one road is not necessarily any better than another.

Emotions play a role in the development of negative stereotypes. Stereotypes based on

### Box 5-3. Levels of Anxiety with Degree of Sensory Perceptions, Cognitive and Coping Abilities, and Manifest Behaviors

| Level of Anxiety | Sensory Perceptions | Cognitive/Coping Ability | Behavior |
|---|---|---|---|
| Mild | Heightened state of alertness; increased acuity of hearing, vision, smell, touch | Enhanced learning, problem solving; increased ability to respond and adapt to changing stimuli<br>Enhanced functioning* | Walking, singing, eating, drinking, mild restlessness, active listening, attending, questioning |
| Moderate | Decreased sensory perceptions; with guidance, able to expand sensory fields | Loss of concentration; decreased cognitive ability; cannot identify factors contributing to the anxiety-producing situation; with directions can cope, reduce anxiety, and solve problems<br>Inhibited functioning | Increased muscle tone, pulse, respirations; changes in voice tone and pitch, rapid speech, incomplete verbal responses; engrossed with detail |
| Severe | Greatly diminished perceptions; decreased sensitivity to pain | Limited thought processes; unable to solve problems even with guidance<br>Cannot cope with stress without help<br>Confused mental state<br>Limited functioning | Purposeless, aimless behaviors<br>Rapid pulse, respirations; high blood pressure; hyperventilation<br>Inappropriate or incongruent verbal responses |
| Panic | No response to sensory perceptions | No cognitive or coping abilities<br>Without intervention death is imminent | Immobilization |

*Functioning refers to the ability to perform activities of daily living for survival purposes.

strong emotions are called prejudices; they are extremely hard to break. The intensity and amount of interaction between people affect the strength of the stereotype. Less emotionally charged stereotypes are more amenable to change. Extreme stereotyping can result in discrimination. **Discrimination** is used to describe situations and actions in which a person is denied a legitimate opportunity offered to others because of bias or prejudice (Kavanaugh, 1991).

If nurses bring their biases with them to the clinical situation, they will distort their perception and prevent client change and growth. To reduce bias in clinical situations, nurses need first to recognize clients as unique individuals, both different from and similar to themselves. Acceptance of the other person needs to be total. Mr. Rogers, the children's television show host, ends his programs by telling his audience, "I like you just the way you are." How wonderful if we, as nurses, could convey this type of acceptance to our clients through our words and actions.

Unconditional acceptance is described by Rogers (1961) as an essential element in the helping relationship. It does not imply agreement or approval because acceptance occurs without judgment. The nurse who uses a nonjudgmental attitude with neutral responses conveys acceptance and develops meaningful client relationships. Exercise 5–8 examines ways of reducing clinical bias.

### Violation of Confidentiality

Confidentiality is breached if conversations are heard by other clients, visitors, or anyone else not involved in the direct care of the client. When conference rooms are unavailable for the sharing

◆ Box 5-4. Nursing Strategies to Reduce Client Anxiety

- Active listening to show acceptance.
- Honesty; answering all questions at the client's level of understanding.
- Clearly explaining procedures, surgery, and policies, and giving appropriate reassurance based on data.
- Acting in a calm, unhurried manner.
- Speaking clearly, firmly (but not loudly).
- Giving information regarding lab tests, medications, treatments, rationale for restrictions on activity.
- Setting reasonable limits and providing structure.
- Encouraging clients to explore reasons for the anxiety.
- Encouraging self-affirmation through positive statements, such as "I will," "I can."
- Using play therapy with dolls, puppets, games.
- Drawing for young clients.
- Using therapeutic touch, giving warm baths, back rub.
- Initiating recreational activities, such as physical exercise, music, card games, board games, crafts, reading.
- Teaching breathing and relaxation exercises.
- Using guided imagery.
- Practicing covert rehearsal.

From Gerrard B, Boniface W, Love B. (1980). Interpersonal Skills for Health Professionals. Reston, VA, Reston Publishing.

of sensitive information among client, nurse, and family, the nurse may pull the curtains around the client's bed, close the door to the client's room, or perhaps ask an ambulatory roommate to leave the room if there is another place on the unit where clients are allowed to congregate.

The advent of computerized client information constitutes a new problem in the confidentiality issue. Once the information is entered into the computer, the nurse may not know under what circumstances it will be accessed. This is discussed in Chapter 23.

There are a few instances in which confidentiality is waived and clients are not allowed to restrict information to persons they approve or to those who have direct contact with their care. These are cases of suspicion of abuse of minors or elders, commission of a crime, or threat of harm to oneself or another person. Courts may also subpoena client records without the client's permission. Apart from these situations, the courts consider all communication between nurse and client as privileged communication.

## Violation of Personal Space

*Personal space* is an invisible boundary around an individual that changes under varying circumstances. The emotional personal space boundary provides a sense of comfort and protection to the person and is defined by past experiences and culture. Davis (1984) described optimal territorial space needed by most individuals living in a Western culture. A person needs 86 to 108 square feet of personal space. Other research has found that 60 square feet is the minimum needed for multiple-occupancy rooms and 80 square feet for

◆ Exercise 5-7. **Identifying Stereotypes**

**Purpose:** To help you identify stereotypes in general and then to identify those you personally hold to be true.

**Procedure:**
1. Make up a list of stereotypes, both positive and negative, with which you are familiar.
2. In small groups, discuss how these stereotypes affect your ability to respond to individual clients.

◆ **Exercise 5–8. Reducing Clinical Bias**

**Purpose:** To identify examples of nursing biases that need to be reduced. Practice in identifying professional stereotypes and in how to reduce them is one component of maintaining high-quality nursing care.

**Procedure:**
Each of the following scenarios indicates a stereotype. Identify the stereotype and how it might affect nursing care. As a nurse, what would you do to reduce the bias in the situation? Are there any individuals or groups of people for whom you would not want to provide care?

**Situation A**
Mrs. Small, an emergency room nurse on night duty, reports to the day shift: "Oh, and a Mr. Johnson came in drunk last night around 3 A.M. He got into a fight and needs a few stitches in his forehead." The head nurse on days learns from Mr. Johnson that he has been sitting and sleeping in the waiting room for the past 4 hours and has not yet seen a physician even though everyone else has been attended to.

**Situation B**
On break, Mrs. Smith complains about the 3-year-old boy to whom she is assigned. "He sure knows when to pour on the tears. There's nothing wrong with him until he sees you, then the tears start, but they wait on him hand and foot."

**Situation C**
Mrs. Daniels, an obstetric nurse who believes in birth control, comments about her client, "Mrs. Gonzales is pregnant *again.* You know, the one with six kids already! It makes me sick to see these people on welfare taking away from our tax dollars. I don't know how she can continue to do this."

**Situation D**
Mrs. Brown, a registered nurse on a medical unit, is upset with her 52-year-old female client. "If she rings that buzzer one more time, I'm going to disconnect it. Can't she understand that I have other clients who need my attention more than she does? She just lies in bed all day long. And she's so fat; she's never going to lose any weight that way."

**Situation E**
Mrs. Waters, a staff nurse in a nursing home, listens to the daughter of a 93-year-old resident. "My mother, who is confused most of the time, receives very little attention from you nurses, while other clients who are lucid and clear-minded have more interaction with you. It's not fair! No wonder my mother is so far out in space. Nobody talks to her. Nobody ever comes in to say hello."

**Situation F**
During a nursing conference, the primary nurse for Sharon Penn, a 16-year-old girl with a 3-year history of diabetes, comments, "I just don't understand why she refuses to take care of herself. She goes off her diet, makes her mother give her insulin shots, never tests her urine or blood glucose, and doesn't care. Doesn't she know she is killing herself? These teenagers today; they never want to take responsibility for themselves."

---

private rooms in hospitals and institutions. Critical care units offer even less square footage.

*Proxemics* is the study of an individual's use of space. Among the many factors that affect the individual's need for personal distance are cultural dictates. In some cultures, people approach each other closely, whereas in others more personal space is required. In most cultures, men need more space than women. People generally need less space in the morning. The elderly need more control over their space, whereas small children generally like to touch and be touched by others. Although the elderly appreciate human touch, they generally do not like it to be applied indiscriminately. Situational anxiety causes a need for more space. Persons with low self-esteem prefer more space as well as some control over who enters their space and in what manner. Usually people will tolerate a person standing close to them at their side more readily than directly in front of them. Direct eye contact causes a need for more space. Placing oneself at the same level, sitting while the client is sitting, for example, or standing at eye level when the client is standing allows the nurse more access to the client's personal space because such a stance is perceived as less threatening. Exercise 5–9 helps identify individual needs for personal space.

Hospitals are not home. Many of the diagnostic and treatment procedures that must be instituted in providing nursing care represent a direct intrusion into the personal space of the client. Frequently, procedures requiring tubes, such as nasal gastric intubation, administration of oxygen, catheterization, and intravenous initiation, restrict the mobility of the client and the client's sense of control over personal territory. When more than one health professional is involved in implementing the procedures, the impact of the intrusion on the client may be even stronger. In many instances, personal space requirements are an integral part of a person's self-image. When a person loses control over personal space, the client may experience a loss of individuality, self-identity, and self-esteem. Consider the issue of respect for personal space in the clinical examples presented in Box 5–5.

When hospitalized clients are able to incorporate parts of their rooms into their personal space, it increases their self-esteem and helps them to maintain a sense of identity. This feeling of security is evidenced when a client asks, "Close my door, please." Freedom from worry about personal space allows the client to trust the nurse and fosters a therapeutic relationship. When invasions of personal space are necessary (e.g., when starting an intravenous catheter on a 2-year-old, performing emergency treatment, or collecting evidence in a rape case), the nurse can minimize their impact by explaining why a procedure is needed or letting a child see the equip-ment. Conversation with clients at such times reinforces their feelings that they are human beings worthy of respect and not just objects being worked on. Advocating for the client's personal space needs is an aspect of the nursing role. This is done by communicating client preferences to the members of the health team and including them in the client's care plan.

Home is not quite home either when the home health nurse, the infusion nurse, or other aides invade the client's personal space in the privacy of the client's own home. Some modification of the nurse's "take charge" behavior is required when giving care in a client's own home.

Nurses should be aware of their own space needs. Nurses who need more space themselves may feel uncomfortable or embarrassed at entering a client's intimate space. Taking into account variations in personal space for both parties in the relationship is important. The same nursing actions that promote privacy and respect for the client's personal space will increase the nurse's sense of space.

## APPLICATIONS
### Steps in the Caring Process

Clayton (1991) described four steps involved in caring. The first is *offering a presence*, during which the nurse introduces his or her purpose in developing a relationship with the client (meeting the client's health needs). The second is *attending*, in which the nurse provides evidence of an intent and ability to care. The third is *affiliating*, in which the client recognizes the value of the offered experience. The fourth is *empowering*, in which the nurse and client gain strength and confidence from the mutual experience while moving toward achievement of client outcomes.

The ability to become a caring person is influenced by previous thoughts, attitudes, and involvement with caring. The person who has received caring is more likely to be able to offer it to others. Caring should not be confused with caretaking. Although caretaking is a part of caring, it may involve giving care to others for the purpose of satisfying the nurse's unmet needs. Caretaking may lack the necessary intentional giving of self. Self-awareness about feelings, attitudes, values, and skills is essential for developing an effective caring relationship.

◆ Exercise 5-9. **Personal Space Differences**

**Purpose:** To identify individual needs for personal space among different client populations.

**Procedure:**
Following is a list of factors affecting personal space. Each has a clinical example. Write another example (clinical or personal) for each factor.

1. *Culture*
Mrs. Hopi, a Native American who is in the intensive care unit for a heart attack, is surrounded by her family and tribe members throughout her stay in the hospital.

Your example: _____

_____

2. *Sex*
Mr. Smith, a retired steel worker, greets his community health nurse with a smile and a gesture to enter his apartment. His ailing wife greets the nurse with outstretched arms.

Your example: _____

_____

3. *Degree of Acquaintance*
The nurse meets Mrs. Parker at the prenatal clinic for the first time. They maintain a distance of 5 feet during the initial interview.

Your example: _____

_____

4. *Time of Day*
Mr. Jones is an 86-year-old man in a nursing home. Every evening before retiring, he prefers to be in bed with the light out before the nurse comes to give him his medications and to say goodnight.

Your example: _____

_____

5. *Age*
Katie Johnson, 17 months old, is always ready to hug her primary nurse when the nurse enters the room.

Your example: _____

_____

6. *Situational Anxiety*
Mrs. Cook just returned from a brain scan, and she is quite anxious about the results. As the nurse attempts to comfort Mrs. Cook by placing her hand on Mrs. Cook's arm, Mrs. Cook snatches her hand away and retorts, ``Just leave me alone.''

Your example: _____

_____

**Discussion:**
Can you think of any other examples of factors relating to personal space?
What is your own preferred space distance? To what do you attribute this preference?
Under what circumstances do your needs for personal space change?

## Reflections on Empowerment

As you think about the concept of empowerment, you might want to reflect on the experiences you have had in which you felt empowered. What was it that made you feel empowered? Another relevant question is, "What groups in society are disempowered, and how might you as a nurse help these individuals feel more empowered?"

## Techniques for Promoting Trust

Sometimes clients "test" a nurse's trustworthiness by sending the nurse on unnecessary errands, asking for unessential care, requesting forbidden items, or talking endlessly on superficial topics. As long as the nurse recognizes testing behaviors, sets clear limits, and defines the nurse's role, it is possible to develop trust.

## Application of Empathy to Levels of Nursing Actions

Nursing actions that facilitate empathy are classified by Gazda (1987) into three major skills: (1) recognition and classification of requests, (2) attending behaviors, and (3) empathetic responses. Two types of requests are for informa-tion and action. These requests do not involve interpersonal concerns and are easier to manage. Another form of request is for understanding involvement, which entails the client's need for empathetic understanding. This type of request requires greater interpersonal skills. It can be misinterpreted as a request for action or informa-tion. The nurse may have to clarify whether the client needs only what he or she specifically asks for or whether further exploration of the mean-ing of the need is necessary.

Attending behaviors facilitate empathy and in-clude an attentive, open posture, responding to verbal and nonverbal cues through appropriate gestures and facial expressions, using eye contact, and allowing client self-expression. They also include offering time and attention, showing interest in the client's issues, offering helpful in-formation, and clarifying problem areas. These responses encourage clients to participate in their own healing.

The third major skill is empathetic response. The nurse helps the client identify emotions that are not readily observable and connect them with the current situation. Using the actions listed in Box 5–2, the nurse uses attending behaviors and nursing actions to express empathy. Verbal

---

**Box 5–5. Clinical Examples of Personal Space Issues for Clients**

1. The nurse places the client on the bedpan without drawing the curtain on a postpartum unit. When the client protests, the nurse states, "Well, we're all girls here."

2. The chief resident comes in with an entourage of interns and medical students. They draw the curtain and the chief resident, standing close to the client, informs the client that his cancer is terminal. The entourage moves on to the next client.

3. Miss Jones has just been brought to the emergency room as a rape victim. Because of the circumstances, she is unable to change her clothes until she has been examined. It is an unusually busy night in the emergency room, and the policy is to practice triage and treat the most serious cases first. Because Miss Jones is not considered an emergency case, it will be some time before she is examined.

4. Dr. Michaels has had an auto accident for which he is receiving emergency treatment by a multidisciplinary team. He is conscious, but no one calls him by name or seems to notice his wife standing outside the door.

5. Barbara Burk has just been admitted to a psychiatric unit. The policy on the unit is to keep all valuables, razors, hand mirrors, and money locked up in the nurse's station. All clients must strip and shower under supervision soon after they arrive on the unit. It was not Barbara's choice to seek in-patient treatment, and she is very scared.

6. Mr. Novack is admitted to the coronary care unit. He is hooked up to a cardioscope so his cardiac condition can be monitored continuously, and nasal oxygen is applied. The defibrillator is located close to his bed. His family is allowed to come in one at a time for 5 minutes once every hour as long as the visits do not interfere with nursing care or necessary treatment procedures.

prompts, such as "Humm," "Uh-huh," "I see," "Tell me more," and "Go on" facilitate expression of feelings. The nurse uses open-ended questions to validate perceptions. Using informing behaviors listed in Box 5–2 enlarges the data base by providing new information. If the client's condition prevents use of familiar communication strategies to demonstrate empathy, the nurse can use alternative strategies. Use of techniques such as validation or touch may demonstrate empathy and help the nurse avoid experiencing frustration (Feil, 1996).

## Reduction of Barriers in Nurse–Client Relationships

Recognition of barriers is the first step in eliminating them, thus enhancing the process of developing a therapeutic professional relationship. Practice with exercises in this chapter should help recognition of possible barriers. Findings from many studies emphasize the crucial importance of honesty and caring, especially listening actively to suggestions and complaints from client and family.

## Respect for Personal Space

Before providing care, the nurse needs to assess the client's personal space needs. A comprehensive assessment includes cultural and developmental factors affecting the client's perceptions of space, how the client reacts to intrusions, how the client defends personal space, and nonverbal behaviors that may indicate loss of territory. All client populations require creative ways of handling personal space. In an attempt to increase the sense of personal space, nurses should decrease close direct eye contact and instead sit beside the client or position the chairs at angles for counseling or health teaching. Clients in intensive care units, where there are many intrusive procedures, benefit from decreased eye contact during certain times, such as when being bathed or during suction, wound care, and changing of dressings. At the same time, it is important for the nurse to talk gently with the client during such procedures and to elicit the client's feedback, if appropriate.

To minimize the loss of a sense of personal space and associated behaviors, the nurse demonstrates a high regard for the client's dignity and privacy. Closed doors for private rest and periods of uninterrupted relaxation are respected. Personal belongings are arranged and treated with care, particularly with very old and very young clients for whom personal items may be highly significant as a link with a more familiar environment. Elderly clients can become profoundly disoriented in unfamiliar environments because their internal sensory skill in processing new information is often reduced. Encouraging persons in long-term facilities to bring pictures, clothing, and favorite mementos is an important nursing intervention with such clients.

### Respect for Personal Space in Hospital Situations

Obviously, there is a discrepancy between the minimum amount of space an individual needs and the amount of space hospitals are able to provide in multiple-occupancy rooms. Therefore, the nurse must recognize individual needs for privacy and implement actions to increase the sense of personal space. Respect for the client's personal space can be accomplished by

- Providing privacy when disturbing matters are to be discussed
- Explaining procedures before implementing them
- Entering another person's personal space tentatively, slowly, and preferably with the person's permission
- Providing an identified space for personal belongings
- Encouraging the inclusion of personal and familiar objects on the client's nightstand
- Decreasing direct eye contact during hands-on care
- Minimizing bodily exposure during care
- Using only the necessary number of people during any procedure
- Using touch appropriately

## SUMMARY

Chapter 5 focuses on six essential concepts needed to establish and maintain a therapeutic relationship in nursing practice: caring, trust, empowerment, empathy, mutuality, and confidentiality. Respect for the client as a unique person is a basic component of each concept. Factors affecting the development of these behaviors, such as level of anxiety, clinical bias, and confidentiality, are described.

Caring is described as a commitment by the nurse that involves profound respect and concern for the unique humanity of every client and a willingness to confirm the client's personhood.

Trust represents an individual's emotional reliance on the consistency and continuity of experience, which are provided by an organized combination of familiar and predictable persons and things. In a trusting relationship with a client, the client perceives the nurse as trustworthy, as a safe person to be with and with whom to share difficult feelings about health-related needs.

Empathy is the ability to perceive accurately another person's feelings and to convey their meaning to the client. Nursing behaviors that facilitate the development of empathy are accepting, listening, clarifying and informing, and analyzing. Each of these behaviors implicitly recognizes the client as a unique individual worthy of being listened to and respected.

Mutuality includes as much shared communication and collaboration in problem solving as the client is capable of providing. To foster mutuality within the relationship, nurses need to remain aware of their own feelings, attitudes, and beliefs.

A related concept is confidentiality: the nurse has an ethical responsibility to respect the client's right to decide who can have access to any information about any aspect of health care or lifestyle. There are limits to confidentiality in the clinical setting. Any information that, if withheld, might endanger the life or physical and emotional safety of the client or others needs to be communicated to the health team immediately. The nurse needs to inform the client what types of information will be shared with other team members.

There are barriers as well as bridges in the establishment of a nurse–client relationship that interfere with the development of a relationship. Anxiety is a vague, persistent, and uncomfortable feeling of impending doom. A mild level of anxiety heightens one's awareness of the surrounding environment, fostering both learning and decision making. Higher levels of anxiety decrease

perceptual ability. The nurse needs to use anxiety- and stress-reduction strategies when clients demonstrate moderate anxiety levels. Severe, sustained levels of anxiety and untreated panic are incompatible with life.

Stereotypes are generalizations representing an unsubstantiated belief that all individuals of a particular social group, race, or religion share the same characteristics. No allowance is made for individual differences within a subgroup. Developing a nonjudgmental, neutral attitude toward a client helps the nurse reduce clinical bias in nursing practice.

Personal space, defined as an invisible boundary around an individual, is another conceptual variable worthy of attention in the nurse–client relationship. The emotional boundary needed for interpersonal comfort changes with different conditions. It is defined by past experiences and culture. Proxemics is the term given to the study of humans' use of space. To minimize a decreased sense of personal space, the nurse needs to demonstrate a high regard for the client's dignity and privacy.

## REFERENCES

Accordino MP. (1997). Relationship enhancement as an intervention to facilitate rehabilitation of persons with severe mental illness. Journal of Applied Rehabilitation Counseling 28(1):47–52.

Anonymous. (1997). Breaking down the barriers to effective communication. Nursing Times 93(2):37–38.

Carkhuff RR. (1969). Helping and Human Relations (Vol. 1). New York, Holt, Rinehart & Winston.

Clarke J. (1992). A view of the phenomenon of caring in nursing practice. Journal of Advanced Nursing 17:1283–1290.

Clayton G. (1991). Connecting: A catalyst for caring. In Chin P (ed.), Anthology of Caring. New York, NLN Press.

Davis J. (1984). Don't fence me in. American Journal of Nursing 84:1141.

Dowrick C. (1997). Rethinking the doctor-patient relationship in general practice. Health & Social Care in the Community 5(1):11–16.

Erikson E. (1963). Childhood and Society (2nd ed.). New York, Norton.

Feil N. (1996). Validation: Techniques for communicating with confused old-old persons and improving their quality of life. Topics in Geriatric Rehabilitation 11(4):34–42.

Gault D. (1983). Development of a theoretically adequate description of caring. Western Journal of Nursing Research 5:313.

Gazda GM. (1987). Foundations of Counseling and Human Services. New York, McGraw-Hill.

Greve P. (1990). Keep quiet or speak up: Issues in patient confidentiality. RN 12:53.

Harrison L. (1990). Maintaining the ethic of caring in nursing. Journal of Advanced Nursing 15:125–127.

Hawks J. (1992). Empowerment in nursing education: Concept analysis and application to philosophy, learning and instruction. Journal of Advanced Nursing 17(5):609–618.

Johns J. (1996). Trust: Key to acculturation in corporatized health care environments. Nursing Administration Quarterly 20(2):13–24.

Kavanaugh K. (1991). Values and beliefs. In Creasia J, Parker B (eds.), Conceptual Foundations of Professional Nursing Practice. St. Louis, Mosby, pp. 187–209.

Kreigh H, Perko J. (1983). Psychiatric and Mental Health Nursing: A Commitment to Care and Concern (2nd ed.). Reston, VA, Reston Publishing Co.

Naish J. (1996). The route to effective nurse-patient communication. Nursing Times 92(17):27–30.

Platt FW. (1995). Conversation Repair: Case Studies in Doctor-Patient Communication. Boston, Little, Brown.

Putnam SM. (1996). Nature of the medical encounter. Research on Aging 18(1):70–83.

Rogers C. (1961). On Becoming a Person. Boston, Houghton Mifflin.

Smith M, Walker M. (1984). Empathy training for nursing students. Journal of the New York State Nursing Association 15:17.

Thompson TL. (1984). The invisible helping hand: The role of communication in the health and social service professions. Communication Quarterly 32(2):148–163.

Wachs JE. (1995). Listening. AAOHN Journal 43(11): 590–592.

## Suggested Readings

Audet MC. (1995). Caring in nursing education: Reducing anxiety in the clinical setting. Nursing Connections 8(3):21–28.

Chinn P (ed.). (1991). Anthology of Caring. New York, NLN Press.

Clay M. (1984). Development of an empathetic interaction skills schedule in a nursing context. Journal of Advanced Nursing 9:343.

Colorado Society of Clinical Specialization in Psychiatric Nursing. (1990). Ethical guidelines for confidentiality. Journal of Psychosocial Nursing and Mental Health 28:43.

Finan SL. (1997). Promoting healthy sexuality. The Nurse Practitioner 22(10–12):79, 62, 54.

Gault D, Leininger M. (1991). Caring: The Compassionate Healer. New York, NLN Press.

Gould D. (1990). Empathy: A review of the literature with suggestions for an alternative research strategy. Journal of Advanced Nursing 15:1167.

Maciorowski L. (1991). The enduring concerns of privacy and confidentiality. Imprint 38:55.

Morse J. (1991). Negotiating commitment and involvement in the nurse-patient relationship. Journal of Advanced Nursing 16:455.

## Electronic Reference

http://www.cios.org/

# 6

# Role Relationship Patterns

### Elizabeth Arnold

**OBJECTIVES**

At the end of the chapter, the student will be able to

1. Define role and role performance
2. Describe the four components of professional role socialization

3. Discuss the professional roles of the nurse
4. Discuss the characteristics of the sick role
5. Apply the nursing process with clients having disturbances in role relationships

---

*Helmer: Remember—before all else you are a wife and mother.*
*Nora: I don't believe that anymore. I believe that before all else I am a human being, just as you are.*

Henrik Ibsen (*A Doll's House*, 1879)

---

This chapter explores the nature and functions of role relationships in the nurse–client relationship. Understanding role relationships as a critical variable in communication is important for both the nurse and the client. How nurses perceive their professional role and their ability to fulfill it has a profound effect on the success of interpersonal communication in the nurse–client relationship. Professional roles help direct therapeutic conversations. They make the relationship safe for the client through role behaviors regarding confidentiality, level of involvement, and competency. On the other hand, role conflicts or role strain that the nurse experiences in the course of completing daily duties can influence the nurse's ability to fully listen and be present for a client, thus compromising the goals of the nurse–client relationship.

Throughout a client's health care experience, the nurse represents a first-line caregiver. Clients' expectations of their nurses are profound and far reaching. Regardless of diagnosis, most clients initially feel dependent on the nurse for guidance and reassurance in a health care system that is complex and often difficult to understand. They invite nurses into the innermost spheres of their lives, almost without question, hoping to find in the nurse a professional who will function as confidante, educational resource, and sounding board.

In times of stress, with its predictable jolt to the self-concept, the nurse listens and supports and does for others what they cannot do for themselves in the health care system. Clients confide their private thoughts and feelings to the professional nurse because they are scared and their sense of self is faltering. They trust that nurses in their professional role will understand and help them regain control over difficult life circumstances. Raudonis and Acton (1997) noted that in health care situations people have special needs and that "the role of the nurse is to discover these needs, from the client's model of the world, and nurture the client towards optimal well-being" (p. 140). It is an awesome responsibility and particularly consequential as nursing moves into the community with less structured opportunities for human health care conversations.

## BASIC CONCEPTS
### Definitions

A *role* is defined as a set of expected behavioral standards established by the society or community to which a person belongs (Creasia, 1991).

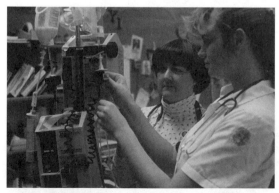

Nurses learn behavioral standards from instructors, nursing staff, and other students. (Courtesy University of Maryland School of Nursing)

Roles represent the social aspects of self-concept. They have performance and relationship expectations. Although roles are socially defined, people implement them differently. For example, two administrators might enact their role on the same unit quite oppositely, one with an autocratic leadership style, the other with a democratic approach. People can have more than one social role simultaneously: a nurse by profession, a spouse, a parent, a daughter, and a lay minister of a church. Roles give meaning and value to life. Exercise 6–1 provides an opportunity for you to explore the role a significant person in your life took in influencing who you are today.

### Related Terms

Related terms also have relevance in the study of role. *Role relationships* include human connections with others. They help define a person's position and status in the community or group. Other people also confirm the value of the role relationship and offer feedback to people as to how successful they are in their role.

---

◆ **Case Example**

Julie is a 15-year-old who has recently been diagnosed with diabetes. You are her primary nurse and will be providing her care and all of her diabetic health teaching. While working with Julie you find that her parents differ in their role relationships with her. Her mother views her illness as possibly caused by her teenage eating habits and conveys an attitude toward Julie that she rarely does anything right and probably will foul up her diabetic care. Her father, on the other hand, is very proud of his daughter's rational acceptance of her illness and believes she probably will be the best patient-learner because she is such a responsible student. How will each of these expectations of role relationship affect Julie's view of herself, her illness, and her ability to care for herself?

---

Role relationships influence communication content and process. Consider your own "role" as a nursing student and how it influences communication content and process. You probably have certain role expectations of your clinical instructor that differ from your expectations of your clients, professional peers, your friends, and significant people in your life. Consciousness of role differences will directly affect the words you select, the spontaneity of your conversation, and

◆ **Exercise 6-1. Role Relations and Self-Concept**

**Purpose:** To demonstrate the influence of the role of significant others on self-concept

**Procedure:**
1. Think of a person who played a role in your development as a person and how you view yourself today. Describe how that person affected you and what he or she did to create that image.
2. Describe how that person's actions and opinions affected your current sense of self. Write your description in a short summary.
3. Each student will share his or her example. The who, how, and what that person did can be written on the chalk-board with short phrases or words.

**Discussion:**
1. What were some of the common factors involving role relationships with significant others that influenced your self-concept?
2. As a nurse, how can you influence a person's self-concept in a positive manner?

the parts of the message you choose to emphasize.

*Role performance* refers to a person's capacity to function in accord with social expectations of a particular role. Perceptions of behavioral standards for role performance differ based on cultural, gender, institutional, and family expectations. People still expect different role behaviors from men and women despite tremendous advances in equal opportunity. The concept of man as breadwinner and woman as caregiver persists today, even though both sexes assume multiple role responsibilities. Different role behaviors are expected of the chief executive officer of a company versus the salaried employee, the oldest child versus the youngest.

*Role transition* describes changes in role expectations that occur as developmental life crises or when unexpected life events such as illness or injury alter role function. For example, a new mother experiences a significant role transition with the birth of her first child, as does a young athlete struck down in a ball game with a spinal cord injury.

*Position* represents a standardized description of a role and associated expectations that makes it understandable to others in the community or group. Social position relates to the status and identity the person holds in the community (Creasia, 1991). The concept of position sometimes plays a role in how helping professionals respond to clients: they sometimes treat clients in high positions differently than those with no

money or low social status. Whereas it is important for the nurse to recognize differences in position as relevant factors in supporting client integrity and self-esteem, nurses need to view all clients as very important persons, treating them all with the same respect and giving them all quality care regardless of position.

*Personal Interpretations of Role*

In 1959, Parsons defined health as "the state of optimum capacity of an individual for the effective performance of his roles and tasks" (p. 10). Today, people's descriptions of themselves and of their feeling of self-worth still reflect role performance more than any other aspect of self-concept. For example, adults evaluate their worth in terms of their work, marriage, parenting, and social roles. For children and adolescents, their social, athletic, and school competencies are primary descriptors of themselves. As older adults reflect back on their lives, personal and professional role performances, both positive and negative, account for most of the memories.

Most people tend to value certain roles over others. These choices have an impact on their commitment and performance. One-sided role development—workaholism, for instance—means that other roles are suppressed or ignored. Neglect of leisure activities leaves an individual with notable life skill deficiencies. When illness, retirement, or adverse circumstances force a person who never developed leisure skills to take a different role in life, the role transition can be difficult. Leisure skills, like work skills, are developed over time.

## Societal Interpretations of Role

Professional roles carry moral, social, and competency expectations. Nurses are expected to act in a professional manner with clients. Because of their position, they cannot engage in questionable financial, sexual, or organizational practices that are incompatible with the moral or professional standards associated with professional nursing. For example, the nurse who is chemically impaired or who administers medication without knowing about the side effects of the drug compromises role behaviors expected of the professional nurse, and occasionally the life of a client. Nurses have a legal and moral obligation to maintain their competency, to work within the scope of their practice as defined in each state's Nurse Practice Act. State nursing boards take legal actions against nurses who fail to meet their professional role responsibilities by suspending or denying their future right to practice.

Social role relationships are recognizable through membership in a community, work responsibilities, cooperative activities, education, and social affiliations. Social customs and performance standards reinforce role relationships. That role relationships and performance matter to people as essential elements of their well-being is evidenced in the emerging symptoms of depression, feelings of emptiness, and even suicidal thoughts when a personal or professional role ceases to exist. Causes of commonly lost role relationships vary among people, but they can include job loss, divorce, retirement, death of a significant person, and chronic or debilitating illness. Nurses always need to be sensitive to the changes in role relationships that even minor illness or injury produces.

One of the major problems people face beyond coping with the physical components of their illness or injury is that of judgments made by society about their fitness to return to former roles, even after successful rehabilitation. People tend to think of the ill person as being less competent or as having maladaptive behavior patterns attributable to the illness but that in reality have little or nothing to do with the illness

(Wynne et al., 1992). Stigmatization of the ill person occurs more frequently when the illness is protracted, recurrent, or seriously role disruptive.

The idea of having a person with an addiction, a brain injury, cancer, acquired immunodeficiency syndrome, stroke, or disfiguring surgery return to a previous work role unfortunately is emotionally difficult for many people in our society. People with such afflictions tend to be treated differently. It is extremely important for the nurse to help clients learn how to respond to subtle discriminatory actions by others and facilitate expression of disappointment and anger when confronted with people's lack of understanding of the client's situation. For example, in his 40s, the head of an academic unit in a university suffered a stroke; residual deficits affected speech. Although he recovered most of his functional ability with intensive rehabilitation, he was relieved of his administrative responsibilities and never was able to regain his former status in the university. University administrators equated his speech difficulties with irreversible cognitive deficits. Despite contradictory evidence in his work performance, they simply could not trust that his rehabilitation was complete. This client recovered from his stroke, but never was able to recover fully from his hurt about the reactivity of others to the changes in his health status.

## Effects of Alteration in Role Performance on Others

Changes in role performance as a result of illness or injury in a client can have a ripple effect on complementary role expectations for other family members. For example, a young mother afflicted with a debilitating disease may no longer be able to fulfill the role of primary caregiver. To compensate for her caregiving deficits, older children in the family may have to assume the role of surrogate parent to younger children. Her husband may have to take on multidimensional responsibilities as breadwinner and primary caregiver for an ailing spouse as well as for the children. Similar role reversals occur for middle-aged adults caught between having to care for their children and for a parent with dementia. These are variables the nurse must consider in planning care.

## APPLICATIONS

### Professional Nurse Role

Current changes in health care create a greater need than ever for professional nurses to have clearly defined roles that provide the basis for nurses to uphold their unique contribution to health care (Chang & Twinn, 1995). *Webster's Dictionary* defines **profession** as a "calling requiring specialized knowledge and often long and intensive academic preparation" and a *professional* as one "characterized by or conforming to the technical or ethical standards of a profession." Box 6–1 presents accepted criteria for a profession. Used by Flexner in 1915 to describe the social work profession, the criteria are equally applicable to nursing. Basically, Flexner believed that a professional is part of an identifiable group and that professional activities are based on a specialized body of knowledge. He held that the activities performed by a professional group are motivated by altruism to provide service to the public. These group-specific activities can be learned through an educational process that is primarily intellectual in nature and practical in its application. The nursing profession upholds its professional standing by ensuring that only qualified individuals are granted the right to practice nursing through licensure.

Today's nurse functions in a high-tech managed health care environment in which the human caring aspects of nursing are easier to over-look. This provides unique challenges to the nurse–client relationship with shorter client contacts, decreased continuity, and lower levels of trust. Yet perhaps the nurse–client relationship and the caring communication that takes place within it will become increasingly important in helping clients feel cared for in a health care environment focused on cost effectiveness and efficient use of time.

Professional role behaviors in the nurse–client relationship include much more than simple caring: they require a sound knowledge base as well as specific technical and interpersonal competencies. On a daily basis, nurses must process multiple, often indistinct behavioral data and have the ability to think through problems critically, without getting lost in detail, in short amounts of time. Through words and behaviors in relationship with other health care providers and clients, nurses provide a distinctive ongoing treatment process in health care situations, with special attention to both the conduct of the therapeutic relationship and skilled nursing actions.

*Professionalism* refers to expectations held by consumers and others within the profession about professional behaviors. These expectations derive from and are responsive to changes in societal norms, advances in education, technology, and the health care system. In 1986, the American Association of Colleges of Nursing published examples of the essential values, attitudes, personal qualities, and professional behaviors associated with the profession of nursing. These examples are presented in Table 6–1.

Professionals are committed to their work and to the development of their profession. Defining the role of the professional nurse in the 21st century is a task that nurses must undertake to strengthen the public's recognition of the nursing profession. Nurses provide essential services to consumers across health care settings. We are the largest work force in the United States and yet we do not always realize our potential or acknowledge our worth. If nursing as a unique profession is to survive in a capitated health care environment marked by blurring of roles and decreased resource allocation, nurses must take a more active part in defining their role, marking their contributions to health care with tangible examples, and developing their profession through membership and support of nursing or-

---

### Box 6–1. Criteria of a Profession

Members share a common identity, values, attitudes, and behaviors.

A distinctive and substantial body of knowledge exists.

Education is extensive, with both theory and practice components.

Unique service contributions are made to society.

There is acceptance of personal responsibility in discharging services to the public.

There is governance and autonomy over policies governing activities of profession members.

There is a code of ethics that members acknowledge and incorporate in their actions.

Table 6-1. **Values, Qualities, and Behaviors Associated with Professionalism in Nursing Practice**

| ESSENTIAL VALUES* | EXAMPLES OF ATTITUDES AND PERSONAL QUALITIES | EXAMPLES OF PROFESSIONAL BEHAVIORS |
|---|---|---|
| 1. Altruism<br>Concern for the welfare of others | Caring<br>Commitment<br>Compassion<br>Generosity<br>Perseverance | Gives full attention to the patient/client when giving care<br>Assists other personnel in providing care when they are unable to do so<br>Expresses concern about social trends and issues that have implications for health care |
| 2. Equality<br>Having the same rights, privileges, or status | Acceptance<br>Assertiveness<br>Fairness<br>Self-esteem<br>Tolerance | Provides nursing care based on the individual's needs irrespective of personal characteristics†<br>Interacts with other providers in a nondiscriminatory manner<br>Expresses ideas about the improvement of access to nursing and health care |
| 3. Aesthetics<br>Qualities of objects, events, and persons that provide satisfaction | Appreciation<br>Creativity<br>Imagination<br>Sensitivity | Adapts the environment so it is pleasing to the patient/client<br>Creates a pleasant work environment for self and others<br>Presents self in a manner that promotes a positive image of nursing |
| 4. Freedom<br>Capacity to exercise choice | Confidence<br>Hope<br>Independence<br>Openness<br>Self-direction<br>Self-discipline | Honors individual's right to refuse treatment<br>Supports the rights of other providers to suggest alternatives to the plan of care<br>Encourages open discussion of controversial issues in the profession |
| 5. Human dignity<br>Inherent worth and uniqueness of an individual | Consideration<br>Empathy<br>Humaneness<br>Kindness<br>Respectfulness<br>Trust | Safeguards the individual's right to privacy<br>Addresses individuals as they prefer to be addressed<br>Maintains confidentiality of patients/clients and staff<br>Treats others with respect regardless of background |
| 6. Justice<br>Upholding moral and legal principles | Courage<br>Integrity<br>Morality<br>Objectivity | Acts as a health care advocate<br>Allocates resources fairly<br>Reports incompetent, unethical, and illegal practice objectively and factually† |
| 7. Truth<br>Faithfulness to fact or reality | Accountability<br>Authenticity<br>Honesty<br>Inquisitiveness<br>Rationality<br>Reflectiveness | Documents nursing care accurately and honestly<br>Obtains sufficient data to make sound judgments before reporting infractions of organizational policies<br>Participates in professional efforts to protect the public from misinformation about nursing |

* The values are listed in alphabetic rather than priority order.
† From American Nurses Association. (1976). Code for Nurses. Kansas City, author.
From American Association of College and University Education for Professional Nursing. (1986). Final Report. Washington, DC, American Association of Colleges of Nursing.

ganizations. Exercise 6–2 is designed to help you focus on your own self-development as a professional nurse.

*Accountability* is one of the distinguishing characteristics of a profession. This term refers to assuming full responsibility for one's actions. Nurses assume accountability for the care they give to clients and for maintaining the necessary knowledge, skills, and competencies to render safe, effective nursing care to clients across health care settings. Exercise 6–3 is designed to help you look at the role responsibilities of practicing nurses.

## Types of Professional Roles

Nurses function in different and sometimes overlapping roles (Box 6–2). New professional roles emerging in the 21st century reflect the expanded advanced practice role of the nurse and include "entrepreneur, recruiter, editor, publisher, ethicist, labor relations expert, nurse anesthetist, lobbyist, culture broker" (Roberson, 1992). Because hospitals no longer are the primary settings for nursing practice, nurse practice roles take place in nontraditional as well as traditional health care settings. Nurses practice in the community, prisons, schools, and homes and with migrant workers in the field. They play an important role in health care of the military, during disasters, and in working with the homeless and medically disadvantaged.

Regardless of the setting and specific application of professional nursing skills, different nursing role functions build on and reflect competence, critical thinking skills, and self-awareness. Interpersonal relationships provide the means by which these components of the professional nursing role interact with each other to provide quality nursing intervention. Box 6–3 identifies professional nursing functions using a nursing process model. Exercise 6–4 helps you to explore the different specialty areas available for professional nurses.

## Role Socialization

*Role socialization* is the "process or set of activities a person uses to gain knowledge, skills, and behaviors in order to participate as a member of a

---

◆ **Exercise 6–2.** **Looking at My Development as a Professional Nurse**

**Purpose:**   To help you focus on your self-development as a professional nurse

**Procedure:**
Write the story of how you chose to become a nurse in a one- to two-page essay (may be done as a homework assignment). There are no right or wrong answers; this is simply your story. You may use the following as guides in developing your story.

1. What are your reasons for choosing nursing as a profession?
2. What factors influenced your decision: people, circumstances, or situations?
3. Describe your vision of yourself as a nurse.
4. What fears do you have about your ability to function as a professional nurse?
5. How do you think being a nurse will affect your personal life?

**Discussion:**
1. In what ways is your story similar to or different from those of your classmates?
2. As you wrote your story, were you surprised by any of the data or feelings?

   Students can discuss some of the realistic difficulties encountered as nursing students both professionally and personally and ways to handle them. Explore through discussion the following:

1. The practices nursing students will need to follow to achieve their vision
2. The types of supports nurses need to foster their ongoing professional development

---

◆ Exercise 6-3. **Professional Nursing Roles**

**Purpose:**   To help the student explore different nursing roles

**Procedure:**
Interview a practicing nurse to obtain the different responsibilities involved in his or her job, the training and credentials required for the position, the client population encountered, the difficult and rewarding aspects of the job, and why the nurse chose a particular area or role in nursing. Write your findings in a short descriptive summary. Questions you might ask follow, but you are also encouraged to create explorative questions.

What made you decide to pursue nursing?
What do you like best about your job?
What would you do in an average workday?
What is the most difficult aspect of your job?
What kinds of preparation or credentials does your position require?
What is of greatest value to you in your role as a professional nurse?
What kinds of clients do you work with?

**Discussion:**
1. Were you surprised by any of your interviewee's answers? If so, in what ways?
2. What similarities and differences do you see in the results of your interview compared with those of your classmates?
3. In what ways can you use what you learned from doing this exercise in your future professional life?

---

particular group" (Doheny et al., 1997). Nursing students learn the professional roles associated with nursing practice through the process of professional socialization. Cohen (1981) identified four goals of professional socialization (see Box 6–4). Entering a nursing education program is somewhat like entering a strange country. The language and customs seem foreign and are not easily understood. Unlike other forms of education, the nursing student must simultaneously adjust to learning new material while starting on-the-job training in which the stakes are high.

Initially, students must learn the pure form of nursing knowledge. They must do this before they can make individualized adaptations in much the same way that one first learns to ride a bicycle and then is able to experiment with more creative applications. The learner is very careful, paying close attention to the facts of nursing and being concerned with knowing the correct policies and procedures governing practice.

The second step in the socialization process

involves internalizing the culture of professional nursing. The nursing faculty and unit preceptors serve as important socializing agents, helping students learn the values, traditions, norms, and competencies of the nursing profession (Neil et al., 1998). As they watch their preceptors, other nurses, and their clinical faculty model desirable nursing behaviors, they begin to emulate similar behaviors. Students add flexibility, autonomy, and creativity to their interpretation of the nursing role as they develop skill and confidence in their professional performance.

Over time, students build a sense of professional identity that enhances their self-esteem as they continue to grow and develop as professionals. Professional identity is evidenced in the nurse's reasoned clinical judgments, in compassionate administering of nursing care, and in competent performance of required psychomotor skills.

The third step in the professional socialization process allows students to tailor nursing interventions to specific client needs. Here nursing

◆ Box 6–2. Professional Nursing Roles

| Role | Role Responsibilities |
|------|----------------------|
| Caregiver | Uses the nursing process to<br>a. Provide complete or partial compensatory care for clients who cannot provide these self-care functions for themselves<br>b. Implement supportive/educative actions to promote optimum health<br>c. Reinforce the natural, developmental, and healing processes within a person to enhance well-being, comfort, function, and personal growth |
| Teacher | Provides health teaching to individual clients and families<br>Develops and implements patient education programs to promote/maintain healthful practices and compliance with treatment recommendations<br>Guides individuals in their human journey toward wholeness and well-being through psychoeducation |
| Client advocate | Protects client's right to self-determination<br>Motivates individuals and families to become informed active participants in their health care<br>Mediates between client and others in the health care environment<br>Acts as client's agent in coordinating effective health care services |
| Manager | Coordinates staff and productivity<br>Delegates differentiated tasks to appropriate personnel<br>Facilitates communication within and among departments<br>Serves on committees to improve and maintain quality of care<br>Makes decisions and directs relevant changes to ensure quality care |
| Evaluator | Sets quality assurance/care standards<br>Reviews records and monitors compliance with standards<br>Makes recommendations for improvement |
| Researcher | Develops and implements research/grant proposals to broaden understanding of important issues in clinical practice and validate nursing theories as a basis for effective nursing practice |
| Consultant | Provides specialized knowledge/advice to others on health care issues<br>Evaluates programs, curricula, and complex clinical data<br>Serves as expert witness in legal cases |
| Case Manager | Administers care for a caseload of clients<br>Coordinates cost-effective care options<br>Monitors client progress toward expected behavioral outcomes<br>Collaborates with other professionals to ensure quality care across health care settings |

students begin to practice the "art" of nursing. To provide high-quality nursing care, nurses need to know themselves well, both personally and professionally, so they can be clear on where and how the professional use of self influences their delivery of client care.

The last step in the student socialization process is an ongoing process in which an individual integrates the nursing role with other life roles. To function as an effective professional, the nurse must be self-directed, be able to live with ambiguity, create and work with alternative choices and diverse systems, and see the creative potential in all human beings, including themselves. Mastering this last step requires discipline and critical self-examination, but it is essential. Having balance in one's life allows nurses to feel creative and energized by their work rather than being overwhelmed by it. Exercise 6–5 offers an opportunity to explore multiple life roles.

## Role Stress

Professionals who give constantly of themselves are at high risk for stress. Nurses work daily with

---

◆ Box 6–3. Nursing Functions Using a Nursing Process Model

1. Interviewing to obtain accurate health assessment data
2. Using all of the senses to assess and validate the health status of clients
3. Developing relevant nursing diagnoses and care plan; referring clients to specialists and religious and community social service agencies if indicated
4. Caring for clients with health care needs to include
   a. Giving partial or wholly compensatory care for clients unable to perform normal self-care functions unassisted
   b. Reinforcing the natural, developmental, and healing processes within a person to facilitate well-being, comfort, function, and personal growth

   c. Teaching and guiding individuals in their human journey toward wholeness and well-being
   d. Motivating individual clients and their families to become informed, active participants in their health care
5. Collaborating with other health care professionals to ensure quality care of clients across clinical settings
6. Evaluating adequacy, appropriateness, effectiveness, and efficiency of treatment programs and quality of nursing care with health care consumers, other health care professionals, and policy makers

---

Adapted from Kelly L. (1992). The Nursing Experience: Trends, Challenges and Transitions. New York, McGraw-Hill, pp. 144–145. Used with permission.

---

complex situations, high in emotional intensity. The professional nursing role demands a commitment that sometimes exceeds the physical, emotional, and psychospiritual resources of an individual nurse. When this occurs, the nurse experiences role stress.

*Role pressures* are external or internal circumstances, capable of change, that interfere with role performance. When role expectations are unclear, the workload is unreasonable, or several role demands occur simultaneously, professional as well as personal relationships suffer. Professional role pressures may be a result of perfectionism or of a confusion and uncertainty about

---

◆ Exercise 6–4. **Exploring a Vision of Professional Nursing**

**Purpose:**   To explore different specialty areas in nursing

**Procedure:**
1. Select a specialty area about which you have an interest in learning more and obtain the American Nurses Association standards of practice for that specialty.
2. Interview a nurse in that specialty area.
3. Write a summary of your impressions of the practice of nursing in that specialty area, describing aspects that are especially important to you.

**Discussion:**
1. Students or student groups can present their summary and discuss aspects of the specialty area that impress them the most.
2. Do you see common threads across clinical specialties?

> ◆ Box 6–4. Steps in the
> Socialization Process
>
> Learn the technology of the profession: the facts, skills, and theory.
> Internalize the professional culture.
> Find a personally and professionally acceptable version of the role.
> Integrate this professional role into all the other life roles.

the nature or validity of one's professional role. The individual nurse may experience simultaneous pressure from clients, the clients' relatives, nursing supervisors, and physicians and can feel overwhelmed when each has different expectations of the nurse's role.

*Role conflict* is defined as an incompatibility between one or more role expectations. This can occur when a nurse feels torn between fulfilling the responsibilities of multiple life roles or when a nurse is asked to perform in ways that compromise client care (e.g., being asked to perform a procedure that is beyond the scope of the nurse's practice or to supervise an unlicensed professional who lacks appropriate training for a treatment). In addition to issues of liability associated with assuming duties without sufficient preparation, the student usually feels very uncomfortable and angry at being put in this position. Other role conflicts can occur with understaffing, having to delegate nursing care to unlicensed personnel, and personal values, even returning to school and having to balance this responsibility with all the others. It is not always easy to make good decisions about putting a 6-year-old child on the school bus and being on time for work.

*Role ambiguity* occurs when roles are not defined clearly. The staff nurse who finds that most of her time is spent on paperwork and little on the direct nursing care specified in her job description may experience frustration, even though the work itself is easy. In all of these situations, the nurse should think about alterna-

---

◆ **Exercise 6–5. Understanding Life Roles**

**Purpose:** To expand your awareness of the responsibilities, stressors, and rewards of different life roles

**Procedure:**
1. Students will think of all the roles they assume in life.
2. Students will write a description of the specific responsibilities, stressors, and rewards related to each role.
3. Students will share some of their roles and their descriptions.

**Discussion:**
As a group, discuss how these different aspects of life roles affect a person's overall functioning.

1. How can this help you to understand your clients better?
2. Discuss what would happen with these roles if you were incapacitated?
3. How might such a situation affect your coping ability?
4. How might it affect others?
5. What roles do you hold in common with other participants in this exercise?
6. What does the learning from this exercise suggest about possible role overload or conflict?
7. Identify one action you could take to reduce the strain of competing life roles.

tive ways to reinforce the reasons he or she entered the profession rather than looking to the institution for answers or abandoning a role relationship that once seemed very important.

*Role stress* is a subjective experience of mental, physical, and social fatigue often accompanied by a loss of meaning related to what previously was important and exciting. Role stress affects the communication process because the nurse expends energy on the conflict rather than on sorting out and resolving underlying issues. Over time, role stress leads to the development of physical, emotional, or spiritual symptoms and burnout. When burnout occurs, nurses lose sight of their personal strengths and in the process lose themselves.

## Self-Awareness in the Professional Role

*Self-awareness* is a necessary precursor to professionalism and absolutely essential in successful implementation of the nurse–client relationship. It is difficult, for example, to remain calm in adverse, unstable clinical situations without a strong sense of self. Yet as an integral part of the most basic struggles, joys, and ambiguities in health care situations, nurses' role in defusing client anxiety is critical. Nurses who are caring yet appear composed give clients confidence in their emotional ability to provide competent care. From professional self-awareness flows the ability to recognize what one needs to do with continuing education, the acceptance of accountability for one's own actions, the capacity to be assertive with professional colleagues, and the capability to serve as a client advocate when the situation warrants it.

In nurse–client relationships, professional self-awareness reflects a balance between personal and professional use of self. The client expects the nurse to act in ways that show the nurse to be a person of feeling without getting caught up in those feelings. At the same time, professional expectations require the nurse to become actively involved with clients without becoming so overidentified with their concerns that it limits emotional objectivity. Exercise 6–6 provides an awareness of personal strengths that can be important buffers in coping with stress.

With coworkers, the key to avoiding the stress related to role performance is to carefully examine your strengths and limitations and what you can realistically accomplish. This self-reflection allows the nurse an opportunity to choose battles that are worth fighting rather than taking a stand on everything or assuming a passive victim role when confronted with conflict. Nurses need to

---

### ◆ Exercise 6-6. **Identifying Personal Strengths**

**Purpose:**  To help you recognize the importance of personal strengths in role development

**Procedure:**
After splitting up into groups of four, write a short summary describing your own strengths and identify how each strength has helped you in life. In the small groups, identify a strength you see in each of the other three students and how you see that it helps that person.

**Discussion:**
In the small groups, share with others the strengths you identified in each individual and how you see that it helps that person.

1. Discuss how your own strengths have helped you in life.
2. Explore the notion of how strengths can be used to improve areas of weakness or deficit.
3. How can this notion be applied in working with clients?
4. Did you learn anything new about yourself or your classmates from this exercise?

define what is important to them and to focus on developing actions that enhance their self-definition. This means saying "what I need and what I want," not "what I don't want or what is wrong with a situation." The solution-oriented nurse is the successful nurse. The next step is prioritizing the activities that truly need intervention and eliminating those that can be delegated or discarded as unimportant in the greater scheme of things. Ask yourself "If this was a year from now, what would happen if I didn't tend to this immediately?" Often this simple inner dialogue can help distinguish significant items from those that are actually nonessential.

Learning to say no to requests that are unrealistic or cannot be handled immediately is an interpersonal communication skill worth developing. Less damage is done when the nurse is able to set realistic expectations and meet them rather than trying to meet everyone's expectations and meeting none.

## Client Role

From the client perspective, loss of or changes in normal roles, role relationships, and role performance are important dimensions of the emotional pain clients experience in health care situations. How well people are able to perform their roles within the family and society influences their reputation within the community and their sense of self-esteem. When illness or injury affects role performance, it also impacts role relationships with others and self-esteem. For example, when lack of physical stamina after a heart attack prevents a woman from fulfilling her customary caregiving roles in the home, she can experience a loss of self-confidence and personal value that can affect her rehabilitation (Arnold, 1997).

The nurse may be the only person who has the expertise and willingness to facilitate discussions of the implications of role changes stemming from altered health status for the client in an objective, compassionate manner. Talking about the meaning of role change is just as important as talking about how to change a dressing or what a physical symptom means. Loss of role, changes in role expectations and performance, and role transitions can occur as a result of age, illness, loss of job or significant person, injury, and mental disorders.

Most people do not assume the sick role voluntarily. Illness or trauma can change an individual's social role from one of independent self-sufficiency to one of vulnerability and varying degrees of dependency on others, a personal role from one of independence to dependence. When clients enter a health care situation, they encounter an interpersonal environment that encourages the development of feelings of anonymity and helplessness. At the hospital door, the client forsakes recognized social roles in the family, work situation, and community, temporarily or permanently. Regardless of how competent the person may be in other life roles, when illness strikes, questions about role performance inevitably arise. Often clients must learn new role behaviors that are unfamiliar and unsettling to previously held self-concepts.

Adjustment to a change in health care status requires a whole new set of coping skills without necessarily having the same social supports. Visitors come, but the routine daily conversations that so many of us take for granted in nourishing the sense of self are limited by visiting hours and lack of availability. Clients clearly need the support of the nurse to incorporate the rapidly changing meaning of the environmental and personal changes encountered in illness into an otherwise basically healthy self-concept.

Differences in perspectives play a major part in determining which illnesses and disorders are recognized as legitimate, the roles clients assume in their health care, and who becomes the culturally assigned expert in promoting, maintaining, and restoring health. For example, some cultures believe that illness is punishment from God or an imbalance of energy that interferes with the body's functioning (Grossman, 1994). These cultural understandings can affect role relationships in health care settings.

Clients are expected to act as participating, cooperative agents in their recovery process. However, an Asian client may appear as a passive recipient of health care, strikingly dependent on family and health caregiver for all guidance and care. Without a clear understanding of this culturally acceptable expression of the sick role, the nurse may respond inappropriately.

### Patient's Bill of Rights

In today's health care environment, clients are considered an integral part of the treatment team. Sometimes, they need to be educated as to their rights and responsibilities as consumers of health care. The American Hospital Association (1992) developed a document that outlines the rights and responsibilities of clients in health care situations (Box 6–5). The nurse, as the client's most direct caregiver, is often in a position to interpret guidelines and to see that the principles of client decision making and treatment choices are integrated in all aspects of the client's care through the nurse–client relationship.

---

### ◆ Box 6-5. A Patient's Bill of Rights

1. The patient has the right to considerate and respectful care.

2. The patient has the right to, and is encouraged to obtain from physicians and other direct caregivers, relevant, current, and understandable information concerning diagnosis, treatment, and prognosis. Except in emergencies when the patient lacks decision-making capacity and the need for treatment is urgent, the patient is entitled to the opportunity to discuss and request information related to the specific procedures and treatments, risks involved, length of recuperation, and medically reasonable alternatives and their accompanying risks and benefits.

3. Patients have the right to know the identity of physicians, nurses, and others involved in their care, as well as the status of the caregivers (e.g., when those involved are students, residents, or other trainees).

4. The patient has the right to make decisions about the plan of care before and during the course of treatment, to refuse a recommended treatment or plan of care to the extent permitted by law and hospital policy, and to be informed of the medical consequences of this action.

5. The patient has the right to have an advance directive (such as living will, health care proxy, or durable power of attorney over health care) concerning treatment or designating a surrogate decision maker with the expectation that the health care institution will honor the intent of that directive to the extent permitted by law and hospital policy. Health care institutions must advise patients of their right to make informed medical choices.

6. The patient has the right to every consideration of privacy. Case discussion, consultation, examination, and treatment should be conducted so as to protect the patient's privacy.

7. The patient has the right to expect that all communications and records pertaining to care will be treated as confidential by the hospital, except in cases such as suspected abuse and public health hazards, when reporting is permitted or required by law.

8. The patient has the right to review records pertaining to medical care and to have the information explained or interpreted as necessary, except when restricted by law.

9. The patient has the right to expect that, within its capacity and policies, a hospital will make reasonable response to the request of a patient for appropriate and medically indicated care and services. The hospital must provide evaluation, service, and referral as indicated by the urgency of the case.

10. The patient has the right to ask and be informed of the existence of business relationships among the hospital, educational institutions, and other health care providers or payers that may influence the patient's treatment and care.

11. The patient has the right to consent or decline to participate in proposed research studies or human experimentation affecting care and treatment or requiring direct patient involvement and to have those studies fully explained before consent.

12. The patient has the right to expect reasonable continuity of care when appropriate and to be informed by physicians and other caregivers of available and realistic patient care options when hospital care is no longer appropriate.

The patient has the right to be informed of hospital policies and practices that relate to patient care, treatment, and responsibilities and to be informed of available resources for resolving conflicts.

## Role Performance as a Nursing Diagnosis

*Role performance* is considered such an important element of a person's self-concept that it warrants its own nursing diagnosis (North American Nursing Diagnosis Association, 1991). How a person functions in social roles, sexual relations with a partner, family roles, and occupational roles are examples of assessment data associated with the nursing diagnosis. The nurse looks for any disruption in the way a person views his or her role performance. In its most extreme forms, this nursing diagnosis can reflect a client's lack of hope about ever having a positive social identity or receiving acceptance from others as a functional member of society. For example, consider the situation of a young athlete who becomes a quadriplegic as the result of an athletic injury or the woman who loses a breast to cancer for whom physical attractiveness is an important part of her self-concept. Here establishing a new sense of role will be particularly important. Assessment data take into consideration the client's developmental stage, available resources and social networks, and the client's understanding of the effect of illness or injury on role performance and relationships.

The nurse analyzes data related to role performance by examining the client's functional performance and satisfaction associated with role responsibilities and relationships. How a client feels about roles and role responsibilities is just as important as the objective data. In an assessment interview, the nurse asks open-ended and focused questions about the client's family relationships, work, and social roles (Box 6–6). Nursing diagnoses related to role performance are provided in Figure 6–1.

### *Supportive Interventions*

Acknowledging the profound sense of loss about changes in role and social identity as normal and helping the client grieve are important dimensions of care that find solace in the nurse–client relationship. Often the nurse's interventions are what makes the difference. Validating the legitimacy of feeling anxious,

---

◆ **Box 6–6. Questions the Nurse Might Ask in Assessing Role Relationships**

**Family**

"Can you tell me something about your family?"

"How would you describe your family unit, for example, age, sex, health status of members?"

"Who assumes responsibility for decision making?"

"What changes do you anticipate as a result of your illness (condition) in the way you function in your family?"

"Who do you see in your family as being most affected by your illness (condition)?"

"Who do you see in your family as being supportive of you?"

**Work**

"Can you tell me something about the work you do?"

"In general, how would you describe your satisfaction with your work?"

"Can you tell me something about how you get along with others on your job?"

"What are some of the concerns you have about your job at this time?"

"Who do you see in your work situation as being supportive of you?"

**Social**

"How do you like other people to treat you?"

"Has your illness affected the way people who are important to you treat you?"

"To whom do you turn for support?"

"If _____ is not available to you, who else might provide social support for you?"

---

hopeless, depressed, or angry helps the client acknowledge the impact of role alteration or loss. Ventilation of normal negative feelings allows a person to put them in perspective. This step in the implementation process often is skipped because at least superficially it seems

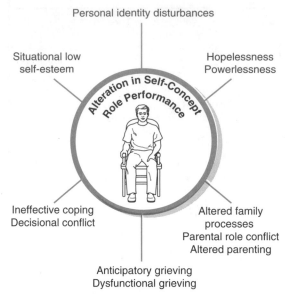

Personal identity disturbances

Situational low
self-esteem

Hopelessness
Powerlessness

Alteration in Self-Concept
Role Performance

Ineffective coping
Decisional conflict

Altered family
processes
Parental role conflict
Altered parenting

Anticipatory grieving
Dysfunctional grieving

Figure 6–1. Nursing diagnosis associated with primary diagnosis: alteration in self-concept.

more logical to resume the task of rebuilding a role identity.

### Developing New Solutions

The next step, helping the client to identify personal strengths and "transferable skills," is an important strategy the nurse can use to help clients change perceptions about role performance. *Transferable skills* are talents and skills a person has that could be used in other productive ways. For example, the ability to analyze, to communicate easily with others, and to solve problems creatively are skills that can be used in a variety of occupations and roles. Yet when people have lost a role, they often feel as though all the talents and skills they ever had associated with that role are lost. Exercise 6–7 gives the nurse practice in identifying transferable skills.

Focusing on alternative options logically follows. Assisting clients to think clearly about the options available instead of the options lost refocuses the client. This intervention does not have to be an either-or issue with the grieving process. The nurse can help the client develop a clearer understanding of realistic goals related

to role performance and the steps needed to achieve them while at the same time supporting natural grieving over a lost role. Support groups assist with practical suggestions and emotional support. Clients identify "just knowing you are not alone" as a major strength of support groups.

Other nursing interventions include providing opportunities for clients to successfully accomplish small tasks and giving meaningful reassurance and positive feedback about efforts and achievements. Relevant client outcomes might include

- Client verbalizes acceptance of changed role.
- Client expresses understanding of role expectations and responsibilities.
- Client develops realistic plans for adapting to changed circumstances.

## SUMMARY

Chapter 6 develops the concept of role relationships as a major influence in nurse–client relationships. A role is defined as a set of behavioral standards and norms established by a society or community group to which a person belongs.

Professionalism is the backbone of the professional nursing role. It consists of values of altruism, aesthetics, autonomy, human dignity, the upholding of moral and legal principles, and faithfulness to truth. Competence, caring, and critical thinking are behavioral outcomes of professionalism.

Professional nursing roles include caregiver, teacher, client advocate, quality of care evaluator, manager, consultant, case manager, and researcher. Professional role behaviors develop through comprehension of the profession's technology, internalization of the professional nursing culture, the finding of an acceptable personal and professional version of the role, and ability to integrate the role into other life roles.

Chapter 6 describes role performance as a significant nursing diagnosis. Assessment and intervention strategies include validating the legitimacy of difficult feelings, identifying personal strengths and transferable skills, focusing on alternative options, and supporting risk-taking behaviors. The nurse can play a significant role in

◆ Exercise 6-7. **Transferable Skills**

**Purpose:** To help you identify the unique skills that can be transferred to other situations

**Procedure:**
1. Think of the one achievement of which you are most proud of.
2. List the strengths or personal actions that went into this accomplishment. For example, ``I was a good swim instructor'' can be recast into personal strengths such as, ``I was a good swim instructor because I was dependable, organized, patient, and persistent.'' ``I am able to relate easily to children,'' and ``I was compassionate with slow learners and was able to inspire others.''
3. Identify the physical, psychological, and psychosocial characteristics that contributed to the accomplishment (e.g., athletic ability, being raised in a large family, ethnic origin).
4. Share your achievement with your classmates.

**Discussion:**
1. How many different aspects of yourself were you able to identify as being a part of your accomplishment?
2. What physical, psychological, and psychosocial characteristics contributed to your achievement?
3. As you listened to the other students' reports, did you think of any other factors present in your situation?
4. Do you see any of these talents or strengths as ``transferable skills'' you might use in other situations?
5. What did you learn about yourself from this exercise?
6. How might you apply what you learned in this exercise to working therapeutically with clients?

helping clients to grieve the loss of old roles and develop satisfying new roles.

## REFERENCES

American Association of Colleges of Nursing. (1986). Values, Qualities, and Behaviors Associated with Professionalism in Nursing Practice. Washington, DC, author.

American Hospital Association. (1992). A Patient's Bill of Rights. Chicago, author.

Arnold E. (1997). The stress connection: Women and coronary heart disease. Critical Care Nursing Clinics of North America 9(4):565–575.

Chang A, Twinn S. (1995). Role determination in nursing— Implications for service provision. Journal of Nursing Management 3(1):25–34.

Cohen H. (1981). The Nurse's Quest for a Professional Identity. Menlo Park CA, Addison-Wesley.

Creasia J. (1991). Professional nursing roles. In Creasia J, Parker B (eds.), Conceptual Foundations of Professional Nursing Practice. St. Louis, MO, Mosby-Year Book.

Doheny M, Cook C, Stopper M. (1997). The Discipline of Nursing: An Introduction (4th ed.). Stamford, CT, Appleton & Lange.

Flexner A. (1915). Is social work a profession? In Proceedings of the National Conference on Social Work, New York, pp 578–581.

Grossman D. (1994). Enhancing your "cultural competence." American Journal of Nursing 94(7):58–62.

Neil K, McCoy A, Parry C, Cohran J, Curtis J, Rausom R. (1998). The clinical experiences of novice students in nursing. Nursing Education. 23(4):16–21.

North American Nursing Diagnosis Association. (1991). Classification of Nursing Diagnoses: Proceedings of the Ninth Conference. Philadelphia, JB Lippincott.

Parsons T. (1959). Definitions of health and illness in the light of American values and social structure. In Jaco E (ed.), Patients, Physicians and Illness. Glencoe, NY, Free Press.

Raudonis BN, Acton G. (1997). Theory based nursing practice. Journal of Advanced Nursing 26(1):138–145.

Roberson M. (1992). Our diversity gives us strength: Comment and opinion. American Nurse 24(5):4.

Wynne L, Shields C, Sirkin M. (1992). Illness, family theory and family therapy: Conceptual issues. Family Process 31:4–17.

# 7

# Critical Thinking: Values and Ethics in Nurse–Client Relationships

## Kathleen Underman Boggs

**OBJECTIVES**

At the end of the chapter, the student will be able to

1. Define terms related to thinking, ethical reasoning, and critical thinking
2. Describe the 10 steps of critical thinking
3. Identify criteria necessary for acquisition of a value

4. Discuss the application of ethics in nurse–client relationships
5. Analyze the critical thinking process used in clinical judgments with clients
6. Apply the critical thinking process to decision making in clinical nursing situations.

*Critical thinking, content knowledge, and practice experience are the three essential components of the development of expertise in clinical judgment.*

Facione & Facione (1996)

◆◆ Chapter 7 examines the role of ethical decision making and critical thinking in clinical judgment. Steps in the critical thinking process used by experienced nurses are discussed. Nurses often face ethical dilemmas in their effort to give quality care to clients. A nurse often has to act in situations with value-laden issues. For example, you may have clients who request abortions or who want "do not resuscitate" ("no" code) orders. Your decisions affect clients' rights and their quality of life. Meeting a client who holds very different values about culture, sexuality, or religion may stir feelings in you that can be destructive in a therapeutic relationship. In the past, the novice nurse learned the process of making clinical judgment by trial and error on the job caring for many clients in a wide variety of challenging situations. Today the focus has shifted to emphasize teaching students how to use a systematic process of critical thinking when making clinical judgments. Use of this process begins with clarification of the issues in a given situation and insight into your own values as well as those of the client.

## BASIC CONCEPTS
### Types of Thinking

There are many ways of thinking about how we think. The mnemonic listed in Figure 7–1 illustrates several of these ways. Students often attempt to use **total recall** just by simply memorizing a bunch of facts (e.g., memorizing the cranial nerves by using a mnemonic such as "On Old

Olympus Towering Tops"). At other times, nursing students rely on developing **habits** by repetitive practice such as practicing cardiopulmonary resuscitation techniques on a Resusci-Annie. More structured methods of thinking such as **inquiry** have been developed in disciplines related to nursing. An example of a method of inquiry with which you are probably familiar is the scientific method. This is a logical but linear method of systematically gaining new information, often by setting up an experiment to test an idea. The nursing process has been developed after this sort of method of systematic steps: assessment before planning, planning before intervention, and so on.

Knowing about your own thinking style is vital not only for your own learning but also because your values impact the quality of relationships you are able to establish with clients. This chapter focuses on only a few of the more important concepts to help you develop your clinical judgment abilities. Specifically, we briefly discuss barriers to thinking and recognizing bias. Completing the exercises will help you develop your skills.

### Barriers

Barriers that decrease a nurse's ability to think critically have been well described in the literature (Alfaro-LeFevre, 1995; Rubenfeld & Scheffer, 1995). **Attitudes** such as "my way is better" tend to interfere with our ability to empower clients to make their own decisions. Our thinking **habits** can also impede communication with clients or families making complex bioethical choices. Examples of such thinking habits are becoming accustomed to having "only one right answer" or selecting only one option. **Behaviors** that act as barriers include automatically responding defensively when challenged, resisting changes, or desiring to conform to expectations. Cognitive barriers such as thinking in stereotypes also interfere with our ability to treat a client as an individual.

We all have a value system developed over our lifetime that has been extensively shaped by our family, our religious beliefs, our years of living, and various other life experiences. Additionally, our education as nurses helps create a set of professional values. Awareness of our own value system is essential in developing an ability to

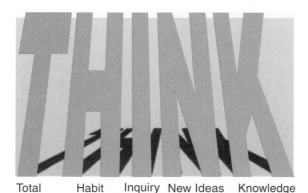

| Total Recall | Habit | Inquiry | New Ideas | Knowledge of Self |

Figure 7–1. Mnemonics can be useful tools.

think critically. Later in this chapter we discuss values and the value clarification process. Of course, clients bring their own set of values, including personal biases, to any interaction. Clients may not even be aware of biases that are actively affecting a current situation. For example, a male client's attitudes toward people of the opposite gender may interfere with his ability to accept advice about his condition or needed changes in lifestyle from female physicians and nurses.

## Ethical Reasoning

Nurses will be faced with a wide variety of ethical dilemmas in their practice. The physician or the agency's ethics committee often is the primary party involved with the client or family in resolving difficult ethical dilemmas. However, on some occasions, the nurse will be called on to make ethical decisions.

According to ethicists, the underlying concepts governing decision making fall into three categories: goal based, duty based, and rights based. The **goal-based model** is utilitarian. It is based on the concept that the "rightness or wrongness" of an action is always a function of its consequences. Rightness is the extent to which performing or omitting an action will contribute to the overall good of the client. Good is defined as maximum welfare or happiness. The rights of clients and duties of a nurse are determined by what will achieve maximum welfare. When a conflict in outcome occurs, the correct action is the one that will result in the greatest good for the majority. An example of a decision made according to the goal-based model is forced mandatory institutionalization of a client with tuberculosis who refuses to take medicine to protect the members of the community.

Decisions made based on the **duty-based model** have a religious-social foundation. Rightness is determined by moral worth regardless of the circumstances or the individual involved. In making decisions or implementing actions, the nurse cannot violate basic duties and rights of individuals. Decisions about what is in the best interests of the client require consensus from all parties involved. Examples are the medical code "do no harm" or the nursing duty to "help save lives."

In considering the **rights-based model**, the be-lief is that each client has basic rights. Our duties as health care providers arise from these basic rights. For example, a client has the right to refuse care. Conflict occurs when the provider's duty is not in the best interest of the client. The client has the right to life and the nurse has the duty to save lives, but what if the quality of life is intolerable and there is no hope for a positive outcome? Such a case might occur when a neonatal nurse cares for an anencephalic infant born without a cerebrum, in whom even the least invasive treatment would be extremely painful and would never provide any quality of life.

On the basis of these concepts, three guiding ethical principles have been developed that can assist us in decision making: autonomy, beneficence, and justice (Fig. 7–2).

**Autonomy**

**Autonomy** is the client's right to self-determination. However, if this right puts others at risk, whose rights take precedence? Exercise 7–1 on autonomy asks you to look at the following cases.

### ◆ Case Example

A pregnant woman's fetus can survive only with surgical intervention. However, the mother refused on religious grounds. The hospital obtained a court order forcing the woman to undergo surgery on her fetus.

### ◆ Case Example

A child was admitted to the Emergency Department after an automobile accident with life-threatening blood loss. The father refused transfusion on religious grounds. The Hospital obtained a court order, and the physician gave the transfusion.

### ◆ Case Example

A 62-year-old woman refused physician-assisted suicide after she was diagnosed with Alzheimer's disease and refused entry into a long-term care facility, deciding instead to rely on her aged, disabled spouse to provide her total care as she deteriorated physically and mentally.

The concept of autonomy has been applied to nursing practice but has some limitations. For

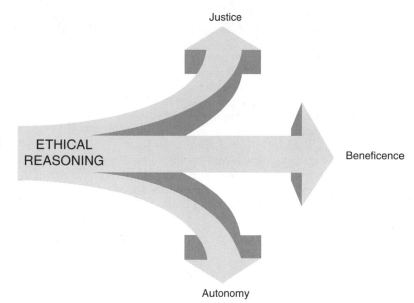

Figure 7–2. Three guiding ethical principles that assist in decision making.

example, a nurse has autonomy in caring for a client but must also follow physician orders and is subject to physician authority. Sometimes ethical issues arise regarding the provision of information to clients. What information should be given to a client and by whom? The following case example helps further illustrate the concept of autonomy.

### ◆ Case Example

Mrs. W, who is 59 years old and has myelogenous leukemia, signed an informed consent for chemotherapy. A nursing instructor was present when Mrs. W was upset and asking about alternative therapies. She asked the nursing instructor to come back and explain these to her daughter-in-law, who reported this to the physician. The physician, in turn, reported the instructor to the State Board of Nursing.

The instructor cited American Nurses Association (ANA) Code for Nurses, which states that the nurse can provide information needed by the client to make an informed decision about his or her medical care. The board judged that the instructor did not have the privilege of functioning autonomously in this situation, that she interfered with the physician–patient relationship, and this constituted unprofessional behavior. Her license was suspended for 6 months. (Benjamin and Curtis, 1981)

### Beneficence

*Beneficence* implies that a decision results in the greatest good or produces the least harm to the

---

### ◆ Exercise 7–1. **Autonomy**

**Purpose:** To stimulate class discussion about the moral principle of autonomy

**Procedure:**
In small groups, read the first three Case Examples (p. 40) and discuss whether the client has the autonomous right to refuse treatment if it affects the life of another person.

**Discussion:**
Prepare your argument for an in-class discussion.

client. This is based of the Hippocratic oath "do no harm." An example is the Christian belief "do not kill," which has been codified into law but has many exceptions. In health care, beneficence is challenged in many situations such as abortion and euthanasia. Currently, some of the most difficult situations involve decisions to withhold treatment. Attempts are made to justify such violations of beneficence in the guise of permitting merciful death. Is there a moral difference between actively causing death and withholding treatment when the outcome for the client is the same death? There are clear legal differences. In most states, a health care worker who intentionally acts to cause a client's death is legally liable. Exercise 7–2 may stimulate thinking about beneficence.

## Justice

*Justice* is actually a legal term. However, in ethics it refers to being fair or impartial. A related concept is equality (e.g., in the just distribution of goods or resources; Thompson & Thompson, 1981). Within the health care arena, this just distribution concept might be applied to scarce treatment resources. As new and more expensive technologies that can prolong life become available, who has a right to them? Who should pay for them? If resources are scarce, how do we decide who gets them? Exercise 7–3 helps students think about this concept of *distributive justice*.

Consider that in Oregon several years ago attempts were made to legislate some restrictions on what Medicaid would pay for. A young boy needed a standard treatment of bone marrow transplant for his childhood leukemia. He died when the state refused to pay for his treatment.

Decisions made based on the principle of justice may also involve the concept of *unnecessary treatment*. Are all operations that are performed truly necessary? Why do some clients receive antibiotics for their viral infections? Are unnecessary diagnostic tests ever ordered just to document that a client does not have Condition X, just in case there is a malpractice lawsuit?

Another justice concept to consider in making decisions is that of *social worth*. Are all people equal? Are some more deserving than others? In the case discussed in Exercise 7–3, if Mr D was 7 years old and the expensive medicine would cure his condition, would these factors affect the decision? Should they? If there is only one liver available for transplant today and there are two equally viable potential recipients, who should get the liver: L, age 54, whose alcoholism destroyed his own liver, or K, age 32, whose liver was destroyed by hepatitis she got while on a life-saving mission abroad?

---

### ◆ Exercise 7–2. **Beneficence**

**Purpose:**   To stimulate discussion about the moral principle of beneficence

**Procedure:**
Read the following case example and prepare for discussion.

◇ Dawn is a staff nurse on 4G. She answers the telephone and receives a verbal order from Dr. Smith, whose voice she does not recognize but who is the physician of record for her client Ms. P. Ms. P was admitted this morning with ventricular arrhythmia. Dr. Smith orders Dawn to administer a potent diuretic, Lasix 80 mg, IV, STAT. This is such a large dose that she has to order it up from pharmacy.

**Discussion:**
Students prepare for in-class discussion.

1. What principles are involved?
2. What would you do if you were this staff nurse?
3. Would it influence your decision if you knew that in a research study 95% of the staff nurses drew up and prepared to administer this dose before the researchers intervened to prevent it?

◆ Exercise 7-3. **Justice**

**Purpose:** To encourage discussion about the concept

**Procedure:**
Read the following case example and answer the discussion questions.

◆ Mr D, age 74, has led an active life and continues to be the sole support for his wife and disabled daughter. He pays for health care with Medicare government insurance. The doctors think his cancer may respond to a very expensive new drug, which is not paid for under his coverage.

**Discussion:**
1. Does everyone have a basic right to health care as well as to life and liberty?
2. Does an insurance company have a right to restrict access to care?

The process of moral reasoning and making ethical decisions has been broken down into steps. Table 7–1 summarizes a model useful for nurses, which was adapted from John Lincourt's model (1998). This model covers the most essential parts of an ethical reasoning process. If the nurse is the moral agent making this decision, he or she must be committed and skillful enough to implement the actions in a morally correct way. Consider the following situation discussed by Veatch and Fry (1987, pp. 84–85).

◆ **Case Example**

Cora is working alone at night with four critical clients on a medical unit. Mrs R, 83, is poststroke and semicomatose. She will inevitably die but now needs suctioning every 10 minutes. Mr J, 47, has been admitted for observation and has been having severe bloody

Table 7–1. **Moral Decision-Making Guide**

| MORAL COMPONENT | DATA | EVALUATION |
| --- | --- | --- |
| Claim | Clear statement of the claim<br>Issues and values are clearly identified | Are values of all parties represented?<br>Who has a stake in the outcome?<br>Are there any ethical conflicts between two or more values? |
| Evidence | List of the grounds, facts, statistics, and so on | Are they true?<br>Relevant? Sufficient? |
| Warrant | Agency policy, professional standards of care, written protocols, legal precedents | Are they general?<br>Are they appropriate? |
| Basis | Identify the moral basis for each individual's claim<br>List backing, such as ethical principle of autonomy, beneficence, or justice | Is the backing recognizable? Impressively strong? |
| Rebuttal | List the benefits and the burdens<br>Weigh them for each alternative in terms of possible consequences for each of the parties involved* | How strong and compelling is the rebuttal argument?<br>Is the decision in accord with or in conflict with the law? |

\* Benefits might include profit for one of the parties. Burden might include causing physical or emotional pain to one of the parties or result in financial burden to them.

stools. Mr H, 52, is a newly diagnosed diabetic with an intravenous drip insulin who requires monitoring of vital signs every 15 minutes. Mr M, 35, is suicidal and has been told today he has inoperable cancer.

1. In deciding how to spend her limited time with these clients, does Cora base her decision entirely on how much good she can do each one?
2. Once she has made a commitment to care for more than one client, in justice what should happen when the needs of these four conflict?

Beneficence can be used to decide on the greatest good for the most clients, but this is a very subjective judgment. Would one of these clients benefit more from the nurse's time than the others?

In using both the ethical decision-making process and the critical thinking process, nurses must be able to tolerate ambiguity and uncertainty (Schank, 1990). One of the most difficult aspects for the novice nurse to accept is that there often is no one "right" answer. Rather, there usually are several options that may be selected, varying in terms of the person or situation. Exercise 7–4 can be used to stimulate discussion of these important issues.

## Values

One important component of both moral reasoning and critical thinking is the ability to identify personal values and to separate these from the professional clinical situation. *Values* are a set of personal beliefs and attitudes about truth, beauty, and the worth of any thought, object, or behavior. They are action oriented and give direction and meaning to one's life (Uustal, 1978). As a noun, a "value" is something that is prized or cherished, like freedom, love, or life. As a verb, "value"

implies action (Uustal, 1980), for example, to fight for something in which you believe. A value represents a way of life and is derived from life experiences. It affects a disposition one has toward a person, object, or idea. Values are almost never isolated but rather are interwoven with each other and with specific life events. They influence each other and are almost always changing. Values continually evolve as an individual matures in the ability to think critically, logically, and morally. Consider the following types of values.

**Conceived Values.** These are conceptions of the ideal (McNally, 1980). These are values that have been taught by one's culture, the ones most talked about in discussions concerning ethics or morality. Examples are such issues as right to life or freedom of speech. These values, although deeply held, have little practical application on a day-to-day basis.

**Operative Values.** These are values an individual uses on a daily basis to make choices about actions. For example, an individual who values honesty would probably give back the extra change that a cashier gave by mistake. When analyzing values, it is important to examine them not only in terms of what a person says but also in terms of what the person does in situations that involve an element of choice (McNally, 1980).

**Value Intensity.** The *intensity* of one's values, or the amount of commitment an individual gives to his or her values, can be measured in several ways. One way intensity can be measured is by the amount of time and energy a person is willing to expend to preserve or act on a value. A nursing student might value high grades and be willing to give up weekend recreational time with friends

---

◆ **Exercise 7–4. Ethical Decision Making**

**Purpose:** To encourage participation in the process of ethical decision making

**Procedure:**
Have students in small groups function as a hospital ethics committee to discuss the cases in this chapter, applying the steps in the moral decision table.

**Discussion:**
Focus discussion on the steps of the process of decision making rather than on finding a "right" answer.

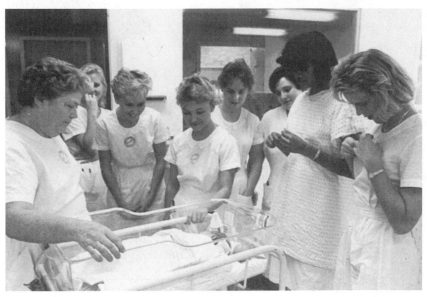

The values people hold often are observed in their interest, involvement, and commitment to people, places, and things. (Courtesy University of North Carolina at Charlotte College of Nursing)

and family to spend more time in the library, whereas another student might choose to party with friends.

Value intensity can also be described by measuring the amount of satisfaction or guilt that is derived from holding onto a particular value. Many times, nursing students hold values that are belittled by their peers. Friends may try to make them feel guilty or foolish for acting on their beliefs. The amount of satisfaction the student gets from staying faithful to his or her value system may determine the level of commitment to it. Strongly held values become a part of a person's self-concept. Exercise 7–5 will assist you in exploring the intensity of your values. When working on this exercise, think about the commitment, the amount of time and energy you are willing to expend, the amount of satisfaction you are willing to give up, and the amount of satisfaction or guilt you obtain from holding onto a value.

**Values Acquisition.** Many of our values are assimilated from family, friends, church, and so on, as we grow. *Values acquisition,* however, is the conscious assumption of a new value. As nursing students advance through their clinical experiences, they take on some of the values of the

nursing profession. Maintaining client confidentiality is an example of a professional value that a nursing student acquires. Exercise 7–6 may help you focus on this concept.

**Cognitive Dissonance.** *Cognitive dissonance* refers to the holding of two or more conflicting values at the same time. If the nurse values a woman's right to choose yet believes that abortion is wrong, then the nurse's values are in conflict. The nurse is experiencing cognitive dissonance. It is important that you become aware of your own values and be sensitive to situations in which they may be in conflict with those of either your client or the health care system.

## Critical Thinking

**Definition.** Critical thinking is purposeful reasoning process that uses specific thinking skills (Bethune & Jackling, 1997). In other words, critical thinking is a method of thinking about thinking. An ability to engage in self-reflective inquiry is required to reflect on one's own thinking process. Besides developing knowledge and skills, the nurse who is a critical thinker needs to develop an attitude of open-mindedness. When you use this method, you improve and clarify your

◆ Exercise 7–5. **Defining Values**

**Purpose:** To help you clarify professional values

**Procedure:**
Complete the following fill-in-the-blank statements:

1. In giving care to an 18-year-old dying client, the most difficult aspect of care for me would be _____.

2. If a client with a diagnosis of cancer asked me to be truthful and tell him his diagnosis, I would _____.

3. If an attractive medical resident asked me out while I was assisting in performing a painful procedure on my client, I would _____.

4. If I was asked to administer a narcotic medication for pain relief to a client who clearly was not having any pain, I would _____.

5. If I was assigned to care for a client with a contagious disease and my employer did not provide protective equipment, I would _____.

6. Before being discharged, a long-term client gives me a very expensive gift. I would _____.

7. If I observed a colleague's unsafe practice, I would _____.

8. If an attractive client asked me out on a date, I would _____.

**Discussion:**
What happens when your personal values are in conflict with your professional values?

---

thinking process so you are more accurately able to solve problems based on available evidence. The process of critical thinking is systematic, organized, and goal directed.

**Characteristics of a Critical Thinker.** Critical thinkers are open-minded, able to consider alternatives, and able to recognize gaps in available information (Alfaro-LeFevre, 1995; Schank, 1990). They clearly recognize that priorities change continually, requiring constant assessment and alternative interventions. An analysis of the decision-making process of expert nurses during interviews conducted by senior nursing students demonstrated that the expert nurses all used the critical thinking steps described in this chapter when they make their clinical judgments (Boggs, 1997). However, they were not always able to articulate specifically the components of their thinking process. The expert nurses organized each input of client information, quickly

distinguishing relevant from irrelevant information. They seemed to categorize each new fact into problem format, obtaining supplementary data and arriving at a decision about diagnosis and intervention. Frequently, they commented about comparing this new information with prior knowledge, sometimes from academic sources but most often from information gained from preceptors. The most striking aspect of the analyses of taped interviews was the constant scanning for new information and constant reassessment of the client situation. This contrasts with the thinking attributed to the novice nurse, who tends to have collections of facts not as efficiently organized into a logical structure. Also, fewer connections are made to past knowledge. Thus, their assessment is generalized and less focused, and they tend to jump too quickly to a diagnosis without recognizing the need to obtain more facts.

◆ Exercise 7–6. **Personal and Professional Value Descriptors**

**Purpose:** To help you identify professional values, to focus on role functions of nursing curricula

**Procedure:**
Mark each of the adjectives in the following word list:

*S,* if you feel it describes yourself

*N,* if you feel it is an ideal characteristic for a professional nurse

*X,* if it is undesirable

Any word may receive more than one mark.

| | |
|---|---|
| _____ Warm | _____ Competent |
| _____ Caring | _____ Solitary |
| _____ Concerned | _____ Efficient |
| _____ Opinionated | _____ Aggressive |
| _____ Reliable | _____ Shy |
| _____ Ambitious | _____ Affectionate |
| _____ Assertive | _____ Thoughtful |
| _____ Intellectual | _____ Skillful |

**Discussion:**
Compare the group of characteristics you feel reflected yourself (*S*) and those you marked only (*N*) nurse.

1. Which attributes labeled *S* might be useful to you in your career?
2. Which attributes marked *N* can be learned?
3. In class, identify the six attributes most frequently identified by class members as reflecting the ideal nurse.
4. With the instructor's assistance, identify curriculum content in your nursing program that may help a student develop these ideal characteristics. Do these curriculum areas include clinical learning experiences?
5. In what other ways could one go about acquiring these values?

# APPLICATIONS
## Solving Ethical Dilemmas in Nursing

Nurses are more frequently dealing with ethical dilemmas in and out of clinical settings. Ethical issues may include anything, ranging from euthanasia to who should receive an organ transplant to caring for a client with acquired immunodeficiency syndrome (AIDS). With the expanded technological advances in health care, there is an ever-increasing need for ethical decisions to accompany these advances. As a result, nurses may feel a growing pressure to be proficient in ethical decision making.

There are three general categories related to ethical issues that nurses are commonly faced with today. These include moral uncertainty, moral or ethical dilemmas, and moral distress. *Moral uncertainty* occurs when the nurse is uncertain as to which moral rules (i.e., values, beliefs, ethical principles) apply to a given situation. For example, should a terminally ill client who is in and out of a coma and chooses not to eat or drink anything be required to have intravenous (IV) therapy for hydration purposes? Does giving IV therapy constitute giving the client extraordinary measures to prolong life? Is it more or less comfortable for the dying patient to maintain a high hydration level? When there is no clear definition of the problem, moral uncertainty develops because the nurse is unable to identify the situation as a moral problem or to define specific moral rules that apply. Strategies that might be useful in dealing with moral uncertainty include using the values clarification process to clarify values, developing a specific philosophy of nursing, and acquiring knowledge about ethical principles.

*Ethical* or *moral dilemmas* arise when two or more moral issues are in conflict. An ethical dilemma is a problem in which there are two or more conflicting but equally right answers. Organ harvesting of a severely brain-damaged infant is an example of an ethical dilemma. Removal of organs from one infant may save the lives of several other infants. However, even though the brain-damaged child is definitely going to die, is it right to remove organs before the child's death? It is important for the nurse to understand that in many ethical dilemmas there is often no single right solution. Some decisions may be "more right" than others, but often what one nurse decides is best differs significantly from what another nurse decides.

The third most common kind of ethical problem seen in nursing today is *moral distress.* Moral distress results when the nurse knows what is "right" but is bound to do otherwise because of legal or institutional constraints. When such a situation arises (e.g., a terminally ill client who does not have a "do not resuscitate" medical order and for whom, therefore, resuscitation attempts must be made), the nurse may experience inner turmoil.

Because values underlie all ethical decision making, nurses must understand their own values thoroughly before making an ethical decision. Instead of responding in an emotional manner on the spur of the moment (as people often do when faced with an ethical dilemma), the nurse who uses the values clarification process as a tool can respond rationally. It is not an easy task to have sufficient knowledge of oneself, of the situation, and of legal and moral constraints to be able to implement ethical decision making quickly. Nurses who have been practicing for years still struggle over ethical dilemmas. Taking time to

examine situations can help the student develop some skill in dealing with ethical dilemmas in nursing.

## Ten Steps in Applying Critical Thinking to the Clinical Decision-Making Process

The following section discusses a procedure for developing critical thinking skills as applied to solving clinical problems. A number of different paradigms illustrate the reasoning process developed by several disciplines. Unfortunately, each discipline has their own vocabulary. Table 7–2 shows that actually we are talking about concepts with which you are already familiar. Table 7–2 contrasts terms used in education, nursing, and philosophy to specify 10 steps to help you develop your critical thinking skills. For example, the nurse performs a client assessment, which in education is referred to as "collecting information" or in philosophy is possibly called "identifying claims."

To help you understand how to apply critical thinking steps, read the following case and then see how each of the steps can be used in making clinical decisions. Components of this case are applied to illustrate the steps and stimulate discussion in the critical thinking process; many more points may be raised.

---

◆ **Case Example**

*Day 1.* Mrs. Vlios, a 72-year-old widowed teacher, has been admitted to your unit. Her daughter Sara lives 2 hours away from her mother, but she arrives soon after admission. According to Sara, her mother lived an active life before admission, taking care of herself in an apartment in a senior citizen's housing development. Sara noticed that, for about 3 weeks now, telephone conversations with her mother did not make sense or she seemed to have a hard time concentrating, although her pronunciation was clear. Admitting diagnosis is dehydration and dementia, rule out Alzheimer's disease, organic brain syndrome, and depression. An IV of 1000 mL dextrose/0.45 normal saline is ordered at 50 drops/hour. Mrs. Vlios's history is unremarkable except for a recent 10-pound weight loss. She has no allergies and is known to take acetaminophen regularly for minor pain.

*Day 2.* When Sara visits her mom's apartment to bring grooming items to the hospital, she finds the refrigerator and food pantry empty. A neighbor tells

Table 7-2. **Reasoning Process**

| GENERIC REASONING PROCESS | DIAGNOSTIC REASONING IN THE NURSING PROCESS | ETHICAL REASONING | CRITICAL THINKING SKILL |
|---|---|---|---|
| Collect and interpret information | Gordon's functional patterns of health assessment | Parties<br>Claim<br>Basis | 1. Clarify concepts<br>2. Identify own values and differentiate<br>3. Integrate data and identify missing data |
| Problem identification | Statement of nursing diagnosis | Statement of ethical dilemma | 4. Collect new data<br>5. Identify problem<br>6. Apply criteria<br>7. Look at alternatives<br>8. Examine skeptically<br>9. Check for change in context<br>10. Make decision |
| Plan for problem solving | Prioritize problems/interventions | Prioritized claims and action plan | |
| Implementation of the plan<br>Evaluation | Nursing action<br>Outcome evaluation | Moral action<br>Moral evaluation | Reflect/evaluate |

her that Mrs. Vlios was seen roaming the halls aimlessly 2 days ago and could not remember whether she had eaten. As Mrs. Vlios's nurse, you notice that she is oriented today (to time and person). A soft diet is ordered, and her urinary output is now normal.

*Day 5.* In morning report, the night nurse states that Mrs. Vlios was hallucinating and restraints were applied. A nasogastric tube was ordered to suction out stomach contents because of repeated vomiting. Dr. X tells Sara and her brother Todos that their mother's prognosis is guarded, she has developed a serious systemic infection, is semicomatose, is not taking nourishment, and needs antibiotics and hyperalimentation. Sara reminds the doctor that her mother signed a living will in which she stated she refuses all treatment except IVs to keep her alive. Todos is upset, yelling at Sara that he wants the doctor to do everything possible to keep their mother alive.

## Step 1. Clarify Concepts

The first step in making a clinical judgment is to identify whether a problem actually exists. Poor decision makers often skip this step. To figure out whether there is a problem, you need to think about what to observe and what basic information to gather. Figuring out exactly what the problem or issue is may not be as easy as it sounds.

**Look for Cues.** Are there hidden meanings to the words being spoken? Are there nonverbal clues?

**Identify Assumptions.** What assumptions are being made?

**Case Discussion.** This case is designed to present both physiological and ethical dilemmas. In clarifying the problem, address both domains.

- Physiological concerns: based on the diagnosis, the initial treatment goal was to restore homeostasis. By Day 5, is it clear whether Mrs. Vlios's condition is reversible?
- Ethical concerns: when is a decision made to initiate treatment or to abide by the advanced directive and respect client's wishes regarding no treatment?
- What are the wishes of the family? What happens when there is no consensus?
- Assumptions: is the diagnosis correct and does the client have dementia, or was her confusion resulting from dehydration and strange hospital environment?

## Step 2. Identify Own Values

Most people do not pay much attention to their values until called on to do so by actions that conflict with their values. For example, what would you do if you witnessed a fellow student cheating on an examination? Some people would immediately call attention to the situation by summoning the exam proctor. Others might tell the proctor after the examination was over. Still others might wait several days and tell the proctor that "some student" was cheating the other day during the examination. Still others might choose not to do anything, believing that cheating will hurt the student in the long run. The ultimate decision on which action is taken often directly relates to the person's value system. Values are a strong determinant in the selections made between competing alternatives. Consider whether the nursing profession holds values regarding this behavior. What if you observed this same student charting that a medicine was given when you know it was not? Exercise 7–7 will give you an opportunity to practice choosing from alternatives and explaining or defending your choices. The exercise demonstrates that many issues require much more thoughtful consideration than most people tend to give them.

### Values Clarification

*Values clarification* is a technique that can help you identify your feelings and sort through, analyze, and prioritize your values. Once there is clarification, an individual is better able to act in a manner consistent with his or her chosen values. Values clarification is a cognitive process that attempts to close the gap between what an individual says and what an individual actually does. The process of values clarification also will be useful in helping you understand and cope better with certain opposing values that your client might possess.

The goal of values clarification is to facilitate self-understanding. The process is dynamic and ongoing, with emphasis on questioning, arguing, and challenging old ideas. The end result of a values clarification process should be increased awareness, empathy, and insight. According to Steele and Harmon (1983), values of paramount importance to an individual should be acted on consistently and predictably. If a value is not acted on with reasonable ease, it may be a value indicator rather than an established value. Acting on a value offers the strongest evidence of the values clarification process.

◆ Exercise 7-7. **Range of Opinion**

**Purpose:** When dealing with controversial topics, people tend to see things as either/or with nothing in between. The following exercise will help you see that there is often a wide range of possible positions on any given issue. This exercise will emphasize the importance of exploring all options before choosing freely.

**Procedure:**
Divide the class into groups of five. Each group is assigned a controversial issue. Sample issues include

Legalization of abortion
Premarital sex
Legalization of marijuana
Legalization of euthanasia

The group then divides the issue into three positions: an ultraconservative stand, a moderate stand, and a liberal stand. Each student selects a stand. A mock debate with a narrator is then initiated.

**Discussion:**
Discuss the result of the debate with spectators from the rest of the class and participants.

An important first step in values clarification is to understand yourself as a person and to know your own personally held values. For example, think about how you would respond if someone of significance to you asked you to steal a watch from an open case in a jewelry store. Would you do it? How about taking a monogrammed towel from a hotel at which you were staying, or claiming charitable donations on your tax return that, in fact, you never made? Exercise 7–8 will help you begin to examine yourself as an individual and as a future professional nurse.

In everyday life, people are faced with situations that require very little thought and only rote actions as well as situations that require a great deal of thought and decision making and carefully planned action. Whether minor or critical, all thoughts, opinions, and ultimate actions are based on consciously or unconsciously held beliefs, attitudes, and values.

During a conflict that involves a values dilemma, people often form opinions prematurely based on their emotional reactions. Their initial reactions usually do not reflect their true beliefs. The ability to make decisions based on values becomes blurred. Often the values underlying decisions are unconscious or difficult to identify, and, as a result, behaviors and attitudes are inconsistent. As a person becomes more involved in a situation, these feelings often change. An individual with a clear sense of values is better able to choose and to initiate responses consistent with his or her value system. Values clarification is a process that is useful in completing this task.

As a nursing student, it is important for you to examine each of the seven steps of the values clarification process to obtain a more comprehensive understanding of how a value is acquired. Once you see how the process works, you can apply it to your own life to identify and understand your own values. This will allow you to apply the values clarification process when trying to understand the value system of your clients. The seven criteria for acquisition of a value are as follows:

• The value must be
  1. Freely chosen
  2. From alternatives
  3. Chosen after careful consideration of each alternative
• There must be
  4. Pride and happiness with the choice
  5. Willingness to make the values known to others

◆ Exercise 7–8. **Values Clarification Grid**

**Purpose:** When learning a new process, it is always helpful to practice before applying it to actual clinical practice. This exercise will help you to integrate all seven steps of the values clarification process into practical nursing applications.

**Procedure:**
On the following grid, write a statement that reflects a belief you have related to a specific nursing application. This statement should reflect an area of conflict or confusion in nursing that you wish to examine. An example might be, ``A nurse should never lie to a patient about anything.'' To the right of this statement, you should then go through the values clarification process step by step, checking as you go along each of the seven steps that reflect your beliefs. In other words, you might choose freely never to be dishonest to a client, but in certain real situations you might not be able to act on this belief and, therefore, cannot check off that point.

The following are examples of conflicts or confusions in nursing on which you may wish to focus.

| | |
|---|---|
| Peer review | Informed consent |
| Accountability | Refusal of care |
| Continuing education | Confidentiality |
| Licensing | Euthanasia |
| Professional organizations | Abortion |
| Patients' rights | Nurses' rights |

Statement: _____

_____

_____.

1. Freely chooses
2. From alternatives
3. Examine consequences
4. Proud
5. Able to disclose
6. Action
7. Acts repeatedly

**Discussion:**
Is your belief a value according to the theory? What steps must you consider more carefully and completely?

---

• It must be acted upon
  6. In response to the choice
  7. In a pattern of behavior consistent with the choice (value is incorporated into the individual's lifestyle)

Exercises 7–9, 7–10, and 7–11 will give you practice in the process of values acquisition.

**Understanding Your Own Values**

Professional values ultimately are an expansion and reflection of an individual's personal values. Many of the things you as a student value may have had an impact on why you decided to become a nurse in the first place. At this time, take a few minutes to contemplate your reasons for

◆ Exercise 7-9. **Professional Values**

**Purpose:** You will learn another way to clarify values.

**Procedure:**
Please indicate your belief in the values presented next by placing the number of the continuum that most closely represents your feelings next to the statement (to be completed before class).

| Strongly disagree | Disagree | Ambivalent | Agree | Strongly agree |
|---|---|---|---|---|
| 1 | 2 | 3 | 4 | 5 |

_____ 1. I should be able to help every client.

_____ 2. The client's needs are more important than mine.

_____ 3. If I make a medication error, I probably should look into a profession other than nursing.

_____ 4. I consider it my responsibility to challenge my client's value system if it does not seem to be in the client's best interest.

_____ 5. I would find it difficult to work with an AIDS client.

_____ 6. If a client's condition is terminal, I believe the choice to use extraordinary measures is not mine to make; it belongs to the family.

_____ 7. I can be most effective with clients who have a similar value system.

_____ 8. It is not possible to express caring without having time to sit down and talk with a client.

_____ 9. I would find it difficult to work with a client who has strict fundamentalist religious beliefs.

_____ 10. I would find it difficult to be empathetic with a child abuser.

_____ 11. Relating to an atheist would be very difficult for me.

_____ 12. Terminally ill and severely handicapped individuals should be allowed to end their own lives.

_____ 13. Severely ill clients should be encouraged to make a living will, which allows the medical and nursing staff to withhold life-saving treatment.

_____ 14. Nurses have an ethical responsibility to tell clients of the limits of confidentiality.

_____ 15. A mentally retarded girl should be given the option to decide whether or not she should be sterilized.

_____ 16. It is acceptable to talk about client problems in a general way as long as the client's name or any identifying information is not included in the discussion.

_____ 17. Consulting with family or outside agencies without the client's permission is appropriate in certain situations.

**Discussion:**
Share responses to exercise in a brief class discussion.

---

◆ **Exercise 7–10. Nurses' Values**

**Purpose:**  To begin to focus thinking on professional role values

**Procedure:**
Read the following statements. Think about each situation carefully. How would you want to respond if you were the primary nurse in the situation?

1. A 40-year-old man tells you of his ongoing extramarital affair. He is very physically and verbally affectionate with his wife when she comes to visit.
2. A gay client tests positive for human immunodeficiency virus, but he does not want to tell his partner because it might jeopardize the relationship.
3. An 8-year-old girl is admitted to the emergency room, immaculately dressed, with many bruises and welts on her arms and legs. Her mother states she was hurt on the playground.
4. You note that your student partner has alcohol on her breath when she picks up her assignments. This has happened on more than one occasion.
5. A client has been told his bone scan shows metastatic lesions. He tells you not to tell his wife because she will just worry.
6. An adolescent client tells you that her friend brought some marijuana to the hospital to help her calm her nerves.
7. A client admitted to the psychiatric unit refuses to take his medication and wants to sign out of the hospital against medical advice.

**Discussion:**
1. How did your answers compare with those of your peers?
2. If you implemented them, what would be the consequences for you and for the client?
3. In what ways did your values enter into your choices?
4. What did you learn about yourself and your preferred value choices from doing this exercise that might help you in your nursing practice?

---

wanting to become a nurse. Next, think about aspects of your life that you value a great deal. Examples might include health, friends, and socialization. Examine the two lists and see whether they have any commonalities.

Values clarification is a valuable tool for the nurse because it serves as a base for helping clients search successfully for and find the values they identify as important. The way your clients respond to the health care system, to their individual diagnoses, or to your therapeutic interventions is influenced by their personal value systems. Unless you are able to identify your client's values and can appreciate the validity of those values, you run the risk of imposing your own values on others rather than modifying, teaching, and working with your client's value system. It is not necessary for your values

and your client's values to coincide; this is an unrealistic expectation. However, whenever possible and appropriate, the client's values should be taken into consideration during every aspect of the nursing process.

The nursing process offers many opportunities to incorporate values clarification into care of the client. During the assessment phase, the nurse can obtain an assessment of the client's values with regard to the health system. For example, the nurse might interview a client for the first time and learn that he has obstructive pulmonary disease and is having difficulty breathing. The client insists on smoking. As the nurse caring for the client, is it appropriate to intervene? If so, to what extent? This is an example of having knowledge that smoking is detrimental to a person's health and, as a nurse,

◆ Exercise 7–11. **Difficult Case Examples**

**Purpose:** To help you develop a practical approach to ethical decision making by understanding your value responses

**Procedure**
The following case studies can be used as discussion catalysts or for role-play situations in order to examine values and to explore possible responses in terms of values only.

1. *Prolongation of life.* Kim is an infant who was born at the gestational age of 25 weeks. She is surviving in the neonatal intensive care unit with major life support systems. Kim's parents are showing increasingly less interest in Kim's progress. One day when you are caring for Kim, the father yells, ``Stop poking and prodding at her! What are you trying to prove by keeping her alive? Turn off those machines.''

2. *Abortion.* Mrs. Smith requested to have amniocentesis to determine whether her fetus would have Tay-Sachs disease. She finds out that the fetus is a girl. Even though it does not have Tay-Sachs disease, she decides to terminate the pregnancy because of her desire to have a boy. Her husband agrees with her decision.

3. *Euthanasia.* An elderly male client is suffering from terminal cancer. He is constantly in a great deal of pain. He says that he has had a good life and does not want his family to suffer. He tells you that he is going to commit suicide. Next consider how you would react if the elderly client was your grandfather.

4. *Refusal to accept blood.* You are an obstetrical nurse. Your client, Mrs. Jones, refuses to receive blood because it is against her religious beliefs. After a difficult cesarean section, she delivers a healthy baby girl. She has lost a great deal of blood and is continuing to hemorrhage. Without a blood transfusion, it is very likely that she will die. She refuses to receive blood.

5. *Sexual advances.* As the nurse, it is your responsibility to care for a very attractive, seductive male (female) client who has had foot surgery. He (she) continues to make subtle sexual advances to you.

6. *Refusal to care for a client.* You are the head nurse on a medical-surgical unit. You have assigned Nurse Brown to care for Mr. Adams, a 28-year-old homosexual who was recently diagnosed as having AIDS. Nurse Brown refuses to care for this patient because she does not want to get AIDS and says she does not like ``that kind of person.''

**Discussion:**
After reading each study, respond to the following questions:

1. What would your reaction be to this situation?
2. What would you do if you were the nurse?
3. What conflicts in values does the situation pose for you?
4. How can you as the nurse respect the integrity of your client's decision when it conflicts with your own value system?
5. In Scenario 3, consider how you would react if the client was your grandfather.
6. In Scenario 6, as head nurse, how would you deal with this situation? How might Nurse Brown use values clarification to deal with this ethical dilemma?

finding the value of health in conflict with the client's value of smoking. In this case, it is important to examine your own values and to try to identify and understand your client's values. Although your values differ, whenever possible you must attempt to care for this client within his realm of value. A client has the right to make decisions that are not always congruent with those of the health care system. These decisions may cause the nurse to feel uneasy unless there is a commitment to respect the rights of the client (Steele & Harmon, 1983).

When identifying specific nursing diagnoses, it is important for the nurse to continue to reflect on his or her own values and on those of the client so that the diagnoses reflect a specific problem and are not biased by the nurse's values. When caring for a client from another culture, diagnoses may involve potential or actual problems. Examples of conflicts indicating differences in values orientation might be spiritual distress related to a conflict between spiritual beliefs and prescribed health treatments or ineffective family coping related to restricted visiting hours for a family in which full family participation is a cultural value.

In the planning phase, it is important to identify and understand the client's value system as the foundation for developing the most appropriate interventions. Care plans that support rather than discount the client's health care beliefs are more likely to be received favorably.

The intervention used identifies values as guidelines for care. The nurse can also use the values clarification process as a therapeutic technique. The process may be used to help clients sort out feelings, identify conflict areas, examine and choose from alternatives, set goals, and act in a manner consistent with their value systems and according to their physical and emotional health. During the evaluation phase, the results of therapeutic intervention can be examined in terms of how well the nursing and client goals were met while keeping within the guidelines of the client's value system.

**Case Discussion.** Identify the values of each person involved.

- Family: Mrs. Vlios signed advanced directive; Sara wants it adhered to; Todos wants it ignored. Why? (Are there religious beliefs? Is there unclear communication? Is there guilt about previous troubles in the relationship?)
- Personal values: what are yours?
- Professional values: The ANA says nurses are advocates for their clients; beneficence means nonmalfeasance "do no harm" but autonomy means the client has the right to refuse treatment. What is the agency's policy? What are the legal considerations?

## Step 3. Integrate Data and Identify Missing Data

Think about knowledge gained in prior courses and during clinical experiences. Try to make connections between different subject areas and clinical nursing practice.

- Identify what data are needed. Situations are often very complicated. It is important to figure out what information is significant to this situation. Synthesize prior information you already have with similarities in the current situation. Conflicting data may indicate a need to search for more information.
- Compare existing information with past knowledge. Has this client complained of difficulty breathing before? Does he have a history of asthma?
- Look for gaps in the information. Actively work to recognize whether there is missing information. What were the vital signs earlier? For a nurse, this is an important part of critical thinking.
- Collect information systematically. Use an organized framework to obtain information. Nurses frequently obtain a client's history by asking questions about each body system. They could just as systematically ask about basic needs.
- Organize your information. **Clustering information** into relevant categories is helpful. For example, gathering all the facts about a client's breathing may help focus your attention on whether or not the client is having a respiratory problem. In your assessment you note rate and character of respirations, color of nails and lips, use of accessory muscles, and grunting noises. At the same time, you exclude information about bowel sounds or deep tendon reflexes as not being immediately relevant to his respiratory status. Categorizing information also helps you notice whether there are missing data. A second strategy that will help you organize information is to **look for patterns.** It has been indicated that experienced nurses intuitively note recurrent meaningful aspects of a clinical situation.

**Case Discussion.** Rely on prior didactic knowledge, clinical experience. Cluster the data. What was Mrs. Vlios's status immediately before hospitalization? What was her status at the time of hospitalization? What information is missing? What additional data do you need?

- Physiology: consider pathophysiological knowledge about the effects of hypovolemia and electrolyte imbalances on the brain, kidneys, vascular system, and so on. What is her temperature? What are her laboratory values? What is her 24-hour intake and output?
- Psychological/cognitive: how does hospitalization affect elders? How do restraints affect them?
- Social/economic: was weight loss a result of dehydration? Why was she without food? Could it be due to economic factors or mental problems?
- Legal: what constitutes a binding advanced directive in the state in which Mrs. Vlios lives? Is a living will valid in her state, or does the law require a health power of attorney? Are these documents on file at the hospital?

## Step 4. Obtain New Data

Once you decide that you need more information, establish an attitude of inquiry and obtain more information. Ask questions, search for evidence, check reference books, journals, the ethics sources on the Internet listed at the end of this chapter, or written professional or agency protocols.

Evaluate conflicting information. There may be time constraints. If a client has suspected "respiratory problems," you may need to set priorities. Obtain data that are most useful or are easily available. It would be useful to know oxygenation levels, but you may not have time to order laboratory tests. However, perhaps there is a device on the unit or in the room that can measure oxygen saturation.

Sometimes you may need to change your approach to improve your chances of obtaining information. For example, when the charge nurse caring for Mrs. Vlios used an authoritarian tone to try to get the sister and brother to provide more information about possible drug overdose, they did not respond. However, when the charge nurse changed his approach, exhibiting empathy, the daughter volunteered that on several past occasions her mother had forgotten what pills she had taken.

**Case Discussion.** List sources from which you can obtain missing information. Physiological data such as temperature or lab test results can be obtained quickly; some of the ethical information may take longer to consider.

## Step 5. Identify the Significant Problem

- Analyze existing information. Examine all the information you have. Identify all the possible positions.
- Make inferences. What might be going on? What are the possible diagnoses? Develop a working diagnosis.
- Prioritize. Which client problem is most urgently in need of your intervention? What are the appropriate interventions?

**Case Discussion.** A significant physiological concern is sepsis regardless of whether it is an iatrogenic (hospital acquired) infection or one resulting from immobility and debilitation. A significant ethical concern is the conflict among family members and client (as expressed through her living will). At what point do spiritual concerns take priority over a worsening physical concern?

## Step 6. Examine Skeptically

Thinking about a situation may involve weighing up positive and negative factors, and differentiating facts that are credible from opinions that are biased or not grounded in true facts.

- Keep an open mind.
- Challenge your own assumptions.
- Consider whether any of your assumptions are unwarranted. Does the evidence available really support your assumption?
- Discriminate between facts and inferences. Your inferences need to be logical and plausible, based on the available facts.
- Are there any problems that you have not considered?

In trying to evaluate a situation, consciously raising questions becomes an important part of thinking critically. At times, there will be alternative explanations or different lines of reasoning that are equally valid. The challenge is to examine your own and others' perspectives for important ideas, complicating factors, other plausible interpretations, and new insights, to see "the big picture" (Jones & Brown, 1993). Some nurses believe that examining information skeptically is part of each step in the critical thinking process rather than a step by itself.

**Case Discussion.** Challenge assumptions about the cause of Mrs. Vlios's condition. For example, did you eliminate the possibility that she had a head injury caused by a fall? Could she have liver failure as a result of acetaminophen overdosing? Have all the possibilities been explored? Challenge your assumptions about outcome: are they influenced by expected probable versus possible outcomes for this client? If she indeed has irreversible dementia, what will the quality of her life be if she recovers from her physical problems?

## Step 7. Apply Criteria

In evaluating a situation, think about appropriate responses.

- Laws: there may be a law that can be applied that can guide your actions and decisions. For example, by law certain diseases must be reported to the state. If you suspect physical abuse, there is a state statute that requires professionals to report abuse to the Department of Social Services.
- Legal precedents: there may have been similar cases or situations that were dealt with in a court of law. Legal decisions do guide health care practices.
- Protocols: There may be standard protocols for managing certain situations. Your agency may have standing orders for caring for a client in respiratory distress, such as administering oxygen per face mask at 5 L/min.

**Case Discussion.** Many criteria could be used to examine this case, including the Nurse Practice Act in the area of jurisdiction, the professional organization code of ethics or general ethical principles of beneficence and autonomy, the hospital's written protocols and policies, state laws regarding living wills, and prior court decisions about living wills. Remember that advanced directives are designed to take effect only when clients become unable to make their own wishes known.

## Step 8. Generate Options and Look at Alternatives

- Evaluate the major alternative points of view.
- Involve experienced peers as soon as you can to assist you in making your decision.
- Use clues from others to help you "put the picture together."

Can you identify all the arguments—pro and con—to explain this situation? Almost all situations will have strong counter-arguments or competing hypotheses.

**Case Discussion.** The important concept is that neither the physician nor the nurse should handle this alone; rather, others should be involved, for example, the hospital bioethics committee, the ombudsman client representative, the family's spiritual counselor, other medical experts such as a gerontologist, psychologist, and the nursing clinical specialist.

## Step 9. Consider Whether Factors Change If the Context Changes

Consider whether your decision would be different if there was a change in circumstances. For example, a change in the age of the client, the site of the situation, or the client's culture may affect your decision.

**Case Discussion.** If you knew the outcome from the beginning would your decisions be the same? What if you knew Mrs. Vlios had a terminal cancer? What if Mrs. Vlios had remained in her senior housing project and you were the home health nurse? What if Mrs. Vlios had remained alert during her hospitalization and refused IVs, hyperalimentation, nasogastric tubes, and so on? What if the family and Mrs. Vlios were in agreement about no treatment?

## Step 10. Make Final Decision

After analyzing available information in this systematic way, a judgment or decision needs to be made. An important part of your decision is your ability to communicate it coherently to others and to reflect on the outcome of your decision for your client.

- Justify your conclusion.
- Evaluate outcomes.

Test out your decision or conclusion by implementing appropriate actions. The critical thinker needs to be able to accept that there may be multiple solutions that can be equally acceptable. In other situations, a decision may need to be made even when there is incomplete knowledge. Be able to cite your rationale or present your arguments to others for your decision choice and interventions.

After you implement your interventions, examine the client *outcomes.* Was your assessment correct? Did you obtain enough information? Did the benefits to the client and family outweigh the harm that may have occurred? In retrospect, do you know you made the correct decision? Did you anticipate possibilities and complications correctly? This kind of self-examination can foster self-correction. It is this process of reflecting on one's own thinking that is the hallmark of a critical thinker.

**Case Discussion.** The most important concept is to forget the idea that there is one right answer to the dilemmas raised by discussion of this case. Accept that there may be several equally correct solutions depending on each individual person's point of view.

**Summarizing the Critical Thinking Learning Process.** The most effective method of learning these steps in critical thinking results from repeatedly applying them to clinical situations. This can occur in your own clinical care. Del Bueno (1994) stated that a new graduate nurse must at a minimum be able to identify essential clinical data, know when to initiate interventions, know why a particular intervention is relevant, and differentiate between problems that need immediate intervention versus problems that can wait for action. Repeated practice in applying critical thinking can help a new graduate fit into the expectations of employers!

Students have demonstrated that critical thinking can be learned in the classroom as well as through clinical experience (Boggs, 1997). Effective learning can occur when opportunities are structured that allow for repeated in-class applications to client case situations, such as using real-life case interviews with experienced nurses, which allows you to analyze their decision-making process. The videotaping described in Exercise 7–12 explains how this is done.

If videotaping or audiotaping is not possible, you may help increase your critical thinking and clinical problem solving skills by discussing the following additional case examples. Remember that most clinical situations requiring decision making will not involve the types of ethical dilemmas discussed earlier in this chapter.

◆ **Case Example
(Farrell & Bramadat, 1993)**

Mr X, age 42 years, has been admitted for surgical repair of his right knee, scheduled for tomorrow. When you enter his room, he complains of being short of breath. Respirations are 22/min and regular. Skin color is pink. Vital signs are normal. Mr X has an anxious facial expression. You stay with him a few minutes to make sure he is oxygenating adequately. After 1 minute, his color is tinged with gray, and respirations are now 30/min and labored.

1. What were you thinking at first?
2. What are you thinking now?
3. How do you sort out this situation?
4. What do you do first (e.g., assess for pain, provide reassurance, administer oxygen, sit him up in bed)?
5. Are you accustomed to doing this?
6. Where did you learn it?

◆ **Case Example
(Jones & Brown, 1993)**

Mr G has terminal cancer. His family defers to the attending physician who prescribes aggressive rescue treatment. The hospice nurse is an expert in the expressed and unexpressed needs of terminal clients. She advocates for a conservative and supportive plan of care.
(A logical case could be built for each position.)

Critical thinking is not a linear process. Analysis of the thinking process of expert nurses reveals that they continually scan the data and simultaneously apply these steps in critical thinking. They constantly reassess the nature of the problem, integrating new data. They continually monitor the effectiveness of their interventions in achieving desired outcomes for their client.

◆ **Exercise 7–12. Interview of Expert Nurse**

**Purpose:** To develop awareness of critical thinking in the clinical judgment process

**Procedure:**
Read the article by S. Corcoran, "Thinking Aloud," and then go out into the community and videotape (or audiotape) a 10-minute interview with a registered nurse who has been in practice at least 4 years. During the interview, have the expert describe an actual client case in which there was a significant change in the client's health status; have the expert describe the interventions and thinking process during this situation. Ask what nursing knowledge, lab data, or experience helped the nurse make his or her decision. You can work with a partner.

**Discussion:**
Each student analyzes the tape using an outline of the 10 steps in Critical Thinking. This should be followed by extensive class discussion in which students first cite examples of each step noted during their review of the taped interview and followed by application to the broad principles. Discussion of steps missed by the interviewed expert can be enlightening as long as care is taken to avoid any criticism of the guest "expert."

## SUMMARY

A nurse's values and critical thinking abilities often have a profound effect on the quality of care given to a client and on the type of interaction that occurs. Individuals acquire values through interactions with others. Professional values are ultimately an expansion and reflection of an individual's personal values. Values clarification helps develop self-understanding.

Functioning effectively within the nurse–client relationship requires knowledge of medical and nursing content, an accumulation of clinical experiences, and an ability to think critically. Every day nurses confront ethical dilemmas and complicated clinical situations that require expertise as a decision maker. The nurse can follow the 10 steps of the critical thinking process described in this chapter as a tool for responding to such situations. Developing skill as a critical thinker is a learned process, requiring repeated opportunities for application to clinical situations. Reflecting on one's own thinking about case example situations provided in this chapter can assist such learning.

## REFERENCES

Alfaro-LeFevre R. (1995). Critical thinking in nursing: A practical approach. Philadelphia, WB Saunders.

Bandman EL, Bandman B. (1995). Critical thinking in nursing. Norwalk, CT, Appleton & Lange.

Benjamin M, Curtis J. (1981). Ethics in Nursing. New York, Oxford University Press.

Bethune E, Jackling N. (1997). Critical thinking skills: The role of prior experience. Journal of Advanced Nursing 26:1005–1012.

Boggs KU. (1997). Addendum to Final Report (CID Grant). Charlotte, NC, UNCC Foundation.

Bowers B, McCarthy D. (1993). Developing analytic thinking skills in early undergraduate education. Journal of Nursing Education 32(3):107–114.

Carnevali DL, Thomas MD. (1993). Diagnostic reasoning and treatment decision making in nursing. Philadelphia, JB Lippincott.

Cascio RS, Campbell D, Sandor MK, et al. (1995). Enhancing critical thinking skills: Faculty-student partnerships in community health nursing. Nurse Educator 20(2):38–43.

Corcoran S, Narayan S, Mooreland H. (1988). Thinking aloud. Heart & Lung 17:463–468.

Cunningham N, Hutchinson S. (1990). Myths in health care ethics. Image 22(4):235.

Del Bueno D. (1994). Why can't new grads think like nurses? Nurse Educator 19:9–11.

Ericksen JR. (1990). Making choices: The crux of ethical problems in nursing. ARON Journal 52(1):394.

Facione NC, Facione PA. (1996). Externalizing the critical thinking in knowledge development and clinical judgement. Nursing Outlook 44(3):129–136.

Farrell P, Bramadat I. (1993). Paradigm case analysis and simulated recall. Clinical Nurse Specialist 4:153–157.

Hanson C, Hodnicki D. (1998). Development of curriculum for FNP education. Presented at the conference of the SREB Kellogg Faculty Fellowship, Atlanta, GA, January 15, 1998.

Hough, MC. (1996). Ethical dilemmas faced by critical care nurses in clinical practice: Walking the line. Critical Care Clinics 12(1):123–133.

Huston CJ, Marquis BL. (1995). Seven steps to successful decision-making. American Journal of Nursing 95(5): 65–68.

Jones SA, Brown LN. (1993). Alternative views on defining critical thinking through the nursing process. Holistic Nursing Practice 7(3):71–76.

Lincourt J. (1998). Private conversation, Philosophy Dept, University of North Carolina, Charlotte, NC.

McNally JM. (1980). Values: Part II. Supervisor Nurse 11:52.

Pederson C, Duckett L, Maruyama G. (1990). Using structured controversy to promote ethical decision making. Journal of Nursing Education 29(4):151.

Rubenfeld MG, Scheffer B. (1995). Critical thinking in nursing: An interactive approach. Philadelphia, JB Lippincott.

Schank MJ. (1990). Wanted: Nurses with critical thinking skills. Journal of Continuing Education in Nursing 21(2):86–89.

Steele SM, Harmon VM. (1983). Values Clarification in Nursing (2nd ed.). Norwalk, CT, Appleton-Century-Crofts.

Thompson JB, Thompson HO. (1981). Ethics in Nursing. New York: Macmillan.

Uustal DB. (1978). Values clarification in nursing: Application to practice. American Journal of Nursing 78:2058.

Uustal DB. (1980). Exploring values in nursing. ARON Journal 31:183.

Veatch RM, Fry ST. (1987). Case studies in nursing ethics. Boston, Jones & Bartlett.

## Suggested Readings

Edwards BJ, Haddad AM. (1988). Establishing a nursing bioethics committee. Journal of Nursing Administration 18:30.

Pence T, Cantrall J. (1990). Ethics in Nursing: An Anthology. New York, National League for Nursing.

## Electronic References

http://lawlib.slu.edu/centers/hlthlaw/links.htm#bioethics (extensive selected Internet resources in health law and policy)

http://www.gen.emory.edu/cgi/bin/MEDWEB/ [MacDonald C. (1995). Guide to moral decision making.]

http://www.nursingworld.org/readroom/position/ethics/etdnr.htm [position statements "do-not-resuscitate decisions" and "foregoing nutrition and hydration" from ANA]

http://www.hortyspringer.com [Patient Care Law]

gopher://gopher.mcw.edu:72/00/bioethics/

http://www.scu.edu/ethics/publications

http://www.nursing.ab.umd.edu [critical thinking scenario]

http://www.gen.emory.edu/CGI/BIN/MEDWEB/search.html

# 8

# The Grief Experience: Life's Losses and Endings

Verna Benner Carson

**OBJECTIVES**

After completing this chapter, the student will be able to

1. Define loss and identify types of losses people face in a lifetime
2. Discuss the concept of grief and its implications for nursing
3. Discuss the contributions of Lindemann and Engel to the work on grief
4. Describe the patterns of grieving
5. Discuss the nurse's role in helping people deal with loss and grief
6. Describe the stages of death and dying
7. Discuss nursing strategies in the care of the dying patient
8. Discuss termination of a nurse–patient relationship
9. Discuss the nurse's role in facilitating termination

*It's as if it just happened. The memories are so vivid—If I close my eyes I can see the waiting room, hear the sounds of the hospital, see the strained faces of other visitors awaiting those precious few moments permitted for visiting an ill loved one. I recall sitting in the waiting room with my family gathered around. I can see the fear and dread in the eyes of my sisters and my dad, my husband and my children, my brothers-in-law, nieces and nephews. We waited in silence—each of us knowing the outcome, but each praying privately that we were wrong. I can remember the expression on the doctor's face as he walked toward us. I knew what he was about to say and for a brief minute even felt sorry for him. How difficult it must be to be the bearer of such painful news. He sat down directly in front of me. I wondered, "why is he singling me out when my family is here?" I listened to him and tried to focus on what he was saying. I couldn't—Instead I focused on the pain that washed over everyone and the tears that started slowly and became torrents. I watched as my father grasped the reality of what was said; I watched his composure melt away like a melting wax candle. I remember all of this. What I can't remember is what the doctor said—except for his final words, "I am so sorry—we did everything we could to save your mother, but I am so sorry, we lost her."*

Anonymous

◆◆◆ Memories—vivid, painful, wrapped in sadness and grief and locked in time. The loss of a loving and loved mother, a moment that leaves a void in the heart that only she could fill. Certainly a loss so significant stands out in our minds forever. However, what about other losses? Do they pale in comparison? Do they share anything in common with the loss of a loved one? Is there something about loss that nurses need to understand, to feel, to appreciate in order to be present to their patients? Let us take a look at loss, the types of losses people experience, the feelings of grief that accompany loss, the phases of grief, the loss and grief that accompany death, and finally a bit about the loss experienced when a nurse–patient relationship comes to an end.

## BASIC CONCEPTS

Loss pervades the life journey; there is no avoiding it. Each person experiences loss as a personal event, and indeed it is. However, the experience of loss is as universal as are the experiences of being born and dying. Losses and the grief experienced as a result of loss are inevitable. No one is exempt. The sorrow that each of us feels whenever we lose something or somebody of significance is repeated many times as we make our way into adulthood. Loss can be an opportunity for growth and transformation, or it can be an obstacle that blocks all future growth and leads to illness. Consider the following normal life events and reflect on the linking theme among all of them.

A 2-year-old leaves his mother for the first time to spend the day at a baby sitter's home while his mother works.

A 3-year-old has to share his mommy with his infant brother.

A 5-year-old separates from his mother to enter kindergarten for the first time.

The family pet dies.

A teenager transfers to a different school.

A grandmother dies.

A couple is granted a divorce.

A nursing student graduates from nursing school.

A young woman receives the news that she has tested positive for the human immunodeficiency virus.

A wife watches as her husband disappears behind the wall of Alzheimer's disease.

A middle-aged man loses his job of 30 years as a result of corporate downsizing.

A nurse leaves his full-time job to return to graduate school.

All of these events are linked by an element

of loss, of saying good-by to what was and beginning anew, of building on the past but of not returning to it. *Loss* is defined as the involuntary separation from something we have possessed and may even have treasured (Jacik, 1996). Box 8–1 lists general assumptions about loss.

Sometimes loss involves ending a relationship through death or separation. In other cases, the loss involves a major change in the relationship that requires the participants to give up former expectations and move on to new ways of relating. In still other cases, the loss involves giving up an old role for a new one. In any event, all losses produce grief, which is characterized by feelings of sadness, a longing for the past, and ambivalence about the future. The feelings associated with various losses differ only in the intensity that they are experienced, as Mark Twain so poignantly expressed: "Nothing that grieves us can be called little; by the eternal laws of proportion a child's loss of a doll and a king's loss of a crown are events of the same size."

Nurses experience loss in their personal relationships as well as in the professional relationships that they develop with clients. The ending of a professional relationship is a special kind of loss and is usually referred to as termination and is discussed later in this chapter. Nurses who have openly acknowledged and shared their feelings of past losses are better prepared to assist their clients. If, on the other hand, nurses have tended to avoid their grief, pushing it out of awareness in their personal lives, their difficulty will be reflected in professional relationships as well. The

---

◆ **Exercise 8–1. The Meaning of Loss**

**Purpose:** To consider personal meaning of losses

**Procedure:** Consider your answers to the following questions:

What losses have I experienced in my life?

How did I feel when I lost something or someone important to me?

How was my behavior affected by my loss?

What helped me the most in resolving my feelings of loss?

How has my experience with loss prepared me to deal with further losses?

How has my experience with loss prepared me to help others deal with loss?

---

more that pain is denied, the deeper it tends to go inside our bodies and souls. The burying of pain only makes it harder to identify, deal with, and ultimately grow beyond. Just as the nurse's past experience with loss and grief impact on present relationships, so to does the client's past experiences with loss and grief bear on current relationships.

Exercise 8–1 will assist you to examine certain aspects of loss in relationships and to look at what loss means to you.

This chapter examines the experience of grief that accompanies life's losses, including termination. You are presented with a theoretical foundation for understanding loss and grief, but equally important you are encouraged to examine how it feels to lose something or somebody of significance. The combination of intellectual comprehension with body and soul "felt" experience leads to a wisdom that allows you to personally deal with loss and grief and to assist clients to do the same.

---

◆ Box 8–1. General Assumptions About Loss

The experience of loss is universal.

Loss involves pain.

Losses that are significant produce emotional upheaval.

Loss requires change and adjustment to situations that are new, uncertain, and unchosen.

Loss can impact many lives.

Adapted from Carson VB, Arnold EN. (1996). Mental Health Nursing: The Nurse-Patient Journey. Philadelphia, WB Saunders, p. 662. Used with permission.

## Grief

Let us first examine the concept of grief, which is also referred to as mourning, and bereavement.

Gyulay (1989, p. 2) defined *grief* as "a journey toward healing and recovering from the pain of a significant loss." This definition includes two major goals: healing oneself and recovering from the loss. The process of achieving these goals is often referred to as grief work. It is probably the most difficult work one does in life. Many who grieve do not come to acceptance, but it is a certainty that the only way to arrive at peace, serenity, recovery, healing, and acceptance is to work through grief. There is no way around it. One must experience the pain of the loss before healing is possible.

Initially, the grieving individual experiences shock, denial, depression, and bargaining in sequence. Then, beyond these initial reactions, the bereaved individual most likely experiences recurring, wavelike, roller coaster–like responses. These responses are not singular experiences that lead easily and predictably to a new stage, but instead move the person along on a rocky, tumultuous course of progress. Grieving feels awful, and the truth is that it continues in some form and level of intensity for a long time. C.S. Lewis (1963), in writing about the death of his wife Joy, stated, "No one ever told me that grief felt so like fear . . . Part of every misery is, so to speak, the misery's shadow or reflection; the fact that you don't merely suffer but have to keep on thinking about the fact that you suffer. I not only live each day in grief, but also live each day thinking about living each day in grief."

## Lindemann's Work on Grief

Lindemann (1944) conducted pioneering work on grieving. He interviewed grieving persons who had lost a relative in the armed forces, persons who had sought psychiatric treatment after the death of a relative, and bereaved victims or relatives of victims who died in the Coconut Grove fire in Boston in the 1940s. From these interviews, he identified patterns of grief, physical symptoms that accompany it, and emotional changes in people who had experienced significant losses. Box 8–2 lists Lindemann's four major observations about grief.

## Engel's Contributions

George Engel (1964) built on the work of Lindemann and identified not only phases of grief but

---

> ◆ Box 8-2. Major Observations About Grief

1. Acute grief is a definite syndrome with both psychological and physical symptoms.
2. Grief may occur immediately after a crisis; it may be delayed; it may be exaggerated; or it may appear to be absent, which is considered pathological grief.
3. Sometimes the typical pattern of grief is distorted.
4. Distorted patterns of grief can be transformed into a normal grief reaction with appropriate clinical interventions.

---

also the components of grief work as well as the psychological disturbances that frequently accompany grief. According to Engel (1964), successful grieving involves three phases: *shock and disbelief*, *developing awareness*, and *restitution*. In the shock and disbelief phase, the person has a need to deny the loss to protect him- or herself from the painful feelings it evokes. The denial usually lasts for a short period of time (minutes to hours to days). During this time, the bereaved person hopes against all hope that some mistake was made, that the loss never really happened. A lengthy period of denial signals an abnormal grief reaction and prevents the person from going forward in the grief process.

In the developing awareness phase, the person realizes the emotional impact of the loss; the loss begins to penetrate consciousness. The bereaved becomes increasingly aware of the anguish created by the loss and has painful feelings of sadness and emptiness. Crying is one of the most evident activities in this phase of grieving. Somatic symptoms (e.g., a choking sensation, inability to eat or sleep, shortness of breath) as well as strong emotional reactions (e.g., anger at the deceased, anger at persons deemed responsible for the loss, extreme helplessness, hopelessness, or guilt) are experienced.

In the restitution phase, the task of mourning begins. In the case of a loss by death, the work of this stage can actually begin with the wake, funeral, and burial. According to Engel, the components of grief work include

1. Freeing oneself from an inordinate attachment to the deceased or to the lost object

2. Readjusting to an environment that no longer includes the deceased or the lost object
3. Undertaking new relationships and social interactions

Engel observed that increased anxiety, depression, insomnia, and tiredness are common psychological disturbances that accompany grief work:

---

*Throughout the year following my mother's death I was aware of a persistent feeling of heaviness—not physical heaviness, but emotional and spiritual. It was as if a dark cloud hung over my heart and soul. I was easily tired with little energy to do anything but the most essential activities, and even those frequently received perfunctory attention. My usual pattern of "sleeping like a log" was disrupted and in its place I experienced uneasy rest that left me feeling as if I had never closed my eyes.*

Anonymous

---

## Patterns of Grieving

Given a choice, many people would prefer not to grieve at all because the process is long, difficult, and emotionally draining. Let us take a look at normal *grieving patterns* and contrast them with those that are abnormal, frequently referred to as complicated grief, morbid grief reactions, the pathological grief syndrome, distorted grief, and unresolved grief.

**Normal Grieving.** The early phase of grieving, marked by disbelief, shock, and dismay, leaves a person feeling dazed, unproductive, and "mechanical" as he or she tries to function. This phase may last for hours, days, or weeks. The person may not remember much of what has happened during that period because of the psychological numbing caused by the loss experience.

**Middle Phase.** The middle phase of grief extends over many months and is acutely painful. This period includes reactions that are more intense in nature. In her book *Living Through Personal Crisis*, Ann Stearns (1984) addressed the

physical expressions of loss. She wrote, "A wide range of marked physical changes can accompany an experience of loss. Not only through tears do we cry out our pangs of grief. Under the stress of what has been unrecoverably lost, our bodies have a dozen ways of weeping with us" (p. 16).

Although what is felt as a person acutely grieves is considered a normal grief reaction, many people will feel that they are crossing over into the realm of mental illness. They may even begin to believe that they have lost their ability to cope and their grasp of reality (Carter, 1989). The fact that the symptoms, feeling, and sensations lose their intensity and become less frequent as time passes is a comfort to most.

**Late Phase.** The late phase of the grief process is characterized by glimmers of hope. Over time, a person experiences new energy for coping, a returning sense of well-being, and a renewed belief in self.

**Complicated Grieving.** Grieving that is incapacitating, unusually long in duration, and involves some disorganized, depressed behaviors falls into the category of complicated grieving. Persons predisposed to this kind of grief reaction are those with a history of

1. Depressive reactions to transitions, crises, or misfortunes
2. Psychiatric problems with periods of hospitalization
3. Substance abuse, especially alcoholism
4. Death of a parent or sibling during childhood or adolescence
5. Prolonged conflict or marked dependency on the deceased person
6. Multiple deaths
7. Posttraumatic stress

Professional help is always required when a person is trapped in complicated grief.

Lindemann (1944) described the characteristics of complicated grieving in the studies he conducted. Calling it "morbid grief reactions," he described the following symptoms:

1. Overactivity or agitation without a keen sense of one's loss
2. Acquisition of symptoms experienced during the last illness of the deceased
3. Exacerbation of a disease of a psychophysio-

logical nature, such as ulcerative colitis, rheumatoid arthritis, or asthma

4. Alteration in relationships with friends and relatives, progressing to complete social isolation
5. Repression of feelings and an absence of emotional display despite the significant loss
6. Lack of initiative or poor decision making, which leads to dysfunctional living patterns (e.g., poor grooming, not cooking or eating, not cleaning self or home)
7. Loss of social status, professional standing, and financial well-being because of unwise or imprudent financial decisions
8. Deterioration into a state of depression marked by agitation, insomnia, feelings of worthlessness, bitter self-accusation, or the need for self-punishment (becoming dangerously suicidal)
9. Extreme hostility toward persons held responsible for the loss

Along with the distorted responses seen in morbid grief reactions, other categories of complicated grief may be seen: absent grief, delayed grief, chronic grief, distorted grief, and converted grief (Wolfelt, 1991).

In *absent grief*, prolonged denial results from psychic numbing, which prevents a person from accepting the reality of a significant loss and from mourning that loss. The person experiencing absent grief is relatively unmoved and psychologically detached as he or she tells the story of the loss that has occurred. Persons actively pursuing an addictive lifestyle or caught in the throes of mental illness are especially prone to exhibit absent grief, even when something or someone very treasured is lost. Absent grief may be present temporarily when uncertainties surround losses, as during wartime, natural disasters, or accidents. In most cases, grieving occurs when doubts are cleared and the extent of the losses is confirmed.

*Delayed grief* involves the postponement of grieving for weeks, months, or years. Delayed grief often can be abruptly ended by subsequent losses or by the losses of others that are similar to one's own ungrieved loss, which may trigger grieving. Sometimes delays in grieving occur out of necessity. *Chronic grief* is a persistent pattern of grieving that tends to be exaggerated and does not reach resolution. It creates disabling symp-

toms, dysfunctional people, and irrational despair. Chronic grief related to death is characterized by attempts to keep the deceased person alive by talking about him or her frequently, maintaining his or her personal things intact, and expecting that the deceased will reenter the mourner's life.

*Distorted grief* is that type of grief that Lindemann called a morbid grief reaction. Anger and guilt are the two emotional expressions that become distorted in this type of grieving. The person is caught up in a state of emotional upheaval that inhibits him or her from effectively carrying out personal responsibilities and activities.

*Converted grief* can be referred to as "somatization disorder." It entails a preoccupation with physical or psychological symptoms that are not linked by the person to his or her loss.

Depression, often seen as a component of both normal and complicated grief reactions, often robs the grieving person of the emotional energy needed to do grief work.

## Nurses' Role

---

*I remember standing next to my mom's bed. We had gone to her room to pay our last respects. A young nurse stood near to me and reached out gently and touched my shoulder. Softly she said, "I'll just stay here with you in case you need something." When I looked at her I saw eyes brimming with tears and a profound sadness on her face. Her presence meant so much; I was grateful for her open expression of sorrow. It confirmed the pain we were all experiencing.*

Anonymous

---

Nurses deal with the grief in others through presence, compassion, and quiet assurance. It is difficult for anyone to remain in a relationship with another whose pain will not go away. This is the challenge for nurses: to remain in relationship to our clients and their loved ones even though we feel inadequate to the task. Our ability to listen and assist those who are grieving to understand their own feelings and behaviors through the use of open-ended statements such as "And then . . .", "Tell me more", "You felt . . .", "How did you do that?", "Who was with you?", "How did you feel?" is sometimes all that is needed to encourage the grieving process. Nurses must be cognizant of the fact that grieving is not a yes or no process, nor is it cut and dried. "Yes, it is true that your loved one has died as a result of acquired immunodeficiency syndrome [AIDS]." "No, he will never come back." These are the only simple realities; beyond these, the grief process is complex.

Nurses can offer assistance in other ways as well. They can provide anticipatory guidance about the process of grief. They can inform the grieving person or family what to expect as far as the intensity and unpredictability of grief; the encompassing nature of grief; that it can leave the grieving individual questioning his or her own mental stability; that the need for support and quiet, compassionate acceptance continues long after most gestures of support have been made and withdrawn. The following quote illustrates some of these characteristics of grief.

*I would think I was doing okay, that I had a handle on my grief. Then without warning, a scent, a scene on television, an innocuous conversation would flip a switch in my mind and I would be flooded with memories of my mother. My eyes would fill up with tears as my fragile composure dissolved. My grief lay right under the surface of my awareness and ambushed me at times and in places not of my choosing.*

Frequently, nurses have opportunities to provide formal and informal teaching about a variety of health-related topics. In the role of teacher, nurses can share simple but effective strategies that others can use to assist someone who is dealing with grief. Box 8–3 lists such suggestions.

Nurses also encounter clients who share information such as: "I never recovered from my son's death" or "I feel like my life ended when my husband died." The client is identifying that grief work was never completed. Grieving that is in-

---

### Box 8–3. Strategies for Helping Someone Deal with Grief

- Prepare meals.
- Provide transportation.
- Provide baby sitting service.
- Help with funeral arrangements.
- Assist with dealing with financial issues.
- Clean home.
- Sit quietly with the grieving person.
- Encourage the person to talk about the deceased or the loss.
- Share a special memory about the deceased with the grieving person.
- Write that memory so that the grieving person can re-read it.
- Weeks and months after the funeral, call and ask how the grieving person is handling his or her grief.
- Avoid giving trite reassurances.
- Accept that your presence is worth more than 1000 words.

---

complete or never attempted at all hangs over the individual and family like a dark cloud, blocking out the sun and resulting in long-term problems such as depression. It is important for the nurse to address this issue, even if the client is seeking help for an unrelated issue. The nurse can suggest a resource like the Grief Recovery Helpline at 800-445-4808. Exercise 8–2: A Personal Loss Inventory could be helpful for both the nurse and the client.

### Reflecting on Personal Experiences with Grief

Nurses are confronted with their own grief as well as the grief of clients and their families and significant others. It is important for nurses to examine their experiences with and feelings regarding grief and loss. How have we handled our grief experiences? Were we able to arrive at acceptance? Did we work our way through grief and not try to sidestep the pain of the loss? How would we cope if we were faced with what our client is facing? This examination is an ongoing one, stimulated by losses in the nurse's personal

---

◆ Exercise 8-2. **A Personal Loss Inventory**

**Purpose:** To provide a close examination of one's history with loss

**Procedure:**
Complete each sentence and reflect on your answers.

The first significant loss I can remember in my life was _____.

The circumstances were _____.

My age was _____.

The feelings I had at the time were _____.

The thing I remember most about that experience was _____.

I coped with the loss by _____.

The most difficult death for me to face would be _____.

I know my grief over a loss is resolved when _____.

---

From Carson VB, Arnold EN. (1996). Mental Health Nursing: The Nurse-Patient Journey. Philadelphia, WB Saunders, p. 666. Used with permission.

---

and professional life. Exercise 8–3 is designed to assist in this process.

## Grief and Loss with Death

Let us now turn our discussion to the process of grief that occurs with death. Death is the ending of all that life holds: successes, failures, relationships, careers, laughter, and pain. Death may come suddenly without warning, or it can stalk a loved one or us over a long period of time. Death seeks the young as well as the old, the rich as well as the poor; it knows no favorites. Yet even though death is a certainty for everyone, we struggle against it, we deny the reality of death, we pretend that it will not touch us; but it does. It touches each of us.

Death is feared; even for those who believe in a spiritual afterlife. There is the fear of the unknown, the fear of losing everyone and everything, the fear of pain; and nurses are not immune from that fear. Nurses cling to life and struggle against death with the same intensity as the clients for whom they compassionately care, yet nurses are called on to rise above their feelings and fears so that they can provide solace and support for the dying person and that person's loved ones. In so doing, nurses must achieve a balance between maintaining their own professional objectivity and psychological well-being and providing the empathy and support needed by their clients.

Death is an event and a process. Once death occurs, it is final. However, death may come slowly over time and the individual, family members, significant others, and health care providers are confronted with the dying process. As Chenitz (p. 454, 1992), a nurse who died from AIDS, so eloquently stated, "Like many people with AIDS, I am not afraid of death. I am afraid of dying. The dying process and how that will be handled is of great concern to me. Everyone is going to die. Death is part of life. However, AIDS brings with it a terrible, painful, often humiliating dying process and that terrifies me." Chenitz's concerns are our concerns. How will we continue to provide compassion, assurance, and competence when we are faced with the dying person's pain, overwhelming losses, and feelings of sadness and anger? Exercise 8–4 can help nurses to explore personal feelings about death.

---

◆ Exercise 8-3. **How Do I Grieve?**

**Purpose:** To examine personal patterns of grief

**Procedure:**
Everyone grieves differently, and each loss may evoke a different grief response. However, over time, each of us develops a pattern for our grieving. Close your eyes and try to remember losses in your life. As you remember, try to recollect the details surrounding each loss. In particular, try to remember the feelings that you experienced. Was there a pattern to your reactions?

When I experience loss, my first reaction is usually _____ .

This initial feeling is replaced by feelings of _____ .

For the first few days after a loss, I would describe my feelings as _____ .

When I think about the ways I have responded to losses, I would describe the way I grieve as _____ .

---

## Stages of Grieving and Death and Dying

Kübler-Ross (1971) provided a framework for understanding the process of dying that is also applicable to the process of grieving. This framework includes five stages: denial, anger, bargaining, depression, and acceptance. This framework is only a rough guide to understanding a client's feelings and behaviors, and not every client exhibits the behaviors of every stage. Some clients may seem to accept the reality of their death from the beginning. Others struggle until the end before finally accepting that death will come. Still others never find acceptance but rather come to a sort of resignation characterized by a negative state of mind. Furthermore, the stages are not neat and orderly. Clients may experience more than one stage simultaneously or may be fixated at a particular stage. However the client deals with the knowledge of his or her dying, it is helpful for the nurses to have a knowledge and understanding of these stages so that they can be a support and not a hindrance to the client (Kellar, 1983).

**Denial.** Frequently, when a client learns that his or her condition is terminal, the initial reaction is one of shock and disbelief. The very thought of one's own death is so overwhelming that a person cannot deal with the feelings generated by such a thought. These feelings can only gradually be allowed into conscious awareness. Consequently, to defend against such terrifying and devastating feelings, the client uses ***denial.*** The client may say things like, "This can't be" or "They must have made a mistake." Kübler-Ross (1971) characterized this stage as the "No, not me" stage.

**Anger.** Increasingly the reality of death makes its way into the client's awareness. Denial no longer works and is replaced with anger, and sometimes rage, as the client reels against the unfairness of the situation. The client's anger is directed to no one in particular but yet spills out toward everyone. The anger is focused on the fact that others have life and health, the very things that the client is losing. Surely no one can argue against the unfairness and cruelty of the client's situation. The client lashes out at family, friends, and staff members. The client is angry that people are oversolicitous and angry that people do not do enough. The client is angry at life and angry with God.

The client feels powerless and alone, and essentially such perceptions are correct. The client is alone with death; no one can die for him or her. No matter how much someone wills it, he or she cannot control death. The enormity of the situation is inescapable. There is no alternative to dying but to die, and the client fights back with all the anger he or she can muster. Kübler-Ross characterized the anger as the "Why me?" stage.

◆ Exercise 8–4. **A Questionnaire About Death**

**Purpose:** To explore your feelings about death

**Procedure:**
Answer the following questions

1. Who died in your first personal involvement with death?

    a. Grandparent or great grandparent
    b. Parent
    c. Brother or sister
    d. Other family member
    e. Friend or acquaintance
    f. Stranger
    g. Public figure
    h. Animal

2. To the best of your memory, at what age were you first aware of death?

    a. Younger than 3 years
    b. Three to 5 years
    c. Five to 10 years
    d. 10 years or older

3. When you were a child, how was death talked about in your family?

    a. Openly
    b. With some sense of discomfort
    c. Only when necessary and then with an attempt to exclude the children
    d. As though it were a taboo subject
    e. Never recall any discussion

4. Which of the following most influenced your present attitudes toward death?

    a. Death of someone close
    b. Specific reading
    c. Religious upbringing
    d. Introspection and meditation
    e. Ritual (e.g., funerals)
    f. Television, radio, or motion pictures
    g. Longevity of my family
    h. My health or physical condition
    i. Other

5. How often do you think about your own death?

    a. Very frequently (at least once a day)
    b. Frequently
    c. Occasionally
    d. Rarely (no more than once a year)
    e. Very rarely or never

◆ **Exercise 8-4. A Questionnaire About Death** *Continued*

6. If you could choose, when would you die?

    a. In youth
    b. In the middle prime of life
    c. Just after the prime of life
    d. In old age

7. When do you believe that, in fact, you will die?

    a. In youth
    b. In the middle prime of life
    c. Just after the prime of life
    d. In old age

8. Has there been a time in your life when you wanted to die?

    a. Yes, mainly because of great physical pain
    b. Yes, mainly because of great emotional upset
    c. Yes, mainly to escape an intolerable social or interpersonal situation
    d. Yes, mainly because of great embarrassment
    e. Yes, for a reason other than those just listed
    f. No

9. What does death mean to you?

    a. The end: the final process of life
    b. The beginning of a life after death; a transition; a new beginning
    c. A joining of the spirit with a universal cosmic consciousness
    d. A kind of endless sleep; rest and peace
    e. Termination of this life but with survival of the spirit
    f. Do not know

10. What aspect of your own death is the most distasteful to you?

    a. I could no longer have any experiences.
    b. I am afraid of what might happen to my body after death.
    c. I am uncertain as to what might happen to me if there is a life after death.
    d. I could no longer provide for my dependents.
    e. It would cause grief to my relatives and friends.
    f. All my plans and projects would come to an end.
    g. The process of dying might be painful.
    h. Other

11. To what extent do you believe that psychological factors can influence (or even cause) death?

    a. I firmly believe that they can.
    b. I tend to believe that they can.
    c. I am undecided or do not know.
    d. I doubt that they can.

*Exercise continued on following page*

◆ **Exercise 8-4. A Questionnaire About Death** *Continued*

12. What is your present orientation to your own death?

    a. Death seeker
    b. Death hastener
    c. Death acceptor
    d. Death welcomer
    e. Death postponer
    f. Death fearer

13. If you had a choice, what kind of death would you prefer?

    a. Tragic, violent death
    b. Sudden but not violent death
    c. Quiet, dignified death
    d. Death in line of duty
    e. Death after a great achievement
    f. Suicide
    g. Homicide victim
    h. There is no ``appropriate'' kind of death

14. If it were possible, would you want to know the exact date on which you are going to die?

    a. Yes
    b. No

15. If your physician knew that you had a terminal disease and a limited time to live, would you want him or her to tell you?

    a. Yes
    b. No
    c. It would depend on the circumstances.

16. What efforts do you believe ought to be made to keep a seriously ill person alive?

    a. All possible efforts should be made (e.g., transplantation, kidney dialysis).
    b. Efforts should be made that are reasonable for that person's age, physical condition, mental condition, and pain
    c. After reasonable care, a natural death should be permitted.
    d. A senile person should not be kept alive by elaborate artificial methods.

17. If or when you are married, would you prefer to outlive your spouse?

    a. Yes, I would prefer to die second and outlive my spouse.
    b. No, I would rather die first and have my spouse outlive me.
    c. Undecided or do not know

18. What effect has this questionnaire had on you?

    a. It has made me somewhat anxious or upset.
    b. It has made me think about my own death.
    c. It has reminded me how fragile and precious life is.
    d. Other effects

**Bargaining.** After clients have vented their anger, they often enter a stage of bargaining with God. Usually, the bargaining takes the form of promises to be a better person in exchange for more time. "If you just let me live until my son's graduation, I'll go to church every Sunday." This stage is reminiscent of childhood days when children frequently plead with their parents. It is almost as though the client is saying, "If God didn't respond to my anger, maybe He'll hear me if I ask very nicely for just a little more time." Kübler-Ross (1971) stated that the client in the bargaining stage characteristically says, "Yes, me, but. . . ."

**Depression.** After the bargaining is complete, the client comes to the "Yes, me" stage. Clients recognize that not only that they will die but also that they will be saying good-by to all that they love. During this stage, clients experience grief as they mourn what they are losing. They cry and gradually retreat to quiet introspection as they work through their losses. In this process, they begin to separate from all that has been their life until finally they no longer need family and friends but only one loved one to sit quietly and wait with them until death comes.

**Acceptance.** The acceptance stage brings peace. Clients are neither happy nor terribly sad. They accept the inevitable. They have brought to closure all of their unfinished business; they have said all the words that need to be said. There is nothing left to do but to be with the people they love and just wait.

## Roles of Nurses Working with Dying Clients

Working with dying clients and their families is an extremely demanding task, but it can be also an emotionally enriching experience for the nurse. Not every nurse can be intimately involved with every dying client and family members. It is hoped that there is at least one nurse available to the client who is able to become involved in the client's pain, to withstand the client's anger, and to help the client in whatever way is needed in this experience of death.

It is this nurse who accepts the client's denial as long as the client needs to use this defense. It is this nurse who can say to the client, "I can see how angry you are, and I wish that I could make

you better." It is this nurse who can assist the client to see that berating family members may not be the best method for dealing with the sense of powerlessness. It is this nurse who communicates a care plan to the rest of the staff so that everyone has an understanding of the client's changing needs. Finally, it is this nurse who helps family members deal with their own grief as they prepare to say good-by.

In planning care for the dying client, the nurse applies the steps of the nursing process (Carson, 1997).

### Assessment

There are a number of important areas for the nurse to assess when working with the dying client, including the client's feelings about death, cultural response to and spiritual beliefs regarding death, life experiences with death, developmental level, role within the family, and support system. All of these factors interact to shape the client's response to death.

The assessment of *feelings* has already been addressed in the discussion of the stage of death and dying. What was not covered was the manner in which clients express their feelings. Most likely, clients will not discuss death in an open and direct way, at least not until they have ascertained that they have a listener who can truly handle this difficult topic. Generally, clients hint about their underlying feelings and concerns. Thus, the nurse must be attuned not only to nonverbal clues that clients communicate but also their use of symbolic language.

Clients may refer to their deaths as a great struggle, "a last train ride," "the biggest fight of my life." The use of symbolic language serves a dual purpose. The first purpose is to avoid the pain associated with the word "death" itself, and the second purpose is to test out the waters so to speak. The client is throwing out bait to a sensitive listener who will give permission to the client to talk about issues of loss, saying good-by, and taking care of unfinished business. The nurse assesses a client's readiness to openly discuss death and, one hopes, responds in a way that says, "You can talk to me. I can't change your situation, but perhaps I can make it less lonely." Sometimes the nurse is the most convenient or the only person who allows the client this freedom.

In assessing the *family's feelings* related to their loved one's death, the nurse must be aware that the family's reaction is not always synchronous with the that of the client. For instance, the client may be ready to openly grieve, but the family is still denying the reality of death. The nurse must also help the family to deal with their feelings so that they can provide empathetic and loving support to the client.

*Culture* plays an important role in how a dying person and family members cope with death, and it behooves the nurse to consider this area, for instance, how grief is expressed is affected by culture. In general, American culture does not encourage or value "falling apart." Instead, what is valued is stoicism and a general denial of grief. It is also important for nurses to examine their own cultural biases so that they are not judgmental toward cultural beliefs and practices that are important to clients and their families. Cultural beliefs about death impact the nurse's role in a number of areas. For instance, culture may dictate such things as (1) the type of care that is given to provide comfort to the dying person; (2) the use of nonprofessional as well as professional caregivers; (3) the understanding of the causes of illness and death; (4) funeral or burial rites; and (5) definition of acceptable sick role behavior and grief responses.

*Spiritual beliefs and religious practices* regarding death are yet another crucial area for the nurse to assess. In doing so, the nurse must differentiate between spirituality and religiosity. Spirituality is a broad concept referring either to a unifying life force or a relationship with a Supreme Being. Religiosity refers to membership in and adherence to the practices of a particular faith tradition or sect. An individual can be very spiritual but not religious. On the other hand, an individual can adhere closely to religious rules and rituals but not have a well-defined relationship either with God or with any unifying life force.

In assessing spiritual needs, the nurse needs to be attuned to clients' verbal and nonverbal behaviors indicative of their feelings and thoughts toward God. Clients may refer to God in a guarded indirect way, they may joke about God, or they may openly plead with God. Their expressions may indicate anger toward God, feelings of abandonment, a belief that death is a way of making retribution to God for wrongdoing or just a seeking of a benevolent God to comfort them in their pain. The Psalms of the Old Testament are replete with all of these themes as David the Psalmist approaches God. Any and all expressions related to spirituality require direct and sensitive intervention either from the nurse or a member of the clergy. Clients are indicating their need to talk about and to God, and this need is as essential for the nurse to address as administering pain medication. The dying process, grief, and death itself herald a spiritual crisis, a crisis of faith, hope, and meaning, the resolution of which is an integral aspect of emerging from grief healed and whole and confronting death with peace and acceptance. Exercise 8–5, "Blueprint for My Life Story," is helpful for nurses to examine the patterns and meaning in their own lives and may be a useful strategy to assist clients to do the same.

Religious practices and rituals are important to clients and may enhance their spirituality. The nurse needs to assess the importance of such rites and facilitate their performance. For instance, a Roman Catholic client may desire to see a priest to receive the Sacrament of Penance, Holy Communion, and the Anointing of the Sick. In such cases, the nurse provides a private environment for the priest and the client and also inquires whether there is anything else that the priest requires, such as a covered table for the placement of religious articles. Although the nurse may not understand the exact meaning of the ritual for the client, the nurse displays reverence and respect toward the client's need for specific religious practices. In addition, the nurse recognizes that facilitating these practices touches the client's inner core and helps him or her to move toward a peaceful death (Jacik, 1996).

*Previous life experiences* with death may also affect clients' attitudes toward their own dying. For instance, if clients have experienced the death of a loved one or a friend who was able to face death with equanimity, they may not view death as something to be feared. On the other hand, if they have watched someone die through a prolonged and painful struggle, they may expect the worst.

The client's *developmental level* is an influencing factor in their attitude toward death. The young child views death entirely differently from the elderly client's view, and this difference cer-

◆ **Exercise 8-5. Blueprint for My Life Story**

**Purpose:** To view life as a whole, integrated process

**Procedure:**
This is a two-part exercise. First, make a single life line across a blank sheet of paper, beginning with your birth. Identify the significant events in your life, and insert on your worksheet the age that you were when the event or moment occurred. When you are finished, answer the following questions:

**Childhood**
1. What was your happiest time as a child?
2. What were your saddest times?
3. What were your chores or responsibilities as a child?
4. What did you hope to become when you grew up?
5. Who were your companions as a child?
6. How did you view your mother? Your father? Your grandparents?
7. How did you feel about your home? Your neighborhood?
8. As a child, who was your most important relationship with?
9. Were boys and girls treated alike in school? In the family?
10. Where was your favorite space?
11. Where did you live as a child?

**Adolescence**
1. What subjects did you like best in school?
2. How and when did you get your first job?
3. Who were your companions as an adolescent, and what did you do with them?
4. Who was your first girlfriend (boyfriend)?
5. Who had the most significant influence on you as an adolescent? In what ways?
6. What was most important to you as an adolescent?
7. Where did you live as an adolescent?

**Adult**
1. What was the best job you ever had? The worst?
2. If you could choose your career again, what would you choose?
3. How did you meet your partner (husband, wife, significant other)?
4. If you have children, when were they born, and what are they like?
5. If you could relive any part of your life, what would it be?
6. What parts of your life are you particularly proud of?
7. Look back over your life; when were you happiest? Saddest?
8. What have you learned about life from the process of living?
9. What was the most exciting part of your life?
10. Who has influenced your life most as an adult?
11. If you could make three wishes, what would they be?

Record your answers in whatever way seems most appropriate to you. Spend some time thinking about the events you have identified on your life line and the answers you have provided in the narrative. Reflect on your life as a whole, with you as the primary actor, producer, and director. Think about ways in which you could write the remaining chapters of your life so they have special meaning to you.

tainly impinges on nursing care. A child younger than 3 years has no clear concept of what death means. By 3 years of age, children begin to play at death, as if it is a game, without any conception of the finality associated with the reality. Very young children react to the anguish and the grief of those around them but are confused as to why everyone is so sad. Preschoolers understand that death involves leaving, but they believe that it is gradual and temporary. Cartoons on television, which frequently depict characters dying and coming back to life, reinforce this belief. Children between 6 and 9 tend to personify death and view it as a person who causes people to die. The older school-age child, 10 to 12 years of age, understands that death is the cessation of bodily life. The adolescent may vacillate between a mature and a childlike attitude toward death.

Adults between 18 and 45 years of age are fully aware of the finality of death, but they tend to believe that only old people die. They are so involved with the tasks of generativity, family, and career that death is not a common thought. Between the ages of 45 and 65 years of age, adults have accepted their own mortality. They have probably already experienced the death of their parents or some of their peers. Adults older than 65 years may view death with several different attitudes. They may see death as a reunion with deceased family members, or they may fear that their deaths will be prolonged and painful and will cause hardship to their children (Carson & Arnold, 1996).

*Family role* is still another area that the nurse needs to assess in relation to the dying client. An unmarried woman with a terminal illness will have different concerns than those of a dying mother; an older widower will have different concerns than those of a newly married young man. Different roles within the family carry with them differing amounts of responsibility. A young mother's death may engender anger and guilt because she feels she is deserting her family. A single person who is dying may also feel anger, but it will probably relate more to a loss of independence.

Last, the client's *support system* also needs to be examined by the nurse. The presence or absence of a loving and supportive family is a determining factor in the client's ability to cope with death. The nurse needs to be aware that the family is subject to all the same feelings and influences regarding death that to which the client is subject. For this reason, the family may need as much support as the client to assist them to be a help to the client. For instance, if a client is expressing anger and is particularly abusive to the spouses, the spouse may be confused and frightened. A situation like this would require some mediation on the part of the nurse not only to help the client deal with his or her anger more appropriately but also to provide the spouse with an understanding of the client's behavior.

## Analysis

The nurse, having made a careful assessment of these areas of concern, analyzes the data he or she has collected and determines the nursing diagnosis for the problems that have been identified. Any or all of the following nursing diagnoses could be appropriate when working with the dying client and family members:

Ineffective coping related to impending death
Coping, potential for growth, related to impending death
Anticipatory grieving related to expected death
Dysfunctional grieving related to expectant death
Fear related to known and unknown factors of expected death
Alteration in self-concept related to death
Spiritual distress related to impending death

## Planning

The care for dying clients and their families requires open and consistent communication among all members of the health team. Usually the nurse coordinates the planning and evaluation of care.

Ideally, one nurse is responsible for the primary care of the client and keeps the rest of the health team members informed of new issues and seeks their input to plan and to evaluate care. This approach prevents fragmentary and inconsistent care and allows the client to be cared for totally.

Although the goals for care would be individualized to particular clients and their families, the following general goals provide a framework for developing more specificity:

1. The client will verbalize feelings of anger.

2. The client will vent anger in appropriate ways.
3. The client will express feelings of grief and loss.
4. The client will explore and evaluate his or her life experiences.
5. The client will identify areas of concern over "unfinished business."
6. The client will express feelings about God in relationship to dying.
7. The client will use religious practices appropriate to his or her beliefs.
8. The client will verbalize a sense of personal order and meaning associated with the dying process.
9. The client will spend private uninterrupted time with his or her family.

### Intervention

In meeting these goals, most of the nurse's interventions will focus on communication. Lindemann (1944) studied dying persons and their families for 30 years and summarized three key components in providing care for them: open, empathic communication; honesty; and tolerance of emotional expression. The following quote from Lindemann succinctly and poignantly identifies these components:

---

*Rely on open communication. Don't fib. The family or the patient always will know if you do, just as children always know. That's number one, and for me it is the basis of helping.*

---

The second important skill is to be able to take the patient's position. Even if what is said seems silly to you, take enough time to hear the patient out, because he may have a very good reason for an attitude that sounds very nonsensical to you at first. So do not brush the client aside. The third skill is not to assume that it is bad for the patient to be sad and miserable and crying for a while. Do not assume that you have to keep everything in the relationship smooth and that the patient must smile. The client may smile just to keep you happy.

Talking about death is not something that comes easily to the nurse. Few schools of nursing actually teach nurses how to converse with the dying client. In addition, nurses are subject to the same societal influences that the client is. These influences paint death as a topic to be avoided at all costs. Nurses frequently feel ill prepared to deal with the emotional turmoil generated by the task. Yet the dying person often has a very strong need to express these feelings; and nurses can be facilitators of this process if they allow themselves to be. Box 8–4 provides guidelines for communicating with terminally ill patients and their families.

In addition to communication, the nurse's other interventions include helping the client to take care of unfinished business, which might involve finalizing a will or taking care of some financial concerns. Providing spiritual care through the use of clergy, the nurse's own interventions of presence, touch, use of prayer, and

---

**Box 8–4. Guidelines for Communicating with Terminally Ill Clients and Their Families**

Avoid rote responses. Each person and family are unique and deserve to be treated as such.

Relate person to person. Show humor as well as sorrow.

Use your mind, eyes, and ears to hear what is said as well as what is not said.

Respect the individual's pattern of communication and ways of dealing with stress. This is not the time to promote change!

Humility and honesty are essential. Be willing to admit that you do not know the answer.

Maintain a sense of calm. This will help the client's sense of control.

Never force the client to talk. Respect the client's need for privacy and be sensitive to the client's readiness to talk.

Let the client lead the discussion to the future. Be comfortable with focusing on the here and now.

Be willing to allow the client to see some of your fears and vulnerabilities. It is much easier to open up to someone who is "human and vulnerable" than to someone who appears to have all the answers.

scripture reading are all important in meeting the identified spiritual needs. A last intervention would be to provide the client and family the privacy necessary to talk and comfort one another, to share thoughts and physical closeness not possible when frequent interruptions by nursing staff occur.

### Evaluation

The evaluation of care of dying clients and their families is an ongoing and continuous process. In some cases, nurses may consider their interventions successful if the client dies in peace surrounded by loved ones. For some clients, though, this kind of death is not possible, and yet this does not mean that the nursing interventions were ineffective. If a client persists in a state of denial until the end, this is the client's right. Although nurses may feel this is not the ideal way to depart from life, it is the client's needs that are paramount in directing care. In general, nursing care of the dying client is successful when the nurse is sensitive to the needs of the client and family and meets those needs in a loving and gentle way. For one client, such care will involve the nurse's quiet presence while the client cries and mourns; for another, it will involve the nurse's faithfulness in light of the client's angry behavior; for still another, it may be the nurse's willingness to pray with him or her for a peaceful death. Death is experienced differently by everyone, and it is the uniqueness of the experience that the nurse attempts to tap into and facilitate.

## Termination: A Special Kind of Loss

*Termination* is used to describe the ending of a professional nurse–patient relationship; it is a special kind of loss and as such involves the experience of grief, especially if the relationship has occurred over time and has involved deep sharing and involvement in the client's life. Although this sense of loss is less likely to occur in the present health care system, which values quick fixes and limited contact between health care professionals and clients, there are settings, such as skilled nursing facilities, rehabilitation hospitals, and state psychiatric facilities, in which long-term relationships can and do develop. Whether the nurse is able to facilitate the ending of a long-term relationship so that it is a growth-producing experience for both participants is greatly influenced by how the nurse has handled losses in the past and whether or not the nurse has resolved the grief experience that accompanied earlier losses. Nurses who have openly acknowledged and shared their feelings of past losses are better prepared to assist their clients (Companiello, 1980).

### Phases of Termination

Terminations are characterized by three developmental phases: denial, grief, and integration. This is similar to what occurs as an individual is faced with grief work. It is important to remember, however, that termination, like grief, is a journey and as such may meander onto paths that do not fit neatly into a stage analysis.

**Denial.** The first phase consists of denial; the individual does not acknowledge either the reality of the loss or the feelings associated with it. Denial is evident when a client repeatedly changes the subject as the nurse tries to discuss termination, or when a nursing student expresses nothing but relief that a long-term relationship is coming to an end. In both instances, denial is being used to ward off painful feelings. The client, by refusing to discuss termination, can avoid focusing on the impending loss. The nursing student, by acknowledging only his or her relief, may be denying feelings of frustration and depression at not being able to be more effective with the client.

**Grief.** When denial begins to break down and is no longer effective at blocking feelings, the person begins the second phase, which is characterized by considerable grief, sadness, and also anger. A client may feel very sad about not being able to see the nurse again and profoundly feels the loss of their relationship, but may simultaneously feel extreme anger toward the nurse for abandoning him or her. Feelings of abandonment and the accompanying anger occur in response to the loss of a relationship, a job, a capability, an ideal, or some highly prized material possession. The fear of abandonment can stimulate an unrelenting rage in persons (e.g., clients) placed in a vulnerable position. The nurse may share this dichotomy of feelings: sadness over the loss but anger at the same time. It is not uncommon for nursing students to feel anger toward an instructor whom they see as responsible for placing them in this painful situation.

The feelings generated by this second phase can be so intense that frequently the client as well as the nurse may want to withdraw from the relationship. The withdrawal can occur either by canceling planned meetings so that there is an actual physical removal from the relationship or by relating on a superficial level so that the withdrawal occurs on an emotional level. The process of withdrawal is a defense against the pain of the loss. The client is saying in effect, "I will abandon you before you have the chance to abandon me." The following example illustrates this.

### ◆ Case Example

On the fifth meeting that Nursing Student Brown had with Mr. James, she reminded him that they only had three more meetings to go before they had to say good-by. When the student asked how Mr. James felt about this, he replied, "Well, that will give me some extra time to do the things I need to do!" [use of denial]. The student told Mr. James that she felt sad about the impending termination and perhaps they could talk about it the next time that they met.

When the time arrived for their sixth meeting, Mr. James was not to be found [withdrawal from the relationship]. When the student inquired as to his whereabouts she was told that he had canceled his clinic appointment for that day. The student decided to call Mr. James to let him know that she had missed him and to remind him of their next meeting. Mr. James arrived for the seventh meeting but he would only discuss the weather and other superficial topics.

In addition to withdrawal from the relationship, other behaviors accompany the sadness of the second phase. Clients may experience a temporary return of disabling symptoms, or they may display indifference. Both of these responses are the client's unconscious attempts to hold on to the relationship. This can be understood in the following way. If the nurse enters the relationship to help the client deal with a particular problem and then the problem intensifies, perhaps the nurse will change his or her mind about terminating the relationship and stay to help the client. The fact is that if the client shows signs of illness or increased dependency, the nurse may feel guilty and find termination extremely difficult. The following example illustrates this point.

### ◆ Case Example

Mrs. Lynch was leaving her position as a diabetic specialist at the community hospital to return to graduate school. She had informed all of her clients of her intended job change months before it was to occur so that she could adequately prepare them for her leaving. As the time drew closer for her to leave her job, she noticed several of her clients were experiencing increasing difficulty with their diabetes control (return of disabling symptoms). Two of the clients had been admitted to the hospital for hypoglycemic episodes. When Mrs. Lynch went to see these clients, they both told her that they did not know how they could manage their diabetes without her support (increased dependency), despite the fact that they had done well for 2 years. Mrs. Lynch was torn between her desire to further her education and her feelings of responsibility to her clients. Mrs. Lynch sought the advice of another colleague, who helped her to recognize that the clients were expressing their difficulties with termination and suggested ways for Mrs. Lynch to help the clients to cope with their feelings in a more constructive way.

**Integration.** The third phase of termination occurs as the client works through the reality of the loss and the feelings of sadness and anger associated with it, and is able to integrate the relationship into other life experiences. This phase may continue even after the nurse and client are no longer seeing each other. As essential as integration is for both participants, it is possible that it may never be completely achieved. To the extent that it is achieved, integration frees both participants from emotional ties and allows them to invest themselves in other relationships and activities. The present relationship has ended, but both the nurse and the client have been enriched by what has transpired between them for new life experiences.

### Problematic Issues

Even in this working-through phase, the feelings of sadness that arise can lead to some problematic issues for the nurse to confront. Gift giving and requests to continue the relationship by exchanging telephone numbers, sending Christmas or birthday cards, or even making visits are the client's last attempt to hold onto the relationship.

Frequently, these behaviors are used during the final meeting between the nurse and the client. It is not uncommon at the end of a meaningful relationship for the participants to wish to exchange gifts as a lasting remembrance of the experience. In a nonprofessional relationship, it would be totally appropriate to exchange gifts. However, in a professional relationship, the issue of gift giving requires closer examination.

Clients sometimes wish to give nurses gifts because nurses have given care to them; the client perceives that the giving has been one way; and they are unable to recognize their own contributions to the relationship. After all, nurses are the listeners; they assist clients with intimate personal tasks; nurses are the doers. The uneven nature of the nurse–client relationship violates a basic characteristic of all human interactions. That is, relationships are characterized by the mutual obligations to give, to receive, and to reciprocate. A gift from the client to the nurse may be an attempt to restore balance and to achieve greater reciprocity between client and nurse. Alternatively, a gift may have other meanings. Examined in this light, gift giving during the termination phase is an especially delicate matter that does not lend itself to absolute caveats but instead invites reflection. There is a difference between a gift given to convey a sincere thank you and a gift given to make the receiver feel guilty about leaving the relationship or even a gift that blocks a critical evaluation of the relationship. These are the issues that the nurse needs to assess. There is no one answer about whether gifts should or should not be exchanged. In fact, if the nurse handled every situation in the same fashion, the nurse would be denying the uniqueness of each nurse–client relationship. Each relationship has its own character and its own strengths and limitations, so that what might be appropriate in one situation would be totally inappropriate in another.

Some nurses are strongly opposed to ever accepting a gift from a client. Sometimes the agency or institution where the nurse is employed has policies prohibiting the accepting of gifts. In any event, regardless of the nurse's personal feelings or the policies of the employing agency, the nurse needs to identify his or her feelings about gift giving before the final interaction with the client. The nurse needs to be prepared to deal with this issue in a gentle and tactful way so that gift giving does not become a stumbling block to a positive termination. An approach that might prove helpful to nurses in refusing gifts is to reflect on all the intangible gifts that the client has given the nurse. The relationship itself, in which the client shares deep feelings and revelations of self, is indeed a beautiful and lasting gift. In turning down a material gift, nurses need to acknowledge the value of all that they have received from a client, thus reinforcing the worth of the client and of the relationship that they shared.

A last word about gift giving responds to the question, "What do I do?" The answer is not simple, but it involves being true to what you know and feel about the client, to assess the meaning of the gesture, and to use judgment in every situation. Most importantly, nurses must give freely of themselves. Exercise 8–6 may help in examining the issue of gift giving.

In addition to giving gifts, some clients will attempt to extend the relationship by requesting the nurse's telephone number or address so that they can "keep in touch." Clients may ask the nurse to either call or visit them. There are two possible explanations for this behavior. The client may not wish to conclude a meaningful relationship with the nurse, or the client may be testing the reliability of the nurse who has said that today is our last meeting.

Termination, as the word implies, should be final. To provide the client with a hint that the relationship will continue is most unfair. It keeps the client emotionally involved in a relationship that has no future. Nurses need to be clear that good-by means just that. This is a very difficult issue for nursing students who either see no harm in telling the client they will continue to keep in contact or who feel they have used the client for their own learning needs and to leave is grossly unfair. However, this perception underestimates the positive things that the client received from the relationship and denies the fact that good-bye, painful as they may be, are a part of life and certainly not new for the client or the nursing student.

## APPLICATIONS
### Nurses' Role in Facilitating Termination

Up to this point, the focus has been on the phases of termination and the feelings and behaviors

◆ Exercise 8–6. **Gift-Giving Role-Play**

**Purpose:** To help students develop therapeutic responses to clients who wish to give them gifts

**Situation:**
Mrs. Terrell, a hospice nurse, has taken care of Mr. Aitken during the last 3 months of his life. She has been very supportive of the family. Because of her intervention, Mr. Aitken and his son were able to resolve a long-standing and very bitter conflict before he died. The whole family is grateful to Mrs. Terrell, particularly his wife, for her special attention to Mr. Aitken.

**Procedure:**

*Role-Play Directions to Mrs. Aitken*
You are very grateful to Mrs. Terrell for all of her help over the past few months. Without her help, you do not know what you would have done. To show your appreciation, you would like her to have a $300 gift certificate at your favorite boutique. It is very important to you that Mrs. Terrell fully understand how meaningful her caring has been to you during this very difficult time.

*Role-Play Directions to Mrs. Terrell*
You have given the Aitken family high-quality care and you feel very good about it, particularly the role you played in helping Mr. Aitken and his son reconcile before Mr. Aitken's death. Respond as you think you might in this clinical situation, given the previous data.

**Discussion:**
1. Discuss the responses made in the role-playing situation.
2. Discuss other possible responses and evaluate the possible consequences.
3. Would you react differently if a client gave you a gift of $200 or a hand-crocheted scarf? If so, why?
4. Are there gifts the clients give a nurse that are intangible? How should these gifts be acknowledged?

---

that a client may exhibit in each phase. The nurse follows the nursing process in selecting appropriate termination strategies. In the assessment process, nurses need to examine their own feelings and reactions to endings in general and in terminating with a particular client. Termination should be mentioned well in advance of the actual ending of relationship. The client needs to be allowed to express feelings related to termination and to discuss the effects of the anticipated loss. Encouraging the client to deal with reactivated feelings from former losses and the nurse's constructive sharing of relevant personal feelings about the relationship and the termination facilitate the process. Together the nurse and client examine the meaning and value of the relationship, including negative as well as positive elements. Finally, there is a mutual evaluation of relationship goal achievement. Follow-up interventions are identified if needed (Koehne-Kaplan & Levy, 1978).

*Assessment*

The nurse needs to assess the client's response to the issue of termination and to be aware of both behavioral and affectional cues that the client communicates when the topic of termination is discussed. If possible, the nurse should ascertain the client's prior experiences with losses and learn how the client has coped with these losses. This information will help the nurse to plan an approach to termination that is individualized to this client.

In addition to assessing the client's feelings, behaviors, and past experiences in regard to termination, nurses must apply the same assessment process to themselves. They need to ask themselves, "In general, how do I feel about saying good-by?" Specifically, "how do I feel about saying good-by to this client?" Nurses need to examine their own reactions to past losses and how those experiences still affect their present behavior. Nurses also need to examine the relationship in terms of goal achievement and strengths and limitations. It is only after examining these issues that nurses can effectively guide the termination process.

### Analysis

Assessment of behaviors and feelings relative to termination provides the nurse with the basis for arriving at a nursing diagnosis. A number of diagnoses are appropriate to the termination process. These include

1. Anxiety related to impending termination of nurse–client relationship
2. Ineffective client coping (return of disabling symptoms) with impending termination of nurse–client relationship
3. Powerlessness related to impending termination of nurse–client relationship
4. Depression and sadness related to impending termination of nurse–client relationship
5. Grieving related to termination of nurse–client relationship
6. Alteration in self-concept related to impending termination of nurse–client relationship

### Plan

From the nursing diagnosis, the nurse derives a plan related to termination and develops objectives. Some of the plans and objectives are mutually decided between the nurse and the client; other aspects of the plan the nurse develops independently.

The nurse's independent responsibilities include planning the best time to inform the client of the termination date. If the relationship is a time-bounded one, in which the nurse knows ahead of time that he or she will have only a certain number of meetings with the client, then termination should be included in the original contract. In subsequent meetings, the nurse

needs to plan times to remind the client of the impending termination date.

If the termination of the relationship is open ended and is determined by the client's achievement of certain goals, then the nurse needs to plan an ongoing evaluation of goals, thus keeping the client up to date on the client's progress. In addition to goal evaluation, the nurse can be planning and informing the client about how much longer they will probably meet. If possible, terminations should never be a surprise.

The nurse must also plan how to deal with his or her own feelings about termination. Sometimes it is enough for the nurse to plan time to think about the issue of termination. At other times and in other relationships, the nurse must plan to talk to a supervisor or a peer about the feelings involved in termination so that these feelings do not interfere with the nurse's effectiveness with the client.

In planning mutually with clients, it is helpful for the nurse to ask clients how they would like to handle termination. Perhaps the client has specific ideas and feelings related to this process, and if so, these ideas and feelings should be included in the plan.

The planning phase also includes the establishment of specific behavioral goals. These goals are derived from the behaviors the nurse has collected and are directly related to the nursing diagnoses. Table 8–1 provides a listing of nursing diagnoses related to specific client goals.

### Interventions

Although the nurse intervenes with actions that are specific to client needs, there are eight general interventions that are appropriate to any planned termination. The first of these is to prepare clients for termination by informing them of the date (contract if possible) and reminding them of this date throughout the relationship. Keeping the date in mind allows clients to become aware of their own feelings, and it allows the nurse and client time to prepare adequately for termination.

The second intervention is to allow clients to express their feelings related to termination. The nurse must be aware of the client's readiness to discuss such feelings. If the client is in the denial phase, the nurse should not force the client to discuss those feelings until he or she is ready.

Table 8-1. **Nursing Diagnoses and Behavioral Goals in the Nurse–Client Relationship**

| NURSING DIAGNOSIS | CLIENT GOAL |
| --- | --- |
| Depression and sadness related to the impending termination of the nurse–client relationship | 1. The client will express feelings of sadness and relate them to termination.<br>2. The client will examine other experiences that have produced similar feelings.<br>3. The client will explore ways of coping with sadness and depression. |
| Grieving related to the termination of the nurse–client relationship | 1. The client will express feelings of loss related to termination.<br>2. The client will explore the positive and negative aspects of the relationship.<br>3. The client will examine how he or she coped with past experiences of loss.<br>4. The client will examine the availability of support to help cope with the loss. |
| Alteration in self-concept related to impending termination of the nurse–client relationship | 1. The client will examine how the relationship affected self-perception.<br>2. The client will examine how the termination affects self-concept. |
| Anxiety related to the impending termination of the nurse–client relationship | 1. The client will report a decrease in anxious feelings related to the discussion of termination.<br>2. The client will display a decrease in behaviors indicative of anxiety (nail biting, foot tapping) when termination is discussed. |
| Ineffective client coping (return of disabling symptoms) related to fear associated with the impending termination of the nurse–client relationship | 1. The client will express feelings of fear related to the impending termination.<br>2. The client will explore the relationship between symptom return and fear.<br>3. The client will identify alternative ways of coping with fear. |
| Feelings of powerlessness related to the impending termination of the nurse–client relationship | 1. The client will express feelings of powerlessness related to impending termination.<br>2. The client will examine related experience that produce similar feelings.<br>3. The client will explore ways to cope with feelings of powerlessness. |

However, the nurse may use interventions that gently confront the denial. A response such as, "It is difficult to talk about saying good-by and certainly easier to talk about the weather, isn't it?" acknowledges the client's denial without a head-on confrontation that may result in the erection of an insurmountable barrier of denial.

The third intervention is to encourage the client to experience and discuss the effects of the anticipated loss. The fourth intervention involves encouraging the client to deal with reactivated feelings from former losses. Questions such as, "As you think about saying good-by to me, are you reminded of other situations when you had to say good-by?", "What experiences are you reminded of when you were confronted with loss?" The fifth intervention involves the nurse's constructive sharing of his or her own feelings about the relationship and the termination. The sixth intervention involves examining the value of the relationship to both the client and the nurse, including both the positive and negative components. The seventh intervention includes mutually evaluating the goals of the relationship. Have goals been accomplished? If not, has progress been made? What work remains to be done?

The last intervention involves helping clients to identify supportive people in family, community, or work situations that can assist them with feelings of loss.

Koehne-Kaplan and Levy (1978) proposed a technique to assist the nurse and client to focus effectively on termination. This technique involves assigning both the nurse and the client homework and is shown in Box 8–5.

Different types of terminations require different strategies. The strategy chosen should correspond to the depth of the relationship. Deep, meaningful relationships require a longer termination, whereas the ending of a short-term relationship is best acknowledged by mutual identification of feelings related to the relationship and summarizing the goal achievement.

Terminations, especially of deep, meaningful relationships, are both here and now experiences and have the capacity to reactivate feelings associated with the earliest losses experienced by an individual, as expressed in the following quote from John Berger.

*When we suffer anguish, we return to early childhood because that is the period in which we first learnt to suffer the experience of total loss. It was more than that. It was the period in which we suffered more total losses than in all of the rest of our life put together. (Berger, 1967, p. 122)*

How an individual is able to handle the feelings aroused by termination provides a good measure of the individual's maturity and psychological well-being. For this reason, termination can be a significant aspect of the nurse–client relationship.

A final suggestion for handling the last interaction between the nurse or client is for both participants to graph or map out their experience, depicting the high and low points of their time together. This technique is helpful in summarizing the accomplishments and the feelings associ-

---

### ◆ Box 8–5. Assignment to Facilitate Termination

1. Before we meet again, I want each of us to take some time to be alone, as much time as we choose but no less than a half-hour. We must plan for this time well so that we ensure we are undisturbed and undistracted.

2. Give careful thought to the place and the time of day you choose for this time alone. Plan well so that nothing deprives you of this time and this time alone is exactly the way you want it to be. Most importantly, spend this time alone. I will do this too.

3. While alone, let yourself reminisce about our relationship. Recall the first session we had together and review historically any moments that come clear to you. Give yourself the luxury of staying with these moments as long as you want. Ask yourself, "What has this experience been for me? What has touched me?" Most importantly, think about you in this relationship and feel whatever feelings come up inside you. I will do this, too.

4. Next, while you are alone, let yourself imagine or fantasize how you want the last session to be. Include as many details as possible. At first, this may be very difficult. Stay with the task, nevertheless, allowing yourself to think and feel whatever comes to you. I will do this too.

5. Having done this imagining, practice this scene. So many of us have never had a satisfactory good-by. Allow thoughts and feelings of previous partings to come to you. How were they? How do you want this one to be? You and I must say good-by. Practice your chosen scene for our parting over and over, changing or modifying until your image of the last session is perfect for you. I will do this too.

From Koehne-Kaplan NS, Levy KE. (1978). An approach for facilitating the passage through termination. Journal of Psychiatric Nursing 16:11. Reprinted with permission.

Table 8-2. **The Nursing Process: One Diagnosis**

| NURSING DIAGNOSIS | GOAL | INTERVENTION | EVALUATION | MODIFICATION |
|---|---|---|---|---|
| Depression and sadness over the loss of the nurse–client relationship | Client will verbally express feeling of sadness related to loss. | 1. Using therapeutic communication skills, the nurse will: Show warmth Display empathy Reflect on client's affect of sadness and ask for client validation | Client acknowledges feeling of sadness but does not want to discuss them at this time. | 1. Look for cues of client readiness to discuss feeling of sadness. 2. Reflect on sadness without pressuring client to discuss until ready. 3. Communicate understanding that feelings are sometimes difficult to discuss. |

ated with the nurse–client relationship (Tilden & Gustafsen, 1979).

Although the last step of the nursing process is generally presented as the evaluation phase, to do so is misleading because evaluation is an ongoing process. The nurse continually evaluates and assesses to determine whether he or she has been accurate in analyzing the client's behaviors and feelings related to termination. If not, then the nurse collects more behaviors and perhaps analyzes the data differently. Likewise, the goals are also continually evaluated not only for goal attainment but also for the appropriateness of the goals to the client's needs.

Interventions are also evaluated in terms of their effectiveness. Did the interventions help the client talk about feelings of sadness and loss? If not, what modification is necessary? Table 8–2 illustrates the complete nursing process applied to one nursing diagnosis.

## SUMMARY

Chapter 8 describes the experience of grief that accompanies life's losses. Although grief and loss are universal experiences, they profoundly impact on us. It is essential for nurses to approach grief and loss both from a theoretical perspective, clearly understanding expected stages and behaviors, and an experiential perspective, understand-

ing their own feelings and responses to loss and grief. This combined perspective provides the nurse with a wisdom that allows him or her to help clients as they grapple with a variety of losses. The nurse is attuned to the issue of loss and unresolved grief and offers therapeutic suggestions to the client and family. Additionally, the nurse is aware of the feelings of grief that can accompany the ending of a meaningful nurse–client relationship. Out of this awareness the nurse plans interventions to facilitate this leave taking. So often, losses and having to say good-by leave us with regrets. We wish we could have said more, given more, and somehow been able to feel less pain. Part of the nurse's role, through compassionate communication, presence, and anticipatory guidance, is to diminish those regrets and to ease the grief of loss. It is both a blessing and a challenge to the nurse to be able to share and participate in a client's deepest and most meaningful life experiences, including the experience of loss.

## REFERENCES

Berger J. (1967). A Fortunate Man: The Story of a Country Doctor. New York: Holt, Rinehart, and Winston.

Carson VB. (1997). Spiritual needs of the caregiver. Seminars in Oncology Nursing 13(4):271–274.

Carson VB, Arnold EN. (1996). Mental Health Nursing: The Nurse-Patient Journey. Philadelphia, WB Saunders.

Carter S. (1989). Themes of Grief. Nursing Research, November/December, 18(6):354–358.

Chenitz WC. (1992). Living with AIDS. In Flaskerud JH, Ungvarski PJ (eds.), HIV/AIDS: A Guide To Nursing Care. Philadelphia, WB Saunders.

Comana MT, Brown VM, Thomas JD. (1998). The effect of reminiscence therapy on family coping. Journal of Family Nursing 4(2):182–197.

Companiello J. (1980). The process of termination. Journal of Psychiatric Nursing Mental Health Services 1(1):29.

Engel G. (1964). Grief and grieving. American Journal of Nursing 64(7): 93–96.

Gyulay JE. (1989). Grief responses. Issues in Comprehensive Pediatric Nursing 12:1–31.

Jacik M. (1996). Loss along the journey. In Carson VB, Arnold EN (eds.), Mental Health Nursing: The Nurse Patient Journey. Philadelphia, WB Saunders, pp. 661–668.

Kellar MH. (1983). What is it like to be dying? Nursing '83 13:65.

Koehne-Kaplan NS, Levy KE. (1978). An approach for facilitating the passage through termination. Journal of Psychiatric Nursing 16:11.

Kübler-Ross E. (1971). What is it like to be dying? American Journal of Nursing 71:54.

Lewis CS. (1963): A Grief Observed. Greenwich, CT, Seabury Press.

Lindemann E. (1944). Symptomatology and management of acute grief. American Journal of Psychiatry 101:141.

O'Neill DP, Kenny EK. (1998). Spirituality and chronic illness. Image 30(3):275–280.

Stearns A. (1984). Living Through Personal Crisis. Chicago, The Thomas Moore Press.

Tilden VP, Gustafsen L. (1979). Termination in the student-patient relationship: Use of a teaching tool. Journal of Nursing Education 18:9.

Wolfelt A. (1991). Toward an understanding of complicated grief: A comprehensive overview. The American Journal of Hospice and Palliative Care Fall:28–30.

## Electronic References

http://dir.yahoo.com/Health/Mental_Health/Bereavement (lists Education and Support Services).

## PART III

# Therapeutic Communication

# 9

# Communication Styles

## Kathleen Underman Boggs

**OBJECTIVES**

At the end of the chapter, the student will be able to

1. Describe the component systems of communication
2. Cite examples of body cues that convey nonverbal messages
3. Identify cultural implications of communication
4. Describe the effects of gender on the communication process
5. Define interpersonal competence
6. Identify five communication style factors that influence the nurse–client relationship

*Communication is a core task in coordinating patient care.*

Anderson and Helms (1998, p. 255).

❖❖ Chapter 9 explores styles of communication as a basis for applying communication skills and strategies in the nurse–client relationship. The clues a client provides through gestures, vocal tones, body movements, and facial expressions help make sense out of the client's words. Sharpening observational skills to gather data needed for nursing assessments, diagnosis, and intervention is of special value to the nurse in planning care for clients. Knowledge of communication styles allows a more client-centered, goal-directed approach to resolving difficult health care issues. Both clients and nurses enter their relationship with their own specific styles of communication. Some individuals depend on a mostly verbal style to convey their meaning, whereas others rely on nonverbal strategies to send the message. Some communicators emphasize giving information; others prioritize conveying interpersonal sensitivity.

## BASIC CONCEPTS
### Metacommunication

*Communication* is a complex composite of verbal and nonverbal behaviors integrated for the purpose of sharing information (Crowther, 1991). Within the nurse–client relationship, any exchange of information between the two individuals also carries messages about how to interpret the communication.

*Metacommunication* is a broad term used to describe all of the factors that influence how the message is perceived (Fig. 9–1). An example is the "play fighting" observed in animals and children. Bateson noted that for an organism to "play" at fighting, it must both appear to be fighting and simultaneously appear not to be actually fighting but merely simulating. This message about how to interpret what is going on is metacommunication (Mitchell, 1991). Metacommunicated messages may be hidden within verbalizations or be conveyed as nonverbal gestures and expressions. The following case example should clarify this concept.

### ◆ Case Example

In their 1997 study, Patch and associates found that there was greater compliance to requests when they were accompanied by a metacommunication message that demanded a response about the appropriateness of this request:

**Student:**   We are trying to encourage community awareness in promoting environmental health and are looking for people to hand out fliers. Would you be willing?

**[metacommunication]:**   I realize that this is a

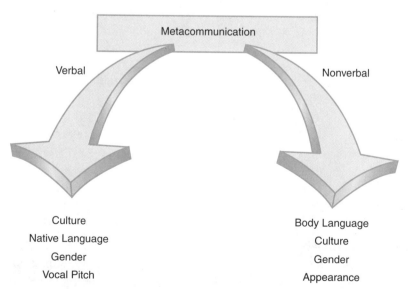

Figure 9–1. Factors in communication styles.

Metacommunication

Verbal                    Nonverbal

Culture                   Body Language
Native Language           Culture
Gender                    Gender
Vocal Pitch               Appearance

strange request seeing that you do not know who I am but I would really appreciate your help. I hope I am not pressuring you, if so please tell me.

Metacommunication in the nurse–client conversation conveys messages about how to interpret meaning through both verbal and nonverbal clues. For example, the nurse conveys a message of caring to her white, middle-class client during their conversation verbally by making appropriate, encouraging responses and nonverbally by maintaining direct eye contact, presenting a smooth face without frowning, and using a relaxed, fluid body posture without fidgeting.

In a professional relationship, verbal and nonverbal components of communication are intimately related. A student studying American Sign Language for the deaf was surprised that it was not sufficient merely to make the sign for "smile," but rather she had to actually show a smile at the same time. This congruence helped convey her message. Some researchers testing language comprehension in primates wear a face mask to avoid inadvertently giving the primate a nonverbal clue from their facial expression.

The nurse nonverbally communicates acceptance, interest, and respect for the client through eye contact, body posture, head nodding at pivotal points in the conversation, and frequent smiling. Studies of nurses' touching of clients has been reported to be perceived both positively as an expression of caring and negatively as a method of control (Mulaik et al., 1991). You need to help the client understand and assimilate the discrepancy so that content can be dealt with directly. For example, when you enter a room to ask Mr. Salsa if he is having any postoperative pain, he says "no" but grimaces and clutches his incision. You comment on the incongruent message, and he admits he is having some discomfort. When nonverbal cues are incongruent with the verbal information, messages are likely to be misinterpreted.

## Verbal Communication

Words are symbols used by people to think about ideas, to share experiences with others, and to validate the meaning of perceptions about the world and one's place in it. Without the use of spoken language, people would be severely limited in their ability to classify and order information in ways that can be understood by self and others. Choice of words is influenced by many factors, including one's age, race, socioeconomic group, educational background, and gender and by the situation in which the communication is taking place.

The interpretation of the meaning of words may vary according to the individual's background and experiences. It is dangerous to assume that words have the same meaning for all persons that hear them. Language is useful only to the extent that it accurately reflects the experience it is designed to portray. Consider, for example, the difficulty an American has communicating with a person who speaks only Vietnamese, the dilemma of the young child with a limited vocabulary trying to tell you where it hurts, or the anguish of the Alzheimer's disease patient who is desperately attempting to communicate, using words that no longer have an understandable meaning.

There are two levels of meaning in language: denotation and connotation. Both are affected by culture (Samovar & Porter, 1985). *Denotation* refers to the generalized meaning assigned to a word, whereas *connotation* points to a more personalized meaning of the word or phrase (Berko et al., 1981). For example, most people would agree that a dog is a four-legged creature, frequently domesticated, with a characteristic vocalization referred to as a bark. This would be the denotative or explicit meaning of the word. When the word is used in a more personalized way, it reveals the connotative level of meaning. "What a dog" and "His bark is worse than his bite" are phrases some people use to describe personal characteristics of a human being rather than a four-legged creature. Translating such phrases for individuals not familiar with their connotation requires explanation of their more personalized meaning. The nurse should be aware that many communications convey only a part of the intended meaning. One should never assume that the meaning of a message is the same for the sender and the receiver until mutual understanding is verified. For example, a 3-year-old child remarked to her mother, who was pregnant at the time, that the mother was getting fat. The mother, assuming the child was referring to changes associated with the pregnancy, launched into an elaborate, theoretically correct explanation of why she was fat. "But, that's not what I meant, Mommy!" her daughter said. "I meant your legs are getting fat." Mother and child were talking to each other, but they were not communicating about the same issue. The best way we can be sure we are getting our message across is to ask for feedback (Telles, 1995).

### Cultural Implications in Spoken Language

According to Giger and Davidhizar (1990b), many nurses lack an understanding of communication principles and the techniques necessary to communicate effectively with clients from backgrounds other than their own. Chapter 11 deals in depth with intercultural communication concepts. Communicating with clients from other ethnic and socioeconomic groups within the American culture also presents some challenges. To communicate as a culturally competent professional, you need to have developed an awareness of the values of a specific client's culture, adapt your style and skills to be compatible with that culture's norms (Campinha-Bacote, 1997).

**Other Cultural Variables.** Language is culturally specific not only to ethnic, geographical, and religious groups but, to a lesser degree, specific occupational and age groups. For example, entering a nursing program entails learning new language sets and new word connotations. The students' initial feelings of being overwhelmed are quite similar to those of any person entering a new and poorly understood culture. Developing an awareness of potential communication differences is the first step toward effective cross-cultural communication. Exercises in Chapter 11 will help develop these skills.

### English as a Second Language

Some people speaking English as a second language say the most difficult aspect is trying to translate expressions for which there is no equivalent English meaning. For others it is the many slang terms, phrases that have double meanings. Many who learn English as an adult continue to think in their native language, translating words into a more familiar dialect before processing in or out. Extra time needs to be allowed for information processing, especially when clients are experiencing emotional tension and are more likely to rely on their native language to assist them in sending and receiving information. Verification of message content is even more essential with clients from different cultural backgrounds to make sure that nuances of language do not get lost. *When speaking with a client who uses English as a second language, allow time between messages.* Use planned spaces of silence, which allow them time to understand your meaning and to prepare a response.

### Slang and Jargon

Different age groups in the same culture may attribute different meanings to the same word. For example, an adult who says, "That's cool" might be referring to the temperature, whereas a teenager might convey his satisfaction by using the term "cool." In health care, the "food pyramid" is understood by nurses to represent the basic nutritional food groups needed for health. However, the term may have limited meaning for individuals not in the health professions.

For successful communication, the words used should have a similar meaning to both individuals in the interaction. An important part of the communication process is the search with the client for a common vocabulary so that the message sent is the same as the one received.

### Pitch and Tone in Vocalization

The oral delivery of a verbal message, expressed through tone of voice and inflection, sighing, or crying, is referred to as ***paralanguage.*** It is important to understand this component of communication because it affects how the verbal message is likely to be interpreted. For example, the nurse might say, "I would like to hear more about what you are feeling" in a voice that sounds rushed, high-pitched, or harsh. The same statement might be made in a soft, unhurried voice that expresses genuine interest. In the first instance, the message is likely to be misinterpreted by the client, despite the good intentions of the nurse; the caring intent of the nurse's message is more apparent to the client in the second instance. Voice inflection suggests mood and either supports or contradicts the content of the verbal message. When the tone of voice does not fit the words, the message is less easily understood and is likely to be discounted. For example, expressing anger in a flat tone of voice as though the matter is of no consequence contradicts the meaning of the message and the intensity of the emotion the individual is feeling. Thus, it is very difficult for the person receiving the message to respond appropriately. A message conveyed in a firm, steady tone is more reassuring than one conveyed in a loud, abrasive, or uncertain manner.

**Vocalization Variations.** Culturally specific modes of emotional expression can sometimes confuse as well as clarify the meaning of a verbal message. The vocal emphasis given to certain sounds and tone modulations is in part culturally determined. In some cultures, sounds are punctuated, whereas in others sounds have a lyrical or singsong quality. Contrast, for example, the vocalization of an Oriental client with that of a German or Spanish client. The vocal inflections are quite different. Nurses need to orient themselves to the characteristic voice tones associated with different cultures to avoid being distracted by them in the process of communication. The tone of voice used to express anger and other emotions varies according to culture and family. For example, it is sometimes difficult for an American nurse to tell when someone from an Indian or Oriental culture is angry because vocalization of strong emotion is more controlled than in most Western cultures. By contrast, a Latin American's vocalization may seem more angry than it is intended to be because of the characteristic Latin emotional intensity of verbal expression. Through repeated interaction with clients, the nurse learns to understand the message the client is trying to communicate. Chapter 11 discusses nonverbal cultural communication in detail.

## Gender Differences in Verbal Communication

Many studies have found differences between men and women in both the content and the process of communication. In health care communication, there is evidence to suggest that more effective communication occurs when the provider of the care and the client are of the same gender (Weisman & Teitelbaum, 1989), although this was not found to be true in other studies (Collier, 1993). In general, men have been shown to use less verbal communication than women in interpersonal relationships (Juang & Tucker, 1991). Among the many gender differences noted in relation to verbal communication is that women tend to disclose more personal information than men. Men, on the other hand, are more likely to interrupt, to use hostile verbs, and to talk more about issues (Cotton-Huston, 1989). In the professional health care setting, women have been noted to use more active listening, using encouraging responses such as "uh-huh," "yeah," and "I see," and to use more supportive words (Bernzweig et al., 1997; Hall et al., 1994).

Studies indicate that women have a greater range of pitch and also tend to use different informal patterns of vocalization than men. Females use more tones signifying surprise, cheerfulness, unexpectedness, and politeness (Cotton-Huston, 1989). Exercise 9–1 should be used to stimulate discussions about whether there is gender bias in communication.

## Nonverbal Communication

The vast majority of person-to-person communication is picked up by monitoring subtle nonverbal communication (Cooper, 1990). The function of nonverbal communication is to give us cues about what is being communicated. Channels for nonverbal communication include facial expression, eye movements, body movements, posture, gestures, touch, and proxemics (Garrud, 1993).

Physicians and nurses use nonverbal communication to build rapport with clients. Observing the client's nonverbal behavior may reveal vital information that will affect the nurse–client relationship. For example, worried facial expression and lip biting may suggest an anxious client. Assessing the extent to which the client uses nonverbal cues to communicate emotions helps you communicate better. Assessment of nonverbal behaviors and their meanings must be verified with the client, because body language, although suggestive, is imprecise. When communication is limited by the client's health state, the nurse

---

◆ Exercise 9–1. **Gender Bias**

**Purpose:** To create discussion about gender bias

**Procedure:**
In small groups, read and discuss the following. Gilloran (1995) listed the following as comments made about care delivery on a geriatric psychiatric unit by staff and students: "male staff tend to be slightly more confident and to make quicker decisions. Women staff are better at the feeling things like (conveying) warmth."

**Discussion:**
1. Were these comments made by male or female staff?
2. How accurate are they?
3. Can you truly generalize any attribute to all "males" and "females"?

---

should pay even closer attention to nonverbal cues. Pain, for example, can be assessed through facial expression, even when the client is only partially conscious (Enlow & Swisher, 1986).

## Proxemics

Proxemics is the use of space, commonly referred to as **body language.** Words direct the content of a message, whereas emotions accentuate and clarify the meaning of the words. Often the emotional component of a message is communicated indirectly through body language. Although there is potential for misreading nonverbal cues, researchers have demonstrated that nonverbal behavior can be correctly used to make accurate inferences about a person (Gifford, 1991).

Generally, nonverbal manifestations of communication are considered useful for expressive and social communication (Harrison, 1989) and may be more reliable than their verbal counterparts. To be effective, nonverbal behavior should be congruent with and reinforce the verbal message. For example, if Mark Beam, RN, smiles as he tells his manager that his assignment is more than he can handle, he negates the seriousness of the message (Raudsepp, 1991). Nonverbal behaviors may be seen as a one-time or occasional occurrence or as part of a generalized pattern of behavior in communication. Knowing the client's usual nonverbal pattern of communication is important in assessing the nature and meaning of changes in behavior.

## Cultural Variations in Nonverbal Communication

Most nonverbal behaviors are culturally specific and contextually bound. They are learned unconsciously through observation of the behaviors of significant people. Sometimes a nonverbal gesture you find acceptable may be perceived as rude in another culture. For example, the nurse meant to signal approval to her Brazilian client by putting thumb and index finger into a circle for "okay," but in Brazil this is considered an obscene gesture! Cultural taboos can inhibit nonverbal behaviors. For example, different cultures have distinct rules about eye contact. Some ethnic clients culturally tend to avoid eye contact when listening and to use it when speaking. The nurse who thinks the African-American or Appalachian client is inattentive to explanations because there is little eye contact during the conversation with the nurse may actually be experiencing a normal, culturally specific nonverbal behavior (Atkinson et al., 1985).

The meaning of *touching* varies across cultures. For example, some Native Americans use touch in healing, so that casual touching may be taboo (Giger & Davidhizar, 1990b). Of course, gender also influences the client's perception of the meaning of being touched. In primary health care, nurses' touch is an important component of assessment. The nurse uses touch to convey caring. Some nurses use "therapeutic touch," harnessing energy fields to promote healing. All nurses caring directly for clients use touch to assist. Their touching contact helps the client walk, roll over in bed, and so on. However, care needs to be taken about when and where on the body clients are touched so that use of touch is not open to misinterpretation (Helm et al., 1997).

### Effects of Gender on Nonverbal Communication

Gender differences in communication have been shown to be greatest in terms of use and interpretation of nonverbal cues (Hyde, 1990). This may reflect gender differences in intellectual style as well as culturally reinforced standards of acceptable role-related behaviors. Women tend to demonstrate more effective use of nonverbal communication and are better decoders of nonverbal meaning (Cotton-Huston, 1989; Keeley-Dyreson et al., 1991). Women tend to use more facial expressiveness, smiling more often, maintaining eye contact, and touching more often (Hall et al., 1994). Wollard's research on Spanish girls' social groups found they tended toward smaller and much more homogeneous social groups compared with the types of groups used by boys (1997). Empirical studies have shown men prefer a greater interpersonal distance between themselves and others. Western men freely use gestures, whereas women are taught at a young age to keep their arms, hands, and legs close to their bodies.

### Interpreting Nonverbal Body Cues and Facial Expressions

*Posture*, rhythm of movement, and gestures accompanying a verbal message are other nonverbal behaviors associated with the overall process of communication. Body stance may convey a message about the speaker. For example, speaking while directly facing a person conveys more confidence than turning one's body at an angle (Duryea, 1991). A slumped, head-down posture and slow movements give an impression of lassitude or low self-esteem, whereas an erect posture and decisive movements suggest confidence and self-control. Rapid, diffuse, agitated body movements may indicate anxiety. Vigorous, directed actions may suggest confidence and purpose. More force with less focused direction in body movements may symbolize anger.

*Eye contact* and *facial expressions* appear to be particularly important in signaling our feelings (Cooper, 1990; Harrison, 1989). Throughout life, individuals respond to the expressive qualities of another's face, often without even being aware of it. Research suggests that individuals who make direct eye contact while talking or listening create a sense of confidence and credi-

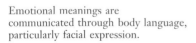

Emotional meanings are communicated through body language, particularly facial expression.

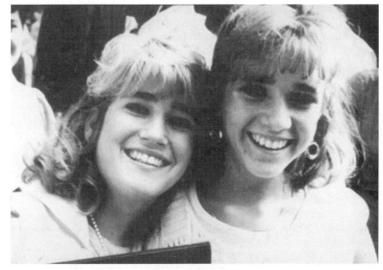

bility, whereas downward glances or averted eyes signal submission, weakness, or shame (Duryea, 1991). We speak of a person as having an open expression or a kind face. Almost instinctively, individuals use facial expression as a barometer of another person's feelings, motivations, approachability, and mood.

*Facial expression* is important in conveying a message. It connects the words presented in the message and the internal dialogue of the speaker. Facial expression either reinforces or modifies the message the listener hears. When the verbal message is inconsistent with the nonverbal expression of the message, the nonverbal expressions assume prominence and generally are perceived as more trustworthy than the verbal content. Mehrabian (1971), in a simulated study of the impact of words, vocalization, and facial expression on the receiver, noted that the power of the facial expression supporting the verbal content far outweighs the power of the actual words.

Six photos of common facial expressions are presented in Figure 9–2. The examples represent global, generalized interpretations of facial expressions. Although facial expression is often a strong indicator of emotional response to a situation, there are exceptions. Some clients control their facial expressions by masking the underlying emotion completely or by expressing it in a different way. A smile may be used to express joy or pleasure, or it may cover other emotions that cannot be expressed. A stoic facial expression and limited affect may hide the intense vulnerability a client is actually feeling when facing a potentially overwhelming situation. In an assessment of facial expression, the nurse notes a *lack* of appropriate facial expression as well as evidence of strong emotion in the facial expression. Because the eyes and corners of the mouth are least susceptible to control, they may provide the most informative data to support or contradict the overall communication picture the client presents.

### ◆ Case Example

A client smiles but narrows his eyes and glares at the nurse. An appropriate comment for the nurse to make might be, "I notice you are smiling when you say you would like to kill me for mentioning your fever to the doctor. It seems that you might be angry with me."

## Clothing as a Nonverbal Message

Everyone is familiar with sayings like "Dress for success." The business world has long noted the role clothing plays in conveying an image of a serious professional. Mangum and associates (1991) surveyed clients, nurses, and administrators to determine whether different styles of nursing uniforms are associated with variations in the professional image of nursing. Findings supported client preference for traditional white uniforms (with nurse caps). Lab coats conveyed a less professional image, as did colored uniforms, scrub clothes, and so on. Most modern nurses have discarded the "dust cap" of previous dress codes. As more men enter the profession of nursing and traditional nursing is replaced by a wider variation in acceptable professional attire, nurses are being defined more by what they do than by what they wear. Exercise 9–2 is designed to help you reflect on nonverbal perceptions of professionalism in the nurse–client relationship.

## APPLICATIONS
## Knowing Your Own Communication Style

The style of communication used by the health provider can influence client behavior, especially their compliance with treatment (Dunbar-Jacob, 1993). Exercises in prior chapters should give you basic skills used in the nurse–client relationship, but you bring your own communication style with you, as does your client. Because we differ widely in our personal communication style, it is important to identify our style and understand how to modify it for certain clients. Personality characteristics influence your style. For example, would you be described as more shy or assertive? One nurse might be characterized as "bubbly," whereas another is thought of as having a "quiet" manner. Just so, clients have various styles. Your two styles need to be compatible. Think about the potential for incompatibility in the following case.

### ◆ Case Example

**Nurse** [speaking in a firm tone]:  Mr. Ruth, it is time to take your medicine!

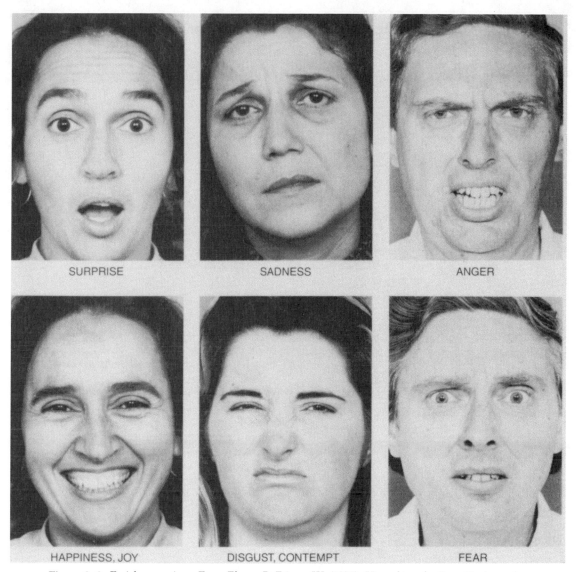

SURPRISE        SADNESS        ANGER

HAPPINESS, JOY        DISGUST, CONTEMPT        FEAR

Figure 9–2. Facial expressions. From Ekman P, Friesen W. (1975). Unmasking the Face. Englewood Cliffs, NJ, Prentice Hall. Used with permission.

**Mr. R.** [complaining tone]:   You are so bossy.

**How Others Perceive You.** Consider all the nonverbal factors that affect a client's perception of you. Your gender, manner of dress, appearance, skin tone, hair style, age, role as a student, gestures, or confident mannerisms may make a difference. Did Exercise 9–2 help you think about this?

The initial step in identifying your own style may be to compare your style with that of others. Ask yourself "What makes a client perceive a nurse as authoritarian or as accepting and caring?" Exercise 9–3 on videotaping may help you to compare your style with that of others. A next step is to develop an awareness of alternative styles that you can comfortably assume if the occasion warrants. Next, it is important to fig-

---

◆ Exercise 9–2. **Nurses' Clothing as Nonverbal Communication**

**Purpose:** To stimulate thinking about nonverbal messages
Clothing communicates a nonverbal message about competence and professionalism to a client, which can influence the nurse–client relationship. Mangum et al. (1991), in describing the conclusions of their study, wrote, "The nurse is judged primarily by what is worn and presented as professional at the bedside" (p. 130).

**Procedure:**
1. Name some of the external symbols of nursing.
2. Take two photographs of yourself: one in uniform and one in some unusual hairstyle and mode of dress. Show the pictures to three strangers, and ask them which one they think you should put on your job resume.

**Discussion:**
1. If you were taking a picture for public relations purposes, how would you dress the nurse?
2. What would different items of clothing suggest about you as a nurse?
3. Are people influenced by skin color, style of hair, dress, and jewelry, for example?

---

ure out whether some other factors influence whether your style is appropriate for a particular client. How might their age, race, socioeconomic status, or gender effect their response to you?

## Interpersonal Competence

Communication is a process through which the nurse can establish a human-to-human relationship and fulfill the purpose of nursing. Through effective communication, the nurse can help individuals and families prevent and cope with the experience of illness and suffering and, if necessary, can assist them in finding meaning in these experiences.

Kasch (1984) proposed that nurse–client communication processes are based on the nurse's interpersonal competence. *Interpersonal competence* develops as the nurse comes to understand the complex cognitive, behavioral, and cultural factors that influence communication. This understanding, together with the use of a broad range of communication skills, helps the nurse interact with the client as he or she attempts to cope with the many demands placed on him or her by the environment.

In dealing with the client in the sociocultural context of the health care system, two kinds of abilities are required. *Social cognitive competency* is the ability to interpret message content

---

◆ Exercise 9–3. **Self-Analysis of Videotape**

**Purpose:** To increase awareness of own style

**Procedure:**
Obtain a partner to role-play the client. Videotape a 5-minute interview with the camera focused on yourself. Topic of the interview could be identifying "health promotion behaviors" and so on.

**Discussion:**
What posture did you use? What nonverbal messages did you communicate? How? Were your verbal and nonverbal messages congruent?

within interactions from the point of view of each of the participants. By embracing the client's perspective, the nurse begins to understand how the client organizes information and formulates goals. *Message competency* refers to the ability to use language and nonverbal behaviors strategically in the intervention phase of the nursing process to achieve the goals of the interaction (Harrison, 1989; Kasch, 1984). Communication skills are then used as a tool to influence the client to maximize his or her adaptation.

## Style Factors Influencing Relationships

Having a knowledge of communication styles is not sufficient to guarantee successful application. The nurse needs to understand the interconnected relationships among intangible aspects of the communicators in the relationship. Box 9–1 lists some communication styles that increase or decrease involvement.

### Responsiveness of Participants

How responsive the participants are affects the depth and breadth of communication. Some clients are naturally more verbal than others. It is easier to have a therapeutic conversation with extroverted clients who want to communicate. The nurse will want to increase the responsiveness of less verbal clients, and there are many ways to enhance communication responsiveness. Verbal and nonverbal approval encourages clients to express themselves. Therapeutic skills and strategies that promote responsiveness include active listening, demonstration of empathy, and acknowledgment of the content and feelings of messages. Sometimes acknowledging the difficulty a client is having expressing certain feelings, praising efforts, and encouraging use of more than one route of communication helps. Such strategies demonstrate interpersonal sensitivity. A responsive care provider has been shown to improve compliance with the treatment regimen and to be preferred by clients themselves (Dunbar-Jacob, 1993; Worchell et al., 1995).

### Roles of Participants

Paying attention to the role relations surrounding the content is just as important as deciphering the meaning of the message (Northouse & Northouse, 1992). The relationships between the roles of the sender and of the receiver influence how the communication is likely to be received and interpreted. The same constructive criticism made by a good friend and by one's immediate supervisor is likely to be interpreted differently, even though the content of both messages may be quite similar and both are delivered in a similar manner. The quality of the relationship will be harmed if the nurse fails to follow through on verbal commitments, fails to pay attention to details, is uncertain or lacks experience, or attempts to reassure without documentation. Many studies, including that of Giannantonio et al. (1995), show that communication between subordinates and their supervisor is far more likely to be influenced by power and style than by gender. When roles are unequal in terms of power, the more powerful individual tends to speak in a more dominant style (Simkins-Bullock & Wildman, 1991). This is discussed in Chapter 22.

### Validation of Individual Worth

Styles that convey "caring" send a message of individual worth that sustains the relationship with the client. For example, in a study of physician providers, a "warm" communication style resulted in more information being shared by the client (Gerbert et al., 1997). Another study of children with birth defects showed that parents want a provider to show caring, to give information, and to allow them time to talk about their own feelings (Strauss et al., 1995).

Confirming responses validate the intrinsic worth of the person. These are responses that affirm the right of the individual to be treated with respect. They also affirm the participant's right ultimately to make his or her own decisions. For example, in a nurse–client relationship, the nurse acts deliberately to accept and confirm the humanity of the client.

Disconfirming responses, on the other hand, disregard the validity of feelings by either ignoring them or imposing a value judgment. Such responses take the form of changing the topic, offering reassurance without supporting evidence, or presuming to know what a client means without verifying the message with the client. In a study of communication interactions between nurses and physicians, Garvin and

### Box 9-1. Behavioral Communication Styles in Nurse–Client Relationships

**To Increase Involvement**

Nurse demonstrates commitment.

- Responds to client as an individual
- Uses close physical distance
- Gives time to the client
- Establishes common ground
- Anticipates needs

Nurse shows perseverance.

- Gets to know client's family
- Follows through on promises and goals

Nurse acts as an advocate.

- Becomes involved
- Connects the client with the system
- Acts as a buffer or go-between
- Adapts or bends rules to meet client's needs

Client tests behavior.

Is nurse a "good person"?

- Tests for dependability
- Evaluates "likability"
- Requests personal disclosures

Is nurse a "good nurse"?

- Obtains information from other clients
- Looks for indicators of empathy
- Evaluates competency
- Tests for ability to keep a confidence

Client makes overtures.

- Acts like "a good patient"
- Is friendly, jokes
- Seeks time with nurse

Client makes decision to trust.

- Conversation content less social, more meaningful
- Relinquishes vigilance

**To Decrease Involvement**

Nurse depersonalizes the client.

- Refers to client by bed number or diagnosis
- Uses formal terms of address
- Has no time to talk

Nurse maintains superefficient attitude.

- Gives impression of business
- Interactions focus on physical care
- Ignores emotional behavior and cues that client wants to discuss difficult questions
- Does not provide meaningful information to client about condition

Nurse does not trust client.

- Suspects ulterior motives
- Keeps client "in the dark"

Client avoids therapeutic relationship.

- Does not self-disclose
- Is late or absent from scheduled meetings or activities
- Focuses conversation on symptoms rather than feelings

Client does not trust the nurse.

- Becomes overly manipulative
- Is demanding

Client expresses discomfort nonverbally.

- Avoids direct eye contact
- Fidgets when conversation "gets personal"
- Refuses to talk
- Turns head or body away from nurse

Kennedy (1988) found that more experienced nurses used more confirming communication than did younger, less experienced nurses. These findings suggest that communication skills are learned.

### Context of the Message

Communication is always influenced by the environment in which it takes place. It does not occur in a vacuum but is shaped by the situation in which the interaction occurs. Taking time to evaluate the physical setting and the time and space in which the contact takes place, as well as the psychological, social, and cultural characteristics of each individual involved, gives the nurse flexibility in choosing the most appropriate context (Weaver, 1984).

## Involvement in the Relationship

Relationships generally need to develop over time because communication changes with different phases of the relationship. In these days of managed care, nurses working with hospitalized clients have less time to develop a relationship, whereas community-based nurses may have greater opportunities. Reexamine the behaviors in Box 9–1 to decide which you could use to increase your client's involvement.

## SUMMARY

Communication between nurse and client or nurse and another professional involves more than the verbalized information exchanged. Professional communication, like personal communication, is subtly altered by changes in pitch of voice and use of accompanying facial expressions or gestures. This chapter explores factors related to effective styles of verbal and nonverbal communication. Cultural and gender differences associated with each of these three areas of communication are discussed. For professionals, maintaining congruence is important. Style factors affecting the communication process include the responsiveness and role relationships of the participants, the types of responses and context of the relationships, and the level of involvement in the relationship. Confirming responses acknowledge the value of a person's communication, whereas disconfirming responses discount the validity of a person's feelings. More nonverbal strategies to facilitate nurse–client communication are discussed in later chapters.

## REFERENCES

Anderson MA, Helms LB. (1998). Comparison of continuing care communication. Image 30(3):255–260.

Atkins CP. (1994). Does genderlect exist? The Clinical Supervisor 12(2):129–141.

Atkinson D, Morten G, Sue D. (1985). Minority group counseling. In Samovar L, Porter R (eds.), Intercultural Communication: A Reader (4th ed.). Belmont, CA, Wadsworth.

Berko R, Wolvin A, Wolvin D. (1981). Communicating: A Social and Career Focus (2nd ed.). Boston, Houghton Mifflin.

Berko R, Wolvin A, Wolvin D. (1988). Communicating: A Social and Career Focus (4th ed.). Boston, Houghton Mifflin.

Bernzweig J, Takayama J, Phibbs C, et al. (1997). Gender differences in physician-patient communication. Archives of Pediatric and Adolescent Medicine 151:586–591.

Brown KC. (1991). Strategies for effective communication. AAOHN Journal 39(6):292–293.

Campinha-Bacote J. (1997). Cultural competence: A critical factor in child health policy. Journal of Pediatric Nursing 12(4):260–262.

Canales M. (1997). Narrative interaction: Creating a space for therapeutic communications. Issues in Mental Health Nursing 18:477–494.

Collier JA, Vu NV, Marcy ML. (1993). Effects of examinee gender, standardized patient gender, and their interaction on standardized patients' ratings of examinees' interpersonal and communication skills. Academic Medicine 68(2):153–157.

Cooper MG. (1990). I saw what you said: Nonverbal communications and the EAP. Employee Assistance Quarterly 5(4):112.

Cotton Huston A. (1989). Gender communication. In King S (ed.), Human Communication as a Field of Study. Albany, State University of New York Press.

Courtney R, Rice C. (1997). Partnership action for healthy communities 22(2):46–48, 54–60.

Crowther D. (1991). Metacommunications: A missed opportunity? Journal of Psychosocial Nursing 29(4):1316.

Dunbar-Jacob J. (1993). Contributions to patient adherence. Health Psychology 12(2):91–92.

Duryea EJ. (1991). Principles of nonverbal communication in efforts to reduce peer and social pressure. Journal of School Health Nursing 61(1):5–10.

Ekman P, Friesen W. (1975). Unmasking the Face. Englewood Cliffs, NJ, Prentice Hall.

Enlow A, Swisher S. (1986). Interviewing and Patient Care (3rd ed.). New York, Oxford University Press.

Garrud P, Chapman IR, Gordon A, Herbert M. (1993). Nonverbal communication: Evaluation of a computer assisted learning package. Medical Education 27:474–478.

Garvin BJ, Kennedy CW. (1988). Confirming communication of nurses in interaction with physicians. Journal of Nursing Education 27:20–30.

Gerbert B, Johnston K, Bleecker T, Bronstone A. (1997). HIV risk assessment: A video doctor seeks patient disclosure. MD Computing 14(4):288–294.

Giannantonio C, Olian JD, Carroll SJ. (1995). An experimental study of gender and situational effects in a performance evaluation of a manager. Psychology Reports 76(3):1004–1006.

Gifford R. (1991). Mapping nonverbal behavior on the interpersonal circle. Journal of Personality and Social Psychology 61(2):279–288.

Giger JN, Davidhizar R. (1990a). Developing communication skills for use with Black patients. ABNF Journal 1(2):33–35.

Giger JN, Davidhizar R (1990b). Transcultural nursing assessment. International Nursing Review 37(1):199–202.

Gilloran A. (1995). Gender differences in care delivery and supervisory relationship. Journal of Advanced Nursing 21:652–658.

Hall JA, Irish JT, Roter D, et al. (1994). Gender in medical encounters: An analysis of physician and patient communication in a primary care setting. Health Psychology 13(5):384–392.

Harrison RP. (1989). Nonverbal communication. In King S (ed.), Human Communication as a Field of Study. Albany, State University of New York Press.

Helm JS, Kinfu D, Kline D, Zappelle M. (1997). Acquisition of a touching style and the clinicians use of touch in physical therapy. Journal of Physical Therapy Education 11(1):17–25.

Hyde JS. (1990). Meta-analysis and the psychology of gender differences. Signs 16(1):55–73.

Juang S, Tucker CM. (1991). Factors in marital adjustment and their interrelationships. Journal of Multicultural Counseling and Development 19(1):22–31.

Kasch CC. (1984). Communication in the delivery of nursing care. Advances in Nursing Science 6:71–88.

Keeley-Dyreson M, Burgoon J, Bailey W. (1991). Human Communication Research 17(4):584–585.

Mangum S, Garrison C, Lind A, et al. (1991). Perceptions of nurses' uniforms. Image 23:127.

Mehrabian A. (1971). Silent Messages. Belmont, CA, Wadsworth, p. 44.

Mitchell RW. (1991). Bateson's concept of metacommunication in play. New Ideas in Psychology 9(1):73–87.

Morse J. (1991). Negotiating commitment and involvement in the nurse–patient relationship. Journal of Advanced Nursing 16:455–468.

Mulaik JS, Megenity J, Cannon R, et al. (1991). Patients' perceptions of nurses' use of touch. Western Journal of Nursing Research 13(3):306–323.

Patch M, Hoang VR, Stahelski AJ. (1997). The use of metacommunication in compliance. Journal of Social Psychology 137(1):88–94.

Patterson J, Zderad LT. (1988). Humanistic Nursing (3rd ed.). New York, Wiley.

Raudsepp E. (1991). Six steps to becoming more assertive. Nursing '91 21(3):112–116.

Samovar L, Porter R (eds.). (1985). Intercultural Communication: A Reader (4th ed.). Belmont, CA, Wadsworth, p. 201.

Samovar L, Porter R (eds.). (1991). Intercultural Communication: A Reader (6th ed.). Belmont, CA, Wadsworth.

Simkins-Bullock J, Wildman BG. (1991). An investigation into the relationships between gender and language. Sex Roles 24(3/4):149–160.

Strauss RP, Sharp MC, Lorch SC, Kachalia B. (1995). Physicians and the communication of bad news. Pediatrics 96(1):82–89.

Telles M. (1995). Good communication skills are crucial for nurses. Nursing News 45(5):4, 9.

Van Buren A, Nowicki S. (1997). Awareness of interpersonal style and self-evaluation. Journal of Social Psychology 137(4):429–434.

Weaver RL. (1984). Understanding Interpersonal Communication. Glenview, IL, Scott, Foresman.

Weisman CS, Teitelbaum MA. (1989). Women and health care communications. Patient Education and Counseling 13(2):183–199.

West C. (1993). Reconceptualizing gender in physician-patient relationships. Social Science and Medicine 36(1):57–66.

Wood I. (1997). Communicating with children in A&E. Accident & Emergency Nursing 5(3):137–141.

Woolard KA. (1997). Between friends: Gender, peer group structure and bilingualism in urban Catalonia. Language in Society 26(4):533–536.

Worchel FF, Prevatt BC, Miner J, et al. (1995). Pediatrician's communication style: Relationship to parents' perceptions and behaviors. Journal of Pediatric Psychology 20(5):633–644.

## Videotape Reference

Dignam J. (1993). Transcultural Perspectives in Nursing. Irving, CA, Concept Media.

## Suggested Readings

Canales M. (1997). Narrative interaction. Issues in Mental Health Nursing 18:477–494.

Kennedy CW, Camden CT, Timmerman G. (1990). Relationships among perceived supervision communication, nurse moral and sociocultural variables. Nursing Administration Quarterly 14(4):38–46.

Raines RS, Hechtman SB, Rosenthal R. (1990). Nonverbal behavior and gender as determinants of physical attractiveness. Journal of Nonverbal Behavior 14(4):253–267.

# 10

# Developing Therapeutic Communication Skills in the Nurse–Client Relationship

Elizabeth Arnold

## OBJECTIVES

At the end of the chapter, the student will be able to

1. Define therapeutic communication
2. Identify the purposes of therapeutic communication
3. Describe the characteristics of therapeutic communication

4. Apply active listening and therapeutic communication strategies and skills
5. Describe selected verbal strategies to facilitate therapeutic communication

*The fundamental fact of human existence is person with person. . . . That special event begins by one human turning to another, seeing him or her as this particular other being, and offering to communicate with the other in a mutual way, building from the individual world each person experiences to a world they share together.*

Stewart, 1986

❖ This chapter describes fundamental principles of therapeutic communication. Communication, often referred to as *relating*, serves as the main point of human contact between two or more people, allowing them to reach common goals through participation in a relationship. In health care settings, the goal of communication is health related, and the focus of communication is on strategies that empower and help people cope more effectively with difficult health related issues.

Stewart (1986) suggested that the quality of the communication process directly influences the character of the relationship. Communication involves interchange of ideas and transmission of feelings between two or more people. People communicate through a variety of verbal and nonverbal modes that includes a combination of means to communicate with each other such as talking and listening, reading, art expression, and writing.

Therapeutic communication takes place within intrapersonal, interpersonal, and physical environments. The intrapersonal environment encompasses a person's internal thought processes, feelings, interpretations of messages, and self-talk about the meaning of message to the individual. The interpersonal environment includes the nurse and client, the health care team, the family, and anyone else involved in the health care of the client. The physical environment in which therapeutic communication actually takes place may be any health care facility or a setting that is not directly health related. As health care delivery moves to a community focus, the physical environment changes; communication will take place in nontraditional care settings: prisons, schools, the client's home, and ambulatory care settings. Although the same principles apply, the nurse will need to modify communication strategies to meet shortened time frames and environ-mental constraints imposed by managed care (Cahill, 1998).

## BASIC CONCEPTS
### Definition

*Therapeutic communication* is a goal-directed, focused form of dialogue used as a tool in health care to promote a client's well-being and positive response to treatment. Tannen (1991) noted that "life is a series of conversations." Therapeutic conversations are similar to those used spontaneously in social communications with several notable distinctions related to purpose, self-disclosure, and focus. In contrast to social conversations, therapeutic conversations have a serious purpose related to the health and well-being of the client. They are designed to help clients learn about their illness and how to cope with it, to comfort dying persons, and to assure them that someone is there to be with them and ease their suffering (Pearson, Borbasi, & Walsh, 1998). Therapeutic conversations help make illness bearable by reinforcing self-esteem and supporting the natural healing powers of a person (Peplau, 1960).

A useful metaphor for understanding the therapeutic communication process is to consider how people play ball. The person who throws the ball (sender of a message) must aim the ball accurately so that it can be caught easily by the receiver. The sender throws the ball with precision, aimed directly at the receiver. The receiver deliberately stands in the proper position to catch it. Once caught, the receiver returns the ball (feedback) to the sender with a similar degree of accuracy and care. When the sender throws a fast ball (abstract vocabulary that the receiver has trouble understanding), curve ball (manipulative or a message with a hidden agenda), or slow ball (vague and tangential messages), the ball (message) catches the receiver off guard and misses the mark.

Effective therapeutic communication is focused on the present situation. Referred to as immediacy, the nurse encourages the client to focus on health-related concerns in the here and now. The nurse not only responds to what the client is saying (catching the ball) but to nonverbal behaviors as well: "I notice that you seem quiet today. Is there something that I can help you with?"

The nurse uses concrete, culturally specific language that matches the client's use of language. Avoiding language that is too medical or global increases the chance of the message being understood and responded to appropriately (Fig. 10–1).

## Purpose of Therapeutic Communication

Ruesch (1961) suggested that the primary purpose of therapeutic communication is to help people cope more effectively as individuals and in relationships with others. Talking aloud about complex problems allows clients and their families to "hear" themselves as they speak of difficult issues and engages clients in a problem-solving process related to health care. The process of receiving objective caring feedback allows people to discover new meaning in personal suffering and to take a fresh look at what is truly important in life. Much more than simply the transfer of information and ideas from one person to another, each therapeutic conversation helps clients realistically sort out priorities and actions they can take to better cope with their specific nursing diagnoses and personal relationship needs (Corey, 1995).

Therapeutic communication is client centered and considers (1) the client's perspective and strengths, (2) readiness to learn, (3) ways of relating to others, (4) physical and emotional condition, and (4) sociocultural norms as relevant factors in planning and implementing communication strategies (Smith Battle, Drake, & Diekemper, 1997). Conversations have defined rules about the nature of the communication and its duration and purpose; the topics focus on specific health care needs.

Therapeutic communication is goal directed and time limited. Both content and process are designed to help nurse and client achieve desired outcomes in an I–thou relationship (Buber, 1970). The relationship provides the flow area in which the communication takes place. Goals are twofold: (1) to provide a safe place for the client to explore the meaning of the illness experience and (2) for the nurse to function as a skilled companion on the illness journey and through communication help the client to achieve well-being (Pearson, Borbasi, & Walsh, 1997).

## Active Listening

### Definition

*Active listening* is a dynamic interactive process in which a nurse (1) hears a client's message, (2) decodes its meaning, and (3) provides feedback to the client regarding the nurse's understanding of the message.

Active listening helps to create a safe environment in which clients can communicate more easily because they feel understood. It is a participatory process and different from simply hearing the client's message. Active listening requires the nurse's full concentration on a client's verbal and nonverbal behavior. The nurse listens not only for facts but also for the attached values, attitudes, and feelings.

Active listening is a cognitive and emotional process that involves taking the original sounds and words and constructing meaning from them. Meanings can differ from what the sender intended because the listener's values, expectations, and experiences impose a perceptual filter on the communicated message. Thus, two people may hear the same conversation and derive entirely different meaning from it. For this reason, frequent validating with the client and self-awareness are essential elements of the therapeutic communication process.

Attending behaviors are nonverbal communication (Box 10–1) such as body posture, gestures, and tears that aid the client in interpreting the message. They accompany the words and accentuate parts of the message. Attending behaviors invite the client to communicate with the nurse, conveying both interest and a sincere desire to understand.

The listening process includes recall and the integration of many factors. Active listening requires critical thinking (see Chapter 7) and choos-

> ### ◆ Box 10-1. Attending Behaviors in the Nurse-Client Relationship
>
> - Erect posture with the upper torso slightly inclined toward the client
> - Direct eye contact
> - Use of open, expansive gestures
> - Minimal encouraging cues
> - Nonverbal cues such as nodding and smiling

ing responses that will aid in gaining a clear understanding of the client's perspective. The listener notes tone of voice, pauses in the conversation, and his or her own intuitive feelings in receiving the message (Metcalf, 1998). The nurse, after listening to the client and observing nonverbal cues, asks the client for feedback that the observations the nurse makes are accurate. Active listening responses promote validation of the client as a person, a critical element in self-esteem, by being able to understand and respond to that person's fears, feelings, and ideas. Feeling confirmed as a person

of worth can be as important as understanding the nursing diagnosis in promoting, maintaining, and restoring the health of an individual.

Previous conversations with the same client and comparisons with other client observations in similar situations can be helpful. For example, is the client's current way of expressing anger about the situation similar or different from previous encounters? Is this a client who habitually complains about care, or is this new behavior? Making such distinctions helps the nurse ask additional questions and draw different conclusions.

Active listening skills result in fewer misunderstandings, effective use of time, and more accurate information. The relationship is stronger because the client feels understood (Straka, 1997). Exercise 10–1 uses principles of active listening in familiar situations.

### Barriers to Active Listening

Barriers to active listening can result from either nurse or client factors. The nurse can become so involved with giving physical care that listening to the client becomes secondary. Alterna-

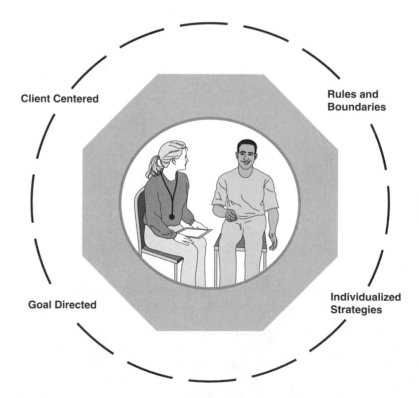

**Client Centered**

**Rules and Boundaries**

**Goal Directed**

**Individualized Strategies**

Figure 10–1. Characteristics of therapeutic communication.

◆ **Exercise 10-1. Active Listening**

**Purpose:** To develop skill in active listening and an awareness of the elements involved

**Procedure:**

1. Students break up into groups of two.
2. Take turns reflecting and describing a significant experience you have had in your life. The sharing partner should describe the details, emotions, and outcome of their experience.

During the interaction, the listening partner

Sits 2 feet away, facing the sharing partner

Makes frequent eye contact

Uses alert body language and attending cues

Pays attention to what is being said (the words) and how it is being expressed (the feelings sharing partner is expressing, e.g., noting variations in tone of voice)

Observes all nonverbal cues

After the sharing partner finishes his or her story, the listening partner indicates his or her understanding by (1) stating in his or her own words what the sharing partner said and (2) summarizing perceptions of the sharing partner's feelings associated with the story and ask for validation. If the sharing partner agrees, then the listening partner can be sure he or she correctly utilized active listening skills.

**Discussion:**
In the large group, pairs of students share their discoveries about active listening. As a class, discuss aspects of nursing behavior that will foster active listening in client interactions.

tively, the client may be too preoccupied with illness, pain, or worry to talk. Sometimes nurses listen only to the parts of the communication that interest them or to those that they assume are relevant. Included in each participant's communicated message are important instructions (metacommunication) about the interpretation of the message. The nurse may hear the content of a message but fail to register the nonverbal contradictions or qualifiers (Crowther, 1991).

In tense situations, or because a situation taps into a nurse's professional insecurity, a nurse's anxiety level can become high enough to obstruct receptive listening. For example, if a client is extremely critical of the nurse's performance, the nurse may have trouble listening fully to the client.

A client's speech patterns, anxiety, or behavioral mannerisms can make it difficult to attend fully or to understand a client's message. Thick accents can interfere with accurate understanding. Some nurses do not ask a client to repeat words for fear of offending the client. This is a mistake. What clients need most is to be under-

stood; caring enough to ask the client to repeat a message aids in this understanding. Other clients do not have a language problem but become increasingly vague when attempting to communicate about emotionally charged material. For example, a client learning of a difficult diagnosis may have trouble talking about it initially. Here the nurse might acknowledge the difficulty talking about the diagnosis; for example, "I think that this must be very difficult for you to absorb. If you would like to talk about it, I would be glad to listen." This simple statement allows the client space to process a highly emotional event while offering assistance. The issue is not that barriers exist, but how to address them effectively.

## Conditions that Influence Communication

### Physical Setting

The physical environment in which a conversation occurs influences ability to effectively communicate. Contrast trying to speak with a close friend in a crowded restaurant versus in a small, intimate restaurant seated at a table apart from other customers. In which setting would you be more likely to express your deep-seated feelings? (See Chapter 4 for suggested conversational settings.)

Where the communication takes place in home care settings is the client's call. Because privacy is a primary communication variable, the nurse should ask "Is there a place we can meet where we won't be disturbed?" Freedom from interruption when discussing private matters enhances the impression that the nurse wants to give full attention to the client. Once a suitable place is determined, the nurse can ask for the family's cooperation in respecting the client's privacy.

The nurse also considers the amount of personal space a client requires for ease of conversation (Hall, 1959). For example, sitting very close to a client who needs more space to feel comfortable can prove highly distracting to the client. The client will not hear the nurse's words because inner tensions created by an invasion of personal space preoccupy the client.

Most therapeutic conversations take place within a social distance. Three to 4 feet is opti-mal. However, clients experiencing high anxiety levels may need more physical space for successful conversation. Culture can dictate distance requirements. Persons from North American, Indian, African-American, Pakistani, and Asian cultures may require greater interpersonal space for successful interaction than Hispanics, Arabs, and southern Europeans (Richmond, Mc-Croskey, & Payne, 1987). Clients experiencing a sudden physical injury or undergoing a painful procedure appreciate having the nurse talk them through the process, in close proximity and possibly using touch. With experience, the nurse learns to gauge the amount of space the client needs. Nonverbal cues such as shifting position, rapid eye movements, and actually moving away slightly offer important cues that the client may need more space (Knapp & Hall, 1992).

Communication is most effective when both participants are positioned so that their eyes are at the same level. It is easier to engage a client lying in bed if you sit in a chair at eye level than if you are standing and the client must look up at you. The next time you are in a client's room, try communicating from a standing position with your eyes looking down at the client; then sit in

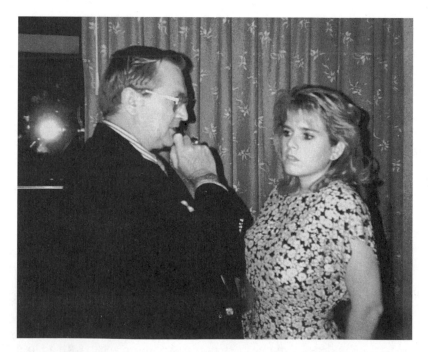

Most conversations take place within a social distance.

a chair facing the client with your eyes at the same level. Notice the differences in the flow of communication. Moving a chair close to the client in a wheelchair enhances communication (Miller, 1990). Whether you are sitting or standing, your posture should be relaxed, and if possible, the upper part of your body should be inclined toward the client. Physical behavioral cues characteristically include the behaviors summarized in Box 10–2.

## Timing

Timing is critical to the success of a therapeutic conversation. The nurse needs to take cues from the client's behavior to determine emotional readiness and available energy. For example, the conversation that takes place during an acute emergency, when a client is in pain, will be different from one that occurs when the client is comfortable or has visitors. Asking a newly diagnosed cancer client about goals reflects a lack of sensitivity to the client's need. The nurse's purpose in asking the question may be legitimate, but the inappropriate timing reflects the nurse's anxiety, and the client is likely to perceive it as remarkably insensitive. Sensitivity of the nurse to the presence of pain, variations in energy levels, and differences in relationship needs under different circumstances enhance communication.

The resistant client needs a different timing approach from the one used with a client who is eager to learn about his or her treatment. In the recovery room, after surgery, the nurse takes into account the client's diminished level of consciousness and lack of physical orientation in choosing appropriate ways to communicate (Severtsen, 1990). Planning for communication during periods when the client is more receptive to the idea and able to participate is time efficient and respectful of the client's needs.

## Personal Factors

Client differences related to socioeconomic status, previous life experience, education level, and occupational status influence the language, attitudes, and format of therapeutic communication. For example, the interpersonally sensitive nurse expresses the same concepts in different words to a homeless person, an adolescent, and an older

---

### ◆ Box 10–2. Physical Behavioral Cues

**Emblems:** gestures or body motions having a generalized verbal interpretation (e.g., handshaking, baby waving bye-bye, sign language).

**Illustrators:** actions that accompany and exemplify the meaning of the verbal message. Illustrators are used to emphasize certain parts of the communication (e.g., smiling, a stern facial expression, pounding the fist on a table). Illustrators usually are not premeditated.

**Affect displays:** facial presentation of emotional affect. Similar to the illustrators just discussed, the sender has more control over their display (e.g., a reproving look, an alert expression, a smile or a grin, a sneer). Affect displays seem to be more pervasive nonverbal expressions of the client's emotional state. They have a larger range of meaning and act to support or contradict the meaning of the verbal message. Sometimes the generalized affect is not related to a specific verbal message (e.g., a depressed client may have a retarded emotional affect throughout the relationship that has little to do with the communicated message).

**Regulators:** nonverbal activities that adjust the course of the communication as the receiver gives important information to the sender about the impact of the message on the sender. Regulators include nodding, facial expressions, some hand movements, looking at a watch.

**Adaptors:** characteristic, repetitive, nonverbal actions that are client specific and of long duration. They give the nurse information about the client's usual response to difficult emotional issues. Sample behaviors include a psychogenic tic, nervous foot tapping, blushing, twirling the hair.

**Physical characteristics:** nonverbal information about the client that can be gleaned from the outward appearance of the person (e.g., skin tone, descriptions of height and weight and relation to body shape, body odor, physical appearance [dirty hair, unshaven, teeth missing or decayed teeth, and so on]).

Adapted from Blondis M, Jackson B. (1982). Nonverbal Communication with Patients: Back to the Human Touch (2nd ed.). New York, Wiley, pp. 9–10. Used with permission.

adult. The words chosen reflect client differences in education and developmental level.

Differences in status or lifestyle between nurse and client are factors to consider. Marked differences in lifestyle may make it more difficult for the nurse to feel comfortable. Understanding the needs of a homeless client or the behaviors of a drug-addicted teenage mother may be difficult for a nurse who has never experienced the stresses associated with these lifestyles (Berne & Lerner, 1992). Although homosexuality is much more acceptable than it used to be, some nurses may find it more difficult to relate to clients with this lifestyle because of personal values and biases. Having a client of high social status or influence can affect communication because the nurse can feel intimidated.

A client making health choices that the nurse finds hard to accept can influence communication. The alcoholic who persists in drinking and the human immunodeficiency virus (HIV)–positive mother who continues to become pregnant discourage the nurse's investment in communicating with these clients. Watching a client make choices that indicate the client has given up also makes therapeutic conversations difficult. For example, an 80-year-old woman with multiple health problems requiring nursing home care may be hard to motivate. Why should she live?

Working with clients who refuse to comply or who have given up is a communication challenge for the nurse. Patience and understanding are key to success (Gorman, 1998). Developing awareness of their personal prejudices and intolerant reactions to people with different characteristics such as obesity, low-level education, aggressiveness, and complaining behavior allows nurses to maintain emotional objectivity with their clients.

## Use of Language

The nurse uses language to help clients connect different parts of their health stories and to let the stories of their lives flow freely. Weingarten (1992) noted that "every conversation creates an opportunity for connection and disconnection; reflection and haste; dialogue and monologue; understanding and misunderstanding; collaboration and instruction; no change and change" (p. 45).

Language is the means by which people organize data about problems and develop problems-solving strategies. Words comfort, challenge, and provide information to clients in distress. Concentrating on issues of greatest importance is most likely to engage the client's attention. Messages that carry mental images of cultural significance to the client are more effective. Using conventional everyday language, keeping in mind the client's developmental and educational level, and speaking in a general spirit of inquiry and concern for the client stimulate trust. Effective verbal messages address core issues in a clear, concise manner and take into account the principles listed in Box 10–3.

People can only absorb so much verbal information at one time. Introducing new ideas one at a time in chunks of simple information allows the receiver to process data more easily. Repeating key ideas and reinforcing information with concrete examples of concepts facilitates understand-

---

◆ **Box 10–3. Guidelines to Effective Verbal Expressions in the Nurse-Client Relationship**

Define unfamiliar terms and concepts.

Match content and delivery with each client's developmental and educational level, experiential frame of reference, and learning readiness.

Keep messages clear, concrete, honest, and succinct.

Put ideas in a logical sequence of related material.

Relate new ideas to familiar ones when presenting new information.

Repeat key ideas.

Reinforce key ideas with vocal emphasis and pauses.

Keep language as simple as possible; use vocabulary familiar to the client.

Focus only on essential elements; present one idea at a time.

Use as many sensory communication channels as possible for key ideas.

Make sure that nonverbal behaviors support verbal messages.

Seek feedback to validate accurate reception of information.

ing and provides an additional opportunity for the client to ask important questions. At the same time, the nurse needs to be alert for nonverbal response cues from the client that support understanding or reflect a need for further attention.

## APPLICATIONS

## Assessment Strategies

### Building Rapport

Communication starts with building rapport in the beginning of a relationship or interview. Building rapport refers to establishing a trusting environment in which the client will feel comfortable sharing information.

For many people, eye contact constitutes an invitation or readiness to interact (Richmond et al., 1987). Similarly, breaking eye contact is sometimes used to indicate nonverbally that the interaction is about to cease. The nurse needs to honor cultural differences in use of eye contact. For example, some cultures, such as Puerto Rican, Japanese, Appalachian, and Native American, favor a more limited use of eye contact in communicating with others than do Western and some Latin American cultures. Withdrawal of eye contact in Western cultures may indicate discomfort, whereas in the first group of cultures mentioned, it might represent deference or respect.

### Observation

The nurse needs to keep in mind that many clients suffer with problems of which they are not consciously aware or are unable to put into words. Besides listening for auditory cues and patterns, the nurse looks for visual indicators of meaning. The nurse takes special notice of the client's facial expression, body movements, posture, breathing rate, and so on as cues indicating either support or nonsupport of the spoken message. For example, the client who verbally declares that he is ready for surgery and seems completely calm may be sending a very different message through the tense muscles the nurse accidentally touches. Cues from the environment (e.g., the half-eaten lunch and noncompliance with treatment) can provide nonverbal clues that a client is in distress. The nurse needs to validate observations for complete accuracy.

Facial expression is a major source of informa-

tion when it is interpreted accurately. Often a person's facial expression indicates whether the person is happy, sad, scared, confident, hostile, annoyed, or pleased. Ekman and Friesen (1975) described guidelines for interpreting facial expressions (Box 10–4) that may be useful in deciphering the nonverbal meaning of facial expression behaviors observed in nursing practice. At the same time, the nurse should verify the meaning of a particular facial expression because certain cultures (e.g., Irish, English, and northern European) demonstrate less facial responsiveness, especially with strangers, and some Asian cultures tend to cover negative emotions with a smile (Dowd, Giger & Davidhizar, 1998). Some people, regardless of culture, smile when they are angry or nervous. Refer back to Exercise 4–1 for practice in identifying nonverbal behavior.

## Asking Questions

Questions are an important form of communication in all phases of the nurse–client relationship and a primary means of obtaining information from a client. The information needed and condition of the client help dictate the number and type of questions. Nurses need to ask enough questions so the client feels the nurse is listening, but not so many that the client feels he or she is being interrogated (Renwick, 1992). Questions fall into three categories: open ended, closed, and circular.

### Open-Ended Questions

An *open-ended question* is similar to an essay question on a test. It is open to interpretation and cannot be answered by "yes," "no," or a one-word response. Such questions are designed to permit the client to express the problem or health need in his or her own words. Open-ended questions are used to

- Assess the client's ability to articulate ideas.
- Elicit the client's thoughts without influencing the direction of an acceptable response.

The wording is important, as is a friendly approach that respects the individual and gives the client as much control as possible in responding. A good starting question is "Can you tell me a little about yourself and why you are here?" Open-ended questions usually begin with "how,"

---

◆ Box 10–4. Facial Expressions Associated with Different Emotions

| | |
|---|---|
| Anguish, distress | Eyebrows down and together, forming "worry triangle"; cheeks stretched and flattened down; corners of lips turned down, eyes without life in them; client may have difficulty looking at nurse |
| Anger, rage | Mouth and jaw firmly set; eyes narrow and alert; facial muscles taut; speech fast; lips curled under and tense; client usually looks directly at nurse with cold, hard stare |
| Guilt, shame | Head down; shoulders slumped; eyes down, avoiding direct eye contact; some twitching of facial muscles; face flushed; client may lick lips |
| Happiness, joy | Face smiling, laughing, life in the eyes; muscles relaxed, stretched upward and outward, nostrils flared; client looks directly at nurse |
| Contempt | Lips pursed, tense with corners turned up; jaw tense; eyes narrowed and focused |
| Interest | Forehead drawn upward; eyes wide open; smiling, mouth open; facial muscles relaxed |
| Fear | Muscles tense; head lowered; eye contact limited, mouth closed |
| Caring | Eyes soft; muscles relaxed, smiling |

Based on Ekman P, Friesen W. (1975). Unmasking the Face: A Guide to Recognizing Emotions from Facial Clues. Englewood Cliffs, NJ, Prentice Hall. Used with permission.

---

"what," "where," "when," "in what way," or "can you tell me about?" The following are examples:

"Can you tell me a little bit about what brought you to the clinic today?"

"What has been most difficult for you regarding. . . ?"

"When would you say you began to feel the helplessness you describe?"

"Can you tell me a little bit about what Dr. Jones has said to you regarding . . . ?"

"Can you tell me about the accident?"

Note that these questions are general rather than specific and open to a variety of answers. Although open-ended questions are desirable in most clinical situations, there are exceptions. Emergencies or other circumstances when information is needed quickly dictate use of focused or closed questions. For example, open-ended questions may not be appropriate to use with a woman in active labor or a new admission to the emergency department. Exercise 10–2 provides an opportunity to practice the use of open-ended questions.

## Focused Questions

A variation of the open-ended question is the *focused question,* which limits the response to a certain informational area but requires more than a "yes" or "no" response. The nurse uses focused questions to obtain data that are more specific. The following are examples:

"Can you tell me any more about the pain in your arm?"

"You mentioned that you had the problem with your back before. How did this problem develop before?"

"Can you give me a specific example of what you mean by . . . ?"

## Closed-Ended Questions

*Closed questions* resemble multiple-choice questions with limited answer options. The answer to a closed-ended question limits expression of the client's feelings, and it may take more questions to obtain the same information. They are useful in emergency situations, when the goal is to obtain information quickly and the client's emotional reactions are of secondary importance.

---

◆ Exercise 10–2. **Asking Open-ended Questions**

**Purpose:** To help develop skill in the use of open-ended questions to facilitate information sharing

**Procedure:**

1. Break up into pairs; one student takes the role of the facilitator and the other the sharer. (If you are in the clinical area, you may want to choose a clinical situation.)
2. As a pair, select a topic; the facilitator begins asking open-ended questions.
3. Dialogue for 5 to 10 minutes on the topic.
4. In pairs, discuss perceptions of the dialogue and determine what questions were comfortable and open ended.

**Discussion:**
As a class, each pair contributes examples of open-ended questions that facilitated the sharing of information. Compile these examples on the board. Formulate a collaborative summation of what an open-ended question is and how it is used. Discuss how open-ended questions can be used sensitively with uncomfortable topics.

---

They also are a quick way to check facts needed for a health assessment. Clients with limited social skills often can respond better initially to closed questions. Examples of close ended questions include

"When was your last tetanus shot?"
"Does the pain radiate down your left shoulder and arm?"
"When was your last meal?"
"Have you had these symptoms before?"

Exercise 10–3 provides experience with assessing types of active listening questions.

### Asking Secondary Questions

Once the nurse has asked preliminary questions about a topic, whether open, focused, or closed, there may be a need to follow up with a secondary question. *Secondary questions* directly relate to the initial data and ask the client to expand on a particular topic. The following are examples:

"Now that we have explored why you are here in the hospital, I wonder whether you could tell me about any other experiences you have had with this problem."
"Now that you have told me about how you handle your diabetic diet in general, can you tell me about any modifications you have to make when you are ill or stressed?"

### Circular Questions

In contrast to linear questions, which explore the descriptive characteristics of a situation, *circular questions* focus on the interpersonal context in which an illness occurs. They are designed to identify family relationships and differences in the impact of an illness on different family members. Circular questions are particularly useful when the family needs to be involved in the client's care. They are categorized as difference, behavioral effect, hypothetical, and triadic types (Box 10–5).

## What the Nurse Listens for

It is essential to explore another's reality before one can be of any help. During an initial interview, the nurse integrates listening skills with questions to understand the client's concerns (McKinney, 1992). Clients bring to an interview attitudes, feelings, and values that must be recognized but are not always apparent to the client. For example, a client newly diagnosed with cancer may be aware of the diagnosis but much less clear about the fear, anger, uncertainty, and resentment that may be underlying emotional themes that will affect treatment compliance. Box 10–6 presents what the nurse should listen for in assessment interviews.

---

♦ **Exercise 10–3. Differences in Active Listening Questions**

**Purpose:**   To help you identify differences in types of listening questions

**Procedure:**
Examine the following questions. Mark those that are open ended with an asterisk (*). Mark a focused question with a plus sign (+). Mark a closed question with a minus sign (−).

Ms. Gai, did you have a productive therapy session?

How do you feel about it now that you've learned that you will be staying at your daughter's house?

What did the doctor say about your lower back pain?

Your tray will be here soon. Are you hungry?

And when you heard that, you felt . . .?

When the physician walked away, you felt rejected?

No one likes to be in pain; can I get you something for it?

In the past when your leg ached, what kinds of things helped?

What do you think about being transferred to a nursing home?

Tell me, what brought you to see the physician today?

Are you having that problem with arthritis in your hand again?

What would you like to discuss today while we take a walk?

How are you?

What happened to you after you fell down?

And then what did you think?

Do you feel like taking your medicine now or later?

---

◇ Box 10–5. Examples of Circular Questions

| Definition | Example |
|---|---|
| Difference type: explores differences between people, between relationships, and between times | "Who is most upset about your father's illness?" "The last time your father was hospitalized, what was most helpful?" |
| Behavioral effect type: explores connections between the effect of one person's behavior on another | "How do you make sense out of the fact that your brother won't visit your father?" "How is your mother handling this?" |
| Hypothetical type: explores possible alternative actions and meanings | "If your father doesn't make it, who will assume responsibility for the care of your mother?" "If you could identify what would be most helpful at this time, what would it be?" |
| Triadic type: explores the person's perception of the relationship between two other people | "If your brother wanted to be supportive to you and your mom, what would he do?" "How does your father respond to his son's lack of interest?" |

Adapted from Loos F, Bell J. (1990). Circular questions: A family interviewing strategy. Dimensions of Critical Care Nursing 9(1):47. Copyright 1990 Hall Johnson Communications, Inc. Reproduced with permission. For further use contact the publisher at 9737 West Ohio Avenue, Lakewood, CO 80226.

---

┌─────────────────────────────────────────┐
◆ Box 10–6. What the Nurse Listens For

- Content themes
- Communication patterns
- Discrepancies in content, body language, and vocalization
- Feelings, revealed in a person's voice, body movements, and facial expressions
- What is not being said as well as what is being said
- The client's preferred representational system
- The nurse's own inner responses
- The effect communication produces in others involved with the client
└─────────────────────────────────────────┘

## Themes

A theme is an underlying feeling associated with concrete facts: powerlessness, fear, abandonment, and helplessness, to cite a few examples. Clients bring their life history to each health care situation, and the manner in which the change in health status affects each individual is unique and reflective of the patient's history as well as the current situation (Ramos, 1992). For example, the client says to the nurse, "I'm worried about my surgery tomorrow." This is one way of framing the problem. If the same client presents his concern as "I'm not sure I will make it through the surgery tomorrow," this changes the focus of the communication from a generalized worry to a more personal one of survival. Alternatively, the client might say "I don't know whether my husband should stay tomorrow for the surgery. It is going to be a long procedure, and he gets so worried." The focus of her concern now includes her relationship with her husband. In each of these communications, concern about the upcoming surgery is expressed. The nurse will want to assess differences in focus accurately and structure responses according to the client's emphasis.

Listening for themes includes understanding what the client is not saying as well as what the person actually reveals. For example, a client may tell you that he is not afraid of his surgery the next day. It is a simple in-and-out procedure, he says, and he plans to be back at work on Monday. At the same time, he is distressed that his girl-friend will not be able to go out with him the night before the operation "to get his mind off the surgery." The mixed message is an important assessment datum.

Emotional objectivity in making sense of client themes is essential. Moving beyond the facts requires critical thinking skills and control of personal feelings and preferences. "Objectivity here refers to seeing what an experience is for another person, not how it fits or relates to other experiences, not what causes it, why it exists, or what purposes it serves. It is an attempt to see attitudes and concepts, beliefs and values of an individual as they are to him at the moment he expresses them—not what they were or will become" (Moustakas, 1974). Exercise 10–4 provides practice in listening for themes.

## Communication Patterns

Communication patterns offer another dimension in designing appropriate responses. Some clients exaggerate information, whereas others characteristically leave out highly relevant detail. Some talk a lot using dramatic language and multiple examples; others say very little. Evaluation of the client's present overall interaction pattern of interaction with others includes strengths and limitations, family communication dynamics, and developmental and educational levels. Culture, role, ways of handling conflict, and dealing with emotions reflect communication patterns. The nurse uses data about client communication patterns as the basis for understanding a client's response to health care and involvement in his or her care. For example, the nurse may give additional cues to the client who has difficulty with verbal expression. Mirroring the client's communication pattern, for example not being blunt with the client whose communication style lends itself to stories or metaphors acknowledges that the nurse has heard and respects the client's communication pattern. Incorporating cultural understanding of communication style also is important (e.g., encouraging use of the client's own words as much as possible).

## Intuitive Communication

Intuitive communication can occur as a personal response from within the nurse. The nurse may feel intuitively that something is amiss, and may

---

◆ **Exercise 10-4. Listening for Themes**

**Purpose:**   To help you identify underlying themes in messages

**Procedure:**

1. Divide yourselves into groups of five students.
2. Take turns telling a short story about yourselves: about growing up, important people or events in your life, significant accomplishments, getting your first job, for example.
3. As each student presents a story, take mental notes of the important themes. Write them down so you will not be tempted to change them as you hear the other students. Notice nonverbal behaviors accompanying the verbal message. Are they consistent with the verbal message of the sharer?
4. When the story is completed, each of the other people in the group shares his or her observations with the sharer.
5. After all students have shared their observations, validate their accuracy with the sharer.

**Discussion:**

1. Were the underlying themes recorded by the group consistent with the sharer's understanding of his or her communication?
2. As other observers related their interpretations of significant words or phrases, did you change your mind about the nature of the underlying theme?
3. Were the interpretations of pertinent information relatively similar or significantly different?
4. If they were different, what implications do you think such differences have for nurse–client relationships in nursing practice?
5. What did you learn from doing this exercise?

**Variation:** students can break up into small groups and each create a clinical scenario in which two or more persons are dialoguing in relation to a situation or health problem. One person is in the helper role. Each group will dramatize their scenario to the larger group. Each student can listen for the emotional and informational themes and write a description of his or her impressions.

---

need to share this sense with the client. If the nurse has no particular personal reason for reacting to the client with anger, fear, or sadness, the inner response may reflect a client's unexpressed feeling. Behavioral reactions that the nurse feels are out of proportion to the situation (e.g., complete calm before surgery, excessive anger, noncompliance or passive compliance with no questions asked, guarded verbalizations, incongruent facial expressions or body language, social withdrawal) are danger signals. Listen to the client, watching nonverbal communication to obtain a full picture. Validating observations for accuracy is important because the nurse's interpretation may not fully represent the client's meaning.

## Focusing

*Focusing* as a communication strategy means that the nurse encourages the client to select one topic over another as the primary focus of discussion. For example, a client with impending surgery for prostate cancer casually mentions that he is afraid of his surgery tomorrow but launches into a lengthy discussion of his family, his job, and so on.

In ordinary circumstances, people have extended time with each other to discuss important issues, but in today's health care delivery, the nurse typically has a short time to gather relevant information and to assist clients in sorting through complex issues. Consequently, the nurse may have to help the client select one topic for discussion among several, keeping other subjects in mind for later exploration. Usually the nurse tries to focus on those issues most relevant to the current situation. To use focusing, the nurse might say to the client, "Mr. Solan, you have given me a lot to think about here, but I would like to hear more about how you are handling the surgery tomorrow. You mentioned that you were feeling afraid, and this is normal. I wonder if we could talk more about this." Note that the nurse focuses on a topic raised by the client rather than a completely unrelated topic. This is called focusing.

Focusing can be an invitation to explore a topic not raised by the client if it is relevant to the client's immediate situation. If in the previous situation the client did not talk at all about the surgery, the nurse might make a general comment about the client's seeming lack of concern and ask for validation that the observation is correct. Expressed as an inquiring observation about behavior occurring in the immediate relationship, this indirect focus strategy usually does not offend. It is essential that the nurse not force a client to focus on an issue that he or she is not yet willing to discuss but rather open the door to the possibility of it being an issue worth exploring. Sometimes nurses feel that it is important for dying clients to speak of death or for those with a new diagnosis of cancer to talk about their response. Although theoretically this may have a therapeutic effect, the nurse must always wait until clients are ready to talk about it. Forcing clients to talk of feelings they do not feel comfortable addressing can be counterproductive; it is not a legitimate use of focusing.

## Therapeutic Listening Responses

Listening responses show the client that the nurse is fully present as a professional partner in helping the client understand a change in health status and the best ways to cope with it. Minimal verbal cues, clarification, restatement, paraphrasing, reflection, summarization, silence, and touch are examples of skilled listening responses (Box 10–7) the nurse can use to guide therapeutic interventions.

### Minimal Cues and Leads

Simple encouraging leads communicate interest. *Minimal cues* through body actions (e.g., smil-

---

◆ **Box 10–7. Listening Responses**

| Listening Response | Example |
| --- | --- |
| Minimal cues and leads | Body actions: smiling, nodding, leaning forward. Words: "mm" or "uh huh," "Oh really," "go on." |
| Clarification | "Could you describe what happened in sequence?" "I'm not sure I understand what you mean. Can you give me an example?" |
| Restatement | "Are you saying that . . . (repeat client's words)?" "You mean . . . [repeat client's words]?" |
| Paraphrasing | Client: I can't take this anymore. The chemo is worse than the cancer. I just want to die.<br>Nurse: It sounds as though you are saying you have had enough. |
| Reflection | "It sounds as though you feel guilty because you weren't home at the time of the accident." "You sound really frustrated because the treatment is taking longer than you thought it would." |
| Summarization | "Before moving on, I would like to go over with you what I think we accomplished thus far." |
| Silence | Briefly disconnecting but continuing to use attending behaviors after an important idea, thought, or feeling. |
| Touch | Gently rubbing a person's arm during a painful procedure |

ing, nodding, and leaning forward) encourage clients to continue with their story. By not detracting from the client's message and by giving permission to tell the story as the client sees it, minimal cues promote client comfort in sharing intimate information. Exercise 10–5 provides an opportunity to see the influence of minimal cues and leads on communication.

## Clarification

**Clarification** seeks to understand the message of the client by asking for more information or for elaboration on a point. The strategy is most useful when parts of a client's communication are ambiguous or not easily understood. Failure to ask for clarification when part of the communication is poorly understood means that the nurse will act on incomplete or inaccurate information.

Clarification responses are expressed as a question or statement followed by a restatement or paraphrasing of part of the communicated message. "You stated earlier that you were concerned about your blood pressure. Can you tell me more about what concerns you?" The tone of voice used with a clarification response should be neutral, not accusatory or demanding. Practice this response in Exercise 10–6.

## Restatement

**Restatement** is an active listening strategy used to broaden a client's perspective or when the nurse needs to provide a sharper focus on a specific part of the communication. Restatement is like bracketing a phrase in a paragraph. It acts as a brief interruption designed to highlight a defined element of a message. Restatement is particularly effective when the client overgeneralizes or seems stuck in a repetitive line of thinking. To challenge the validity of the client's statement directly could be counterproductive.

---

### ◆ Exercise 10–5. **Minimal Cues and Leads**

**Purpose:** To practice and evaluate the efficacy of minimal cues and leads

**Procedure:**

1. Initiate a conversation with someone outside of class and attempt to tell the person about something with which you are familiar for 5 to 10 minutes.
2. Make note of all the cues that the person puts forth that either promote or inhibit conversation.
3. Now try this with another person and write down the different cues and leads you observe as you are speaking and your emotional response to them (e.g., what most encouraged you to continue speaking).

**Discussion:**
As a class, share your experiences and observations. Different cues and responses will be compiled on a board. Discuss the impact of different cues and leads on your comfort and willingness to share about yourself. What cues and leads promoted communication and what inhibited sharing?

**Variation:** this exercise can be practiced with a clinical problem simulation in which one student takes the role of the professional helper and the other takes the role of client. Perform the same scenario with and without the use of minimum encouragers.

**Questions for Discussion:**

What were the differences when encouragers were not used? Was the communication as lively?

How did it feel to you when telling your story when this strategy was used by the helping person?

---

◆ Exercise 10–6. **Using Clarification**

**Purpose:** To develop skill in the use of clarification

**Procedure:**
Write a paragraph related to an experience you have had. Place all the paragraphs together, and then pick one (not your own) and develop clarification questions for the selected paragraph.

**Discussion:**
Share with the class your chosen paragraph and the clarification questions you developed. Discuss how effective the questions are in clarifying information. Other students can suggest additional clarification questions.

---

Repeating parts of the message in the form of a query serves a similar purpose without raising defenses. Restating a self-critical or irrational part of the message focuses the client's attention on the possibility of an inaccurate or global assertion. Restatement should be used sparingly and only as a point of emphasis. Otherwise it can sound stilted.

### Paraphrasing

*Paraphrasing* is a response strategy designed to help the client elaborate more on the cognitive part (content) of a verbal message. The nurse takes the original message and transforms it into his or her own words without losing the meaning. The paraphrase statement is shorter and a little more specific than the client's initial statement so that the focus is on the core elements. Presented as a tentative statement, the paraphrase listening response invites but does not force a specific answer. Paraphrasing is particularly useful in the early stages of a relationship or when the client is raising a troublesome topic for the first time. It is also valuable in checking whether the nurse's translation of the client's words is an accurate interpretation of the message. Exercise 10–7 is designed to help students understand the difference between paraphrasing and reflection. Exercise 10–8 provides practice in paraphrasing.

### Reflection

*Reflection* as a listening response focuses on the emotional overtones of a message. This listening response helps the client clarify important feelings and experience them with their appropriate intensity in relation to a particular situation or event.

When the nurse uses reflection as a listening response, it gives a client permission to *have* feelings. Often clients are relieved to find that having conflicting emotions is a normal response in new and unfamiliar circumstances. Timing is critical in the use of reflection. Reflective listening responses have more impact if they are used sparingly to accentuate only the important themes. Reflection is most useful when the nurse uses it in a compound sentence that connects the feeling with the appropriate content (Charkhuff, 1983; Cormier, Cormier, & Weisser, 1984); for example, "It sounds as though you feel _____ because _____ ."

Sometimes nursing students feel they are putting words into the client's mouth when they "choose" an emotion from their perception of the client's message. This would be true if they were choosing an emotion out of thin air, but not when the nurse empathetically considers the client's situation and does not go beyond the data the client presents. Reflection is different from interpretation in that it simply puts into words the feelings a nurse hears in the client's comments without either adding or subtracting from them. Exercise 10–9 gives practice in using reflecting responses.

### Summarization

*Summarization* is an active listening skill used to review content and process. Here the nurse reduces a lengthy interaction or discussion to a few succinct sentences. A summary statement is

◆ **Exercise 10-7. Practice in Differentiating Paraphrasing and Reflection**

**Purpose:** To practice use of paraphrasing and reflection as listening responses

**Procedure:**

1. The class forms into groups of three students each. One student takes the role of client, one the role of helper, and one the role of observer.

2. The client shares with the helper a recent health problem he or she encountered and describes the details of the situation and the emotions experienced. The helper responds with the use of paraphrasing and reflection in a dialogue that lasts at least 5 minutes. The observer records the statements made by the helper. At the end of the dialogue, the client writes his or her perception of how the helper's statements affected the conversation, including that comments were most helpful. The helper write a short summary of the listening responses he or she used, with comments on how successful they were.

**Discussion:**

1. Share your summary and discuss the differences in using the techniques from the helper, client, and observer perspective related to influencing the flow of dialogue, helping the client feel heard, and the impact on the helper's understanding of the client.

2. How could you use this exercise to understand your client's concerns?

3. Were you surprised by any of the summaries?

Participants A and B will hold a discussion on why A chose to be a nurse or some other important decision or event in A's life. Participant B may respond to A only with a paraphrasing response. Participant C will act as observer.

At the end of 5 minutes, C shares his or her observations.

Then for the next 5 minutes, C acts as the protagonist in describing his or her first day on the clinical unit or the first day in a nursing course. Participant from A responds to C with paraphrase while B acts as observer.

After 5 minutes, the process may be repeated with another scenario to give C the chance to practice the paraphrase response.

Discuss the difficulties in trying to paraphrase the statements of clients.

Did the paraphrased statement encourage you to continue? Did you feel more understood as a result of hearing the listener's response? What did you learn personally from this exercise about paraphrasing as a listening response?

---

particularly useful before moving on to a different topic area. Summarization pulls several ideas and feelings together. The ideas may relate to the same interaction or to different ones. Exercise 10–10 gives practice in summarization.

## Silence

Silence, used deliberately and judiciously, is a powerful listening response. It allows the client to think, and it is often beneficial for the nurse to step back momentarily and process what he or she heard before responding. Too often a quick response addresses only a small part of the message or gives the client an insufficient opportunity to formulate a complete idea fully. A short silence to get in touch with one's personal anxiety aroused by a client's response is appropriate before responding. On the other hand, long silences become uncomfortable. The silent pause should be just that, a brief disconnection followed by a verbal comment.

Silence can accent an important point in a verbal communication. By pausing briefly after presenting a key idea and before proceeding to the next topic, the nurse encourages the client to notice the most important elements of the communication.

When a client falls silent, it can mean that something has touched the client profoundly.

◆ Exercise 10-8. **Practicing Paraphrasing**

**Purpose:** To practice paraphrasing as an active listening response

**Directions:**
For each statement, write one appropriately rephrased sentence.

1. ''I'm on a diet but I seem to be gaining a lot of weight even though I usually try to stick to it faithfully.''

Appropriately paraphrased example
''You want to lose weight, but your diet isn't working?''
*Inappropriate:* ''You can't stick to your diet?''

2. ''I need an operation but can't take the time to have it until my business is doing better.''

*Appropriate paraphrase*

_____

_____

3. ''The doctor just told me I have cancer, but I'm not sure what he means.''

*Appropriate paraphrase*

_____

_____

◆ Exercise 10-9. **Practicing the Use of Reflecting Responses**

**Purpose:** To practice the use of reflection as a listening response

**Procedure:**

1. May be done alone or in any size class group.
2. Read the following situation.
   Jamie, age 7, is dying of a chronic respiratory condition. His small stature and optimistic sense of humor have made him a favorite on the unit. Jamie's mom breaks down crying one day, saying to you ''I try to do good, to help out on the unit these last 4 weeks. Why is God punishing me this way? I can't take much more of this staying here constantly, watching Jamie struggle for every breath. Only his intravenous fluids and oxygen keep him alive. Sometimes I think it would be better to stop them and let him die in peace.''
3. Write appropriate nurse responses that reflect back to the mother your perception of the feeling underlying her statements.
4. Write other responses that reflect your perception of her feelings.
5. Combine the responses to attain an appropriate reflection of content and feeling. It may be easier to do this exercise for each sentence in the situation.

**Discussion:**

1. Was it more difficult to use reflection as a communication strategy? If so, why?
2. What did you personally learn from this exercise?

---

◆ **Exercise 10-10. Practicing Summarization**

**Purpose:**  To provide practice in summarizing interactions

**Directions:**

Choose a partner.

For 5 minutes, discuss, in pairs, a medical ethics topic such as euthanasia, heroic life support for the terminally ill, or "baby Doe" decisions to allow malformed babies to die if the parents so desire.

After 5 minutes, both must stop talking until Participant A has summarized what B has just said to B's satisfaction and vice versa.

**Discussion:**

After both partners have completed their summarization, discuss the process of summarization, answering the following questions:

Did knowing you had to summarize the other person's point of view encourage you to listen more closely?

Did the act of summarizing help clarify any discussion points? Were any points of agreement found? What points of disagreement were found?

Did the exercise help you to understand the other person's point of view?

What should an effective summary contain? Is it hard to summarize a long conversation?

How did you determine which points on which to focus in your summarization?

---

Respecting the client's silence and sitting without breaking the mood can be important in sharing the meaning of the communication. Clients often marvel at the nurse's willingness to sit quietly and without awkwardness in their moments of silence. Practice in this skill is developed in Exercise 10–11.

## Touch

Touch, the first of our senses to develop, represents a person's first experience in communicating with another human being. Usually experienced as a nurturing, validating form of communication, touch remains a vital form of communication throughout life. It is a powerful listening response when words would break a mood or verbalization would fail to convey the empathy or depth of feeling between nurse and client (Nelson, 1998). A hand tenderly placed on a frightened mother's shoulder or a gentle squeeze of the hand can speak far more eloquently than words in times of deep emotion, whether sad or joyful. Clients in pain, those who feel repulsive to others because of altered appearance, lonely and dying clients, and those experiencing sensory deprivation or feeling confused respond positively to the nurse who is unafraid to enter their world and touch them (Miller, 1990).

Touch can deepen the meaning of language. When combined with words (e.g., in a back rub), touch tends to enhance the feeling of comfort. Holding a small child or placing your hand in another's during a painful procedure is as important a means of communication in the therapeutic relationship as knowing the right words to say.

People vary in their comfort with touch as a listening response. All cultures have norms about how people should touch each other and when touching is appropriate. Cultural competence requires an understanding of the meaning of touch to clients from different cultures. Additionally, some people enjoy being touched and experience it as a human connection. Other clients will shrink from such closeness or will misinterpret its meaning. How individuals interpret the meaning of touch depends also on such factors as its duration, intensity, and the body part touched. Here, as in other aspects of the relationship, the nurse uses professional judgment about the use

◆ Exercise 10–11. **Therapeutic Use of Silence**

**Purpose:** To experience the effect of the use of silence as a listening response

**Procedure:**

1. Two people act as Participants A and B.
2. Participant A plays the role of the nurse and Participant B is a healthy, ambulatory 80-year-old female (or male) client in an extended-care facility, having been placed there against her will by her family, who is moving to another state.
3. Participant B's role is to describe feelings (shock) at being institutionalized and to discuss the slow adjustment to new surroundings and new companions, describing both the positive and the negative aspects.
4. Participant A's objective is to make at least three deliberate efforts to use silence during the conversation (as a therapeutic device to encourage Participant B's consideration of life and problems).

**Discussion:**
After 15 minutes of role-playing, have a general discussion to share feelings about the effective use of silence.

of the strategy and its possible interpretation by the client. Before reaching out to a client with touch, the nurse needs to assess the client's receptiveness. Observation of the client will provide some indication, and the nurse may need to ask for validation. If the client is paranoid, out of touch with reality, verbally inappropriate, or mistrustful, touch is contraindicated as a listening response.

## Verbal Responses

Verbal responses are communications the nurse uses to relate in a significant way to a client: to teach, to encourage, to provide information, to gather information, to move a client in a certain direction toward goal achievement. Active listening and verbal responses are inseparable from each other. Ideally, they support one another and

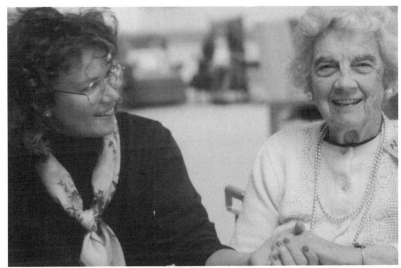

Touch can be an important form of communication. (Courtesy of the University of Maryland School of Nursing)

provide a more complete picture. In making a verbal response, the nurse gives or changes the perspective on a health-related topic.

Most clients are not looking for brilliant answers from the nurse but rather for feedback and support that suggests a compassionate understanding of their particular dilemma. No matter what level of communication exists in the relationship, the same questions arise: "Who am I?" "What is the meaning of my current experience?" "How can I cope with what is happening to me?" The same needs—"hear me," "touch me," "respond to me," "feel my pain and my joys with me"—are identifiable as basic underlying themes. Simple communication strategies to help clients feel understood include

- Allowing the client enough time to answer questions
- Informing the client of what the nurse is going to do and why
- Asking the client what his or her feelings were about what is happening (Duldt, 1991)

Verbal responses provide guidance and information to help clients assume responsibility for their health and well-being. With shorter time frames for actual client contact, nurses need to use verbal communication to connect with clients as partners from the first encounter in (1) developing a mutually agreed-on focus for intervention based on client data, (2) identifying and integrating client strengths to plan and implement treatment objectives, and (3) using environmental supports and community resources to enhance treatment.

Verbal strategies include framing responses, metaphors, humor, confirming responses, reframing, providing relevant feedback, and validation, all of which are designed to strengthen coping abilities of the client alone or in relationship with others. Although described individually for purposes of description in this chapter, in real practive the nurse will integrate more than one even in a single intervention. As with active listening responses, the nurse uses observation, validation, and patterns of knowing to gauge the effectiveness of verbal interventions. On the basis of the client's reaction, the nurse may have to use simpler language, use a different strategy, and in whatever way is needed adjust verbal re-

sponse so that the client can fully understand the message.

## Mirroring Depth in Verbal Response

Regardless of content, the nurse's verbal responses should match the client's message in level of depth, meaning, and language (Johnson, 1980). The client needs to lead the way to any exploration of deeper feeling. If the client makes a serious statement, the nurse should not respond with a flip remark. Likewise, a superficial statement does not warrant an intense response. Responses that encourage a client to explore feelings about limitations or strengths at a slightly deeper but related level of conversation are likely to meet with more success.

## Matching Response with Verbal Content

Verbal response should neither expand nor diminish the meaning of the client's remarks. Notice the differences in the nature of the following responses to a client:

**Client:**  I feel so discouraged. No matter how hard I try, I still can't walk without pain on the two parallel bars.

**Nurse:**  You want to give up because you don't think you will be able to walk again?

At this point, it is unclear that the client wants to give up so the nurse's comment expands on the client's meaning without sufficient data. Although it is possible that this is what the client means, it is not the only possibility. The more important dilemma for the client may be whether her efforts have any purpose. The next response focuses only on the negative aspects of the client's communication.

**Nurse:**  So you think you won't be able to walk independently again.

In this statement, the nurse ignores the client's perception of a connection between her efforts and the result, thus potentially diminishing the client's meaning. In the final response example, the nurse addresses both parts of the client's message and makes the appropriate connection. The nurse's statement invites the client to validate the nurse's perception.

**Nurse:** It sounds to me as if you don't feel your efforts are helping you regain control over your walking.

## Using Appropriate Vocabulary

The final match needed for successful communication is use of appropriate vocabulary. Using jargon or language that is beyond the client's educational level and experiential frame of reference generally means that little information will be retained. Unless the client is able to associate new ideas with familiar words and ideas, the nurse might as well be talking in a different language. More often than not, clients will not tell the nurse that they do not understand a verbal response for fear of offending the nurse or revealing personal deficits. Talking down to a client or giving information that fails to take into account the client's previous experiences also tends to fall on deaf ears. Frequent validation with the client related to content can help reduce this problem.

Format is another factor to consider for full understanding. Some clients need a straightforward, concrete format. Others respond favorably to more imaginative formats. Observation, really listening to the client's mode of expression and cultural understanding of language nuances and meaning, helps the nurse select an appropriate format. Here is where the nurse uses artistry in choosing the most appropriate communication strategies for building and maintaining rapport.

## Using Metaphors

*Metaphor* is a therapeutic communication strategy in which one idea or object substitutes for another in a way that implies their similarity (Billings, 1991). A metaphor introduces a new perspective and provides the client with a foundation for learning new ways of functioning. Everyday metaphors such as "happy as a lark," "pain in the neck," "sharp as a tack," and "pillar of strength" demonstrate how a short phrase can convey a mental picture without needing fuller explanation. Metaphors form the basis for many children's stories. In *The Tale of the Velveteen Rabbit*, the reader understands the process of becoming real through the metaphor of a young boy and his toy rabbit.

The nurse can use metaphor as a statement, "If you give a man a fish, you feed him for a day; if you teach a man to fish, you feed him for life," or as a short story. For example, with a noncompliant client, the nurse might say "Now suppose that I wanted to lose weight. I go to the best dietitian, who tells me that I need to change my eating habits, eat low-fat foods, and exercise to lose weight. I thank her profusely but don't follow any of her advice. What chance do you think I would have of losing weight?"

## Reframing Situations

Bandler and Grinder (1997) defined **reframing** as "changing the frame in which a person perceives events in order to change the meaning (p. 1). Meaning and behavioral responses are so interrelated that when the meaning changes a person's responses and behaviors also change. The meaning of an event acts as a perceptual frame that guides subsequent action. For example, clients who look at a glass as half empty as those who look at it as half full will approach the same situation differently.

Steps in the reframing process call for the nurse to discover a positive or useful element in the client's situation (Pesut, 1991). To illustrate, receiving a diagnosis of terminal illness is devastating, but once a person gets over the initial shock of the diagnosis, it can be reframed as a "gift" in that it gives the individual the opportunity to take advantage of the moment and to connect with significant people they might have taken for granted otherwise. Here the nurse might ask a seriously ill client whether the illness has brought him closer to a family member or has caused him to contact a distant friend.

Reframing strategies emphasize client strengths. For example, the nurse might ask the client to identify coping strategies that have worked in the past and suggest that these transferable skills such as persistence and creativity can be used in a different way in the current situation. The new frame must fit the current situation and be understandable to the client. Otherwise it will not work. This means that the nurse should consider the reframe from several different perspectives and choose the one most likely to have the strongest impact.

Reframing a situation is helpful when blame is a component of a family's response to the client's illness. For example, the reason a person fails to take medication or continues to drink alcohol may have little to do with a desire to annoy or punish significant others. Helping a family to see these behaviors as client symptoms for which they cannot assume responsibility helps the spouse or child reframe the situation as one they cannot control and leads to needed detachment.

## Using Humor

Humor is a powerful communication technique when used with deliberate intent for a specific therapeutic purpose. McGhee's (1985) definition of humor is as follows: "the mental experience of discovering and appreciating ludicrous or absurdly incongruous ideas, events, or situations" (p. 6).

The surprise element in humor can cut through an overly intense situation and reframe it. Humor reframes an impossible situation by putting it into perspective. Once a person can appreciate the many absurdities and incongruities of life, the spirit lifts. Humor has the capacity to encourage a sense of intimacy, acceptance, and warmth, which can reduce emotional distance in the nurse–client relationship (Lynch & Anchor, 1991). Laughter helps create natural highs by increasing the presence of $\beta$-endorphin, a neurotransmitter agent known to stimulate positive chemical changes in the body that encourage healing (Cousins, 1976). For all of these reasons, humor plays an important role in therapeutic communication.

A good joke creates a distraction, but it needs the proper context. Humor is most effective when rapport is well established and a level of trust exists between the nurse and client. A shared joke becomes a bond and in some cases almost a password in well-established relationships (McGhee, 1998). When humor is used, it should focus on the idea, event, situation, or something other than the client's humanity. Humor that ridicules is not funny.

Occasional use of humor is more effective than constant use. Constant use of humor can lead the client to minimize personal recognition of serious issues. It is up to the nurse to maintain the appropriate level of intensity and heightened interpersonal awareness in the relationship to help clients meet health goals. The following factors contribute to the successful use of humor:

• Knowledge of the client's response pattern
• An overly intense situation
• Timing
• Geared to the client's developmental level

Before using humor, the nurse needs to collect enough data on the client to have a working knowledge of how a humorous remark or joke might be received. Some clients respond well to humor; others are insulted or perplexed by it. They may not see it as appropriate or culturally acceptable in a helping relationship. Small children cannot relate to humor as well as adults because of their concrete thinking. Adolescents respond enthusiastically to some types of humor and can be emotionally devastated by other humorous remarks, particularly if the comments directly relate to them as persons.

Professional judgment in the use of humor is critical to its success. Humor is less effective when the client is tired or emotionally vulnerable. However, it is an effective tool to introduce therapeutic change when the client is emotionally immobilized. Depending on level of anger, humor can reduce aggression or tension in ways that a serious comment cannot. If the client is very frustrated or on the verge of losing control, however, humor may be inappropriate intervention. Instead, the client may need structure and calming support.

## Confirming Responses

**Confirming responses** are statements designed to validate the client and enhance self-esteem. They respect and support the uniqueness of a client's experience. For example, the nurse might say to a mother reluctant to leave her small child, "I can see that it is hard for you to say goodnight to your little boy, knowing that he does not understand why you have to leave. Is there anything I can do to make it easier for you?" To the client who tells the nurse, "I know it is silly to worry about general anesthesia with one-day surgery. I don't know why I am so uptight about it," the nurse might say, "No, it is not silly; many people worry about anesthesia. Can you tell me more about what worries you?" With each confirming response, the nurse acknowledges the legitimacy of the client's feelings and invites the client to explore further the meaning of the message.

Disconfirming responses, in contrast, are

those statements that contradict, minimize, or deny the client's feelings. They tend to lower the client's self-esteem and limit full disclosure (Heineken, 1982). Examples of disconfirming responses are provided in Box 10–8.

## Giving Feedback

Feedback is a special form of communication in which a person responds to messages or behavior. Verbal feedback provides, through words, the receiver's understanding of the sender's message and personal reaction to it. Nonverbal feedback registers the other's reaction to the sender's message through such facial expressions of surprise, boredom, or hostility. Other nonverbal feedback can occur through behaviors such as leaving a situation or shutting down verbally.

Verbal feedback, if offered in a supportive way, can have a profound impact on behavior. Helpful feedback is *descriptive* in nature. By simply describing one's reaction to a behavior and avoiding any evaluation of it, the receiver is free to use or discard the feedback. The following

nursing responses demonstrate two types of feedback to a diabetic client.

**Nurse:** I was disappointed when you didn't ask any questions about rotating sites for your insulin injection.

**Nurse:** You should have asked questions about rotating sites if you didn't understand it.

With the first response, the nurse expresses the nature of the relationship and a personal reaction to the client's noncompliance. The client does not feel judged. The second response places all of the responsibility for noncompliance on the client. The nurse assumes that it is lack of understanding that precipitated the noncompliance, which may or may not be true. The client is likely to respond negatively, so that response does not further the goal of compliance.

Effective feedback is *specific* rather than general. Telling a client he or she is shy or easily intimidated is less helpful than saying, "I noticed when the anesthesiologist was in here that you didn't ask her any of the questions you had about your anesthesia tomorrow." Precise information

---

### Box 10–8. Disconfirming Responses that Block Communication

| Category of Response | Explanation of Category | Examples |
|---|---|---|
| False reassurance | Using pseudocomforting phrases in an attempt to offer reassurance | "It will be okay." "Everything will work out." |
| Giving advice | Making a decision for a client; offering personal opinions; telling a client what to do (using phrases such as "ought to," "should do") | "If I were you I would . . ." "I feel you should . . ." |
| False inferences | Making an unsubstantiated assumption about what a client means; interpreting the client's behavior without asking for validation; jumping to conclusions | "What you really mean is you don't like your physician." "Subconsciously, you are blaming your husband for the accident." |
| Moralizing | Expressing your own values about what is right and wrong, especially on a topic that concerns the client | "Abortion is wrong." "It is wrong to refuse to have the operation." |
| Value judgments | Conveying your approval or disapproval about the client's behavior or about what client has said using words such as "good," "bad," or "nice" | "I'm glad you decided to." "That really wasn't a nice way to behave." "She's a good patient." |
| Social responses | Polite superficial comments that do not focus on what the client is feeling or trying to say; use of clichés | "Isn't that nice?" "Hospital rules, you know?" "Just do what the doctor says." "It's a beautiful day." |

about an observed behavior can suggest a solution. The client is more likely to respond with validation or correction, and the nurse can provide specific guidance.

*Timing* of feedback is crucial for effectiveness. Generally, feedback given as soon as possible after a behavior is observed is most effective. Other factors such as a client's readiness to hear feedback, privacy, and the availability of support from others need to receive consideration.

Feedback should be *appropriate* to the needs of the situation and the client. For example, a very obese mother in the hospital was feeding her newborn infant 4 ounces of formula every 4 hours. She was concerned that her child vomited a considerable amount of the undigested formula after each feeding. Initially, the nursing student gave the mother instructions about feeding the infant no more than 2 ounces at each feeding in the first few days of life, but the mother's behavior persisted and so did that of her infant. The nursing student then began to assess the mother's experience by asking questions and discovered that the mother's mother had fed her 4 ounces right from birth with no problem. As a new mother, this woman felt that she should follow her mother's guidelines. By considering the mother's past experience, the nurse was able to provide the educative support that allowed the client to see her infant as a unique human being and to feel comfortable and confident in feeding him.

*Avoid generalities and pick your battles wisely.* Not all feedback is equally relevant. Nor is it always equally accepted. The benchmark for deciding whether or not feedback is appropriate is to ask, "Does the feedback advance the goals of the relationship?" and "Does it consider the individualized needs of the client?" If the answers are "no," the feedback may be accurate but inappropriate for the moment.

*Usable* feedback is perceived as interest and concern. In contrast, providing feedback about behaviors over which the client has little control only increases the client's feelings of low self-esteem and leads to frustration. For example, telling a cardiac client in the hospital with his second heart attack that "you should have known better than to go back to work so soon" is feedback the client already knows and cannot use in his present situation. Similarly, it is not useful to

tell a 350-pound client, "You should lose some weight." Most obese client are acutely aware of their weight problem.

Effective feedback is *clear*, *honest*, and *reflective*. Feedback supported with realistic examples is believable, whereas feedback without documentation is perceived by many clients as lacking in credibility. To illustrate from your nursing school experience, if you were told that you would have no trouble passing any of the exams in nursing school, you would wonder whether the statement was true. However, if your instructor said, "On the basis of past performance and the fact that your score on the entrance exams was high, I think you should have little problem with our tests as long as you study," you probably would have more confidence in the statement.

Assumptions stated as facts are difficult for the client to respond to. When the nurse tells the client "I know what you mean" without asking the client whether the communication or situation has the same meaning for both, the nurse may be completely wrong. Feedback is relevant only when it addresses the topics under discussion and does not go beyond the data presented by the client. Switching the topic or focus of the conversation in the middle of a stream of thought tends to bring communication to a dead halt or to leave it at a superficial level.

### ◆ Case Example

A nursing student had a client with pancreatic cancer who was in considerable pain, so that even shaving required effort almost beyond his endurance. It was one of the first days of spring, and the weather was bright and sunny. The client said to the nurse, "I wish I were dead; there is nothing to live for." The nurse responded, "It's such a beautiful day. At least that should have some meaning."

In this example, the nurse's answer reflected personal anxiety rather than the client's statement of anguish. With a complete switch in topic to one that had no connection with the ongoing subject, the nurse was ignoring the client's emotional needs and focusing on her own. In tense situations, it is not hard to make such a communication error. The nurse who recognizes her own discomfort as the basis for making such a switch might apologize to the client, acknowledge her own discomfort, and refocus the conversation back onto the client's needs.

Feedback sometimes can have a surprise twist leading to an unexpected conclusion, as shown in the following example.

### ◆ Case Example

It was Jovan's third birthday. There was a party of adults (his mother and father, his grandparents, his great uncle and aunt, and me (his aunt), because Jovan was the only child in the family. While we were sitting and chatting, Jovan was running around and playing. At a moment of complete silence, Jovan's great uncle asked him solemnly:

**Uncle:** "Jovan, who do you love the best?

**Jovan:** "Nobody!"

Then Jovan ran to me and whispered in my ear:

**Jovan:** "You are Nobody!" (Marjanovic-Shane, 1996, p. 11)

### Asking for Validation

Validation is a special form of asking for feedback from a client based on the principle that *meanings are in people, not in the words themselves.* Clients differ in how they respond to a message, and these variations influence the ways they understand and use language. Validation is a way of checking out the accuracy of the message received by the nurse or of confirming that the message sent by the nurse was received by the client in the manner intended. Asking the client

"How do you feel about what I just said?" or "I'm curious what your thoughts are about what I just told you" gives the client an opportunity and the interpersonal space to express his or her feelings.

If the client does not have any response, the nurse might follow up the inquiry with a simple statement suggesting that the client can respond later. For example, the nurse might say "Many people do find they have reactions or questions about [the issue] after they have had a chance to think about it, and I would be glad to discuss them with you if you find you have some later on." Taking the time to ask for validation helps clients feel that the nurse genuinely cares about their feelings and fosters clients' sense of being full participants in their care (Heineken, 1998). Simply asking clients whether they understand what was said is not an adequate method of validating message content. Nurses need to rephrase or verbally reflect back to the clients their perceptions of what they hear and observe for complete accuracy.

### ◆ Case Example

Mr. Brown (to nurse taking his blood pressure): I can't stand that medicine. It doesn't set well (grimaces and holds his stomach).
Nurse: Are you saying that your medication for lowering your blood pressure upsets your stomach?
Mr. Brown: No, I just don't like the taste of it.

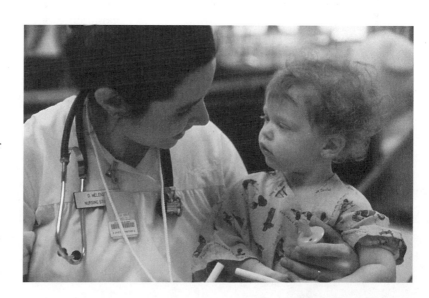

Whether you are sitting or standing, your posture should be relaxed and, if possible, the upper part of your body should be inclined toward the client. (Courtesy of the University of Maryland School of Nursing)

Sometimes validation occurs in the client's behavior rather than through words.

### ◆ Case Example

After a diabetes diet instruction class, Mr. Oxam questions the nurse as to whether the potato served him at lunch was an equivalent exchange for the toast he ate at breakfast. The nurse has behavioral evidence that the client has a basic understanding of the concepts related to food exchanges in diabetic diets. However, Mr. Oxam may need further information and practice to make concrete applications in his life.

Validation is a useful strategy to reinforce information and to ask clients about changes in their behavior that enhances compliance or reasons for noncompliance. Here validation takes the form of tactful inquiry coupled with observational data.

### ◆ Case Example

Jane Smith has been coming to the clinic to lose weight. At first she was quite successful, losing 2 pounds per week. This week, however, she has gained 3 pounds. The nurse validates the change with the client by simultaneously seeking additional information:

**Nurse:**   Jane, over the past 6 weeks you have lost 2 pounds per week, but this week you gained 3 pounds. There seems to be a problem here. Let's discuss what might have happened and how we can get back on track with your goal of losing weight.

In using this strategy as query, the nurse describes the observed client *behavior*, remains nonjudgmental in asking for the client's *perceptions* of the behavioral change, and reaffirms the original treatment goal. Box 10–9 presents a summary of the different therapeutic interviewing skills presented in this chapter as they apply to the phases of the nurse–client relationship.

## When Face-to-Face Communication Is Not Possible

Ideally, all communication should involve face-to-face contact. When this is not possible, nurses should consider how their words might be interpreted. The number of behavioral cues decreases as communication becomes removed from direct interpersonal contact. Telephone calls represent a more distant way of communicating, whereas written communication is the most detached form of interpersonal contact. Even so, a written message is better than nothing when the interests of the relationship warrant it. A note can provide closure for the nurse and comfort for the client. There may be times, for instance, when a nurse must end with a client because of a sudden transfer without being able to say good-by or when a client dies on an off shift and the nurse would like to share thoughts with the family. Writing a note at least acknowledges the meaning of the relationship. When writing notes, consider the relevance of indirect communication cues such as the formality of the message, typed versus handwritten notes, and the nature of the closing remarks in drafting it.

### Communicating by Telephone

Frequently, it is the nurse who calls the family when a client is near death or has died. When placing a call, the nurse first clarifies that the person on the other end of the line is the correct significant other. Addressing the client's significant other by name centers the person. It is important to explain who you are and the reason for your call at the outset. Details are not given at this time (Buckman, 1992). The nurse keeps communication simple while providing clear directives as to the next step. In calling a client's responsible significant other, the nurse might use the following format: "Hello, is this Mr. Peters? My name is Judy Cooper, and I am a nurse at Bayley Hospital. Your son has been in an accident and was admitted to our emergency room. I know this must be a terrible shock to you, and I think it is important for you to come to the hospital as soon as possible. Are you familiar with the route to the hospital?"

If the family directly asks whether the client has died, the nurse needs to answer truthfully. Other details are better discussed once the family has arrived on the unit. Nurses should make every effort to deliver bad news in person. If the family wants details over the telephone, the nurse

### Box 10–9. Interviewing and Relationship Skills

| Phase | Stage | Purpose | Skills |
|---|---|---|---|
| Orientation phase | Rapport and structuring | To build a working alliance with the client | Basic listening and attending; information giving |
| Assessment, engagement, and beginning active intervention phase | Gathering information, defining the problem, identifying strengths | To determine how the client views the problem and what client strengths might be used in their resolution | Basic listening and attending; open-ended questions, verbal cues, and leads |
| Planning, active intervention phase | Determining outcomes: what needs to happen to reduce the self-care demand?; where does the client want to go? | To find out how the client would like to be; how would things be if the problems were solved? | Attending and basic listening; influencing; feedback |
| Implementation, active intervention phase | Explaining alternatives and options | To work toward resolution of the client's self-care demand | Influencing; feedback balanced by attending and listening |
| Evaluation, termination phase | Generalization and transfer of learing | To enable changes in thoughts, feeling, and behaviors. To evaluate the effectiveness of the changes in modifying the self-care demand. | Influencing; feedback; validation |

Adapted from Ivey A. (1983). Ivey's five stage model of interviewing. In Ivey A (ed.), Intentional Interviewing and Counseling. Monterey, CA, Brooks/Cole; Richmond V, McCroskey J, Payne S. (1987). Nonverbal Behavior in Interpersonal Relations. Englewood Cliffs, NJ, Prentice Hall. Used with permission.

can respond with a simple statement, "As soon as you come in, we will be able to tell you everything that happened and will be able to answer your questions. Our experience is that being able to answer your questions directly in person is best." If the family member insists, the nurse can give only the most basic information and should conclude the brief explanation with the request that it would be better to discuss the events in person. Learning the details of a serious injury or the death of a relative with the direct support of hospital staff is more comforting than imagining things. Nursing personnel can interpret baffling medical data and provide practical advice regarding the next steps in caring for the client and the family. If the client has died, the nurse represents an anchor and calming presence in the face of an overwhelming crisis (Jacob, 1991). Having an opportunity to see the client in death and being able to say good-by in person are important to families. It allows natural closure on an important relationship.

Telephone communication is an important link for clients as periodic informational telephone calls to enhance family involvement in the long-term care of clients. Over time, some families lose interest or find it too painful to continue active commitment. Interest and support from the nurse reminds families that they are not simply nonessential, interchangeable parts in their loved one's lives. Their input is important. Strategically timed telephone calls designed to inform, not blame, reinforce and sustain the family–client connection. The call also serves as a reminder that the nurse is a resource to the family member as well as the client during difficult times. Chapter 19 discusses handling ongoing informational telephone calls in stressful situations.

## SUMMARY

This chapter discusses basic therapeutic communication strategies the nurse can use with clients across clinical settings. Application of communication strategies should fit the purposes of the relationship and the communication style of the nurse. The nurse uses clarification to obtain more information when data are incomplete. Restatement is appropriate when a particular part of the content is needed. Paraphrasing addresses the content or cognitive component of the communication. Reflection is a technique used more specifically to get at the underlying feelings or the affective part of the message. Silence gives the client additional opportunity to clarify thoughts and to process information. Touch is a nonverbal strategy that underscores verbal understanding or is used in place of verbal expression when words would fail as a response to the depth of feeling expressed by the client. Summarization integrates the content and feeling parts of the message by rephrasing two or more parts of the message.

Open-ended questions give the nurse the most information because they allow clients to express ideas and feelings as they are experiencing them. By contrast, focused and closed questions narrow the range of possible answers. They are most appropriate in emergency clinical situations when precise information is needed quickly.

The nurse uses verbal communication strategies that fit the client's communication patterns in terms of level, meaning, and language. Other strategies include use of metaphors, reframing, humor, confirming responses, feedback, and validation. Feedback provides a client with needed information.

## REFERENCES

Bandler R, Grindler J. (1997). Reframing. Palo Alto, CA, Science and Behavior Books.

Berne M, Lerner HM. (1992). Communicating with addicted women in labor. American Journal of Maternal Child Nursing 17(1):22–26.

Billings C. (1991). Therapeutic use of metaphors. Issues in Mental Health Nursing 12:1–8.

Blondis M, Jackson B. (1982). Nonverbal Communication with Patients: Back to the Human Touch (2nd ed.). New York, Wiley.

Buber M. (1970). I and Thou. New York, Scribner.

Buckman R. (1992). How to Break Bad News: A Guide for Health Care Professionals. Baltimore, Johns Hopkins University Press.

Cahill J. (1998). Patient participation—a review of the literature. Journal of Clinical Nursing. 7(2):119–128.

Charkhuff R. (1983). The Art of Helping (5th ed.). Amherst, MA, Human Resources Development Press.

Corey G. (1995). Theory and Practice of Counseling and Psychotherapy (5th ed.). Monterey, CA, Brooks/Cole, p. 240.

Cormier L, Cormier W, Weisser R. (1984). Interviewing and Helping Skills for Health Professionals. Monterey, CA, Wadsworth.

Cousins N. (1976). Anatomy of an illness. New England Journal of Medicine 295(26):1458–1463.

Crowther DJ. (1991). Metacommunications: A missed opportunity? Journal of Psychosocial Nursing and Mental Health Services 29(4):13–16.

Dowd S, Giger J, Davidhizar R. (1998). Use of Giger and Davidhizar's Transcultural Assessment Model by health professions. International Nursing Review 45(4):119–122.

Duldt B. (1991). I-Thou in nursing: Research supporting Duldt's theory. Perspectives in Psychiatric Care 27(3):5–12.

Ekman P, Friesen W. (1975). Unmasking the Face: A Guide to Recognizing Emotions from Facial Clues. Englewood Cliffs, NJ, Prentice Hall.

Gorman M, Devine J. (1998). What to do when your patient uses illicit drugs. American Journal of Nursing 98(3):54.

Hall E. (1959). The Silent Language. New York, Doubleday.

Heineken J. (1982). Disconfirmation in dysfunctional communication. Nursing Research 31(4):211–213.

Heineken J. (1983). Treating the disconfirmed psychiatric client. Journal of Psychosocial Nursing 21(1):21–25.

Heineken J. (1998). Patient silence is not necessarily client satisfaction: Communication problems in home care nursing. Home Health Care Nurse 16(2):115–120.

Jacob S. (1991). Support for family caregivers in the community. Family and Community Health 14(1):16–21.

Johnson M. (1980). Self disclosure: A variable in the nurse-client relationship. Journal of Psychiatric Nursing 18(1):17–20.

Knapp M, Hall J. (1992). Nonverbal Communication in Human Interaction. Fort Worth, TX, Holt, Rinehart & Winston.

Loos F, Bell J. (1990). Circular questions: A family interviewing strategy. Dimensions of Critical Care Nursing 9(1):47.

Lynch T, Anchor K. (1991). Use of humor in medical psychotherapy. In Anchor K (ed.), Handbook of Medical Psychotherapy. Lewiston, NY, Hogrefe & Huber.

Majanovic-Shane A. (1996). Propositional Model of Meaning Construction. Available from http://www.geocities.com/Athens/2253/modelll.html.

McGhee M. (1985). Humor. In Snyder M (ed.), Independent Nursing Functions. New York, Wiley.

McGhee P. (1998). Rx laughter. RN 61(7):50–53.

McKinney S. (1992). The nurse who listened. Nursing 22(5):71.

Metcalf C. (1998). Stoma care: Exploring the value of effective listening. British Journal of Nursing 7(6):311–315.

Miller C. (1990). Understanding the psychosocial challenges of older adulthood. Imprint 37(4):67–69.

Moustakas C. (1974). Finding Yourself: Finding Others. Englewood Cliffs, NJ, Prentice Hall.

Nelson J. (1998). Personal touch. Nursing Standard 12(36):18.

Pearson A, Borbasi S, Walsh K. (1997). Practicing nursing therapeutically through acting as a skilled companion on the illness journey. Advanced Practice Nursing Quarterly 3(1):46–52.

Pearson A, Borbasi S, Walsh K. (1998). Practicing nursing therapeutically through acting as a skilled companion on the illness journey. Advanced Practice Nursing Quarterly 3(1).46–52.

Peplau H. (1960). Talking with patients. American Journal of Nursing 60(7):964–966.

Pesut D. (1991). The art, science, and techniques of reframing in psychiatric mental health nursing. Issues in Mental Health 12(1):9–18.

Ramos MC. (1992). The nurse-patient relationship: Theme and variation. Journal of Advanced Nursing 17(4): 196–206.

Renwick P. (1992). Teaching the use of interpersonal skills. Nursing Standard 7(9):31–34.

Richmond V, McCroskey J, Payne S. (1987). Nonverbal Behavior in Interpersonal Relations. Englewood Cliffs, NJ, Prentice Hall.

Ruesch J. (1961). Therapeutic Communication. New York, Norton, p. 32.

Severtsen BM. (1990). Therapeutic communication demystified. Journal of Nursing Education 29(1):190–192.

Smith Battle, Drake MA, Diekemper M. (1997). The responsive use of self in community health nursing practice. Advances in Nursing Science 20(2):75–89.

Stewart J (ed.). (1986). Bridges Not Walls (4th ed.). New York, Random House.

Straka DA. (1997). Are you listening? Have you heard? Advanced Practice Nursing 3(2):80–81.

Tannen D. (1991). You Just Don't Understand: Women and Men in Conversation. New York, Balantine.

Weingarten K. (1992). A consideration of intimate and non-intimate interactions in therapy. Family Process 31:45–59.

# 11

# Intercultural Communication

Elizabeth Arnold

---

**OBJECTIVES**

At the end of the chapter, the student will be able to

1. Define culture and describe related terminology
2. Discuss the concept of intercultural communication

3. Apply the nursing process to the care of the culturally diverse client
4. Discuss characteristics of selected cultures as they relate to the nurse–client relationship

---

*If we are to achieve a richer culture, rich in contrasting values, we must recognize the whole gamut of human potentialities, and so weave a less arbitrary social fabric, one in which each diverse human gift will find a fitting place.*

Mead (1988)

---

❖❖❖ The focus of Chapter 11 is on intercultural communication. Culture is primarily a social concept. The U.S. population is changing, and health care consumers increasingly are people of color. Recent estimates indicate that by the year 2000, more than 25 percent of the American population will consist of people of color and will include approximately 6 million more immigrants (U.S. Department of Health and Human Services [DHHS], 1991). Nurses will need to interact with clients from many different backgrounds who speak many different languages. They will have to respond to the emergence of new roles for men and women; far-ranging economic uncertainty; and increases in the number of single-parent families, the elderly population, and the poverty-stricken population. Each of these social changes adds to the diversity of the health care consumer. Communication competence with culturally diverse clients requires appropriate ways of speaking to the clients and knowledge of culturally congruent ways to manage intercultural health care events (Smith, 1998).

## BASIC CONCEPTS

### Definition

Madeleine Leininger (1977), a nurse theorist, defined *culture* as "a common collectivity of beliefs, values and shared understandings and patterns of behavior of a designated group of people." Culture provides the community with its strength and vitality. It is an abstract human structure with many variations in meaning (Westbrook & Sedlacek, 1991). Each cultural community develops fundamental standards of behavior that differentiate those who "belong" and those who are outsiders. Personal patterns of emotional expression, language, child-rearing practices, values, rules, and even physical objects such as dress and equipment trace their origin to cultural experience. They contribute to the development of a cultural world view that includes the individual's perceptions of his or her relationship with the larger community (Sue, 1978).

Differences in cultural expectations, ways of being in the world, and meanings help with understanding atypical individual behavior patterns in health care. For example, in some cultures, when a family member becomes ill, the entire family camps out in the hospital. As Shweder (1991) noted, "When people live in the world differently, it may be that they live in different worlds" (Exercise 11–1).

Children learn about the culture into which they are born from their parents; culture is a *learned social experience*. Culture grounds their life experience and connects an individual to the larger community. A person within the culture is respected and treated as an equal, whereas one who is not a part of the culture is treated with misgivings and suspicion. When one culture supports certain behavior standards that conflict with those of the dominant culture, a person's behavior can appear dysfunctional when, in fact, it is quite appropriate from a transcultural perspective (McGoldrick & Rohrbaugh, 1987).

### ◆ Case Example

Mohan is an Asian nursing student trying to cope in an American society characterized by autonomy, self-assertiveness, and self-disclosing responsiveness. By contrast with American students, Mohan seems nonaggressive and does not always act in his own best interest. Sometimes he is late for class, and he is guarded, by American standards, in what he reveals about himself. Viewed from an Asian perspective, Mohan's behavior is not at all unusual. In India, the individual does not seek personal attention. Each person is part of the larger cosmos and seeks to blend harmoniously with traditions and the community. Achievements count, but it is culturally incorrect to view them as part of a personal identity (Kakar, 1991).

## Cultural Terminology

### Multiculturalism

*Multiculturalism* describes a heterogeneous society in which several diverse cultural world views can coexist with some general ("etic") characteristics shared by all cultural groups and some ("emic") perspectives that are unique to a particular group. A multicultural perspective "implies a wide range of multiple groups without grading, comparing, or ranking them as better or worse than one another and without denying the very distinct and complementary or even contradictory perspectives that each group brings with it" (Pederson, 1991a, p. 4). In today's global social environment, its rapidly changing demographics,

◆ Exercise 11-1. **Meaning of Culture**

**Purpose:** To help students appreciate the many dimensions of culture

**Procedure:**
Frequently, the attitudes, feelings, and understandings people have about a culture are found in the words they associate with that culture.

1. Think about the word ``culture'' and write down all of the words and phrases you can think of in response to the word. There are no right or wrong answers.
2. Assign a negative (−) sign to the words you perceive might have a negative value. Assign a positive (+) sign to the words you perceive might have a positive value. Do not assign any value to words you perceive as being without a value.
3. Share your results with the other members of your class group.

**Discussion:**
1. Were you surprised at any of the words that popped into your mind?
2. What does your list tell you about your attitudes and feelings about culture?
3. In what ways were your words and phrases similar to or different from those of your classmates?
4. In what ways did your answers reflect your own cultural background?
5. How could you use the information you gained from this exercise to provide culturally congruent care?

and an increasingly interdependent world economy, the term *multiculturalism* fits most community definitions of culture (Exercise 11–2).

## Acculturation

*Acculturation* is used to describe the process by which a person consciously learns and accepts the values of a new culture. Because culture is a socially learned process, it also is an adaptive process. Cultural behaviors change as people within a culture come in contact with "outsiders" and blend their cultural beliefs with those outside the original culture. For example, the adult children of a second-generation Vietnamese living

◆ Exercise 11-2. **Recognizing Components of Group Culture**

**Purpose:** To help students appreciate the cultural components of everyday life

**Procedure:**
1. Each student is to attend some type of group or community activity.
2. Observe as many behaviors, norms, rules, dress, membership commonalities, roles, and so on as possible.
3. Write a descriptive summary of the group you observed that portrays an image of the group to others. Include what you have learned about the culture of this group and what might you be careful about in order to communicate effectively in this group

**Discussion:**
1. Each student will share observations with the group and address the cultural components that are unique to this group.
2. Discuss how different cultural components impact on communication.
3. How should the nurse incorporate cultural awareness into communication?

in America are likely to develop ease with the English language and customs as they live longer in the United States and to use American customs to guide their behavior rather than more traditional values.

As the social environment and biological needs of a people change, so do the traditional forms of the culture. For example, as Thailand becomes more westernized, with more people moving to the cities, the children are less likely to demonstrate loyalty to traditional Thai values that worked with agrarian economy but are less useful in an urban society. On the other hand, the roots of cultural behavioral standards run deep and can influence behavior, even over generations in the new culture (Exercise 11–3).

## Subculture

*Subculture* is defined as an ethnic, regional, or economic group of people joined by distinguishing characteristics that differentiate the group from the predominant culture or society (Samovar & Porter, 1988). Usually the subculture speaks the same language and can trace its roots equally well as coming from the same geographical location as the predominant culture. Examples of subcultures in the United States include Amish, Appalachians, Jehovah's Witnesses, Hare Krishnas, the homeless, and migrant workers. Although the cultural differences of these groups might not seem pronounced, meaningful communication can be difficult because the communication of subcultures reflects the cultural meaning the groups attach to the content of a message.

## Cultural Diversity

*Cultural diversity* describes the fact that there are differences among cultural groups. Diversity is becoming the norm in our society rather than the exception. It can include variables such as nationality, ethnic origin, gender, educational background, geographical location, economic status, language, politics, and religion (Pederson, 1991b).

Diversity occurs within the same community (e.g., age and differences in the work culture of management and employees). Situations that are culturally significant to adolescents and young adults may not have the same meaning to their grandparents, and vice versa. Such gaps also occur within a work culture. Differences in cultural expectations for the physician, social worker, ward clerk, nurse, and physical therapist can affect decision making and task allocation in health care settings.

Although the fact that people differ from one another is not a deterrent to communication, it is essential that nurses understand, acknowledge, and respect these differences in the nurse–client relationship as being a part of a unique human being. Having this understanding can mean the difference between success and failure in providing effective nursing care (Napier, 1998).

---

◆ **Exercise 11–3. Family Culture Experiences**

**Purpose:** To help students appreciate how culture is learned

**Procedure:**
1. Identify and describe one family custom or tradition. It can relate to special family foods, a holiday custom, a child-rearing practice, or any other special tradition.
2. Describe the custom or tradition in detail.
3. Talk with a family member about how this family tradition originated in your family.
4. Discuss how this custom or tradition has changed over time.
5. Describe how this family tradition has affected your family functioning.

**Discussion:**
1. Share your family tradition with your classmates.
2. As a class, discuss how differences in family culture can influence health.
3. Discuss how knowledge of family customs can influence communication and health care promotion.

## Cultural Relativism

**Cultural relativism** refers to the belief that cultures are neither inferior nor superior to one another, and that there is no single scale for measuring the value of a culture. Furthermore, within a culture there are many variations in behaviors and in how individuals interpret their cultural heritage. In fact, there may be more individual differences among members of the same culture than among dissimilar cultures. Bromwich (1992) noted that "an artist, of any race or sex or ethnic identity, has more in common with other artists, however remote, than with other members of the same . . . 'cultural' group." This point has implications for the nurse–client relationship in that the individualized needs of the client should determine the degree to which cultural variations require modifications of the treatment plan. For some clients, the modifications mandated by culture will be extensive; for others, an understanding of sensitive issues is sufficient. Customs, beliefs, and practices must be understood in context and according to the needs of each client (Cochran, 1998).

## Ethnicity

**Ethnicity** is defined as a personal awareness of certain symbolic elements that bind people together in a social context. The word "ethnic" derives from the Greek word *ethnos*, meaning "people." An **ethnic group** is a social grouping of people who share a common racial, geographic, religious, or historical culture. In contrast to culture, which does not always involve a conscious awareness of norms and symbols, ethnicity is a chosen awareness and commitment to a cultural identity. In the United States, common ethnic groups include African-American, Native American, Hispanic, Asian, Indian, Jewish, Irish, Italian, and Amish.

Ethnic identity is an important part of a person's self-identity and can play an important role in how a client interprets symptoms and responds in a clinical setting. For example, an Orthodox Jewish client cannot ring the emergency bell or turn on the lights during the Sabbath period. This client will require special food and food preparation techniques to feel comfortable.

Ethnicity is not the same as race, a common overgeneralization. Race refers to differences in biological characteristics such as color of the skin, facial features, and hair texture. As people from different racial groups intermarry, they assume cultural and physical characteristics of both racial groups. Although we label a person by virtue of race as belonging to a particular ethnic group, this is not always valid. A person from Jamaica can have dark skin and other biological characteristics of African-American descent and yet have no geographical link whatsoever to Africa. Is this person really an African-American? Is the cultural identification linked to Africa or Jamaica?

## Ethnocentrism

**Ethnocentrism** refers to a belief that one's own culture is superior to others (Leininger, 1977). Taking pride in one's culture is appropriate, but when a person fails to respect the pride that other people from a different culture take in their ethnic identity, it is easy to develop prejudice, which can be highly destructive to a relationship (Thiederman, 1986). The deadly extremes of ethnocentrism were apparent in the Nazi persecution of the Jews in the name of the Aryan race during Hitler's regime. Similar persecutions for ethnic reasons are ongoing today in parts of Europe and the Middle East.

Ethnocentrism—the belief that certain groups of people are inferior—happens on a smaller scale with the physically or mentally disabled, the urban poor, the homeless, persons with acquired immunodeficiency syndrome (AIDS), and certain minority groups. Age and racial discrimination are subtle forms of ethnocentrism that add to the feelings of devaluation and inferiority experienced by minority members of a dominant culture. Consider the following example in which one health-related characteristic results in the judgment that the man possessing it is not as worthy as others.

### ◆ Case Example

I knew a man who had lost the use of both eyes. He was called a "blind man." He could also be called an expert typist, a conscientious worker, a good student, a careful listener, a man who wanted a job. But he couldn't get a job in the department store order room where employees sat and typed orders which came over the phone. The personnel man was impatient to get the interview over. "But you are a blind man," he kept saying and one could almost feel his silent assumption that somehow the incapability in one aspect made the man incapable in every other. So blinded by the label was the interviewer that he could not be persuaded to look beyond it. (Lee, quoted in Allport, 1982)

When the stereotyped label corresponds to undesirable personal traits in the eyes of the dominant cultural expectation, whether the deviation from the norm has a cultural, physical, or psychological origin, the person is at a distinct disadvantage because of the implied negative value judgments. To counteract this tendency, Allport (1982) suggested using ethnic labels as adjectives rather than nouns. Thus, the nurse would speak of the "person of color" rather than "the African-American." Recognizing implied value judgments and taking the time to be sensitive to the subtle interpretations of value-laden ethnic terms in conversation can prevent misunderstanding and hurt feelings. To provide quality care for clients from different cultures, the nurse must make a conscious effort to see each client as a unique individual with many complex characteristics, one of which happens to be different from those of the majority norm (Doswell & Erlen, 1998). Exercise 11–4 makes it easier to see the prevalence of stereotypes. Exposure to different cultures allows for a different perception of cultural differences and the universality of humanness.

◆ **Case Example**

Mara has a stereotyped view of Hispanic people. Her mother distrusts Hispanic people and has told her that Hispanic people are low class and lack initiative. Without having had exposure to Hispanic people, Mara's ideas reflect her mother's teaching and bear very little resemblance to reality. Her college roommate is Hispanic. As the roommates exchange experiences, they develop a shared history, quite different from Mara's experience. Mara finds that her roommate is not so different from herself. Her roommate comes from a socioeconomic background similar to her own and is one of the best students in the class. Mara's knowledge and attitude toward Hispanic people change dramatically.

## Intercultural Communication

Samovar and Porter (1988) defined *intercultural communication* simply as a communication in which the sender of an intended message is a member of one culture and the receiver of the message is from a different culture. Different languages create and express different personal realities. Many experts note that language has four primary functions: (1) to direct actions, (2) to interpret the meaning of events and situations, (3) to connect past experiences with the present through imagination, and (4) to establish and maintain relationships with people. These functions are woven into the fabric of every culture.

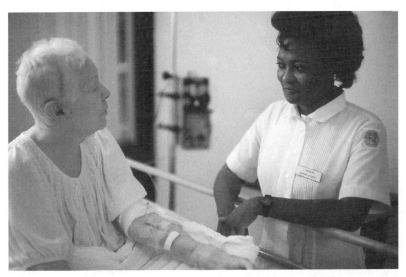

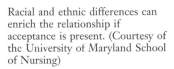

Racial and ethnic differences can enrich the relationship if acceptance is present. (Courtesy of the University of Maryland School of Nursing)

◆ Exercise 11-4. **Exploring Stereotypes**

**Purpose:** To help students examine stereotypes and their impact on communication and relationships

**Procedure:**
The first part of this exercise should be written outside of class, anonymously, to encourage honest answers. The following list represents some of the groups in our society that carry familiar value-laden stereotypes.

| | |
|---|---|
| American Indians | people on welfare |
| African-Americans | teenage mothers |
| Asiansr | AIDS victims |
| Hispanics | migrant workers |
| Homosexual men | the elderly |
| Lesbians | people with sensory deficits |
| The homeless | mentally ill persons |

1. Write down the first three words or phrases that come into your mind regarding each of these groups.
2. Make a grid to show stereotypes. Use three columns, with each cultural group. On the vertical column at the left, list positive, neutral, and negative connotations at the top.
3. As a class group, take the collected words and phrases and decide whether they represent one or more culturally specific connotations. Place each word or phrase under the appropriate column for each group. Use an *X* to indicate repetitive words or phrases.

**Discussion:**
For each cultural group, consider the following:

1. Why do you think people believe that this cultural group possesses these characteristics?
2. What were the common themes of these groups? Did certain groups have more negative than positive responses? If so, how would you account for this?
3. In what ways did this exercise help you to think about your own cultural socialization process?
4. Did this exercise cause you to question any of your own assumptions about culturally different values?
5. From your view, what implications do these stereotypes hold for providing appropriate nursing care?
6. How can you use this exercise in your future care of culturally different populations?

Adapted from Eliason M, Macy N. (1992). A classroom activity to introduce cultural diversity. Nurse Educator 17(3):32–35. Used with permission.

People name objects, situations, events, qualities, and feelings in their own language symbols. Language helps people understand the motivations of others and to make theirs known to others (Grasska & McFarlane, 1982; Scott, 1991). People tell each other what is socially acceptable behavior and reinforce adaptive behavior. Thus, cultural differences in language affect every aspect of the behavior and relationships that occur between nurses and their clients and can function as a major barrier to mutual understanding (Geissler, 1991a).

It is not unusual for a client and a family member for whom English is a second language to revert to their native language in times of stress (Thompson et al., 1990). Conversation slows because the person is trying to have two conversations, one with the interviewer and one within him- or herself about the meaning of the message. Although the client uses American words and phrases, they are translated into, and processed in, the client's native language. Sometimes it is difficult for the nurse to appreciate this double cognitive processing because the responses are in English, and the nurse is aware only that the client seems to be taking more time than usual. Subtle but important language differences also can color the meaning of words and change their understanding. For this reason, it is essential for the nurse to use clear, precise language and to avoid slang and clichés with clients who display limited English skills. Asking the right questions, providing verbal cues, and allowing more time for clients with limited language skills to answer conveys interest and respect; this kind of communication also helps decrease unnecessary anxiety. Exercise 11–5 addresses the issue of language barriers.

◆ **Case Example**

A nursing student from the Philippines said she was thoroughly confused by her instructor's slang expression, "I want to touch base with you." The student did not know how to respond, because her literal translation of the sentence did not express its meaning to her. Had the instructor said, "I would like to talk with you," the student would have known how to respond.

Intercultural communication is more than simply an issue of language translation. Cultural interpretations of illness, behaviors, and symptom expressions are important considerations, as are issues related to traditions about treatments, family hierarchy, and decision making. Sometimes the cultural differences are striking, involving language, dress, diet, and behavioral styles that are completely foreign to the nurse. At other times, variations are more subtle, involving the

---

◆ **Exercise 11–5. Understanding Language Barriers**

**Purpose:**  To help students understand the role of language barriers

**Procedure:**

*Situation 1*
Lee Singh is a 24-year-old Korean patient who speaks no English. She was admitted to the maternity unit and has just delivered her first child, a 9-pound infant. It was a difficult labor because the infant was so big. Lee Singh speaks no English. The initial objectives of the health care providers are to help the client understand what is happening to her and to help her become comfortable with her baby.

*Situation 2*
Jose Perot is a 30-year-old Hispanic male who was admitted to the emergency department with multiple injuries after a car accident. His family has been notified, but the nurse is not sure they understand what has happened. They have just arrived in the emergency room.

1. Break up into two groups of four or five students. Each group acts as a unit. The groups role-play Situation 1 and reverse roles for Situation 2.
2. The client group should completely substitute bogus words that only they understand for the words they would normally use to communicate in this situation. The bogus words should have the same meaning to all members of the client group.
3. The health provider group must figure out creative ways to understand and communicate with the client group.

**Discussion:**
1. In what ways was it different being the client and being the health provider group?
2. What was the hardest part of this exercise?
3. In what ways did this exercise help you understand the frustrations of being unable to communicate?

meaning of a gesture, the interpretation of a remark, consciousness of space and time, or the relationship of the person to the larger community. An educated nurse consciously incorporates knowledge of the client's culture into every interaction, particularly in health teaching (Lester, 1998).

## APPLICATIONS

### Assessment

A culturally relevant assessment starts with clients' reality. Leininger (1991) developed a sunrise model that provides a framework for areas of concern (Fig. 11–1). By letting clients tell their story and asking reflective questions to ensure understanding, the nurse learns to make sense of the cultural context of the health care need. Self-awareness of cultural blind spots reminds the nurse that people are different despite belonging to a certain cultural or minority group. Not all clients from the same ethnic or cultural group share the same understandings of their illness or expectations for treatment. Treating ethnic minority clients as though they follow the same norms does not recognize the individual uniqueness of each client.

The way a client presents symptoms can reveal which aspects of the client's complaints are culturally acceptable and how the client's culture permits their expression. For example, Latin culture populations describe their pain and symptoms with dramatic body language and emotional words, whereas Asian and Pacific Islands cultural norms mandate controlled emotional expression (Giger & Davidhizar, 1991). Being able to recognize that a behavior may be characteristic of a culture rather than "abnormal behavior" places a nurse at an advantage in relating effectively and therapeutically with clients from differing cultures.

Nurses need to ask their clients what they think caused their illness or injury. Health care professionals sometimes mistakenly assume that illness is a single concept, but illness is a complex personal experience, strongly colored by cultural norms, values, social roles, and religious beliefs (Deetz & Stevenson, 1986). For example, some lower income, rural African-Americans who are not integrated into the predominant culture consider illness from a natural and unnatural perspective. Natural illness occurs because the individuals have not protected themselves sufficiently from the forces of nature. Unnatural illness happens when the person receives a "hex" from bad spirits, usually of a supernatural nature. Clients who believe in an unnatural origin for their illness often require the services of a folk healer in addition to medical treatments as part of their treatment process (Campinha-Bacote, 1992).

Some illnesses carry negative cultural values. For example, in Chinese cultures, it is more acceptable for an individual to have venereal disease than to have tuberculosis; physical explanations for behavioral symptoms are acceptable, but psychological explanations are denied outside the family circle (Kleinman, 1980). Some illnesses can not be treated for cultural reasons. Vaccinations for smallpox cannot be given in some parts of India because smallpox is considered a god in rural areas.

### Cultural Assessment Sequence

One method nurses use to understand the needs of clients from a different culture is a cultural assessment (Rosenbaum, 1991). The data base should include the information presented in Box 11–1. A cultural assessment consists of three progressive interconnecting elements: (1) a general assessment, (2) a problem-specific assessment, and (3) the cultural details needed for successful implementation of the care plan. This structure represents a logical way of organizing relevant cultural data and is easy for the client to follow. Exercise 11–6 provides practice with cultural assessment.

The general assessment provides the nurse with an initial regular appraisal of care issues that potentially could affect health care delivery. Common areas of cultural variation include client responses to pain, the need for privacy and body exposure, eating preferences and style, consciousness of space and time, isolation and quiet, the number of people involved in decision making, hygiene practices, religious and healing rituals, eye contact, and touch (Guarnaccia, 1998). Most people find comfort in sharing their culture with others and appreciate the nurse who asks. Usually clients will not volunteer such information without being asked.

The second stage of the cultural assessment

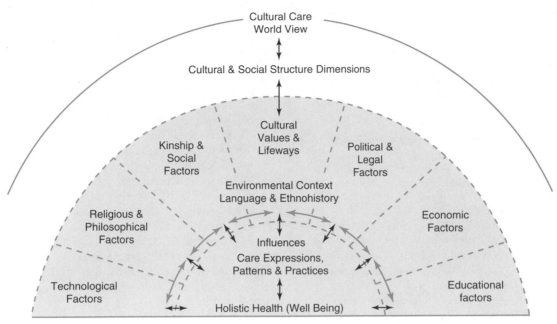

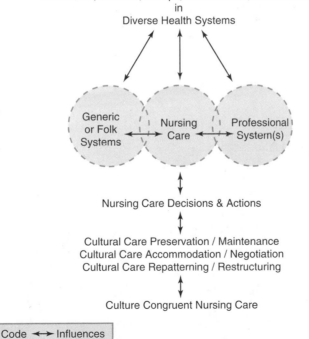

Figure 11–1. Leininger's sunrise model to depict the theory of cultural care diversity and universality. (From Leininger M. (ed.) (1991). *Cultural Care Diversity and Universality: A Theory of Nursing.* National League for Nursing. Sudbury, MA, Jones and Bartlett Publishers. Reprinted with permission.)

◆ Box 11-1. Data Base for the Culturally Diverse Client

Information should focus on

1. Patterns or lifestyles of an individual or group
2. Specific cultural values, norms, and experiences of a client (or group) regarding the health and caring behavior of his or her culture
3. Cultural taboos or myths
4. The world view and ethnocentric tendencies of an individual (or group)
5. General features the client (or group) perceives as different from, or similar to, other cultures in or near his or her environment
6. The health and life care rituals and rites of passage to maintain health and avoid illness
7. Folk and professional health-illness systems
8. Detailed caring behavior and nursing care for self and others
9. Indicators of cultural changes and acculturation processes influencing health care

Adapted from Leininger M. (1978). Transcultural Nursing. New York, Wiley, pp. 88–89. Used with permission.

is problem specific. Here the nurse gathers data related to the condition or problem for which the client is seeking treatment. Culture plays a role in cause, presentation, and treatment. Sickle cell anemia is found almost exclusively among African-Americans, and Tay-Sachs disease is a genetic disorder unique to the Jewish community. Cystic fibrosis is found in Caucasian children. In cases of tuberculosis reported for children, 83 percent occurred in ethnic minorities (U.S. DHHS, 1991).

Drug responses vary across cultures. For example, it has been documented that Asians have a tendency to metabolize drugs more slowly and thus achieve a higher therapeutic effect with smaller doses of medication (Keltner & Folks, 1992; Lin et al., 1986).

Using a specific cultural assessment allows the nurse to place a particular client problem or need within its unique cultural context, to understand it, and to educate the client. Sample questions are found in Box 11-2.

The final phase of the cultural assessment focuses on the specific cultural details needed for client acceptance of treatment plans. It is a way to engage the client as an active coparticipant in the treatment process. For example, if diet is a major part of the treatment protocol, the nurse elicits information about cultural diet preferences and works with the client to include rele-

◆ Exercise 11-6. **Cultural Assessment**

**Purpose:**  To help students identify cultural assessment data

**Procedure:**
1. Select a specific ethnic culture, and using Leininger's model, interview someone from that culture. Information about different cultures can be found in the literature and on the Internet, or perhaps you have had personal experience with the ethnic culture you are describing.
2. Write a short report on that culture, including a discussion of values, traditions, health care beliefs, nutrition, death rituals, and so on.
3. Share your written report with your classmates.

**Discussion:**
1. Discuss each ethnic culture and the common characteristics of the cultural group.
2. What important values did you uncover?
3. Discuss how the cultural value of a particular ethnic group impacts health care.
4. Discuss how the nurse can best meet the needs of culturally diverse clients while respecting their cultural identity.

---

┌─────────────────────────────────────┐

◆ **Box 11-2. Sample
Assessment Questions**

- Can you tell me something about the reasons you are seeking health care for . . . ?
- Can you tell me something about how a person in your culture would be cared for if they had a similar condition?
- Have you been treated for a similar problem in the past? (If the client answers yes, more information about the precise nature of treatment is elicited.)
- Can you tell me what people in your culture do to remain healthy?
- Can you tell me something about the foods you like and how they are prepared?
- Are there any special cultural beliefs about your illness that might help me give you better care?

└─────────────────────────────────────┘

vant foods whenever possible in a therapeutically restricted diet.

## Nursing Diagnoses

We currently do not have nursing diagnoses that specifically address the culturally imposed difficulties our clients experience in the dominant culture health care system. Current nursing diagnoses related to the communication difficulties of the culturally diverse client include (1) impaired verbal communication related to cultural differences, (2) impaired social interaction related to sociocultural dissonance, and (3) noncompliance related to a patient's value system: beliefs about health and cultural influences (North American Nursing Diagnosis Association [NANDA], 1989; Geissler, 1991b). Although these diagnoses are in current use, they often fail to inform the nurse fully of the complexity of the cultural issues that led to the diagnosis and should be used with caution. As Geissler (1991a) noted, each of these diagnoses has features that imply a negative clinical judgment about the person. For example, in the first diagnosis, is communication impaired because a person cannot speak the language, or is the nurse equally impaired because of a similar lack of knowledge about the client's language? Impairment implies a disability. In what ways, then, does "impaired verbal communication" ac-

tually describe the communication problem of the culturally diverse client?

The second diagnosis has similar problems. Is the social isolation experienced by the culturally diverse client truly an impairment, or should this diagnosis be described differently, perhaps as an impairment of the larger society? The third diagnosis assumes that the client is being noncompliant. Yet this client may be acting according to deeply held cultural beliefs. To comply with Western medical protocols would place the client at odds with personal cultural values. Thus, the nursing diagnosis, while providing words about the client's difficulty, may not be usable as a valid descriptor. Knowing the cultural implications of the client's behavioral response, should the nurse still assume that the client is noncompliant and try to change the client's behavior? If you as a professional nurse wanted to make these diagnoses culturally congruent, how would you change their wording?

## Factors in Planning
### Language Barriers

Clients from different cultures frequently identify language barriers as the most frustrating aspect of cultural diversity. They feel helpless, even desperate, when they cannot express their thoughts and feelings to someone who must be able to understand their meaning in order to help them. The nurse needs to assess the extent of language barriers and to explore what it means to the client. Acknowledging language difficulties and trying to find creative ways to share experiences are important for the client's acceptance of the nurse.

Strategies the nurse can use include using pictures and developing "flash cards" with commonly used hospital terms such as pain, medicine, bathroom, can't sleep, hungry, hot, cold, doctor, and so on, with the words in the client's language written beside them (Thompson et al., 1990). Learning a few specific words related to the client's health care in the client's language and teaching the client some simple English words to express health needs also help. Refer to Exercise 11–5 for help in experiencing language differences.

### Defining Role Relations

Cultural customs may require role relationships to be more formal, with well-defined boundaries and clearly verbalized expectations. For example, Asian clients respond best to a formal relationship. They favor an indirect communication style characterized by polite phrases and marked deference (Tsui & Schultz, 1988). Typically, the client waits for the information to be offered by the nurse as the authority figure. This behavior does not mean that the Asian client is timid, passive, or unwilling to participate in the treatment process. It simply is a cultural characteristic that needs to be acknowledged, respected, and accounted for in developing an individualized plan of care for a client exhibiting such culturally determined behavior.

On the other hand, Hispanic clients need a more personal, informal interpersonal format to feel comfortable. They respond best to a health professional who is open, warm, and willing to respond to personal questions (Pagani-Tousignant, 1992).

In some minority cultures, there is an unspoken tendency to view health professionals as authority figures, treating them with deference and respect but disregarding their advice. This value is so strong that a client frequently will not question the nurse or in any way indicate mistrust of this authority figure's counsel. Such clients simply will not follow the nurse's recommendations or will withdraw from treatment. Careful attention to the flow of the ethnic client or family's concerns helps to prevent this situation.

## Level of Family Involvement

Level of family involvement is another issue. For example, the degree of family involvement among Asian, Hispanic, and African-American cultures is apt to be much greater than the norm in the United States. Within these cultures, the extended family is the basic social unit. Health problems affecting one family member have direct implications for all other members of the family. In most instances, the number of potentially involved caregivers is correspondingly larger than in the main culture. Moreover, there also is a sex-linked hierarchy; the oldest male is the final authority on family matters in Asian and Hispanic cultures. For this reason, the nurse might address the husband first, even if another adult family member is the actual client. Identifying and including all those who will be taking an

active part in the care of the client from the outset recognizes the communal nature of family involvement in health care. For the Native American client, this may include many members of an immediate tribe or its spokesperson.

### Time Orientation

Orientation to time and to time pressures differs in certain cultures depending on whether it is past, present, or future oriented. In the United States, "time is money," and people are very concerned about exact time frames for appointments, taking medications, and so on. Present-oriented time does not consider the commitment to a future appointment as important as attending to what is happening in the moment. Giger and Davidhizar (1991) noted that "a common belief shared by some African-Americans and Mexican-Americans is that time is flexible and events will begin when they arrive" (p. 105). Some flexibility with time schedules for nursing care procedures should be factored into the care plan for these clients.

## Intervention
### Using Culturally Based Teaching

Cultural differences affect a nurse's teaching and coaching functions. A useful teaching sequence for culturally diverse clients follows the guidelines for the mnemonic *LEARN: L*isten, *E*xplain, *A*cknowledge, *R*ecommend, and *N*egotiate (Campinha-Bacote, 1992, p. 11). With this process, the nurse listens carefully to the client's perspective on his or her health problem, including (1) cause, (2) expectations for treatment, and (3) information about family and others who traditionally are involved in the client's care. Once the nurse has a clear understanding of the client's perception of the problem, the nurse can explain his or her understanding of it, using simple, concrete terminology and can ask for validation that this perspective is correct.

After this discussion, the nurse can acknowledge the differences and similarities between their perceptions. The information serves as a basis for planning interventions, with the nurse making specific recommendations to the client and negotiating a mutually acceptable treatment approach (Campinha-Bacote, 1991, 1992).

Throughout the negotiation process to determine goals and the means to achieve them, the nurse is respectful of the client's right to hold different cultural views. If family members traditionally are involved in decision making, they should be made an integral part of the relationship at each step in the process. The same information given to the client is shared with the family. Otherwise, the treatment process is likely to fail, no matter how worthy the intervention.

Specific teaching strategies can enhance culturally based recommendations. For example, incorporating storytelling as a teaching strategy is likely to facilitate success with the Native American client who is used to learning in this manner (Moody & Laurent, 1984). Providing a maternity client with booklets about breast-feeding written in her native language is a small, yet meaningful gesture. The offering is tangible evidence of the nurse's acknowledgment of cultural differences. Box 11–3 provides general teaching guidelines for use with culturally diverse clients.

---

◆ Box 11–3.

General Communication Guidelines for Interacting with Culturally Diverse Clients

Use the same sequence and repeat phrases, expanding on the same basic questions.

Speak slowly and clearly, and use concrete language the client can understand. Make the sentence structure as simple as possible.

Encourage the client by smiling and by listening. Provide cues such as pictures and gestures.

Avoid the use of technical language, and choose words that incorporate cultural terms whenever possible.

Allow enough time, and do not assume that simply because the client nods or smiles the communication is understood.

Identify barriers to compliance such as social values, environment, and language.

Help the client develop realistic, culturally relevant goals.

Incorporate culturally specific teaching formats. For example, use an oral or storytelling format with clients who have oral teaching traditions.

Close with cultural sensitivity: "I've really learned a lot today about [restate highlights]. Thanks for sharing with me."

---

## Use of Interpreters

Federal law mandates the use of a trained interpreter according to standards established by the Joint Commission on Accreditation of Hospitals and criteria published under Title VI of the Civil Rights Act for clients who cannot communicate because of language differences. In many cases, a family member speaks both the native language and English, or it is possible to communicate in a more limited way. Having someone act as an intermediary, who can communicate with the client and who can understand the subtle nuances of the culture, often bridges the language gap (Newhill, 1990). When interpreters are necessary, they should be chosen with care, keeping in mind differences in dialects as well as the sex and social status of the interpreter and the client, if this is likely to be an issue.

## Applications to Special Populations

Some basic concepts about the traditional characteristics of the larger minority groups living in the United States are included in this chapter. In no way are they intended to be all inclusive or completely descriptive of the culture. It also seems essential to emphasize that not everyone associated with a particular culture demonstrates the same characteristics or has the same desire for an ethnic identity. The nurse needs to use the basic information about different cultures as a basis for inquiry and must engage the client as the primary resource in learning the best ways to provide culturally congruent care for each individual.

## African-American Clients

African-Americans account for 12 percent of the U.S. population, making it the largest minority group in the nation (U.S. DHHS, 1991). They are referred to as blacks, Afro-Americans, or African-Americans. For many African-Americans, their ethnic culture traces back to slavery and deprivation. The vestiges of this heritage are evidenced in a seriously disproportionate level of poverty, with its attendant social and health problems, and a visible need for further efforts to ensure equal opportunity for this

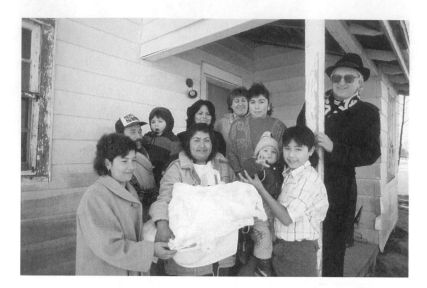

Nurses interact with clients from many cultural backgrounds.

group. A smaller group emigrated from other countries such as Haiti and Jamaica.

Lower income African-American clients statistically are less likely to use regular health services because of subtle and overt discrimination that have been a part of their lives for as long as they can remember and because of cost. African-Americans tend to rely on informal helping networks in the community, particularly those associated with their church, until a problem becomes a crisis and use of folk-healing measures is common.

Establishing trust is a critical element for success with African-American clients, who are more willing to participate in treatment when they feel respected and are treated as partners in their health care. Allowing these clients to have as much control over their health care as possible helps reinforce personal strengths and enhances their self-concept. This is a useful strategy with any client who feels oppressed and stigmatized by the health care system. Understanding the reasons behind a client's hostility and mistrust of the health care provider allows the nurse to be more patient and proactive.

### Health Care Concerns

Health care concerns of African-Americans cover a variety of social and physical diseases. The rate of AIDS, homicide, and drug abuse—social diseases associated more with poverty and substandard living conditions than ethnicity—are significantly higher for black than for white Americans. African-Americans are subject to higher rates of hypertension, adolescent pregnancy, diabetes, and stroke. If you are a black male, you have a significantly greater chance of developing cancer and of dying from it (U.S. DHHS, 1991).

In the traditional African-American culture, disease is thought to occur because of a lack of harmony with nature. Voodoo is still practiced in some rural communities.

### ◆ Case Example

Ms. Jones was a 56-year-old African-American who was brought by her family to the psychiatric emergency service of a large city hospital. She claimed that she had been poisoned by her husband's lover. After a psychiatric examination, Ms. Jones was given the diagnosis of delusional disorder–jealous type. She was admitted to the inpatient psychiatric unit and started on a neuroleptic medication. However, the diagnostician failed to conduct a culturological assessment, which would have revealed that Ms. Jones felt she was experiencing voodoo illness. A more culturally relevant treatment would have included consultation with a folk healer (Campinha-Bacote, 1992).

### Family

The family is the rallying point of the African-American's social life. Loyalty to the extended family is a dominant value, and family members rely on each other for support (Sterritt & Pokorny, 1998). African-American families stick together in times of trouble, and it is not uncommon for an entire entourage of family visitors to camp out in the hospital waiting room during a serious illness.

Many low-income African-American children grow up in extended families because one or both parents cannot assume child care responsibilities, and grandparents take the role of primary caregiver. As a result, generational boundaries are not always clear-cut. Decision making is largely matriarchal in low-income families. Women often become the heads of their families because of racial discrimination and limitations imposed by the U.S. Department of Health, Education, and Welfare on the presence of the father in the home. This is not true of the large black middle class. These individuals are more likely to have intact families and to enjoy high socioeconomic and professional status in their communities. Their health care behaviors more closely resemble those of the dominant culture.

## Religion

Most African-Americans are Christian. The black Muslim religion is a strict fundamentalist religion, favored by some African-Americans, that strongly endorses ethnic identity through dress and actions. The church plays a central role in black culture. For centuries, it served as the primary social, economic, and community life center. It continues to provide a strong resource in times of stress, to affirm and inspire the black community. Black political leaders, for example, Jesse Jackson, Ralph Abernathy, and the late Martin Luther King, Jr., also are church leaders. Because of the central meaning of the church in African-American life, incorporating the appropriate clergy in treatment plans is a useful strategy. Likewise, readings from the Bible and gospel hymns are sources of support during hospitalization.

## Hispanic-American Clients

Spanish-speaking Americans are the second largest minority group in the United States (U.S. DHHS, 1991). They usually identify themselves as Hispanic-Americans or Latinos. Mexican-Americans are referred to as Chicanos. Typically, Hispanic clients identify their country of origin, for example, Puerto Rico, Colombia, and San Salvador, in their self-description.

Hispanic clients typically uses the formal health care system only as a short-term, problem-solving strategy. They like to keep their problems within the family, so talking with a "stranger" is difficult. In a health care situation, the Hispanic client needs to develop *confianza* (trust) in the health care provider and frequently will ask personal questions to establish the bonding necessary for disclosure. This practice is not based on a desire to invade the nurse's privacy but rather is the normal way the Hispanic client establishes an acceptable context for conversation (Pederson, 1988). Consequently, if asked, the nurse might provide simple information about marital status, number of children, or other nonintrusive data.

Hispanic clients living in rural areas rely on *curanderos* (local folk healers and herb doctors) for most of their medical advice. The curandero uses a combination of healing practices, medicines, and herbs to cure illness. They often view physical diseases and the treatments used to cure them as being related to dietary practices. It is important to determine whether the client ascribes to the hot and cold theory of treating illness. For example, many Hispanic clients view arthritis as a "cold" disease that should be treated with "hot" foods such as cornmeal, garlic, alcohol, coffee, onions, and chili peppers. "Hot" diseases such as constipation, diarrhea, or ulcers would be treated with "cold" medication, such as bicarbonate of soda and milk of magnesia (Cowell, 1988).

## Health Care Concerns

Health care concerns of particular relevance to the Hispanic population are teenage drug abuse, adolescent pregnancy, lack of preventive and of prenatal health care, and a higher incidence of human immunodeficiency virus (HIV) infections in women and children than in the white population. Heart disease and cancer are the most frequent causes of death in the United States. Hispanic immigrants believe that illness can be the result of a great fright (*susto*) or falling out of favor with God. Hispanic women may be reluctant to express their private concerns in front of their children, even adult children.

## Family

The family is the center of the Hispanic client's life and serves as a primary source of emotional support. Hispanic clients are "family members first, and individuals second" (Pagani-Tousignant, 1992, p. 10). Social interactions, often on a daily basis, take place among the nuclear and extended family and a few close friends. Close friends are considered a part of the family unit. In the Hispanic culture, cooperation is more important than competition, and competitive situations are avoided whenever possible.

Sex roles are relatively rigid, and it is very important that the male remain in control of his feelings (*machismo*). Hispanic men are trained from early childhood not to show their feelings, particularly to a strange woman. Hispanic women are socialized to serve their husbands and children without question (*la sufrida*, or the long-suffering woman) (Pagani-Tousignant, 1992). The nurse needs to be sensitive to the role of these cultural beliefs in treatment situations.

## Religion

Hispanic clients are usually deeply religious; the predominant religion is Catholicism. They view illness and suffering with a fatalistic acceptance having religious overtones (*si Dios quierre*, or if God wishes). The relationship between God and the individual is a close, intimate one. In fact, the relationship is so close that it is acceptable for individuals to experience visions and dreams in which God or the saints speak directly to the individual. In many Western cultures, such behaviors might be labeled as hallucinations, and psychiatric treatment might be recommended.

## Asian-American Clients

The third most common minority group in the United States is Asian. Pagani-Tousignant (1992) noted that there are more than 32 ethnic groups comprising the cultural community of Asians and Pacific Islanders. Traditionally, the Asian client exercises significant emotional restraint in communication. It is hard to tell what Asian persons are truly thinking or feeling because, typically, their facial expressions are not as flexible and their words are not as revealing as those people in the dominant culture. For this reason, the nurse can underestimate or neglect the Asian client's suffering. Asking the client about pain and suggesting possible feelings are helpful interventions. The Asian client also appreciates a clinician who is willing to provide advice in a matter-of-fact, concise manner.

## Health Care Concerns

Health care concerns specifically relevant to this population include a higher than normal incidence of tuberculosis, hepatitis B, and some forms of cancer (U.S. DHHS, 1991). The Asian client traditionally perceives illness as an imbalance of yin and yang. In this ancient representation, yin is the female force containing all the elements that represent darkness, cold, and weakness. Yang represents the male elements of strength, brightness, and warmth. Acupressure and herbal medicines are among the medical practices used by Asian clients to reestablish the balance between yin and yang. The influence of Eastern health practices and alternative medicine are increasingly incorporated into the health care of all Americans.

The following is a case example of an Asian client in an American hospital.

### ◆ Case Example

A young Vietnamese woman, Mrs. N., gave birth to a healthy boy. During labor, the mother was smiling and said nothing. Seemingly, the labor process caused her no stress. The father remained at the hospital during the labor but assumed a passive role, entering the delivery room only to translate some instructions to his wife. On the postpartum unit, Mrs. N. refused to take her medications with the ice water offered to her. She seemed reluctant to get out of bed other than to use the bathroom, and she refused to eat. Despite a smiling, polite posture during most of her postpartum course, she became visibly upset when the nurse brought her baby to her and made pleasing remarks about the infant (Hollingsworth et al., 1980).

To the casual observer, Mrs. N.'s behavior was perplexing. However, if the nurse viewed the same behaviors from a transcultural perspective, they made complete sense. Mrs. N.'s composure during her labor and her politeness during postpartum were cultural responses dictated by the cultural need to remain stoic. In Vietnam, the newborn is bathed and clothed before the father has contact with it. This custom explains Mr.

N.'s behavior in exiting the delivery room quickly and not spending initial time with his newborn infant.

Mrs. N.'s postpartum behavior has cultural meaning. The Vietnamese view childbirth as disturbing the balance between yin and yang (hot and cold) in the body. Only the body part to be examined can be exposed, and only in private. Mrs. N.'s refusal of medications was related to a fear of disturbing the balance between yin and yang in her body. Likewise, her poor eating pattern can be explained by this humoral imbalance. Only certain foods, such as chicken, rice, and pork, are thought to be "warm" foods. Postpartum women do not traditionally eat salads. Vietnamese women traditionally avoid early ambulation because of a belief that too much movement will prevent their distended internal organs from resuming their prepregnancy state. Finally, the nurse's enthusiasm in recognizing her new infant was unacceptable to Mrs. N. because of a cultural belief that should a spirit overhear the comments and find the child desirable, the spirit might attempt to steal it away.

This case example demonstrates the importance of cultural knowledge in implementing nursing care. No more time needs to be expended, but planning would be practical and simple, with clear attention given to the cultural implications of each intervention. Although this case example may seem extreme, subtle misunderstandings and problems can occur in any nursing situation in which the nurse and client are not of the same ethnic background.

### Family

The family is crucial and all encompassing, with adult members of the family living together in the same household even after marriage. The family may consist of (1) father, mother, and children; (2) nuclear family, grandparents, and other relatives living together; or (3) a broken family in which some family members are in the United States and other nuclear family members are still living in their country of origin (Gelles, 1995). There is family pressure on younger members to do well academically, and family members assume a great deal of responsibility for each other, including financial assistance. Sons have a higher value than daughters, and sex roles are well defined; the male is viewed as the breadwinner and the female is designated the caretaker. In contrast with many other societies, the elders in an Asian community are highly respected and well taken care of by younger members of the family (Pagani-Tousignant, 1992).

### Communication

The Asian client views the nurse as an authority figure. In the Asian culture, a person must show complete respect for authority figures. It is almost impossible for the Asian client to argue or disagree with the nurse. Consequently, the nurse has to ask open-ended questions and clarify issues consistently in every interaction. If the nurse uses questions that require a yes or no answer, the answer may reflect the client's polite deference rather than an honest response. Explaining treatment as problem-solving facts, asking the client how things are done in his or her culture, and working with the client to develop a culturally congruent solution usually is most effective (McLaughlin & Braun, 1998).

Asian men may have a difficult time disclosing personal information to a female nurse unless the nurse explains why the data are necessary for care, because in serious matters women are not considered as knowledgeable as men. Asian clients may be reluctant to be examined by a person of the opposite sex, particularly if the examination or treatment involves the genital area. Many Asians consider the head the repository of the soul, so that touching the head is seen as damaging the equilibrium of the soul. For this reason, it is useful to explain the reason for touching the head before doing so (Santopietro, 1981).

### Religion

The three major religious groups in Asian culture are Hinduism, Sikhism, and Islam. Religious beliefs are tightly interwoven into the social fabric of everyday life and affect every aspect of it. Hindus are required to pray regularly, and they are devoted to the ideals of pacifism, reincarnation, and a God who can be worshiped in many forms. There is a well-defined caste system that is important because what a person is and does in this life affects life after reincarnation (Abrahams, 1985). Hindus are vegetarians because it is against their religion to kill living creatures. Sikhism is a reformed variation of Hinduism in which women have more rights in domestic and community life.

Islam is the world's fastest growing religion, and it is found predominantly in Southeast Asia. The Muslim religion is a way of life in which an individual submits entirely to Allah and follows Allah's basic rules about everything from personal relationships to business matters, including personal matters such as dress and hygiene. In the end, Allah decides whether a person has been successful in following the rules and whether the person will be allowed to enter paradise, and there are rituals that must be followed in death. Islam has some strong tenets that affect health care, an important one being that God is the ultimate healer. There can be no physical contact between a woman and a man who is not her husband. Physical modesty is a high value.

## Native American Clients

Although Native Americans represent the smallest of the major ethnic groups in the nation, there are almost 400 tribes in the United States. Very few Native Americans still dwell on Indian reservations (Pagani-Tousignant, 1992). Native Americans living in or around Alaska refer to themselves as Alaska natives. Those living in other states prefer the label American Indian (U.S. DHHS, 1991).

### Health Care Concerns

Health concerns of particular relevance to the Native American population are unintentional injuries, of which 75 percent are alcohol related—suicide, cirrhosis, alcoholism, and obesity. Juvenile diabetes is a major problem, and the death rate from the disease is significantly higher than it is in the white population. It is estimated that 95 percent of American Indian families are affected directly or indirectly by alcohol abuse (U.S. DHHS, 1991).

### Communication Patterns

As an ethnic group, the Native Americans are much more comfortable with long periods of silence than other groups. Native Americans are private persons who respect the privacy of others. They are less likely to speak of their feelings and prefer to talk about the facts rather than the accompanying emotions. Native American clients respond best to health professionals who stick to the point and do not engage in small talk. They are suspicious of interviewers who ask many questions, and they are hesitant to volunteer information about anyone other than themselves. For this reason, it is better to ask questions in short sessions rather than all at once and to ask each person directly for information. Native Americans live in the present and have little appreciation of time commitments, which can be a problem in health care delivery. Calling the client before making a home visit or to remind the client of an appointment is useful.

### Family

The family is highly valued by the Native American. Sex roles are less rigid than in other cultures, and family boundaries are extended to include people who are not blood related. For example, it is not unusual for a child to have several mothers and siblings who are not related but are considered a part of the person's family. The nurse may need to include these people in care planning because they can be a very important social support to the Native American client (Long & Curry, 1998). Tribal identity is maintained through regular powwows and other ceremonial events. Both men and women feel an obligation to promote tribal values and traditions through their crafts and traditional ceremonies.

### Religion

The religious beliefs of Native Americans are strongly linked with nature and the earth, with use of symbols and metaphors to explain and make sense of reality. Inanimate objects such as rocks and the elements of weather are imbued with spiritual qualities. If a person is in harmony with the supernatural forces in the universe, the person will not experience disease. Illness is viewed as an imbalance, a punishment from God for some real or imagined imbalance with nature; it is believed to be divine intervention to help the individual correct evil ways. In some cases, recovery is likely to occur only after the client is cleansed of the "evil spirits." Native Americans view death as a natural process, but they fear the power of dead spirits and use numerous tribal rituals to ward them off.

Because person and nature are one and the

same, most healing practices are strongly embedded in religious beliefs. Native Americans may seek medical help from their tribal elders and *shamans* (highly respected spiritual medicine men and women). The shaman uses spiritual healing practices and herbs to cure the ill member of the tribe (Pagani-Tousignant, 1992).

### Culture of Poverty

There are enough differences in the cultural world view of those who fall below the poverty line to warrant special consideration of their needs in the nurse–client relationship. The culture of poverty is characterized by acute deprivation. The poor generally are disadvantaged educationally. They do not have the same access to the health care system and preventive health care because of cost and availability. The poor who seek health care are also subject to long waits and sometimes very rude treatment by health professionals who do not seem to want to help. Consequently, health-seeking behaviors among the poor and homeless tend to be crisis oriented. Medical help is sought only when a person is acutely ill and is discontinued when obvious symptoms disappear. The nurse needs to use a crisis-oriented approach for greatest impact.

**Health Care Strategies**

In our society, being poor means being powerless. Many poor people experience virtually no control over meeting their basic needs, things that most of us take for granted such as food,

housing, and clothing or the chance for a decent job and the opportunity for education. Often they have experienced violence rather than social justice as the means to provide their fundamental needs. Consequently, the idea that they can exercise choice in their lives and make a difference in their health care is not part of their world view. They look to and expect others to take responsibility and to make things better. Poor people often do not take the initiative simply because their life experiences tell them they cannot trust that their own efforts will produce any change. This is a very difficult but important cultural concept for nurses to incorporate into their relationships with people of poverty. The nurse must take a proactive, persistent, and patient-oriented approach to understanding and working with this population (Minick et al., 1998). Communication strategies that acknowledge, support, and empower the poor to take small steps to independence are most effective. Exercise 11–7 provides practice with a practical application of cultural differences.

## Evaluation

Evaluation of goals achieved in a transcultural nurse–client relationship should include answers to such questions as the following: Were the learning activities culturally specific and sufficient to produce the desired outcome? Is the client satisfied with the outcome? What cultural modifications are needed to provide the client with the content and process the client needs to

---

◆ **Exercise 11–7. Applying Cultural Sensitivity to Nursing Care**

**Purpose:** To familiarize you with culture-specific elements of nursing care for several populations

**Procedure:**
This can be done in small, even-numbered groups rather than as an individual exercise.

1. Each student creates a clinical scenario based on a client from a cultural group. Be creative, and write a situation in which ethnicity or cultural factors present in the client's nursing needs.
2. Trade scenarios with another student, and write how you would incorporate cultural needs and strategies into their care plan.
3. Each student presents the final case scenario with the care plan he or she developed.

**Discussion:**
The group will discuss additional ways to incorporate cultural needs into nursing care.

achieve the objectives? The nurse needs to reflect on any potential biases that may have gotten in the way of providing culturally congruent care.

## SUMMARY

Chapter 11 explores intercultural communication that takes place when the nurse and client are from different cultures. Culture is defined as a common collectivity of beliefs, values, shared understandings, and patterns of behavior of a designated group of people. It needs to viewed as a human structure with many variations in meaning.

Multiculturalism describes a heterogeneous society in which diverse cultural world views can coexist with some general (etic) characteristics shared by all cultural groups and some (emic) perspectives that are unique to a particular group. Combining the two perspectives provides the multicultural perspective. Related terms include cultural diversity, cultural relativism, subculture, ethnicity, ethnocentrism, and ethnography. Each of these concepts broadens the definition of culture. Intercultural communication is defined as a communication in which the sender of a message is a member of one culture and the receiver of the message is from a different culture. Different languages create and express different personal realities.

A cultural assessment is defined as a systematic appraisal of beliefs, values, and practices conducted to determine the context of client needs and to tailor nursing interventions. It is composed of three progressive, interconnecting elements: (1) a general assessment, (2) a problem-specific assessment, and (3) the cultural details needed for successful implementation.

Knowledge and acceptance of the client's right to seek and support alternative health care practices dictated by culture can make a major difference in compliance and successful outcome. Health care professionals sometimes mistakenly assume that illness is a single concept, but illness is a personal experience, strongly colored by cultural norms, values, social roles, and religious beliefs. Interventions that take into consideration the specialized needs of the culturally diverse client follow the guidelines for *LEARN: L*isten, *E*xplain, *A*cknowledge, *R*ecommend, and Negotiate.

Some basic thoughts about the traditional characteristics of the larger minority groups (African-American, Hispanic, Asian, Native American) living in the United States relating to communication preferences, perceptions about illness, family, health, and religious values are included in the chapter. The culture of poverty is discussed.

## REFERENCES

Abrahams J. (1985). Asian expectations. Nursing Times 81:44–46.

Allport G. (1982). The language of prejudice. In Eschholz P, Rosa A, Clark V (eds.), Language Awareness (3rd ed.). New York, St. Martin Press.

Atkinson DR, Morten G, Sue S. (1989). Counseling American Minorities: A Cross-Cultural Perspective (3rd ed.). Dubuque, IA, William C. Brown.

Bromwich D. (1992). Politics by Other Means: Higher Education and Group Thinking. New Haven, CT, Yale University Press.

Campinha-Bacote J. (1991). Community mental health services: A culturally specific mode. Archives of Psychiatric Nursing 5(4):229–235.

Campinha-Bacote J. (1992). Voodoo illness. Perspectives in Psychiatric Care 28(1):11–16.

Carmichael C. (1985). Cultural patterns of the elderly. In Samovar L, Porter K (eds.), Intercultural Communication: A Reader. Belmont, CA, Wadsworth.

Castaneda C. (1974). The Teachings of Don Juan: A Yaqui Way of Knowledge. New York, Touchstone.

Cochran M. (1998). Tears have no color. American Journal of Nursing 98(6):53.

Cowell D. (1988). Proceedings from the meeting of the National Institutes of Health, "Cultural Implications of Health Care," Washington, DC.

Deetz S, Stevenson S. (1986). Managing Interpersonal Communication. New York, Harper & Row.

Doswell W, Erlen J. (1998). Multicultural issues and ethical concerns in the delivery of revising care interventions. Nursing Clinics of North America 33(2):353–361.

Geissler EM. (1991a). Nursing diagnoses of culturally diverse patients. International Nursing Review 38(5):150–152.

Geissler EM. (1991b). Transcultural nursing and nursing diagnoses. Nursing and Health Care 12(4):190, 192, 203.

Gelles R. (1995). Contemporary Families. Thousand Oaks, CA, Sage.

Giger J, Davidhizar R. (1991). Transcultural Nursing: Assessment and Intervention. St. Louis, Mosby-Year Book.

Grasska MA, McFarlane T. (1982). Overcoming the language barrier: Problems and solutions. American Journal of Nursing 82(9):1376–1379.

Guarnaccia P. (1998). Multicultural experiences of family caregiving: A study of African American, European American, and Hispanic American families. New Directions in Mental Health Services 77:45–61.

Hollingsworth AO, Brown LP, Brooten DA. (1980). The refugees and childbearing: What to expect. RN 43:45–48.

Kakar S. (1991). Western science, Eastern minds. Wilson Quarterly 15(1):109–116.

Keltner N, Folks D. (1992). Culture as a variable in drug therapy. Perspectives in Psychiatric Care 28(1):33–36.

Kleinman A. (1980). Patients and Healers in the Context of Culture. Berkeley, University of California Press.

Klinman A, Eisenberg L, Good B. (1978). Culture, illness and care. Annals of Internal Medicine 88:251.

Leininger M. (1977). Cultural diversities of health and nursing care. Nursing Clinics of North America 12(1):518.

Leininger M. (1978). Transcultural Nursing. New York, Wiley, pp. 88–89.

Leininger M. (1991). Transcultural nursing: The study and practice field. Imprint 38(2):55, 57, 59.

Lester N. (1998). Culture competence. A nursing dialogue. American Journal of Nursing 98(8):26–33.

Lin K, Poland R, Lesser I. (1986). Ethnicity and psychopharmacology. Culture, Medicine and Psychiatry 10:151–165.

Long C, Curry M. (1998). Living in two worlds: Native American women and prenatal care. Health Care for Women International 19(3):205–215.

McGoldrick M, Pearce J, Giordano J (eds.). (1982). Ethnicity and Family Therapy. New York, Guilford Press.

McGoldrick M, Rohrbaugh M. (1987). Researching ethnic family stereotypes. Family Process 26:89–99.

McLaughlin L, Braun K. (1998). Asian and Pacific Islander cultural values: Considerations for health care decision-making. Health & Social Work 23(2):116–126.

Mead M. (1988). Sex and Temperament in Three Primitive Societies. New York: William Morrow & Co.

Minick P, Kee C, Borkat L, Cain T, Oparah-Iwobi T. (1998). Nurses perceptions of people who are homeless. Western Journal of Nursing Research 20(3):356–369.

Moody LE, Laurent M. (1984). Promoting health through the use of storytelling. Health Education 15(1):8–10, 12.

Napier B. (1998). Diversity and aging. Cultural understanding. Home Care Provider 3(1):38–40.

Newhill C. (1990). The role of culture in the development of paranoid symptomatology. American Journal of Orthopsychiatry 60(2):176–185.

North American Nursing Diagnosis Association. (1989). Taxonomy I Revised—1989 with Official Diagnostic Categories. St. Louis, MO, author.

Pagani-Tousignant C. (1992). Breaking the Rules: Counseling Ethnic Minorities. Minneapolis, MN, The Johnson Institute.

Pederson P. (1988). A Handbook for Developing Multicultural Awareness. Alexandria, VA, American Association for Counseling and Development.

Pederson P. (1991a). Introduction to the special issue on multiculturalism as a fourth force in counseling. Journal of Counseling and Development 70:4.

Pederson P. (1991b). Multiculturalism as a generic approach to counseling. Journal of Counseling and Development 70:6–11.

Rosenbaum J. (1991). A cultural assessment guide: Learning cultural sensitivity. Canadian Nurse 87(4):32–33.

Samovar L, Porter R. (1988). Approaching intercultural communication. In Samovar L, Porter R (eds.), Intercultural Communication: Reader (5th ed.). Belmont, CA, Wadsworth.

Santopietro M. (1981). How to get through to a refugee patient. RN 44:43–48.

Scott JK. (1991). Alice Modig and the talking circles. Canadian Nurse 87(6):25–26.

Shweder RA. (1991). Thinking Through Cultures. Cambridge, MA, Harvard University Press, p. 23.

Smith L. (1998). Concept analysis: Cultural competence. Journal of Cultural Diversity 5(1):4–10.

Sterritt P, Pokorny M. (1998). African American caregiving for a relative with Alzheimer's disease. Geriatric Nursing 19(3):127–128, 133–134.

Sue D. (1978). World views and counseling. Personal and Guidance Journal 56:458–462.

Thiederman SB. (1986). Ethnocentrism: A barrier to effective health care. Nurse Practitioner 11:52, 54, 59.

Thompson WL, Thompson TL, House RM. (1990). Taking care of culturally different and non-English speaking patients. International Journal of Psychiatry in Medicine 20(3):235–245.

Tripp-Reimer T, Afifi L. (1989). Crosscultural perspective on patient teaching. Nursing Clinics of North America 24(3):613–619.

Tripp-Reimer T, Friedl MC. (1977). Appalachians: A neglected minority. Nursing Clinics of North America 12(1):41–54.

Tsui P, Schultz G. (1988). Ethnic factors in group process: Cultural dynamics in multiethnic therapy groups. American Journal of Orthopsychiatry 58(1):136–142.

U.S. Department of Health and Human Services. (1991). Healthy People 2000: National Health Promotion and Disease Prevention Objectives (DHHS Publication No. PHS 91-50212). Washington, DC, U.S. Department of Health and Human Services.

Westbrook F, Sedlacek W. (1991). Forty years of using labels to communicate about nontraditional students: Does it help or hurt? Journal of Counseling and Development 70:20–28.

# 12

# Communicating in Groups

## Elizabeth Arnold

### OBJECTIVES

At the end of this chapter the student will be able to

1. Define group communication
2. Identify the differences between primary and secondary groups
3. Discuss factors that influence group dynamics

4. Identify the stages of group development
5. Apply group concepts in clinical settings
6. Contrast different types of groups in health care settings

*He knew intuitively how to be understanding and acceptant. . . . This kind of ability shows up so commonly in groups that it has led me to believe that an ability to be healing or therapeutic is far more common in human life than we might suppose. Often it needs only the permission granted by a freely flowing group experience to become evident.*

Rogers, 1972

❖❖ Chapter 12 focuses on group communication in health care settings. At its most basic level, group communication is an integral form of communication in family, social, and work relationships and strongly influences a person's physical, emotional, and social development through the modeling and feedback a person receives in these relationships (Hawkins, 1998). Lewin (1951) observed that "the *person* we are does not happen in isolation, but rather takes place as the result of exposure to the attitudes and habits of the social groups to which we belong."

Group communication skills are an important dimension of professional growth in professional nursing. Think of the nurses you know who are recognized for their expertise in professional work situations. Are they not also people who raise important issues in work groups and are skilled in group communication? In work settings, groups represent an effective mechanism for discussing staff issues, effecting change, and establishing new work policies. Interdisciplinary health professionals work as a group to provide consistent and collaborative interactions for effective health care delivery (McGinley et al., 1996).

Nurses use group formats to provide information and emotional support for clients and their families in a variety of health care settings ranging from preventive care to rehabilitation (Zahniser & Coursey, 1995). Educational groups are important resources in primary prevention and provide a safe environment to learn information about an illness or treatment protocol. Therapy groups help clients learn more effective coping skills and achieve personal growth. Support groups foster creative problem solving and provide community-based opportunities for people with serious health care problems to interact with others experiencing the same kinds of problems (Agapetus, 1996). As managed care limits interactions with health care professionals, support groups become increasingly important as a tool for people to share information about a specific illness, coping strategies, and resources (Yalom & Yalom, 1990).

## BASIC CONCEPTS
### Definition

A group is not simply a collection of people but rather a collection of people who elect to be together because of a common cause, activity, purpose, or goal. A **group** is defined as (1) a gathering of two or more individuals (2) who share a common purpose and (3) meet over a substantial time period (4) in face-to-face interaction (5) to achieve an identifiable goal. Every group is a unique. Groups develop a culture or personality, reflecting each group's unique behaviors. Relationships among members are interdependent, so that each member's behavior influences the behavior of other group members. Group cultures develop through shared images, values, and meanings that over time become the stories, myths, and metaphors about the group and how it functions.

## Primary and Secondary Groups

Groups are categorized as primary or secondary groups. *Primary groups* are more spontaneous and linked to the values of an individual. Characterized by an informal structure and social process, group membership is either automatic (e.g., family) or is freely chosen because of a common interest such as scouting, religious, or civic groups. Primary groups are an important part of a person's self-concept, revealed in self-descriptions such as "I am Jamie's mother." A study of the number and types of groups to which a person belongs provides valuable data about values and interests. Exercise 12–1 presents an idea of the role groups play in a person's life.

*Secondary groups* are not spontaneous. They differ from primary groups in structure and purpose; they have a planned, time-limited association, a prescribed structure, a designated leader, and a specific identified purpose. When the group achieves its goals, the group disbands. Examples include focus groups, therapy groups, discipline specific work groups, interdisciplinary health care teams, and educational groups. People join secondary groups for one of three reasons: (1) to meet personally established goals, (2) to develop more effective coping skills, or (3) because it is required by the larger community system to which the individual belongs.

## Concepts Related to Group Dynamics

*Group dynamics* is used to describe the communication processes and behaviors occurring dur-

◆ Exercise 12-1. **Role of Group Communication**

**Purpose:** To help students gain an appreciation of the role group communication plays in their lives

**Procedure:**

1. Write down all of the groups in which you have been a participant (e.g., family, scouts, swim team, and community, religious, work, and social groups).
2. Describe the influence membership in each of these groups had on the development of your self-concept.
3. Identify the ways in which membership in different groups was of value in your life.
4. Identify the primary reason you joined each group. If you have discontinued membership, specify the reason.

**Discussion:**

1. How similar or dissimilar were your answers from those of your classmates?
2. What factors account for differences in the quantity and quality of your group memberships?
3. How similar were the ways in which membership enhanced your self-esteem?
4. If your answers were dissimilar, what makes membership in groups such a complex experience?
5. Could different people get different things out of very similar group experiences?
6. What implications does this exercise have for your nursing practice?

ing the life of the group. Individual and group characteristics combine with each other to achieve a group purpose. Group dynamics are an important influence on the success of goal achievement and member satisfaction (Fig. 12–1).

## Individual Characteristics

**Commitment.** Commitment connotes responsibility and involvement. Successful groups consist of members who are motivated to fulfill their responsibilities as group members. Members attend meetings through choice and feel a sense of responsibility for the well-being of other group members. They achieve personal satisfaction from contributing to the group goal, which acts as reinforcement for further engagement. By contrast, lack of commitment results in group apathy and rarely is the group task accomplished. The leader can increase group commitment by (1) preparing members for the group before starting the group, (2) allowing time to process possible resistance, and (3) making group participation a matter of interest and benefit to individual members. In Exercise 12–2 member commitment is discussed.

**Functional Similarity.** Yalom (1985) described *functional similarity* as meaning that group members have enough common intellectual, emotional, and experiential characteristics to interact with each other and to carry out the group objectives. Some real-life examples illustrate the concept. Medication groups require a certain level of cognition because their goal is to provide education related to taking medication. The Alzheimer's disease victim, lacking the cognitive ability to acquire new information, generally does not benefit from such groups. A highly educated older adult placed in a group of young adults with limited verbal and educational skills is a misfit. In each case, the "different" member became a group casualty. In another group with clients having similar issues, the outcome might have been quite different.

*The Ugly Duckling*, a children's fairy tale of a baby swan trying to gain acceptance in a group of ducks, presents the dilemma of being different. Final acceptance and a sense of community came

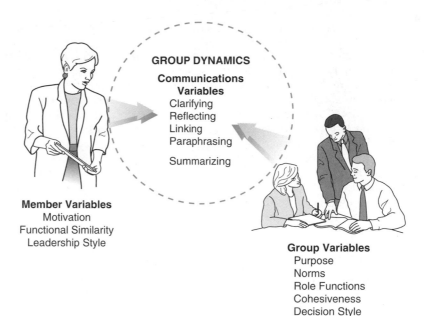

Figure 12–1. Factors affecting group dynamics.

**Member Variables**
Motivation
Functional Similarity
Leadership Style

**Group Variables**
Purpose
Norms
Role Functions
Cohesiveness
Decision Style

---

◆ Exercise 12–2. **Member Commitment**

**Purpose:**  To help you understand the connection of personal commitment to group dynamics

**Procedure:**

1. In small groups of three to five students, think of a group to which you belonged and would characterize as being successful.
2. What did you do in this group that contributed to its success?
3. What made this group easier to commit to than other groups to which you belonged? Be as specific as you can be about the factors that enhanced your commitment.
4. Have one student act as scribe and write down the factors that increased commitment to share with the rest of the class.

**Discussion:**

1. What are the common individual themes that emerged from the discussion?
2. Discuss the relationship of commitment to success.
3. Did commitment emerge as a major factor related to goal achievement?
4. Did commitment emerge as a major factor related to personal satisfaction?
5. What factors emerged as important variables in personal commitment?
6. How could you use what you learned in this exercise in client groups?

when the swan recognizes and is recognized by the larger group as no longer "one of a kind." Careful selection of group members based on their capacity to derive benefit from the group and to add to the discussion is a critical individual variable in successful groups.

Functional similarity should not be confused with similarity of interpersonal communication style. Whereas it is important that group members speak enough of a common language to understand each other, differences in interpersonal styles help clients learn a broader range of behavioral responses. Having different ways of looking at things help ensure a more lively discussion and a more productive outcome.

## Group Variables

**Purpose.** A group's purpose establishes the rationale for the group's existence. It provides direction for membership decisions, development of group norms, and type of communication required to meet group goals. For example, if a group's purpose relates to medication compliance, the interventions would be educational. This purpose is quite different from a therapy group's purpose, focused on improved interpersonal functioning, with insight-oriented interventions. Common group purposes are presented in Box 12–1.

**Norms.** *Group norms* are the behavioral standards expected of group members. Norms facilitate goal achievement because they provide the needed predictability for effective group functioning. For example, think of how a class group

would operate if there were no behavioral standards. Suppose your instructor did not set a class agenda or provide expectations for student behavior. How satisfied would you be if students as well as the instructor did not hold you accountable for behaviors so that all might learn? What would it be like if you did not know what behaviors were needed to achieve a grade of A versus a C. Groups develop unspoken rules that shape the behaviors that a group will and will not tolerate. These norms reflect the values of its members. Some norms are universal standards, and others are specific to a particular group's dynamics.

UNIVERSAL GROUP NORMS. *Universal norms* are behavioral standards foundational to the success of group life. Examples include confidentiality, regular attendance, and a willingness to share with others. Unless group members can trust that personal information revealed in the group will not be shared outside the group setting (confidentiality), the necessary trust will not develop. As with individual therapeutic relationships, some information about behaviors of individual clients may need to be shared with the health care team. If this is the case, members should understand beforehand what information will be shared and with whom.

Because the value of most groups depends on members sharing with each other, this is a prerequisite for group interaction. Regular attendance at group meetings is also critical to goal achievement. Without a commitment of attendance from each member, a group becomes an

---

### ◆ Box 12–1. Identifying Group Purpose

| Type of Group | Opportunities |
|---------------|---------------|
| Therapy | Reality testing, encouraging personal growth, inspiring hope, strengthening personal resources, developing interpersonal skills |
| Support | Giving and receiving practical information and advice, supporting coping skills, promoting self-esteem, enhancing problem-solving skills, encouraging client autonomy, strengthening hope and resiliency |
| Activity | Getting people in touch with their bodies, releasing energy, enhancing self-esteem, encouraging cooperation, stimulating spontaneous interaction, supporting creativity |
| Education | Learning new knowledge, promoting skill development, providing support and feedback, supporting development of competency, promoting discussion of important health-related issues |

unstable means of promoting dialogue and action. Thus, repeated unexcused absences are not acceptable regardless of the reason; this is a universal norm.

GROUP-SPECIFIC NORMS. *Group-specific norms* emerge from the combined expectations, values, and needs of group members. Although group members initially look to their leader to model important norms, other members will assume a more active role in defining and modifying behavioral standards as group trust evolves. Examples include the degree of individual risk taking, decision making, toleration of humor and anger, focus on task or process, and level of leader control. For instance, some groups are characterized by blunt provocations designed to strip away a person's defenses, forcing members to confront their feelings. In other groups, confrontations are presented with tact and sensitivity. Once formed, norms are difficult to change, although circumstances no longer warrant their existence. Exercise 12–3 will help you develop a deeper understanding of group norms.

**Cohesiveness.** *Cohesiveness* refers to value a group holds for its members and their investment in being a part of the group (Yalom, 1985). Cohesiveness enhances commitment because people are willing to work harder to achieve individual and group goals when they value other group members and want to be a part of the group. Cohesiveness can develop from the appeal other group members personally hold for the individual, the significance of the group task, or the values and goals held by the group. Cohesiveness parallels the sense of mutuality and rapport that develops in successful one-to-one therapeutic relationships (Budman et al., 1989).

Norms that encourage open expression of feelings, acceptance, and mutal support enhance cohesiveness as does feeling valued by others. This, in turn, stimulates self-disclosure and a willingness to take interpersonal risks.

Caring for each other is strong outcome evidence of cohesiveness. The sense of human interdependency and community that develops within a group helps people who feel alienated to reconnect with others socially (Dallam & Manderino, 1997). Communication principles that enhance

---

◆ Exercise 12–3. **Identifying Norms**

**Purpose:**  To help identify norms operating in groups

**Procedure:**

1. Divide a piece of paper into three columns.
2. In the first column, write the norms you think exist in your class or work group. In the second column, write the norms you think exist in your family. Examples of norms might be as follows: no one gets angry, decisions are made by consensus, assertive behaviors are valued, missed sessions and lateness are not tolerated.
3. Share your norms with the group, first related to the school or work group and then to the family. Place this information in the third column.

**Discussion:**
Discussion could focus on the following questions:

1. Were there many similarities between the norms you think exist in your school or work group and those others in the same group had on their list?
2. Were there any ``universal'' norms on either of your lists?
3. Were you surprised either by some of the norms you wrote down when you thought about it or with those of your classmates?
4. Did you or other members in the group feel a need to refine or discuss the meaning of the norms on your list?
5. How difficult was it to determine implicit norms operating in the group?

the development of cohesiveness are found in Box 12–2. Research suggests that cohesive groups experience more personal satisfaction with goal achievement and that members of such groups are more likely to join other group relationships (Brilhart & Galanes, 1997).

**Group Think.** Cohesiveness carried to an extreme results in **group think,** a term used to describe a group dynamic in which loyalty to the group and approval by other group members become so important that members are afraid to express conflicting ideas and opinions for fear of being excluded from the group. The group exerts pressure on members to act as one voice. Critical thinking and realistic appraisal of issues get lost (Janis, 1971; Rosenblum, 1982). The symptoms of group think are outlined in Figure 12–2.

**Group Role Positions.** People assume roles in groups that influence their communication and the responses of others. A person's role position in the group corresponds with the status, power, and internal image that other members in the group have of the member. Group members usually have trouble breaking away from roles they have been cast in despite their best efforts. For example, people will look to the "helper" group member for advice even when that person lacks expertise or needs the group's help him- or herself. Other times, group members "project" a role position onto a particular group member representing a hidden agenda or unresolved issue for the group as a whole (Gans & Alonso, 1998). For example, a monopolizer in a group is difficult to tolerate. Group members may resent the mo-

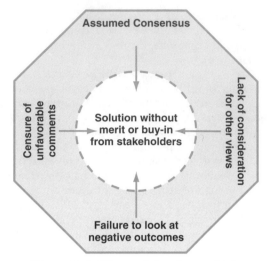

Figure 12–2. Characteristics of group think.

nopolization, but this person can become the repository for group anger or may serve a useful purpose for the group by diverting attention away from other member's equally critical issues. If the group as a whole seems to scapegoat, ignore, defer to, or consistently idealize one of its members, this group phenomenon can signify a group projection. Exercise 12–4 considers group role position expectation.

Some group members, because of the force of their personalities, emerge as dominant forces in a group. Groups often give power to the group members who best clarify the needs of the other group members or move the group toward goal achievement. These are not always the group members making the most statements. A person can make few but very meaningful comments. What seems important is the ability to reflect and deliver the dominant thinking of a group in a concise, direct manner.

### ◆ Case Example

Al is a powerful leader in a job search support group. Although he makes few comments, he has an excellent understanding of and sensitivity to the needs of individual members. When these are violated, Al speaks up and the group listens. His observations are always on target, and because he has the respect of the other group members, his opinions are influential in shaping the behaviors of other group members.

---

### ◆ Box 12–2. Communication Principles to Facilitate Cohesiveness

1. Group tasks are within the membership's range of ability and expertise.
2. Comments and responses are nonevaluative; they are focused on behaviors rather than on personal characteristics.
3. The leader points out group accomplishments and acknowledges member contributions.
4. The leader is empathetic and teaches members how to give feedback.
5. The leader sanctions creative tension as necessary to goal achievement.

◆ Exercise 12-4. **Headbands: Group Role Expectations**

**Purpose:**

1. To experience the pressures of role expectations
2. To demonstrate the effects of role expectations on individual behavior in a group
3. To explore the effects of role pressures on total group performance

**Procedure:**

1. Break the group up into a smaller unit of 10 to 15 members. In a large group, a small group performs while the remaining members observe.
2. Make up mailing labels or headbands that can be attached or tied around the heads of the participants. Each headband is lettered with directions on how the other members should respond to the role. Examples:

Comedian: laugh at me.

Expert: ask my advice.

Important person: defer to me.

Stupid: sneer at me.

Insignificant: ignore me.

Loser: pity me.

Boss: obey me.

Helpless: support me.

3. Place a headband on each member in such a way that the member cannot read his or her own label, but the other members can see it easily.
4. Provide a topic for discussion (e.g., why the members chose nursing, the women's movement) and instruct each member to interact with the others in a way that is natural for him or her. Do not role play but be yourself. React to each member who speaks by following the instructions on the speaker's headband. You are not to tell each other what the headbands say, but simply to react to them.
5. After about 20 minutes, the facilitator halts the activity and directs each member to guess what his or her headband says and then to take it off and read it.

**Discussion**

Initiate a discussion, including any members who observed the activity. Possible questions are as follows:

1. What were some of the problems of trying to ``be yourself'' under conditions of group role pressure?
2. How did it feel to be consistently misinterpreted by the group: to have them laugh when you were trying to be serious or ignore you when you were trying to make a point?
3. Did you find yourself changing your behavior in reaction to the group treatment of you, withdrawing when they ignored you, acting confident when they treated you with respect, giving orders when they deferred to you?

Adapted from Pfeiffer J, Jones J. (1977). A Handbook of Structured Experiences for Human Relations Training, Vol. VI. LaJolla, CA, University Associates Publishers. With permission.

**Role Functions.** Role functions differ from the positional roles group members assume. Bennis and Shephard (1948) described role functions as behaviors members use to (1) move toward goal achievement (*task functions*) and (2) ensure personal satisfaction (*maintenance functions*). A healthy balance between task and maintenance functions increases group productivity. When task functions predominate to the exclusion of maintenance functions, member satisfaction decreases, and there is less investment in the goal. Alternatively, groups in which maintenance functions override task functions do not always reach their goals and eventually will cease to exist. Group life flourishes, but little is accomplished.

Members do not confront controversial issues, and the creative tension needed for successful group growth does not occur.

Within the group, a person may assume several different roles, although most people tend to gravitate toward one versus the other. Task and maintenance role functions found in most successful small groups are given in Box 12–3. Exercise 12–5 gives practice in identifying task and maintenance functions.

Bennis and Shephard (1948) also identified nonfunctional role functions in a group. **Self-roles** are roles a person uses to meet self-needs at the expense of other member needs, group values, and goal achievement. Self-roles, identi-

---

◆ **Box 12–3. Task and Maintenance Functions in Group Relations**

**Task Functions: Behaviors Relevant to the Attainment of Group Goals**

Initiating: identifies tasks or goals; defines group problem; suggests relevant strategies for solving problem

Seeks information or opinion: requests facts from other members; asks other members for opinions; seeks suggestions or ideas for task accomplishment

Gives information or opinion: offers facts to other members; provides useful information about group concerns

Clarifies, elaborates: interprets ideas or suggestions placed before group; paraphrases key ideas; defines terms; adds information

Summarizes: pulls related ideas together; restates key ideas; offers a group solution or suggestion for other members to accept or reject

Consensus taking: checks to see whether group has reached a conclusion; asks group to test a possible decision

**Group Maintenance Tasks: Behaviors that Help the Group Maintain Harmonious Working Relationships**

Harmonizing: attempts to reconcile disagreements; helps members reduce conflict and explore differences in a constructive manner

Gate keeping: helps keep communication channels open; points out commonalties in remarks; suggests approaches that permit greater sharing

Encouraging: indicates by words and body language unconditional acceptance of others; agrees with contributions of other group members; is warm, friendly, and responsive to other group members

Compromising: admits mistakes; offers a concession when appropriate; modifies position in the interest of group cohesion

Standard setting: calls for the group to reassess or confirm implicit and explicit group norms when appropriate

*Note.* Every group needs both types of functions and needs to work out a satisfactory balance of task and maintenance activity.

---

After Rogers C. (1972). The process of the basic encounter group. In Diedrich R, Dye HA (eds.), Group Procedures: Purposes, Processes and Outcomes. Boston, Houghton Mifflin. Used with permission.

◆ Exercise 12–5. **Task Versus Maintenance Functions**

**Purpose:** To help you identify task versus maintenance functions

**Procedure:**

1. Break up into groups of eight students each.
2. Choose a topic to discuss (e.g., how you would restructure the nursing program; nursing and the women's movement; the value of a group experience; nursing as a profession).
3. Two students should volunteer to be the observers.
4. The students discuss the topics for 30 minutes; observers use the initial of each student and the grid below to mark with a tick (///) the number of times each student uses a task or maintenance function.
5. After completion of the group interaction, each observer shares his or her observations with the other group members.

**Task Functions:**

Initiating _____

Information seeking _____

Clarifying _____

Consensus _____

Testing _____

Summarizing _____

_____

_____

**Maintenance Functions:**

Encouraging _____

Expressing _____

Group feeling _____

Harmonizing _____

Compromising _____

Gate keeping _____

Setting standards _____

**Discussion:**

1. Was there an adequate balance between task and maintenance activity?
2. What roles did different members assume?
3. Were the two observers in agreement as to members' assumptions of task versus maintenance functions? If there were discrepancies, what do you think contributed to their occurrence?
4. What did you learn from this exercise?

fied in Box 12–4, detract from the group's work and compromise goal achievement by taking time away from group issues and creating discomfort among group members.

**Leadership.** Leadership is defined as "inter-personal influence, exercised in situations and directed through the communication process, toward the attainment of a specified goal or goals" (Tannenbaum, Wechsler, & Massarik, 1988). Two basic assumptions support the function of

---

**◆ Box 12–4. Nonfunctional Self-Roles**

| | |
|---|---|
| Aggressor | Criticizes or blames others, personally attacks other members, uses sarcasm and hostility in interactions |
| Blocker | Instantly rejects ideas or argues an idea to death, cites tangential ideas and opinions, obstructs decision making |
| Joker | Disrupts work of the group by constantly joking and refusing to take group task seriously |
| Avoider | Whispers to others, daydreams, doodles, acts indifferent and passive |
| Self-confessor | Uses the group to express personal views and feelings unrelated to group task. |
| Recognition seeker | Seeks attention by excessive talking, trying to gain leader's favor, expressing extreme ideas, or demonstrating peculiar behavior. |

Developed from Benne KD, Sheats P. (1948). Functional roles of group members. Journal of Social Issues 4(2):41–49. Used with permission.

---

group leadership: (1) group leaders have a significant influence on group process, and (2) most problems in groups can be avoided or reworked productively if the leader is aware and responsive to the needs of individual group members, including the needs of the leader.

Effective leadership requires adequate preparation, professional leadership attitudes and behavior, responsible selection of clients, and use of a responsible scientific rationale for determining a specific group approach. Beginning practitioners with knowledge of group dynamics can lead discussions, educational sessions, and some types of activity groups. Additional training and supervision are needed to lead a psychotherapy group effectively. Educational group leaders need to have expertise on the topic for discussion. Self-awareness of values, possible biases, and interpersonal limitations are important qualifications for all group leaders. Characteristics of effective and ineffective groups are presented in Box 12–5.

Effective leaders are good listeners. They are competent and are able to convey warmth and understanding. Effective leaders adapt their leadership style to fit the changing needs of the group. Effective group leaders are committed to the group goals and to supporting the integrity of group members as equal partners in meeting these goals. Effective group leaders have a clear understanding of their skills and limitations. Such knowledge allows the nurse to choose to explore new roles or to use previously untapped skills.

**TYPES OF LEADERS.** The *designated* leader in most health care settings is a health professional with training in group dynamics and process. *Emergent leaders* are informal leaders who emerge from the group membership and are recognized by other group members as powerful and often having equal status with the designated leader. Ideally, group leadership is a shared function of all group members; many emergent leaders and each member contribute to the overall functioning of the group (Brilhart & Galanes, 1997). Exercise 12–6 is designed to help you develop an understanding of the leadership role.

**Decision Making.** Group decision making often yields a better product than individual solutions for three reasons. First, the knowledge, skills, and resources of all participants are available to influence the solution; group members build on one another's ideas. Second, because so many different perspectives are available in group thinking, it is more likely that positive and negative consequences of each solution will be considered. Third, if the decision is to be implemented by a group rather than an individual, including those affected by the solution in the decision-making process ensures ownership and greater likelihood of compliance. Each decision-making approach will have different consequences for the group.

**STEPS IN THE DECISION-MAKING PROCESS.** The steps in group decision making parallel those described in Chapter 4. First, the group considers the nature of the problem and the amount of

## ◆ Box 12–5. Characteristics of Effective and Ineffective Groups

| Effective Groups | Ineffective Groups |
|---|---|
| 1. Goals are clearly identified and collaboratively developed. | 1. Goals are vague or imposed on the group without discussion. |
| 2. Open, goal-directed communication of feelings and ideas is encouraged. | 2. Communication is guarded; feelings are not always given attention. |
| 3. Power is equally shared and rotates among members, depending on ability and group needs. | 3. Power resides in the leader or is delegated with little regard to member needs. It is not shared. |
| 4. Decision making is flexible and adapted to group needs. | 4. Decision making occurs with little or no consultation. Consensus is expected rather than negotiated based on data. |
| 5. Controversy is viewed as healthy because it builds member involvement and creates stronger solutions. | 5. Controversy and open conflict are not tolerated. |
| 6. There is a healthy balance between task and maintenance role functioning. | 6. One-sided focus on task or maintenance role functions to the exclusion of the complementary function. |
| 7. Individual contributions are acknowledged and respected. Diversity is encouraged. | 7. Individual resources are not used. Conformity, the "company man," is rewarded. Diversity is not respected. |
| 8. Interpersonal effectiveness, innovation, and problem-solving adequacy are evident. | 8. Problem-solving abilities, morale, and interpersonal effectiveness are low and undervalued. |

## ◆ Exercise 12–6. Clarifying Personal Leadership Role Preferences

**Purpose:**  To help you focus on how you personally experience the leadership role

**Procedure:**
Answer the following questions briefly:

1. What do you enjoy most about the leadership role?
2. What do you like least about the leadership role?
3. What skills do you bring to the leadership role?
4. What are the differences in your functioning as a group member and as a group leader?

**Discussion:**

1. What types of transferable skills did you find you bring to the leadership role? For example, are you an oldest child, did you organize a play group, did you teach swimming to retarded children in high school, are you a member of a large family?
2. Were some of the uncomfortable feelings "universal" for a majority of the group?
3. What skills would you need to develop in order to feel comfortable as a group leader?
4. What did you learn about yourself from doing this exercise?

time and level of resources available to resolve it. Then the group brainstorms all possible solutions. Initially, the group gives equal weight to all proposed solutions, the only stipulation being that the solution must relate to the problem under discussion. Once the group generates sufficient ideas, group members begin to analyze potential alternatives and narrow their selection to the most promising ones. Group members consider the consequences of the refined alternatives and the impact on all of the people (stake holders) who will be affected by the solution. The actual selection of the most promising solution is the outcome of the decision-making process. Further refinements occur as the solution gets implemented.

## Concepts Related to Group Process

**Group process** refers to the structural development of the group, its life cycle. Groups follow progressive stages of development that parallel the developmental stages of individual relationships. Each phase of group development has its own set of tasks that build and expand on the work of previous phases. Phases overlap, and the group can return to an earlier stage of development as it faces crises or as membership changes. Tuckman's (1965) theory of small group development provides an uncomplicated theoretical framework for examining group process at different stages in the life of the group. He described four stages: forming, storming, norming, and adjourning.

Group process also describes the order in which topics are brought up and how the group responds to them both verbally and nonverbally. For example, expecting a newly formed group to move directly into problem resolution without first going through the necessary introductory stages of building trust can cause needless frustration and conflict. Having knowledge of group process helps the leader to recognize the conflict emerging in the storming phase of group development as a normal and necessary stage rather than as resistance on the part of individual members. Viewed in this way, the interventions are likely to be compassionate and productive.

## APPLICATIONS
## Comparison Between Group and Individual Communication

Group communication shares many of the characteristics of individual communication. The acceptance, respect, and understanding needed in individual relationships are essential components of effective group communication. Similar communication strategies of using open-ended questions, reflecting, paraphrasing, asking for clarification, linking, and summarizing are also important in group communication. Minimal cues in the form of eye contact with speakers and other group members, leaning forward, nodding, and smiling encourage sharing in groups. Allowing for pauses when it looks as though people are thinking is particularly important in groups. Usually it is anxiety provoking but worthwhile to wait. Pauses serve a similar purpose of bracketing information and allowing think time. The group leader can use a variety of listening responses to respond to a client's statements, each of which can elicit a different focus.

### ◆ Case Example

*Group member:* I hate my work. No matter how hard I try, I can't please my boss. I'd quit tomorrow if I could.
*Leader:* I'm not sure I quite understand your situation; could you tell me more about it? [Asking for clarification]
*Leader:* From what you say, it sounds as though you are feeling desperate. [Reflecting]
*Leader:* You're so unhappy with what is going on at work that you are thinking of quitting? [Paraphrasing]

As in individual relationships, the nurse links ideas with feelings and periodically summarizes member contributions, but there is an important distinction. Instead of linking ideas with feelings, the leader links together common themes of two or more members.

### ◆ Case Example

*Member:* I feel like giving up. I've tried to do everything right, and I still can't seem to get good grades in my classes.

*Leader:* I wonder if the discouragement you are feeling is similar to Mary's disenchantment with her job and Bill's desire to throw in the towel on his marriage.

Periodically, the leader summarizes or asks members to summarize the group's activities with an observational statement about the group dynamics for that session. For example, the nurse might say, "Today it seems as though we covered a lot of ground in finding useful strategies to reduce stress." Alternatively, the nurse might invite group members to respond: "We're almost out of time; I wonder if any of you have any final comments you'd like to make."

Although there are similarities, there are also important differences between individual and group communication strategies. Communication is more complex as each member brings to the group a different set of perspectives, perceptions of reality, communication styles, and personal agendas. Many people find it more difficult to express themselves in a group initially, and the leader may need to help them feel more comfortable. Because the focus is on group interaction rather than the I–thou communication of individual therapeutic relationship, the leader might ask other group members for their reaction rather than give a personal response.

---

◆ **Case Example**

**Martha:** I was upset with last week's meeting because I didn't feel we made any progress. Everyone complained, but no one had a solution.
**Leader:** Would anyone like to respond to what Martha just said?

---

A summary of suggestions for group communication feedback is presented in Box 12–6.

## Leader Tasks in the Life Cycle of a Group

Figure 12–3 depicts the life cycle of groups. Descriptions of the tasks follow.

### Before the Group Begins: Assessment and Planning

Before the group begins, the group leader considers the most effective structural framework for the group, given its purpose and goals. Foremost is the question, "What is the purpose of this group?" A well-defined group purpose gives direction to member selection and the establishment of group goals. Purpose dictates the group structure and format. A group's purpose can be educational, therapeutic, or supportive or designed to work on a particular problem or issue.

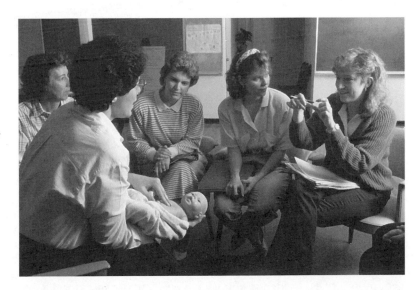

Groups offer a special forum for learning and emotional support. (Courtesy of the University of Maryland School of Nursing)

For example, a medication group would have an educational purpose. A group for parents with critically ill children would have a supportive design, and a therapy group would have a therapeutic expectation. Exploration of personal experience would be limited and related to the topic under discussion in an education group. In a therapy group, such probing would be encouraged.

## Defining the Goals of the Group

Group goals reflect the purpose of the group but differ in that they provide information about the therapeutic outcome a group hopes to attain through its efforts. For example, a group goal might be that the "group members will demonstrate knowledge of the actions and side effects of their medications." Group goals need to be achievable, measurable, and within the capabilities of group membership. Identifying a group goal helps the leader determine the time frame and type of membership needed to achieve the group objectives. Evidence of goal achievement justifies the existence of group and increases client satisfaction.

## Matching Client Needs with Group Goals

Matching group goals with client needs is essential. The leader needs to ask is, "How will being in this group enhance a client's health and well-being?" When there is a good match and clients have the capacity to contribute to the group, members develop commitment and perceive the group as having value. When this is not the case, the group experience can be destructive. For example, clients with serious verbal difficulties, significant memory deficits, or limited tolerance for cooperative behaviors do best in group situations specially geared to meet their needs. Placing such a client in a therapy group in which group participation requires high-level cognitive processing would be inappropriate. "Patient mix difficult for the group" was the most frequently mentioned perceived barrier to nurse-conducted groups in a study completed by Van Servellen et al. (1991).

## Types of Group Membership

The leader needs to decide whether the group will have a closed or an open membership and whether the group goals are better achieved with a homogeneous or heterogeneous membership. *Closed groups* have a defined membership with an expectation of regular attendance and time commitment, usually at least 12 sessions. Group members may be added, but their inclusion depends on a fit with group-defined criteria. Most psychotherapy groups fall into this category. *Open groups* do not have a defined membership other than that imposed by the purpose and goals of the group. Anyone can attend. Individuals come and go depending on their needs so that one week the group might consist of 2 to 3 members and the next week 15 members. Norms are of necessity much looser. Most community support groups in the community have open membership.

Another way of determining group membership is using homogeneous versus heterogeneous membership. *Homogeneous* groups have a common denominator pertaining to all members of the group such as a diagnosis (e.g., breast cancer support group) or a personal characteristic (e.g.,

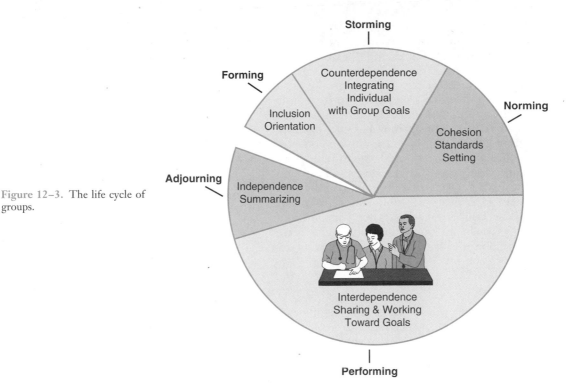

Figure 12–3. The life cycle of groups.

gender or age). Research indicates that such groups benefit clients who are coping with issues of exclusive importance to a particular group (e.g., a women's group focused on women's issues) (Prehn & Thomas, 1990). Psychotic clients and those with a specific diagnostic behavioral focus such as eating disorders or drug addiction, Alcoholics Anonymous, ostomy clubs, Compassionate Friends, Alzheimer's disease family support groups, and gender-specific consciousness-raising groups are familiar examples of homogeneous groups.

*Heterogeneous* groups may represent a wide diversity of human experience and problems, consisting of members who vary in age, gender, and psychodynamics. Most psychotherapy and insight-oriented personal growth groups have a heterogeneous membership (Bertcher & Maple, 1985). Educational groups held on inpatient units (e.g., medication groups) typically are heterogeneous related to educational background, age, gender, and so on.

## Creating the Appropriate Environment

Complete privacy and freedom from interruptions are key considerations in selecting an appropriate site for group activity. The group should be conducted in a quiet, open space, apart from the mainstream of activity. The room should be neither too hot nor too cold and large enough to accommodate all participants comfortably. Holding meetings in the same room each time fosters continuity and trust. A sign on the door indicating the group is in session prevents unwelcome intrusions.

Seats should be comfortable and arranged in a circle so that each member has face-to-face contact with other members and clear access to the facial expressions and nonverbal cues that accompany member communication. Being able to see and respond to several individuals at one time is essential to effective group communication (see Fig. 12–1).

The number of sessions, time of day, and frequency of meetings depend on the type of group and the group goals. For example, a work group might meet twice a month, whereas a therapy group might meet weekly. Support groups meet as frequently as once a week or as infrequently as once a month. An educational group might meet for one to eight sessions and then disband.

Although the length of a group session may vary, most groups meet for 60 to 90 minutes on a regular basis with established agreed-on meeting times. Having a time that does not conflict with the members' other obligations and that is conveniently schedules enhances group participation. Groups that begin and end on time help create an atmosphere of trust and predictability.

### Determining Appropriate Group Size

The purpose and goals of the group will influence the number of members needed. In general, therapy and personal growth groups consist of six to eight members. With this number of people there is sufficient time and space to express feelings and get feedback. The group is large enough to contain a diversity of opinions and ideas, yet small enough to permit intimate connection with all of the other members. Generally, therapy groups should not have fewer than five members. With less than this number, interaction tends to be more limited and if one or more members are absent, the group interaction can become intense and uncomfortable for the remaining members. Educational groups are traditionally larger than therapy groups. Twelve to 20 members is common, but because the focus is on relating to the presentation of a speaker, the level of interaction is not as important as it is in a therapy group.

## Conducting a Pregroup Interview

If the group has a therapeutic purpose, the leader may want to meet with the prospective member before first meeting. The purpose of this interview is to explain the goals of the group, assess the client's suitability for placement in the group, describe the type of commitment needed, and structure an opportunity for the client to ask questions. The description of the group and of its members is kept short and simple. The nurse asks potential clients what they hope to obtain from the group experience and the kinds of issues they wish to explore. Using this approach, the nurse has a better idea of client expectations and is better able to correct misperceptions. The leader allows ample time for questions and comments.

## Forming Phase

The initial phase of group development is the forming phase. When the group has just formed, members experience much anxiety (Jacobson, 1989). The basic need of members is acceptance. Time and effort must be given to developing commitment and trust before the actual work of the group takes place. Getting to know each other and finding common threads in personal experience seem to be important aspects of beginning group life that cannot be short changed without having a serious impact on the evolving effectiveness of the group (Yalom, 1985).

### Developing Trust

People enter group relationships as strangers to each other. Communication is superficial, and trust is at a surface level, as members get to know one another. Regardless of the importance of the identified task, the emphasis in the beginning is on getting to know other group members, their interpersonal boundaries, and their basic orientation to the sharing of responsibility, collaborative decision making, and control. Here are some common initial questions of members:

- Will I be accepted for who I am as a person in this group?
- Can I really say what I feel? What happens if I am honest with my feelings?
- Will I be expected to perform, or can I just be myself in this group?
- Am I enough like the other members to feel comfortable participating?
- Can I count on the leader to establish norms that respect my uniqueness as a person?

The leader takes an active role in helping the group members feel acceptance. The leader might initially ask the members to introduce themselves and give a little of their background or their reason for coming to the group. Either the leader or the person who looks most at ease can start the introduction. This can be followed by a general leading question if appropriate to the group focus. "As we begin, I would like to ask each of you, "What does . . . [stress, having a baby, a diagnosis of cancer, being in this group] mean to you?" or "I'm sure everyone here has a different mental image of what a therapy [support, educational] group is like. I wonder if you would be willing to share your perceptions." Finding that others have the same fears and perceptions decreases anxiety. Clients need to be educated about the nature of the group process and the behaviors required to achieve group goals.

The group leader's role is to facilitate group interaction. In the first session, the group leader identifies the purpose and goals of the group and allows ample time for questions. Although members may know the purpose ahead of time, taking the time to verbalize the purpose allows group members to hear it in the same way. Sometimes members' responses and questions related to purpose or goals provide important information to individual group members as well as to the group's leader. Next, the leader clarifies how the group will be conducted and what the group can expect from the leader and other members in achieving group goals. Knowing what to expect helps to reduce anxiety.

◆ **Case Example**

**Nurse leader (prenatal group):** I will be giving you information about taking the best care of yourself before the baby comes and what to expect during labor and delivery. This is a special time, and the more you know about yourself and your baby, the more you will get out of the group experience. It is very important that you ask questions and provide your ideas as we go along.

### Fostering Mutual Identification (Universality)

Identification with others is an important element in the formation of bonds (Eibl-Eibesfeldt, 1975). As people talk about themselves, their hopes, and fears, other group members hear the echo in their own experience. They both understand and feel understood when this occurs. Knowing that you are not alone and other people have the same fears and reactions helps put difficult health issues in perspective (Brandman, 1996). The leader may start with asking clients to talk about their expectations (e.g., by saying, "It's useful at the start of a group to have an idea of what each of you would like to get out of the group. I'd like to start with Jack and ask what each of you hopes to get out of being here"). In addition to enhancing mutual identification among members, this strategy also gives the leader an opportunity to correct misperceptions about group goals. As members develop a growing group identification, content and process issues tend to carry over from one group session to another. There is a developing sense of continuity within the group, as the group begins to assume active responsibility for its own functioning.

### Establishing the Group Contract

The group leader develops a working agreement with group members that specifies the time and place of meetings, the nature of the group interaction, and behavioral expectations of members with respect to behavior. The group contract becomes a shared commitment to and with the group.

The leader identifies universal behavioral norms, such as confidentiality, attendance, and mutual respect (Corey & Corey, 1990); group-specific norms are negotiated as the group matures. From the beginning, nurse group leaders model an attitude of caring, objectivity, and integrity in their communication with group members.

## Storming Phase

Once people feel comfortable with each other, a transitional stage in group development follows in which people strive to understand themselves and other group members at a deeper level. Referred to as the storming phase, group members cope with power and control issues. People use testing behaviors to elicit boundaries, communication styles, and personal reactions from other members and from the leader. Such behaviors might include disagreement with the group format, the topics for discussion, the best ways to achieve group goals, and certain member contributions compared with other member offerings. Although this stage is uncomfortable, it leads to the development of group norms and thus is a very important stage in group development.

The leader plays an important role in the storming phase by accepting differences in group member perceptions as normal and growth producing and by balancing group forces when one member threatens to sabotage group efforts or becomes the target of group reaction. For example, the leader can follow a different opinion made by a member with a statement such as "That is a good point," "That comment is right on target with the next issue we need to take up," or "Thank you for clarifying your position." The group leader models effective group behaviors and directly confronts sabotage behavior with statements that deal with behavior rather than motivation.

### ◆ Case Example

**Leader:** As I understand it, you agree with John that he should take his medication when he needs it, but you don't think he is paying enough attention to the times when his symptoms are getting out of control. Is that correct?

In this way, the participants are challenged to express differences, and the leader demonstrates an appropriate way to word statements of disagreement. Focusing on the positive comments of members and linking the constructive themes of members are effective modeling behaviors.

The group leader can also ask for group input, a particularly useful strategy when one group member is monopolizing the conversation. For example, the nurse might reflect out loud in the group, "I wonder if others in the group share Bob's reservations"; or "How would other group members respond to what Bob is saying?" Looking in the direction of positive group members as the statements are made also encourages member response. It is important for the group leader to remain nonreactive and to redirect provocative remarks back to their maker or to the group; for example, "Bill, I wonder if you might be able to tell us a little more about how you personally feel about this project without bringing anyone else into it."

If a member continues to monopolize the conversation, the leader can respectfully acknowledge the person's comment and refocus the issue within the group. "I appreciate your thoughts, but I think it would be important to hear from other people as well. What do you think about this, Jane?" or "That sounds like a strong position on _____ . I'm wondering if others agree or disagree."

Members who test boundaries through sexually provocative, overly flattering, or insulting remarks need to have limits set promptly: "That behavior isn't appropriate in the group. Our purpose as a group is to help each other, and your behavior is preventing that from happening." Resolution of this stage may be seen in the willingness of members to take stands on their personal preferences without being defensive and in accepting the comments of other members. Gradually, the group will begin to seek compromises: "I think we should consider our first proposal" or "Maybe we should consider a number of options before we decide on this." When such comments are made, the group is ready to establish group norms, which are needed for the group to reach its goals.

## Norming Phase

As the group enters the norming phase, feedback becomes more spontaneous, and group members begin to share more responsibility for the leadership of the group. Out of the conflict and newfound cooperation, behavioral standards emerge that will help the group achieve its task. Group members exchange more personal information about each other and begin to think more about the task at hand. Common agreement develops about the behavioral standards expected if the group is to achieve its goals. Individual goals become aligned with group goals. Once the group norms are established, the group holds members accountable and challenges individual members who fail to adhere to them. When this occurs, the leader can help the erring member see that it is because he or she is important to the functioning of the group that this matters.

## Performing Phase

Most of the group's work is accomplished in the performing phase. Cohesiveness develops to a stronger degree, so that the group is freed to work on issues as they relate to the accomplishment of group goals. Working together on a project or participating in another person's personal growth allows members to experience one another's personal strengths and the collective caring of the group. Therefore, there is an esprit de corps and a possibility of affirmation. Affirmation is an abstract feeling that people experience as feeling validated, respected, and cared about as persons. The experience of affirmation occurs unexpectedly and emotionally rather than intellectually. Affirmation usually occurs in a way one never would have anticipated, yet it normally exceeds one's fondest expectations. Of all the possibilities that can happen in a group, feeling affirmed and respected is most highly valued by group members.

## Termination Phase (Adjourning)

The final phase of group development is termination or adjournment, which ideally occurs when the group members have achieved desired outcomes. The leader encourages the group members to express their feelings about one another as significant group members and their perception of personal contributions to attainment of identified objectives. Each member can do this in turn, perhaps ending with the leader, who adds his or her own personal observations and feelings. Any concerns the group may have about an individual member or suggestions for future growth can be stated, and there is a constructive purpose in making such statements. By waiting until the group ends to share closing comments, the leader has an opportunity to soften or clarify previous comments, to connect cognitive and feeling elements, and to summarize the group experience. The leader needs to remind members that the norm of confidentiality does not end with the completion of the group. Exercise 12-7 considers closure issues.

## TYPES OF THERAPEUTIC GROUPS

"Therapeutic as it applies to group relationships doesn't always mean having to do with treatment of emotional and behavioral disorders but rather having as a broad purpose increasing people's knowledge of themselves and others" (Corey & Corey, 1987). Support groups for mentally healthy individuals who are seeking personal growth or emotional support are considered in the broad category of therapeutic groups. Psy-

---

◆ **Exercise 12-7. Group Closure, Expressing Affection**

**Purpose:** To experience summarizing your feelings about each other
Time: 45 minutes

**Procedure:**

1. Focus your attention on the group member next to you, and think about what you like about the person, how you see him or her in the group, and what you might wish for that person as a member of the group.
2. After 5 minutes, your instructor will ask you to tell the person next to you to use the three themes in making a statement about the person. For example, "The thing I most like about you in the group is . . ."; "To me you represent the . . . in the group"; and so on.
3. When all of the group members have had a turn, discussion may start.

**Discussion:**

1. How difficult was it to capture the person's meaning in one statement?
2. How did you experience telling someone about your response to him or her in the group?
3. How did it feel being the group member receiving the message?
4. What did you learn about yourself from doing this exercise?
5. What implications does this exercise have for future interactions in group relationships?

choeducational, parenting, and medication groups have a therapeutic purpose because they empower people to take self-responsibility for important aspects of their health and well-being.

In a group, a client can feel a deep sense of identification with other members who are dealing with issues that are similar to the one that concerns the client (Goldstein, Alter, & Axelrod, 1996). The group becomes a valued resource (*cohesiveness*). The social contact and support that clients experience with other group members who are in the same predicament as they are and who have the same supposedly unacceptable feelings provide a different perspective of self that simply is not available in a one-to-one interpersonal relationship (Kreidler & Carlson, 1991). Within a natural, safe setting, the person can hear and see from the experiences of others that he or she is not unique or alone, that difficulties can be resolved. Feeling understood by peers who are struggling with similar issues (*universality*) helps people feel tremendous relief that the struggle is not unique or incomprehensible to others. Having a regular, safe place to talk about problems helps. A woman undergoing chemotherapy in a breast cancer support group expressed the value of the group experience as

I'm hopeful that this treatment will work, but I'm also dealing with the fact that I might not make it. But I can't talk with my husband about it because he doesn't want to see me cry. Mom has had enough. I have to keep a stiff upper lip with my friends and children because they can't handle my talking about dying. They think I'm giving up. I'm not, but I need to talk about it with someone who understands. I have no one to turn to. . . . This group is my lifeline.

Therapeutic groups offer a structured format that encourages a person to experience his or her natural healing potential (*instillation of hope*), and other group members reinforce individual group member resolve. When six other people are supportive and understanding and, even more important, when they think there are solutions a client may have overlooked, it is difficult to deny the warmth and obvious caring that can foster hope. Sharing intimate feelings with one another (*catharsis*), coupled with the respect others have for the worth and uniqueness of the individual, strengthens personal resources (*self-responsibility*) and stimulates creative solutions to a problem.

Therapeutic groups provide reality testing. People under stress lose perspective. Loss of perspective compromises effective problem solving because the problem seems too big to manage. In groups, other group members usually scrutinize a member's global statements and gently suggest alternative explanations. They rarely accept universal statements at face value and can say things to the client that friends and relatives are afraid to say for fear of offending the client.

### ◆ Case Example

**Client:** I have been worthless since I had this heart attack. I can't do anything anymore.
This global statement represents a real and pervasive feeling, but the statement reveals little else about the remaining capabilities of the individual. It probably is not true that the person has lost all value. In a group, others might challenge the validity of this client's statement.

**Nurse:** I can appreciate that the shock of having a heart attack can leave you feeling off balance, but I wonder how others see your situation.
Generally, other group members will give the client specific feedback that offers insights the client has not considered. Coming from peers in similar circumstances, the feedback has a special credibility. After discussion, the client might develop a more specific problem-centered statement (self-understanding) that accurately reflects his or her situation.

*Client:* Six weeks ago, I had a heart attack. I feel worthless because my activities are restricted.

Individuals tend to act in groups as they do in real life. The group provides a mirror with which clients can learn how others perceive them and can learn more adaptive responses (Brandman, 1996). When situations cannot be changed, therapeutic groups help clients accept that reality and move on with their lives. They empower clients, providing needed emotional reinforcement and comfort for clients through the supportive framework of caring words and caring actions (Dobrof et al., 1990). A hidden benefit of the therapeutic group experience is the opportunity for clients to experience giving as well as receiving help from others. A satisfaction in helping others enhances self-esteem (*altruism*). Finding value as a resource and making a difference in someone else's life is particularly beneficial for clients who, in the throes of their own misfortune, feel they have little to offer others (Murphy, 1975).

In a number of studies, clients ranked their group therapy as one of the most valuable components of their treatment protocol (Hoge & McLoughlin, 1991). The goals of psychotherapy directly relate to personal growth and the modification of maladaptive interpersonal behaviors. Clients are expected verbally to share personal feelings, develop insights about personal behaviors, and practice new and more productive interpersonal responses. Psychotherapy groups proliferate in outpatient mental health centers as a primary form of treatment for many clients and are used in inpatient settings for treatment of the seriously mentally ill.

## Therapeutic Groups in Psychiatric Settings

Because of personnel shortages, nurses without advanced degrees frequently lead or colead unit-based group psychotherapy with clients who are experiencing major psychiatric illness (Clarke, Adamoski & Joyce, 1998). Because they frequently spend the most time with psychotic clients, they are in an excellent position to develop effective, formal group relationships with them and to understand their painful conflicts. For the hospitalized psychotic client, life becomes incomprehensible, without meaning. Group therapy offers a safe place for exploring the client's natural healing processes (Birckhead, 1984). The client can re-experience life differently through the eyes of the nurse leader and the conversations that take place in the group, even though limited and halting.

Leading a group with psychotic members is anxiety provoking. The leader needs to take an active role and a proactive approach. Before each session, the nurse may need to remind group members individually of the meeting. It may appear to the leader that psychotic clients are not willing to attend. More often, this is not the case; their seeming reluctance is part of the passivity that characterizes psychotic clients in interpersonal situations. Holding the group session in the same room at the same time is particularly important for the psychotic client, who relies on structural cues despite being seemingly oblivious to them.

A flexible, proactive leadership approach is needed. Spontaneous sharing among group members is not the rule, at least in the early stages of group development. If a topic is not forthcoming from the group, the leader can introduce a relevant, concrete, problem-centered topic and elicit discussion about how group members view the issue or have handled a similar problem. Patience, using minimal encouragers, and helping people feel comfortable by acknowledging each and every contribution help. Over time, the conversation will increase. Offering refreshments in the group session is appropriate with regressed clients because it represents another form of nurturance that enhances socialization.

A primary goal of the leader in group psychotherapy with clients suffering from a major psychiatric illness is to understand each person as a unique human being with needs disguised as symptoms. If the person chooses to use delusions, repetitive questions, or schizophrenic images in speaking, the nurse can try to "decode" the psychotic message by uncovering the underlying theme and translating it into understandable language. Sometimes other members will translate the message if called on by the nurse leader. The leader might say to the group, "I wonder if anyone in the group can help us understand better what John is trying to say." At other times, the leader decodes the message: "I wonder if your fear that the Martians are coming and will destroy you has anything to do with your parents' visit tomorrow?" Changes in physical appearance are noted. For example, one client, after being told she was attractive, appeared at the next meeting wearing make-up.

As with any chronic illness, the seriously mentally ill client suffers setbacks and remission of symptoms. Understanding that this is a dynamic of the illness and not a resistant response to group interaction is essential. It is important to recognize how difficult it is for the psychotic client to tolerate close interaction and how necessary it is to do so if the client is to succeed in the outside environment. With patience and a genuine regard for each client, the nurse can treat inevitable regressions as temporary setbacks capable of being reversed.

Because the demands of leadership are so intense with psychotic clients, coleadership is recommended. Cotherapists can share the group process interventions, offset negative transference from group members, and provide useful feedback to each other. In addition, cotherapy provides additional opportunities for modeling cooperative behaviors in healthy relationships, so frequently missing in the psychotic client's interpersonal experience. If there is more than one leader, every group session should be processed immediately after its completion.

## Therapeutic Groups in Long-Term Settings

Nurses frequently lead therapeutic groups in long-term settings. They provide a chance for the elderly to get together in a structured format designed to encourage interaction. They provide needed stimulation for people who have much more limited resources to draw from for social interaction. A balance of stimuli is needed to arouse but not overwhelm the elderly client. When making referrals or organizing such groups, the nurse should match the purpose of the group with the client's level of functional ability. For example, groups aimed at increasing insight would not be appropriate or helpful for clients who are confused. Here are some of the different therapeutic groups available to the elderly.

**Reality Orientation Groups.** Used most often with the confused elderly client, reality orientation groups help clients maintain contact with the environment and reduce confusion about time, place, and person. Such groups are usually held each day for approximately a half hour, and the focus of the discussion is on the immediate environment; when possible the group is led by the same person. The nurse uses props such as a calendar, a clock, and pictures of the seasons to stimulate interest. The group should not be seen as an isolated activity; what occurs in the group needs to be reinforced throughout the 24-hour period. For example, on one unit, the nurses placed pictures of the residents in earlier times on the door to their bedroom.

**Resocialization Groups.** Because of their step-by-step structure, resocialization groups are quite useful for withdrawn, elderly clients. Resocialization groups focus on providing a simple social setting for clients to experience basic social skills again. For example, a group might settle around a table with silverware and simple foods. The nurse would provide modeling and guidance to make basic conversational requests for food. Resocialization groups are used with clients who might not be able to get involved with a remotivation group but who need companionship and involvement with others. Improvement of social skills contributes to an improved sense of self-esteem. Although the senses and cognitive abilities may diminish in the elderly, basic needs for companionship, interpersonal relationships, and a place where one is accepted and understood remain the same throughout the life span.

**Remotivation Groups.** Remotivation groups have a more directed focus. They are helpful in counteracting the isolation and apathy resulting from long-term institutionalization. Remotivation groups are deliberately designed to stimulate thinking about activities required for everyday life. Originally developed by Dorothy Hoskins Smith for use with chronic mental patients, remotivation groups represent an effort to reach the "unwounded areas of the patient's personality, i.e., those areas and interests that have remained healthy."

Nurses, nursing students, and nonprofessional staff with an understanding of group dynamics and interest in the elderly can lead such groups. Typically composed of 10 to 15 members, remotivation groups focus on everyday topics such as the way plants or trees grow, or they might consist of poetry reading or art appreciation. Visual props engage the participant and stimulate more responses.

The steps the leader takes with remotivation groups, presented in Box 12–7, are easy to follow, and the project is rewarding to those nurses willing to take the time.

**Reminiscence Groups.** Reminiscence groups offer powerful sources of self-esteem for cognitively intact, elderly clients. Kovach (1991) described reminiscence as "a cognitive process of recalling events from the past that are personally significant and reality based." Sharing past achievements with others in a group helps the person remember personal life experiences that can be integrated into the individual's current self-concept. The knowledge that one has lived a meaningful life and has been loving and loved enhances self-esteem.

> ◆ Box 12–7. Steps for Conducting Remotivation Groups
>
> 1. Provide an accepting environment and greet each member by name.
> 2. Offer a bridge to reality by discussing topics of interest, such as news items and historical items.
> 3. Develop topic with group members through the use of questions, props, or visual aids.
> 4. Encourage members to discuss the topic in relation to themselves.
> 5. Express verbal appreciation to members for their contributions, and plan the following session.

Nurses sometimes worry that the recalled memories will be unpleasant. Sometimes the memories are indeed bothersome or anxiety provoking, but the reminiscence group can help the individual rework in a positive way unresolved issues from the past and integrate them into the present reality. Research also supports the fact that for most people reminiscences are pleasant and ego enhancing (Hyland and Ackerman, 1988). Topics most likely to stimulate positive self-esteem include those that confirm personal meaning and those that validate personal capabilities and strengths (Kovach, 1991).

The leader guides the group in telling their story, asking questions and pointing out common themes to stimulate further reflections. Members create for themselves a shared reality by revealing to one another what life has meant and can be for them and in the process reconnect with sometimes forgotten parts of their life that held meaning for them.

## Therapeutic Activity Groups

Activity groups are often overlooked as a legitimate form of therapeutic group, yet they account for the majority of nurse-led group modalities in psychiatric inpatient settings (Van Servellen et al., 1991). More frequently found in extended-care, mental health, or rehabilitation health care settings than in acute care or community hospitals, they offer clients a variety of self-expressive opportunities through creative activity rather than through words. The nurse may function as group leader or as a support in encouraging client participation.

- Occupational therapy groups allow clients to work on individual projects or to participate with others in learning life skills. Examples are a cooking or activities of daily living group. Other clients go to the occupational therapy area to make such items as ceramics or leather-tooled objects. Tasks are selected for their therapeutic value as well as for client interest. Life skills groups use a problem-solving approach to interpersonal situations.
- Recreational therapy groups offer opportunities to engage in leisure activities that release energy and provide a social format for learning interpersonal skills. Some people never learned how to build needed leisure activities into their lives.
- Dance therapy groups, originally developed by Marion Chase, are a form of group therapy in which participants can experience movement in a safe environment. Dance therapy provides companionship without demands, and physical movement shared with others often prompts conversation about its meaning.
- Art therapy groups encourage clients to reveal feelings through drawing or painting. Such groups can focus on individual artwork, which is then described by each member, or on a combined group effort in the form of a mural. Psychological interpretations of artwork require advanced preparation in art therapy, but nurses can assist by modeling health behaviors that can be useful to the entire group. Often clients will be able to reveal feelings through expression of color and abstract forms that they initially cannot talk about.
- Poetry and bibliotherapy groups select readings of interest and invite clients to respond to literary works. Sluder (1990) described an expressive therapy group for the elderly in which the nurse leader first read free verse poems and then invited the clients to compose group poems around feelings such as love or hate. Members were asked to describe the feeling in a few words, and the contributions of each member were recorded. Clients writing free verse poems and reading them in the group followed this activity. In the process of developing their poetry, clients got in touch with their personal creativity.

• The nurse can lead an exercise group to stimulate body movement and group interaction. Usually the nurse models the exercise behaviors, either with or without accompanying music. This type of group works well with chronically mentally ill clients.

## Community Support Groups

Support groups provide emotional and practical support to clients and their families who are experiencing chronic illness, crises, or the ill health of a family member. Community support groups are led informally by group members rather than professionals, although frequently a health professional acts as an adviser. The meetings are free and open to anyone with a specified diagnosis or problem. Examples of familiar support groups are found in Box 12–8.

Members attend when they wish to and are not penalized for nonattendance. Support groups rarely have a formal ending, and group member-ship is not conditional on personality characteristics or interpersonal suitability. Nurses are encouraged to contact support group networks in their community to become informed of the countless groups available to clients and their families (see Exercise 12–8). Referral to community-based support groups will become increasingly important as cost containment continues to drive health care delivery.

Nurses frequently lead support groups on the unit. Examples of support groups for family members are Alzheimer's disease support groups for family caregivers, support groups for clients with a specific diagnosis (e.g., cancer, acquired immunodeficiency syndrome, learning disabilities), aftercare groups for families of former clients who are having emotional difficulties, parent groups, and bereavement groups. A suggested format for leading a support group is presented in Box 12–9.

## Educational Groups

Educational groups are used in community and hospital settings to help clients develop skills in taking care of themselves (Schilling et al., 1995). They also provide families of clients with serious or chronic illness with the knowledge and skills they need to care for their loved ones.

Educational groups are reality based and focus on the present situation (Esplen, Touer, Hunter, et al., 1998). They are time-limited group applications; for example, the group might be held as four 1-hour sessions over a 2-week period or as an 8-week, 2-hour seminar. Examples of primary prevention groups are childbirth education, parenting, stress reduction, and professional support groups for nurses working in critical care settings. Suitable adolescent groups include those that deal with values clarification, health education, and sex education as well as groups to increase coping skills, such as avoiding peer pressure to use drugs (Griffith, 1986).

Medication groups are an excellent example of educational group formats used in hospitals and community clinics. Clients are taught effective ways to carry out a therapeutic medication regimen while learning about their disorder. A typical sequence would be to provide clients with information about (1) their disorder, (2) purpose of the medication, (3) how long before the medi-

---

### Box 12–8. Examples of Mutual Aid Support Groups in the Community

Alcoholics Anonymous

Al-Anon

Adult Children of Alcoholics

Anorexia nervosa and bulimia support groups

Chemically Dependent Anonymous

Chronic Pain Outreach

Compassionate Friends (bereaved parents of dead children)

Emotions Anonymous

Make Today Count

Men to End Spouse Abuse

Narcotics Anonymous

Neurotics Anonymous

On Our Own

Overeaters Anonymous

Parents Anonymous (parents of child abuse victims)

Parents Club of Children with Asthma

Seasons: Suicide Bereavement

Threshold: Alliance for the Mentally Ill

Tough Love (parents of teenagers)

United Ostomy Association

◆ Exercise 12-8. **Learning About Support Groups**

**Purpose:** To provide direct information about support groups in the community
Time: homework assignment

**Procedure:**

1. Contact a support group in your community. (Ideally, students will choose different support groups so that a wide variety of groups is shared.)
2. Identify yourself as a nursing student and ask for information about the support group, the time and frequency of meetings, the purpose and focus of the group, how a client joins the group, the types of services provided, who sponsors the group, issues the group might discuss, and fee schedules, for example.
3. Write a two-paragraph report including the information in Procedure 2, and describe your experience in asking for the support group information.

**Discussion:**

1. How easy was it for you to obtain information?
2. Were you surprised by any of the informants' answers?
3. If you were a client, would the support group you chose to investigate meet your needs?
4. What did you learn from doing this exercise that might be useful in your nursing practice?

cation will take effect, (4) what to look for with side effects, (5) when to call the physician, (6) what to do when they do not take the medication as prescribed, (7) what to avoid while on the medication (e.g., some medications cause sun sensitivity), (8) tests needed to monitor the medication. The nurse would present the didactic material in an informal manner, starting with what clients already know about their disorder and the medication. Giving homework and materials to be read between sessions can be helpful if the medication group is to last more than one session. The group leader allows sufficient time for questions and, by encouraging an open informal discussion of the topic, engages individual members in the group activity.

## Focus Discussion Groups

Focus discussion groups are used for a variety of purposes in health care by both health care providers and consumers. They provide group input that is useful to caregivers in planning health care for particular populations. Through discussion of a specific topic, clients learn more about health care issues affecting them and have the opportunity to reflect on their own perceptions (Laube & Wieland, 1998). Careful prepara-

tion, formulation of relevant questions, and use of feedback ensure that personal learning needs are met. Functional elements appropriate to discussion groups are found in Box 12–10.

Group leadership is divided equally among the group members. Discussion groups in which only a few members actively participate are disheartening to group members and are limited in learning potential. Because the primary purpose of a discussion group is to promote the learning of all group members, other members are charged with the responsibility of encouraging the participation of more silent members. Allowing enough interpersonal space for dialogue to occur and asking for but not demanding the reluctant member's opinion encourage communication.

Sometimes when more verbal participants keep quiet the more reticent group member begins to speak. It is just as important to learn when to stop talking as it is to present material. Cooperation, not competition, needs to be developed as a conscious group norm in all discussion groups. Characteristics of effective and ineffective listening habits in discussion groups are found in Box 12–11.

Discussion group topics use prepared data and

---

◆ Box 12–9. Sample Format for Leaders of Support Groups

| Steps | Sample of Statements |
|---|---|
| 1. Introduce self. | "I am Christy Atkins, a staff nurse on the unit, and I am going to be your group facilitator tonight." |
| 2. Explain purpose of the group. | "Our goal in having the group is to provide a place for family members to get support from each other and to provide practical information to families caring for Alzheimer's disease victims." |
| 3. Identify norms. | "We have three basic rules in this group. (1) We respect each other's feelings. (2) We don't preach or tell you how to do something. (3) The meetings are confidential; everything of a personal nature stays in this room." |
| 4. Ask each member to identify self and something about his or her situation. | "I'd like to go around the room and ask each of you to tell us your name and something about your situation." |
| 5. Link common themes. | "It seems as if feeling powerless and out of control is a common theme tonight. What strategies have you found help you to feel more in control?" |
| 6. Allow time for informal networking (optional). | Providing a 10-minute break with or without refreshments allows members to talk informally with each other. |
| 7. Provide closure. | "Now I'd like to go around the room and ask each of you to identify one thing you will do in the next week for yourself to help you feel more in control." |

---

◆ Box 12–10. Elements of Successful Discussion Groups

| Element | Rationale |
|---|---|
| Careful preparation | Thoughtful agenda and assignment establish a direction for the discussion and the expected contribution of each member. |
| Informed participants | Each member should come prepared so that all members are communicating at relatively the same level of information and each is contributing equally. |
| Shared leadership | Each member is responsible for encouraging the participation of more silent members and for adhering to the agenda. |
| Relevant questions | Focused questions keep the discussion moving toward the meeting objectives. |
| Useful feedback | Thoughtful feedback maintains the momentum of the discussion by reflecting different perspectives of topics raised and confirming or questioning others' views. |

◆ Box 12-11. Characteristics of Effective and Ineffective Listening Habits in Discussion Groups

| 10 Keys to Effective Listening | The Bad Listener | The Good Listener |
|---|---|---|
| 1. Find areas of interest. | Tunes out dry subjects | Opportunizes; asks, "What's in it for me? |
| 2. Judge content, not delivery. | Tunes out if delivery is poor | Judges content, skips over delivery errors |
| 3. Hold your fire. | Tends to enter into argument | Does not judge until comprehension is complete |
| 4. Listen for ideas. | Listens for facts | Listens for central themes |
| 5. Be flexible. | Takes intensive notes using only one system | Takes fewer notes; uses four or five different systems, depending on speaker |
| 6. Work at listening. | Shows no energy output; fakes attention | Works hard, exhibits active body state |
| 7. Resist distractions. | Is easily distracted | Fights or avoids distractions, tolerates bad habits, knows how to concentrate |
| 8. Exercise your mind. | Resists difficult expository material; seeks light, recreational material | Uses heavier material as exercise for the mind |
| 9. Keep your mind open. | Reacts to emotional words | Interprets color words; does not get hung up on them |
| 10. Capitalize on face: thought is faster than speech | Tends to daydream with slow speakers | Challenges, anticipates, mentally summarizes, weighs the evidence, listens between the lines to tone of voice |

Sperry Corporation. (1988). Your listening profile. In Cathcart R, Samovar L (eds.), Small Group Communication: A Reader (5th ed.). Dubuque, IA: William C. Brown, p. 382. Reprinted with permission of Unisys Corporation.

group-generated material. New information is integrated with more established data. This new information requires the client to synthesize data into a relevant whole rather than simply parroting major themes and topics. Before the end of each meeting, the leader or a group member should summarize the major themes developed from the content material.

## SUMMARY

Chapter 12 looks at the ways in which a group experience enhances clients' abilities to meet therapeutic self-care demands, provides meaning, and is personally affirming. The rationale for providing a group experience for clients is described. Group dynamics include individual member commitment, functional similarity, and leadership style. Group concepts related to group dynamics consist of purpose, norms, cohesiveness, roles, and role functions. Communication variables such as clarifying, paraphrasing, linking, and summarizing build and expand on techniques used in individual relationships.

Group processes refer to the structural phases of group development—forming, storming, norming, performing, and adjourning—as described by Tuckman (1965). In the forming phase of group relationships, the basic need is for acceptance. The second phase of group development, referred to as the storming phase, focuses on issues of power and control in groups. Behavioral standards are formed in the norming phase that will guide the group toward goal accomplishment. The group becomes a "safe" environment in which to work and express feelings. Once this occurs, most of the group's task is accomplished during the performing phase. Feelings of warmth, caring, and intimacy follow; members feel affirmed and valued. finally, when the group task is completed to the satisfaction of the individual members, or of the group as a whole, the group enters a termination (adjourning) phase.

Different types of groups found in health care include therapeutic, support, educational and discussion focus groups.

## REFERENCES

Agapetus L. (1996). Yalom's model applied to an outpatient better breathers group. Journal of Psychosocial Nursing and Mental Health Services 32(12):11–24.

Bennis W, Shepherd H. (1948). Functional roles of group members. Journal of Social Issues 4(2):41–49.

Bertcher H, Maple F. (1985). Elements and issues in group composition. In Sundel M, Glasser S, Vinter R (eds.), Individual Change through Small Groups. New York, Free Press.

Birckhead L. (1984). The nurse as leader: Group psychotherapy with psychotic patients. Journal of Psychosocial Nursing 22(6):24–30.

Brandman, W. (1996). Intersubjectivity, social microcosm and the here-and-now in a support group for nurses. Archives of Psychiatric Nursing 10(6):374–378.

Brilhart J, Galanes G. (1997). Effective Group Discussion (9th ed.). New York, McGraw-Hill.

Budman S, Soldz S, Demby A, et al. (1989). Cohesion, alliance and outcome in group psychotherapy. Psychiatry 52:339–350.

Clarke D, Adamoski E, Joyce B. (1998). Inpatient group psychotherapy: The role of the staff nurse. Journal of Psychosocial Nursing and Mental Health Services 36(5):22–26.

Corey G, Corey M. (1987). Groups: Process and Practice (2nd ed.). Monterey, CA, Brooks/Cole.

Corey G, Corey M. (1990). Groups: Process and Practice (3rd ed.). Monterey, CA, Brooks/Cole.

Dellam S, Manderino M. (1997). Free to be peer group supports patients with MPD/DD. Journal of Psychosocial Nursing and Mental Health Services 35(5):22–27.

Diedrich R, Dye HA (eds.). (1972). Group Procedures: Purposes, Processes and Outcomes. Boston, Houghton Mifflin.

Dobrof J, Umpierre M, Rocha L, Silverton M (1990). Group work in a primary care medical setting. Health and Social Work 15(1):32–37.

Eibl-Eibesfeldt I. (1975). Ethology: The Biology of Behavior. New York, Holt, Rinehart & Winston.

Esplen M, Touer B, Hunter J, et al. (1998). A group therapy approach to facilitate integration of risk information for women at risk for breast cancer. Canadian Journal of Psychiatry 43(4):375–380.

Gans J, Alonso A. (1998). Difficult patients: Their construction in group therapy. International Journal of Group Psychotherapy 48(3):311–326.

Goldstein J, Alter C, Axelrod R. (1996). A psychoeducational breavement support group for families provided in an outpatient cancer center. Journal of Cancer Education 11(4):233–237.

Griffith LW. (1986). Group work with children and adolescents. In Janosik EH, Phipps LB (eds.), Life Cycle Group Work in Nursing. Monterey, CA, Wadsworth.

Hawkins D. (1998). An invitation to join in difficulty: Realizing the deeper promise of group psychotherapy. International Journal of Group Psychotherapy 48(4):423–438.

Hoge M, McLoughlin K. (1991). Group psychotherapy in acute treatment settings: Theory and technique. Hospital and Community Psychiatry 42(2):153–157.

Hyland D, Ackerman A. (1988). Reminiscence and autobiographical memory in the study of the personal past. Journal of Gerontology 43(2):35–39.

Jacobson L. (1989). The group as an object in the cultural field. International Journal of Group Psychotherapy 39(4):475–497.

Janis I. (1971). Groupthink. Psychology Today 5:43–46, 74–76.

Kovach C. (1991). Reminiscence: Exploring the origins, processes, and consequences. Nursing Forum 26(3):14–19.

Kreidler MC, Carlson RE. (1991). Breaking the incest cycle: The group as a surrogate family. Journal of Psychosocial Nursing and Mental Health Services 29(4):28–32.

Laube J, Wieland V. (1998). Nourishing the body through use of process prescriptions in group therapy. International Journal of Eating Disorders 24(1):1–11.

Lewin K. (1951). Field Theory in Social Sciences. New York, Harper & Row.

McGinley S, Baus E, Gyza K, et al. (1996). Multidisciplinary discharge planning: Developing a process. Nursing Management 27(10):55, 57–60.

Murphy G. (1975). Group psychotherapy in our society. In Rosenbaum M, Berger M (eds.), Group Psychotherapy and Group Function. New York, Basic Books.

Prehn R, Thomas P. (1990). Does it make a difference? The effect of a women's issues group on female psychiatric inpatients. Journal of Psychosocial Nursing 28(11):34–38.

Rogers C. (1972). The process of the basic encounter group. In Diedrich R, Dye HA (eds.), Group Procedures: Purposes, Processes and Outcomes. Boston, Houghton Mifflin.

Rosenblum EH. (1982). Groupthink: One peril of group cohesiveness. Journal of Nursing Administration 12(4):27–31.

Schilling R, El-Bassel N, Haden B, Gilbert L. (1995). Skills training groups to reduce HIV transmission and drug use among methadone patients. Social Work 40(1):91–101.

Sluder H. (1990). The write way: Using poetry for self disclosure. Journal of Psychosocial Nursing 28(7):26–28.

Tannenbaum R, Wechsler I, Massarik F. (1988). Leadership: A frame of reference. In Cathcart R, Samovar L (eds.),

Small Group Communication (5th ed.). Dubuque, IA, William C. Brown.

Tuckman B. (1965). Developmental sequence in small groups. Psychological Bulletin 63:384.

Van Servellen G, Poster E, Ryan J, Allen J. (1991). Nurse-led group modalities in a psychiatric inpatient setting: A program evaluation. Archives of Psychiatric Nursing 5(3):128–136.

Yalom I. (1985). The Theory and Practice of Group Psychotherapy (3rd ed.). New York, Basic Books.

Yalom V, Yalom I. (1990). Brief interactive group psychotherapy. Group Psychotherapy Psychiatric Annal 43:440–407.

Zahniser J, Coursey R. (1995). The self-concept group: Development and evaluation for use in psychosocial rehabilitation settings. Psychiatric Rehabilitation Journal 19(2):59–64.

# 13

# Communicating with Families

Elizabeth Arnold

---

**OBJECTIVES**

At the end of the chapter, the student will be able to

1. Define and describe family
2. Identify theoretical frameworks used to study family communication and family dynamics

3. Apply the nursing process in caring for the family as client
4. Identify selected communication strategies to use in interacting with families

*I know I'm hot tempered like my father, but still I believe it's important to remember relatives' birthdays with cards the way my mother always did. My interest in world affairs comes from her, but I learned from my father how to unwind from gardening. His pride in a paycheck made me want always to have one of my own. Her pride in a tastefully furnished home gave me a yen for interior decorating.*

McBride (1976)

Chapter 13 addresses communication issues specific to families. and presents an overview of common problems nurses encounter as they communicate with families. From the moment a person enters a family through birth or adoption, significant family members guide the person's ideas, influence his or her decisions, and teach him or her how to be human. Families provide both the context and process in the formation and support of human experience. Some family therapists believe that "the family of origin is the most powerful force in organizing and framing later life experiences and choices" (Framo, 1992, p. 128). Like them, hate them, or ignore them, families are the single most important variable in our early development. Although people later marry and create new family groups, family of origin values and patterns continue to influence their lives. Nurses interact with families in many areas of practice. Whether obtaining an adequate assessment, accompanying a patient to surgery, or enlisting the family to support the coping of an ill member, nurses often find themselves relating to the family as much as to the identified client. Sometimes the entire family becomes the client as nurses expand their ideas of practice and appropriate units of care. Understanding family communication and learning how to communicate with families is different and more demanding than communicating with individuals. Whereas most nursing education focuses on dealing with an individual client, the nurse needs to add family communication to the repertoire of nursing skills. Functions of family communication are presented in Box 13–1.

## BASIC CONCEPTS
### Definitions

Whall (1990) defined *family* as "a self-identified group of two or more individuals whose associa-

> ### Box 13–1. Functions of Family Communication
>
> A tool to help children learn about the environment
> A way to communicate rules about how family members should think and act
> A tool for family conflict resolution
> A tool for nurturing and developing self-esteem
> A primary mode to transmitting cultural values and traditions
> A means of expressing emotions within the family unit

tion is characterized by special terms, who may or may not be related by bloodlines or law, but who function in such a way that they consider themselves to be a family" (p. 52). Strong emotional ties and durability of membership characterize family relationships. The family is the earliest and most important place where people learn about how to relate to others and to the world around them.

### Family Structure

The family is a social system and structure refers to the way a family is organized: its composition and interpersonal and subsystem boundaries. Minuchin (1974) defined family structure as "the invisible set of functional demands that organizes the ways in which family members interact" (p. 51). Over the life of a family, structure does not remain the same, although a certain structural continuity is maintained. Structural roles are relatively enduring, maintained by covert rules that influence communication. Family composition changes as new members are added or leave the immediate family circle.

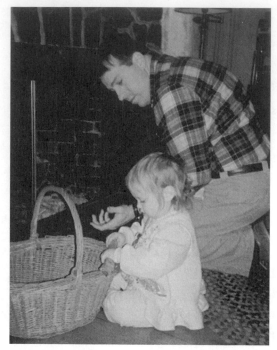

Young children learn the family rules for communication from their parents.

A variety of structural forms define the family unit, as presented in Box 13–2. The common idea of a traditional American family living in a household with mother, father, and two children is outdated and to some extent was always a myth. Today, however, there are so many more combinations of people living together and calling themselves family that Wright and Leahey (1994) simply stated that a "family is who they say they are" (p. 40).

Knowing about differences in family structure helps the nurse plan the most effective strategies. For example, single-parent families must accomplish the same developmental tasks as two-parent families but, in many cases, without support of the other partner or equal financial resources (Mailick & Vigilante, 1997). Children in biological and blended families have a different life experience based on differences in family structure. Box 13–3 displays some of the differences between biological and blended families. Issues for blended families include discipline, money, use of time, birth of an infant, death of a stepparent,

inclusion at graduation, marriage, and so on. Health care decision making in divorced families marked by conflict may have to take into account more than one set of circumstances and role relationships in arriving at what is best for the child. Communication with divorced families needs to acknowledge the different relationships and modes of family behavior in ways that include the perspectives of all family members. Exercise

---

### ◆ Box 13–2. Forms of Family Units

**Nuclear:** a father and mother, with one or more children, living together but apart from both sets of their parents.

**Extended:** nuclear family unit's combination of second- and third-generation members related by blood or marriage but not living together

**Three generational:** any combination of first-, second-, and third-generation members living within a household

**Dyad:** husband and wife or other couple living alone without children

**Single parent:** divorced, never married, separated, or widowed male or female and at least one child; most single-parent families are headed by women

**Stepfamily:** family in which one or both spouses are divorced or widowed with one or more children from a previous marriage who may not live with the newly reconstituted family

**Blended or reconstituted:** a combination of two families with children from one or both families and sometimes children of the newly married couple

**Common law family:** an unmarried couple living together with or without children

**No kin:** a group of at least two people sharing a nonsexual relationship and exchanging support who have no legal or blood tie to each other

**Polygamous family:** one man (or woman) with several spouses

**Gay:** a homosexual couple living together with or without children

**Commune:** more than one couple living together and sharing resources

**Group marriage:** all individuals are "married" to one another and are considered parents of all the children

◆ Box 13-3. Structural Developmental Differences between Biological and Blended Families

| Biological Families | Blended Families |
|---|---|
| Family is created without loss. | Family is born of loss. |
| There are shared family traditions. | There are two sets of family traditions. |
| One set of family rules evolves. | Family rules are varied and complicated. |
| Children arrive one at a time. | Instant parenthood of children at different ages occurs. |
| Biological parents live together. | Biological parents live apart. |

13–1 provides you with the opportunity to learn more about different family structures.

*Family Function*

*Family function* is a broad term used to describe how a family normally interacts with each other to achieve identifiable goals. The term can include family activities such as protecting, socializing, working, or reproducing. One way of assessing how a family functions is by looking at role expectations within the family system; for example, who is the breadwinner, who assumes care giving functions, and who makes decisions? Are these responsibilities shared? Do gender, individual characteristics, or critical events determine role expectations?

◆ Exercise 13-1. **Positive and Negative Family Interactions**

**Purpose:** To examine the effect of different family interactions

**Procedure:**
Answer the following questions in a brief essay:

1. Do you remember a situation in dealing with a client's family that you felt was a positive experience? What characteristics of that interaction made you feel this way?

_____

_____

_____

2. Do you remember a situation in dealing with a client's family that you felt was a negative experience? What characteristics of that interaction made you feel this way?

_____

_____

_____

**Discussion:**
Compare experiences, both positive and negative. Were there connections between things that made you uncomfortable and your own family upbringing? If so, what are the implications of this in your nursing parctice?

Family functioning is viewed on a continuum ranging from optimal function to disintegration as a family unit. Bowen (1985) described families as more or less healthy according to their level of differentiation and the amount of anxiety that is present in the family. Psychologically healthy families should have moderate degrees of cohesion, coordination, and adaptability in most family functions (Green & Werner, 1996).

Challenges to the functioning of the family system can include expected normative crises such as divorce, retirement, marriage, or remarriage or placement of an elderly parent in a nursing home. Alternatively, the challenge can relate to unexpected disruptions such as sudden job loss, trauma, or the untimely death of an important or conflictual family member (Walsh, 1996). The nurse will want to assess the family's functioning in the current nursing situation as well as inquire about past patterns.

## Family Process

A process is a phenomenon that occurs over a period of time. The term *process* implies change, but within every change there are often patterns and connections with events in the past that are likely to recur. Family members continually create shared meanings as their interactions unfold over time, and family process describes the predictable and repetitive interaction patterns of families. For example, Mother always watches Johnnie's behavior very closely. Johnnie gets upset with her attention and complains to Dad. Dad goes to Mother and complains that she is too harsh with Johnnie. Mother backs off for a while but soon resumes her attention. These patterns communicate meanings to family members about the world and their place in it.

The tracking of these processes originated from communications theory. Because family communication takes place within ongoing relationships, the relational aspects of communication become more important than in other types of communication. In the midst of enduring relationships within family systems, styles and forms of communication develop that become patterns, which are repeated. These patterns can be identified as interaction sequences that have typical starting points and follow a predictable sequence of interaction (Watzlawick et al, 1967). Typically, members of the family know their place within the pattern and jump in at the appropriate place whenever the sequence starts. Some patterns can be helpful to the family, such as a pattern that nurtures or offers support. Others can be destructive, such as a pattern in which one member consistently loses out in decision making (Exercise 13–2).

Family communication not only conveys a message, it provides information about family relationships in terms of power, affection, and control. For example, if a child balks about doing chores and the mother says, "That's okay, I'll do that for you," the message that is communicated is that the child is in the protection or care of the mother. If the mother instead says, "I'll help

---

◆ **Exercise 13-2. Family Structures and Processes**

**Purpose:** To develop an awareness of the different structures and processes within families

**Procedure:**
Each student will attempt to spend time with a family other than their own family of origin. (Family can be any two or more persons of relation.) Students should observe the communication patterns, roles, and norms of the family and write a descriptive summary of their experience. How do you think this family would cope with one of the members becoming ill? Think about how this family differs from your own regarding structure and process.

**Discussion:**
Each student will share experiences with the group. Identify how families are different and similar. What are some of the coping strategies that you predicted based on observations? Discuss how the nurse can interface with families and assist them with coping.

you learn how to do this," the message that is communicated is that the child is capable of caring for him- or herself with some help. Playing the part of the "competent husband" or "comforting wife" may become a shared meaning for a couple that each partner adheres to expectantly and behaviorally.

A *double-bind communication* is a communication that sends two conflicting messages at once. For example, a mother who says, "Come here, I love you" to a child and yet remains rigid and cold when the child approaches is sending conflicting messages. Not only is the child in a double bind because he or she is unable to respond to both messages, but the communication usually includes an unspoken message: "Don't comment on how incongruent this communication is."

Early theories on family communication suggested that any family member's behavior, no matter how "crazy," could be understood if one understood the family's communication rules. Some people interpreted this to mean that faulty family communication "caused" mental illness. We now know that psychological illness is linked to biological causes. However, family interactions can influence how an individual responds to symptoms. Today the focus is on exploring the appropriate expression of negative and positive emotions on health and well-being and its effect on supporting dependent members, spouses, self-esteem, and family satisfaction.

## Family Communication

The ability to communicate effectively is essential to all aspects of family functioning because communication is an integral part of daily living. Family communication is defined as the transactional process of sharing information and creating meanings within a family system. It occurs on several different levels. As in individual communication, there is a literal meaning of a message transmitted through words (content) and a relationship level (metacommunication). Metacommunication gives direction about how the receiver should interpret the message and helps explicate the relationship between the communicators.

Family communication can be direct or indirect. Direct communication helps individual members understand the meaning of the communication. The content and the metacommunication match. Satir (1972) referred to this type of communication as "leveling." Indirect communication is less likely to be easily understood. The content and the relational aspects of the message clash, or the message is delivered in an indirect way through another family member, who may or may not want to be involved. For example, in one family, the only way to complain about something may be for the mother to talk to the son, who will then talk to the father. This communication may always be done in a derogatory way so that the father is blamed for what is happening.

Communication styles within the family are further defined as symmetrical or complementary exchanges. *Symmetrical relationships* are interactions in which each person has equal power and the exchanges mirror each other: "Do you want to go to the movies, Honey?" and she replies, "Yes, I'd like that." In contrast, *complementary relationships* involve unequal distribution of power: "I would like to go to the movies," and she replies, "Okay, I will get ready." Symmetrical and complementary exchanges demonstrate family values, roles, and power. Functional family communication involves both types of exchanges. For example, a complementary form of communication might be appropriate between parent and child, whereas symmetrical exchanges are more likely to occur between husband and wife.

### Functional Versus Dysfunctional Family Communication

In any family, there is no such thing as completely functional or completely dysfunctional communication. The communication is usually a mixture of the two, and so may be viewed on a continuum from healthy to less healthy communication. *Functional communication* is direct communication. The message is clear enough that the receiver is able to understand both the literal meaning of the message and the emotional interpretations implied within the message. Functional communication is based on valid assumptions that are supported by evidence and confirmed through feedback. Prerequisites of fully functional communication are trust in the other's intention and a firm sense of self. Each person uses "I" statements and takes full responsibility for his or her part of the conversation. In contrast, dysfunctional communication distorts the message based on unspoken rules that govern the communication. For example, some families have strong family values that pressure members into agreeing with each other totally. A unified opinion is the only acceptable one in this type of family. Differences are viewed as threatening because they may lead to conflict (a peace-agree family) or because they increase awareness that people are separate individuals. Other families may operate using "family myths," which are shared distorted ideas about the way the world or the family operates. For example, "Our family is better than other families and is above obeying societal rules."

## Dysfunctional Sending of Messages

**Dysfunctional communication** usually includes the use of *assumptions*, with the speaker taking for granted that he or she knows what the receiver is feeling or thinking and that the receiver understands the sender's message without validation. **Dysfunctional sending** occurs when part of or the entire message fails to express the truth or is expressed in such a way that the receiver experiences it as a personal attack. In either case, responding to the message is difficult. *Speaking for the other* occurs when one family member assumes that he or she knows what the other member wants without validating it. For example, a mother might say to a teacher, "Billy's father and I think that will be a good idea." Use of *generalizations* is another trap in family communication: "You're always messy" or "You never listen to me."

Unclear expression of feelings sends the feelings underground or leads to resentment and hurt. For example, *sarcasm, silent resentment,* or *expression of hurt as anger* is hard to decipher. Communications that contain messages that are *judgmental* are also dysfunctional. "You should do this" implies that the sender knows what is good and anything else is bad.

## Dysfunctional Receiving

**Dysfunctional receiving** leads to a breakdown in communication. The receiver may *fail to listen,* *disqualify* what is sent, *respond with negativity,* or *fail to validate* the message. Disqualification involves failure to attend to the important parts of the message, such as evading an important issue or making a response that is tangential to the conversation. A "yes but" message sends a message that the receiver disagrees with the message but does not want to say so directly. Negativity includes being defensive, insulting, attacking, or rebuffing ("Tell me again how I get to the car dealer" or "I'm not going to repeat myself"). Failing to validate or to explore the meaning of a message, giving advice prematurely, and cutting off communication terminates the message that is sent and leads to unclear communication and negative feelings.

In general, **dysfunctional communication** tends to occur in families in which at least some family members suffer from chronically low self-esteem. Rather than risk the anger or disapproval of family members, individuals communicate in ways that restrict their individuality and growth of family members. On the other hand, family members who are self-centered will expect all decisions and family events to revolve around them. This focus on one's own needs to the exclusion of those of others communicates the message that "You are less important, less worthy, or less powerful than I am."

## Comparison of Family and Individual Relationships

Therapeutic relationships with families are similar to individual relationships in that the relationship will proceed through certain stages, including engagement, a working phase, and a termination phase. The nurse uses the nursing process to help establish therapeutic relationships with families just as he or she does with individuals. However, incorporating family values and mutuality into the care-planning process is more important if the nurse expects to empower the family to participate in the care.

Families are unique, just as individuals are, affected by their culture, age, gender, and economics as to how they respond. Having a comprehensive understanding of the way families operate is necessary for the nurse to be able to work with them effectively. Families need to tell their experience of the client's illness or injury, which may be different from how the client is experiencing it. For example, grandmother may be very upset at being placed in a nursing home after fracturing her hip. However, this placement may need to occur for reasons that are family oriented, not individual determined. The nurse will need to understand the family's position as well as the client's situation in order to be helpful. Exercise 13–3 examines coping strategies among families.

## Theoretical Frameworks for Family Assessment

Thinking about a family as a system is such a common approach that many other approaches actually combine their way of thinking about families with a systems perspective (Barker, 1998). Von Bertalanffy (1968) described certain principles applicable to all systems in his general systems theory:

1. A system is a unit in which the *whole* is greater than the sum of its parts.
2. Certain *rules* govern the operation of such systems.
3. Every system has a *boundary* that is somewhat open or closed.
4. Boundaries allow exchange of information and resources into (*inputs*) and outside (*outputs*) the system.
5. *Communication* and feedback mechanisms between parts of the system are important in the function of the system.
6. *Circular causality* helps to explain what is happening better than linear causality. A change

in one part of the system leads to change in the whole system.
7. Systems operate on the principle of *equifinality;* that is, the same endpoint can be reached from a number of starting points.
8. Systems are made up of *subsystems* and are themselves parts of *suprasystems.* Subsystems describe relationships among family member units such as siblings, spousal, child–parent subsystem. The suprasystem represents the larger context of community. Bowen's family systems theory is used widely by nurses as an application of general systems theory for examining family communication.

### Bowen's Systems Theory

Bowen's systems framework uses natural systems theory to describe the nature of family interaction. It is one of the most fully developed theories of family functioning (Innes, 1996). Family systems evolve with time and circumstances similar to the evolution of biological organisms. Bowen viewed the family as an emotional system in which energy from its emotional process impacts on every member in it. Individual family members react to each other in predictable and reciprocal ways. Each family member has a role in the family goal of preserving the stability of the family system and reducing tension to a workable level. Bowen contended that within the family are "interlocking relationships . . . that are governed by the same counterbalancing life forces that operate in all natural systems" (Kerr & Bowen, 1988, p. ix). Until one family member

---

◆ Exercise 13–3. **Family Coping Strategies**

**Purpose:**  To broaden awareness of coping strategies among families

**Procedure:**
Each student is to recall a time when their family experienced a significant crisis and how they coped. Did the crisis cause a readjustment in roles? Did it create tension and conflict, or did it catalyze turning to one another for support? Look at individual members' behavior. What would have helped your family in this crisis? Write a descriptive summary about this experience.

**Discussion:**
Each student shares their experience. Coping strategies and helpful interventions will be compiled on the board. Discuss the differences in how families respond to crisis. Discuss the nurse's role in support to the family.

is willing to challenge the functionality of the emotional system by refusing to play his or her reactive part, the emotional energy fueling a family's rigid dysfunctional communication pattern persists.

Differentiation of self within the system is the primary means of changing family process. *Self-differentiation* is a term used to describe the capacity to stay involved in one's family without losing one's identity. Bowen (1985) believed that "the level of differentiation is the degree to which oneself fuses or merges with another self in a close emotional relationship" (p. 200). A person who is self-differentiated is able to think, feel, and act for himself as a separate person without getting caught up in the emotionality of the family system. This person has the courage to define self without having to disengage from the family unit (Bohlander, 1995). Personal energy is directed toward changing the self rather than others. A self-differentiated family member simultaneously respects the rights of self and others.

Bowen (1985) described family process as occurring through a *multigenerational transmission process*, by which a family passes germane ways of behaving and communicating from generation to generation. For example, family patterns of alcoholism, abuse, or depression are threads of emotional energy that persist over generations and continue to exert powerful pressures on current family functioning. As you explore a family genogram, you may discover that all of the women in the family married men who womanized or that the pattern of divorce is consistent over many generations. Family rules such as "family comes first" or "appearances are the only thing that counts" can operate so strongly within a family that they dominate family functioning even when they do not fit current family circumstances. When family members buy into these maxims without considering whether they have relevance for themselves as individuals and partners in new relationships, their communication tends to be "less flexible, less adaptable, and more emotionally dependent on those about them" (Bowen, 1985, p. 362).

Another key concept is the *family projection process*. Bowen understood this to mean that when family tensions become too elevated, a family may unconsciously try to reduce its anxiety by projecting it on to one of its members. Examples of the projection process include the family hero, the dysfunctional child, and the family scapegoat. Rather than viewing the created role as a family dynamic to reduce anxiety, the family acts as if a single family member has certain characteristics that are alien to an understanding of the family unit.

Bowen suggested looking for *emotional cutoffs* within the family, defined as a situation in which family members break off contact with family members. Cutoffs require emotional energy that is not always recognized and typically is dysfunctional.

The reasons for the cutoff vary, ranging from very serious (e.g., sexual abuse) to illogical when viewed objectively (e.g., feeling snubbed by a relative). Sometimes other family members not directly involved in the original cutoff have no idea why it exists.

Making contact with cut-off parts of the family allows family members to create new relationships and roles within their family. For most people, even contemplating contacting people that they do not know is frightening. However, exploring family connections beyond what is usual for you broadens your personal perspective of yourself in ways that allow most people to have more fluid and enriching relationships that also extend beyond the family unit.

Triangles are a critical element in Bowen's theory (Glasscock & Hales, 1998). They are present in every family. A *triangle* is a three-person emotional system that begins when there is tension between two members. A third person or object is brought in to stabilize the two-person relationship. For example, the mother feels that the father is not paying enough attention to her. She calls her son at college on a daily basis and complains that she is very lonely. The father never hears of her discontent, but the son feels resentful that he is expected to fill the gap. The father feels bitter because he thinks his wife prefers talking with the son than with him. Typically, in any triangle, two people are close and the third person is in a more distant position. In a triangle, there are always unspoken feelings that need to be addressed with the odd person out in the triangle. One side of the triangle usually includes conflict or emotional tension. Attempting to map the primary or most influential triangles in the family is a part of describing the family relationships.

A systems perspective recognizes that change in one part of the family system affects the entire family. For example, the alcoholic has the drinking problem, but the problem usually becomes the organizing principle in the family. When the alcoholic stops drinking, other family members do not know how to behave. A systems perspective does not look for causes but instead seeks information about what the family is willing to consider in coming up with a viable solution acceptable to both client and family. The goal of viewing families as an interconnected system makes nursing care more difficult to plan and perform, but in the final analysis it is a more accurate and efficient way to think about families.

## Duvall's Developmental Framework

Another way of looking at families is through a developmental framework. According to Duvall (1958), families are primarily formed to promote the growth and development of their members. Her stage developmental model proposes that the family as a unit engages in a developmental process of growth, aging, and change over its life span. Developmental tasks associated with each stage must be achieved if the stage is to be negotiated successfully. The better equipped a family is to meet its tasks, the more successful is family development.

Duvall outlined eight stages of the family life cycle and the specific tasks to be accomplished in each stage. Family stages, as presented in Box 13–4, are defined by the age of the oldest child. For example, a family with two children aged 6 and 2 would be considered a school-age family. A family in the launching stage typically has a young adult who is preparing to leave home; the family must complete the developmental tasks of releasing the young adult while maintaining a supportive home base. Simultaneously, they must re-establish the relationships and structure within the family to adjust to the missing member.

In the cycle of family development, the transition from one stage to the next is the critical period, and successful completion of current critical phases is determined to some extent by the completion of earlier tasks.

Duvall (1958, p. 336) identified nine family characteristics indicative of successful family development. She suggested that the family must be able to establish and maintain

1. An independent home
2. Satisfactory ways of earning and spending money
3. Mutually acceptable patterns in the division of labor
4. Continuity of mutually satisfying sexual relationships
5. An open system of communication
6. Workable relationships with relatives
7. Ways of interacting with the larger social community
8. Competency in childbearing and child rearing
9. A workable philosophy of life

Duvall's framework is useful in assessing the types of normal developmental stressors families face at different points in the life span. Developmental milestones tell the nurse about possible concerns and suggest ways to adapt interventions to meet the needs of families experiencing them. Criticism of the model is that her framework focuses on the two-parent traditional family form that no longer is fully descriptive of many modern families. More children grow up in single-parent families. As people live longer, the time when the youngest child leaves home coincides with assuming increased responsibilities for elderly parents.

## Satir's Interactional Model

Satir (1976) believed that "communication is to relationship what breathing is to maintaining life." Satir suggested that healthy communication is *open, clear, direct,* and *congruent.* She referred to healthy communication as **leveling,** in which the interaction is emotionally honest and congruent. This communication style is integrated, flowing, and alive. Messages are simply and unambiguously stated. The content and metacommunication match. They are directed to the person who needs to receive the message rather than through someone else.

Satir (1991) described four dysfunctional ways people communicate when they are under stress:

---

### ◆ Box 13–4. Duvall's Eight-Stage Family Life Cycle and Family Developmental Tasks

| State Family Life Cycle Stage | Family Development Tasks |
| --- | --- |
| I. Beginning families (married couples without children) | Establishing a mutually satisfying marriage; adjusting to pregnancy and the promise of parenthood; fitting into the kin network |
| II. Child-bearing families (oldest child birth through 30 months) | Having, adjusting to, and encouraging the development of infants; establishing a satisfying home for both parents and infant(s) |
| III. Families with preschool-age children (oldest child 2 1/2–6 years of age) | Adapting to the critical needs and interests of preschool-age children in stimulating, growth-promoting ways; coping with energy depletion and lack of privacy as parents |
| IV. Families with school-age children (oldest child 6–13 years of age) | Fitting into the community of school-age families in constructive ways; encouraging children's educational achievement |
| V. Families with teenagers (oldest child 13–20 years of age) | Balancing freedom with responsibility as teenagers mature and emancipate themselves; establishing postparental interests and careers as growing parents |
| VI. Families launching young adults (first child leaving home through last child leaving home) | Releasing young adults into work, college, marriage with appropriate rituals and assistance; maintaining supportive home base |
| VII. Middle-age parents (empty nest to retirement) | Rebuilding the marriage relationship; maintaining kin ties with older and younger generations |
| VIII. Family during retirement and aging (retirement) | Adjusting to retirement; closing the family home or adapting it to aging; coping with bereavement and living alone |

From Duvall EM. (1977). Marriage and Family Development. Glenview, IL, Addison Wesley Educational Publishers, pp. 144, 179. Reprinted by permission of Addison Wesley Educational Publishers.

---

1. Agreeing with what is being said despite reservations (placating)
2. Attributing responsibility for problems to others and not taking personal responsibility (blaming)
3. Intellectualizing about a problem and leaving out the emotional components (superreasonable)
4. Using irrelevant responses instead of dealing directly with the issue (irrelevant)

Healthy families have developed successful ways to *negotiate conflict* and send messages that affirm others' worth and that *promote self-esteem*. Box 13–5 lists Satir's (1976) five freedoms described as the foundation for promoting self-esteem in family members.

---

### ◆ Box 13–5. The Five Freedoms

To see and hear what is here instead of what should be, was, or will be

To say what one feels and thinks instead of what one should

To feel what one feels instead of what one ought

To ask for what one wants instead of always waiting for permission

To take risks in one's own behalf instead of choosing to be only "secure" and not rocking the boat

## Theoretical Models of Family Coping

### McCubbin's Crisis Model of Coping

The way in which a family responds to a crisis helps identify its coping pattern. Hill's work in 1949 led to the formulation of the A-B-C-X crisis model of family coping. A (the event) interacts with B (resources) and with C (family's perception of the event) to produce X (the crisis). The family responds with a course of adjustment involving disorganization, recovery, and a subsequent level of reorganization. McCubbin and colleagues (1982) expanded this model in a double A-B-C-X model that adds concepts of *pileup* of demands, *family system resources*, and *postcrisis* behavior to the original model (Fig. 13–1).

McCubbin's systems model says that for successful coping to occur, the family must be able to (1) develop internal conditions for family orga-

nization and communication, (2) promote member independence and self-esteem, (3) maintain family bonds of coherence and unity, (4) develop social supports within the community, and (5) control the impact of the stressor on the family unit.

In 1993, McCubbin and associates extended the C factor in the double A-B-C-X model to describe family schemata, emphasizing a relativistic view of life and a willingness to accept less than perfect solutions as a path to resilient coping. Resilient families are those with high degrees of bonding and flexibility.

Knowledge of a family's coping pattern enables the nurse to understand the client's health problems in its larger context, and provides a solid base for developing family-based nursing diagnoses amenable to nursing intervention. The understanding that family coping is a process that changes over time can be communicated to the family as it is helped to make decisions.

The key to helping families cope is the percep-

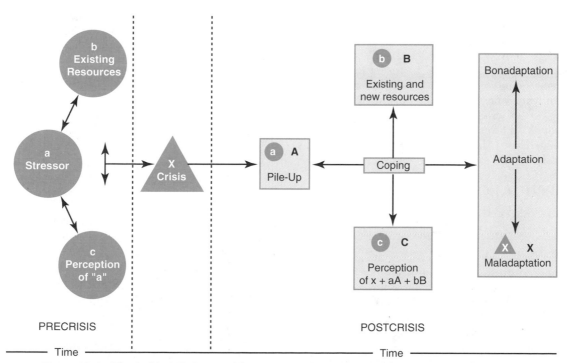

**Figure 13–1.** The double A-B-C-X model. (From McCubbin H, Cauble AE, Patterson J. (1982). Family Stress, Coping, and Social Support. Springfield, IL, Charles C Thomas, p. 46. Courtesy Charles C Thomas, Publishers.)

tions the family has of the event, individually and as a group. Individual family members do not respond equally to a change in the health of one of its members. The death of an infant, for example, can be a different experience for mother, father, sibling, and grandparent despite the common crisis event. Individual members may use different coping styles or behaviors to deal with the stress. The goal of nursing intervention is to strengthen the family as a functional unit in their response to difficult health situations.

## Family Resilience

Walsh (1996) suggested that "the concept of family resilience offers a useful framework to identify and fortify key processes that enable families to surmount crises and persistent stresses" (p. 261). Family resiliency is more likely to occur in a healthy family atmosphere of warmth and affection. Emotional support for individual family members and reasonable, clear-cut limits provide the foundation for positive coping strategies. Having at least one supportive person in your immediate environment who believes in you and can provide emotional support can offset a negative family climate. This person can be a grandparent, family friend, or leader in a community agency. Other strategies to foster family resiliency include encouraging collaboration among family members, reinforcing teamwork and sharing of experiences, and referring to support groups. The concept of resilience is closely aligned with that of using personal and family strengths in responding to crisis.

## APPLICATIONS
## Assessment
### Indications for Family Assessment

Healthy People 2000 considers the family as an important resource in health promotion and disease prevention. Families introduce their members early in life to health values and choices that will influence their health throughout life. Illness is usually a family event rather than an individual one.

Assessment of relevant family experiences provides a way of understanding the client within a social environmental context that surrounds

and supports his or her recovery. Box 13–6 lists sample indicators for family assessment. The nurse has the opportunity to understand the family's perception of the health problem or need, which may or may not be quite different from that of the client. Additionally, the family's willingness and capacity to develop options that are helpful in resolving the health care concern are of major importance.

The nurse may want to collect identifying information or demographic data about the family. Collecting data about the family's physical environment, such as the presence of accident hazards, for example, in terms of window screens, plumbing, or cooking facilities, may help the nurse plan care that matches or supplements family resources and identify potential health problems. Community resources and facilities available to the family should also be noted. Box 13–7 displays a sample family assessment tool developed by nursing students for outpatient cardiac rehabilitation.

### Family Assessment Tools

Families have unique identities that cannot be understood when one thinks about only the pieces. The familiar adage "the whole is greater than the sum of its parts" means there is some-

---

◆ **Box 13–6. Indicators for Family Assessment**

Initial diagnosis of a serious physical or psychiatric illness/injury in a family member

Family involvement and understanding needed to support recovery of client

Deterioration in a family member's condition

Illness in a child, adolescent, or cognitively impaired adult

A child, adolescent, or adult child having an adverse response to a parent's illness

Discharge from a health care facility to the home or an extended-care facility

Death of a family member

Health problem defined by family as a family issue

Indication of threat to relationship (abuse, neglect, anticipated loss of family member)

## ◆ Box 13-7. Family Assessment for Client Entering Cardiac Rehabilitation

### Family Assessment
### Coping/Stress

Who lives with you? _____

_____

How do you handle stress? _____

_____

Have you have any recent changes in your
    life (e.g., job change, move, change in marital
    status, loss) _____

_____

Whom do you rely on for emotional support? ____

_____

Who relies on you for emotional support? _____

_____

How does your illness affect your family
    members/significant other? _____

_____

Are there any health concerns of other family
    members? _____

_____

If so, how does this affect you? _____

_____

### Communication/Decision Making

How would you describe the communication
    pattern in your family? _____

_____

How does your family address issues/concerns? ____

_____

Can you identify strengths/weaknesses within the
    family? _____

_____

How do the strengths/weaknesses affect you? _____

_____

Are family members supportive of each other? ____

_____

How are decisions that affect the entire family
    made? _____

How are decisions implemented? _____

_____

### Role

What is your role in the family? _____

_____

Can you describe the roles of other family
    members? _____

_____

### Value Beliefs

What is your ethnic/cultural background?

_____

What is your religious background?

_____

Are there any particular cultural/religious healing
    practices in which you participate?

_____

### Leisure Activities

Do you participate in any organized social
    activities? _____

In what leisure activities do you participate? _____

_____

Do you anticipate any difficulty with continuing
    these activities? _____

_____

If so, how will you make the appropriate
    adjustments? _____

_____

Do you have a regular exercise regimen? _____

### Environmental Characteristics

Do you live in a rural, suburban, or urban area? __

_____

What type of dwelling do you live in? _____
Are there stairs in your home? _____
Where is the bathroom? _____
Are the facilities adequate to meet your needs? ____
If not, what adjustments will be needed? _____

_____

*Box continued on following page*

---

**◆ Box 13–7. Family Assessment for Client Entering Cardiac Rehabilitation** *Continued*

How do you plan to make those adjustments? _____

_____

Are there any community services provided to you
    at home? (explain) _____

_____

Are there community resources available in your
    area? _____
_____

Do you have any other concerns at this time? _____

_____

Is there anything that we have omitted? _____

Signature _____ (must be completed
    by RN) Date/Time _____

Developed by Conrad J, Williamson J, Mignardi D. (1993). University of Maryland School of Nursing.

---

thing more to a family than simply adding characteristics of individual members. Parameters that are often assessed include family processes, roles, communication, division of labor, decision making, boundaries, styles of problem solving, and coping abilities. Some widely used family assessment tools are discussed next.

## Genograms

A *genogram* is a family diagram that records information about family members and their relationships for at least three generations (McGoldrick and Gerson, 1985). Genograms make it easier for a clinician to keep in mind the family members, patterns, and significant events that are important in the family's care. The picture of the family that is presented on the genogram helps the observer think about the family systematically and over time. Sometimes when a larger picture is presented, connections between events and relationships become clearer and can be viewed in a more objective way.

Typically, the genogram is constructed in the first or a very early session and revised, as new information becomes available. There are three parts to genogram construction: (1) mapping the family structure, (2) recording family information, and (3) delineating family relationships.

A diagram of family members placed in each generation is drawn using horizontal and vertical lines. Symbols used to represent pregnancies, miscarriages, marriages, deaths, and so on are presented in Figure 13–2. Males are placed on the left of the horizontal line and females on the right. Placing the oldest sibling on the far left and progressing toward the right represents birth order. In the case of multiple marriages, the earliest is placed on the left and the most recent on the right.

Family information presented on the genogram includes ages, birth and death dates for all family members, geographical location, occupations, and educational levels. Critical family events and transitions such as moves, marriages, divorces, losses, and successes are recorded. Family members' physical, emotional, and social problems or illnesses are identified. Relationship patterns are identified as fused, close, distant, cut off, or conflictual on the diagram. Seeing the relationship on the diagram can be quite useful for clients and their families. Often relationships take the form of triangles that are more easily presented on a genogram than talked about without having this assessment tool. An example of a family genogram is presented in Figure 13–3.

In addition to providing assessment information, the process of collecting and recording information for the construction of a genogram serves as a way for the interviewer and family to connect in a personal but emotionally safe way. Asking other family members for missing information can foster the development of new relationships and stimulate feelings of belonging. The genogram also provides the interviewer with information about how the members of the family think about family problems and interact with other members. Beginning to record information on a genogram can serve to detoxify issues or reduce anxiety about the family problem. The nurse joins the family and helps to normalize and

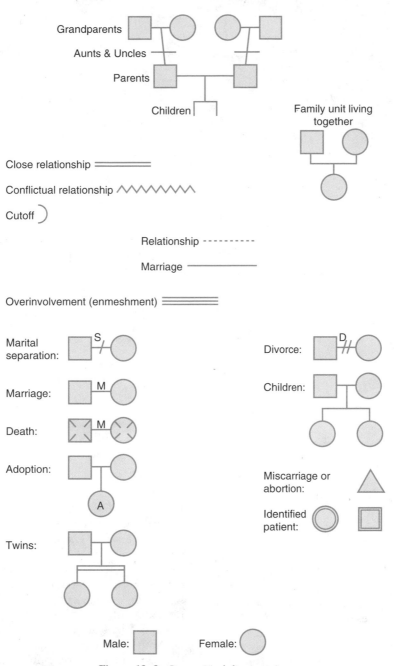

Figure 13–2. Generational diagramming.

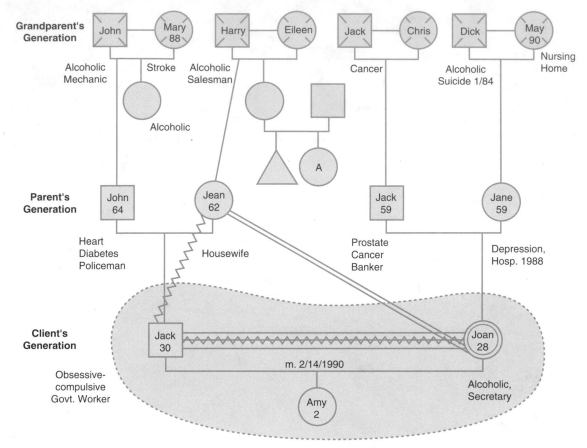

**Grandparent's Generation**

John — Mary 88

Harry — Eileen

Jack — Chris

Dick — May 90

Nursing Home

Alcoholic Mechanic    Stroke    Alcoholic Salesman

Cancer

Alcoholic Suicide 1/84

Alcoholic

A

**Parent's Generation**

John 64

Jean 62

Jack 59

Jane 59

Heart Diabetes Policeman

Housewife

Prostate Cancer Banker

Depression, Hosp. 1988

**Client's Generation**

Jack 30

Joan 28

m. 2/14/1990

Obsessive-compulsive Govt. Worker

Amy 2

Alcoholic, Secretary

Figure 13–3. Basic family genogram.

reframe problems so that they are viewed in a larger context. This type of interaction helps someone to step back and think about an issue in a calmer way. Exercise 13–4 provides practice with developing a family genogram.

**Family Time Lines**

Time lines are another way of diagramming family life events and patterns. Horizontal events occur in the present and include such milestones as marriages, illnesses, or the births. Family patterns that occur through multigenerational transmission are represented as vertical lines. They may be patterns of early death, marriage at an early age, high educational level, and so on (Fig. 13–4). This diagram is useful in looking at how the family history and concurrent life events interact with the current health concern.

**Ecomaps**

*Ecomaps* are a means of diagramming a family member's relationship with external resources. They define the current life space of the family in concrete terms (Hartman, 1978). Here an inner circle in the middle of the page, labeled with the family's name, represents the family. Smaller circles outside the family circle represent other significant people, agencies, and social institutions that affect a family's well-being and ability to cope. Lines are drawn from the inner family circle to outer circles indicating the strength of the contact and relationship. Straight lines indicate relation, with widening of the line used to indicate the strength of the relationship. Dotted lines suggest fragile relationships. Stressful relationships are represented with slashes placed

---

◆ Exercise 13–4. **Family Genogram**

**Purpose:** To learn to create a family genogram

**Procedure:**
Students will break into pairs and interview one another to gain information to develop a family genogram. The genogram should include demographic information, occurrence of illness or death, as well as relationship patterns for three generations. Use the symbols for diagramming in Figure 13–2 to create a visual picture of the family information. Write a short description of what it was like for you to obtain information from someone else regarding their family.

**Discussion:**
Each person will display their genogram and discuss the process of obtaining information. Discuss strategies for obtaining information expediently yet sensitively and tactfully. Discuss how genograms can be used in a helpful way with families.

---

through the relationship line. Directional arrows indicate the flow of the relational energy.

## Recognizing Families at Risk

Not all families act in the best interests of their members. Marital discord, parental mental illness, overcrowded housing conditions, and limited parenting skills place children at risk for faulty development (Hawley & DeHaan, 1996). Abuse of family members, violence, substance abuse, neglect, and dysfunction are on the increase as families become more and more stressed while trying to cope with the demands of today's world. The nurse must also be able to recognize families who are providing unsafe environments for their members. Referring families to professionals able to deal with these complex problems and notifying protective service authorities when necessary are other roles of nurses who work with families. Nurses are considered reporting agents in most states and, therefore, are required by law to report suspicion of child physical or sexual abuse to child protection agencies.

## Obtaining Client Data from the Family

To plan effective care, it is also crucial for the nurse to gain an understanding of the entire context in which a person lives. Sometimes the client is unable to provide accurate information needed for appropriate nursing intervention. For example, when the client is unconscious or has an altered mental status, the family may be the only source of data. Other times, the information obtained from the family provides a more complete picture.

Information about the nature of family support is also necessary. For example, nursing interventions will differ for a client whose family is very supportive and for one whose family is unavailable and has few resources during the experience of recovering from surgery. Family participation in data assessment is therapeutically empowering and enhances the therapeutic relationship (Mailick & Vigilante, 1997).

### Family Interview

Interviewing families can be more difficult than interviewing an individual client. For a nurse unfamiliar with this situation, it can be intimidating. After all, the family has been together for a long time and has a history together that gives even the most dysfunctional family strength and a collective power. On the other hand, interviewing families can be a rich source of information and a path to establishing relationships that are fulfilling and meaningful for both the nurse and family members. Paying attention to the family's use of metaphor and the meaning they attribute to their life experience facilitates communication (Bruner, 1990).

Families might first be seen in the hospital, clinic, community setting, or their own home. Seeing families in their own environment is pref-

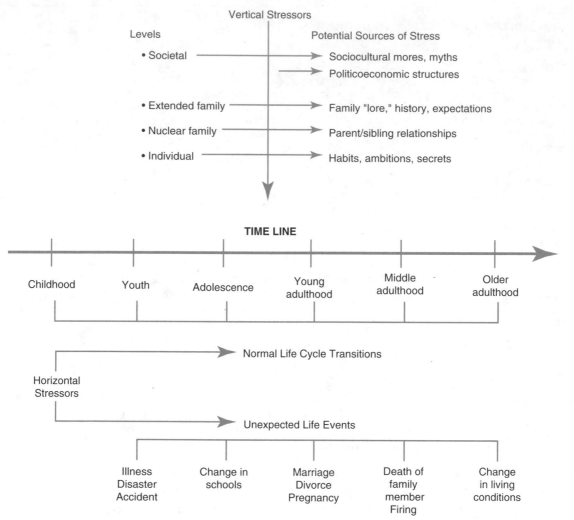

**Figure 13-4.** Learning activity. Develop a comprehensive assessment of your family composed of three-generational family genogram and identification of vertical and horizontal stressors.

erable, of course, because the nurse can observe firsthand the physical and environmental conditions as well as the way the family members act with each other on their own turf. Ideally, the nurse will plan the first meeting to include an explanation of his or her role with the family and what the initial meeting will cover. Exercise 13–5 focuses on the nurse's role with family issues.

**Engaging the Family.** Everyone has been in an interpersonal situation in which things just do not seem to "click." For the nurse–family relationship to be successful, there must be some connection between the nurse and the family that encourages the family to want to continue the relationship. This usually happens when the nurse can communicate respect and empathy to the family. Families know when the nurse is sincere in demonstrations of acceptance and regard for family values. The nurse who truly enjoys working with families in the community will be able to communicate this to families when he or she is not anxious. Families who feel they can trust a nurse will respond by letting the nurse into their private family world.

◆ Exercise 13-5. **Communication Skills with Families**

**Purpose:** To develop communication with families

**Procedure:**
Each student will work with a family related to a specific problem. This can be a current or previous situation for the family. Talk with the family about the problem, and learn how they have dealt with the problem and their perception of the problem and its impact on their family. Try to include all members.

Write a descriptive summary of your experience, including a self-evaluation. Evaluate the experience with the family as well specifically for feedback regarding your approach. Did they feel you were too intrusive or not assertive enough? Did you validate all members' perceptions and perspectives? Did you clarify information and feelings? Did you remain nonjudgmental and objective? Did you respect the family's values and beliefs without imposing your own? Did you assist the family in clarifying and understanding the problem in a way that could lead to resolution?

**Discussion:**
Students share their experience and the feedback they received from the family. Discuss the obstacles encountered when communicating with families. Discuss strategies to facilitate goal-directed communication and resolution of problems. How can nurses best provide support to families? How could families learn to use leveling most of the time? How does one influence this in one's own family?

**Clarifying Purpose.** The first meeting usually needs to be an information-gathering session. For most families, the issues that are of concern are too complex to be dealt with in one meeting. Letting the family know at the outset that the visit will be a time to gather information and to define their concerns is important so that realistic expectations of the visit can be kept.

**Clarifying Boundaries.** The nurse will want to be clear about the boundaries of the nursing encounters. How much time will be spent and when? Where will the interview take place? Who will be present? Are there conditions that are unacceptable to either nurse or family that must be spelled out? For instance, it is common in some cities for nurses to encounter families in which drugs or guns are part of daily life. If this is suspected, the nurse should have some plan about her presence within this home.

**Setting Limits.** For inexperienced nurses, the desire to have families appreciate them and cooperate with them can backfire. Families may test what the nurse is willing to do or may be so overwhelmed and looking for help that they make inappropriate or unrealistic demands. Sometimes families ask for time, money, rides, or assistance with tasks that they could do them-

selves. Sometimes families are just so emotionally distraught that they seek relief from their uncomfortable feelings by placing unrealistic hopes on the nurse. The nurse tries to develop a relationship with a family that inspires their trust. Agreeing to demands that are unrealistic or uncomfortable for the nurse will eventually erode that relationship. Starting at the very first contact nurses need to learn to be comfortable identifying and stating their limits to the family.

## Identifying Family Strengths

Otto (1963) proposed that families possess strengths as a group that can enhance family unity and function. The nurse should look for physical, emotional, and spiritual factors present in the family that can help them experience the current health alteration as potentially growth producing for the entire family. Strengths also can include family motivation, interests, and financial resources. By reinforcing meaningful and clear communication, flexibility in family function and rules, and healthy child-rearing practices, the nurse can optimize family strengths to reduce the impact of difficult health care issues. As families use their inherent strengths and combine their use with external resources, they achieve greater success in problem solving and commitment to family goals (Mailick & Vigilante, 1997).

## Planning

Once a family assessment has been completed, the nurse analyzes the data and summarizes the family's needs. Sometimes individuals within the family are the target of nursing interventions.

Box 13–8 presents selected family diagnoses with defining characteristics.

Working with a family requires that the nurse be aware of the importance of mutual goal setting. Sometimes the family's perception of the problems or its determination of priorities is very different from the nurse's determination. Empowering a family eventually to help itself (Dunst et al., 1988) requires that the nurse negotiate a plan of care that first addresses the family priorities. Setting realistic and achievable goals helps to

---

**◇ Box 13–8. Defining Characteristics of Selected Family Diagnoses**

### Altered Family Processes

The state in which a family that normally functions effectively experiences a dysfunction. Families with this diagnosis are those in which the family system or family members are described as follows:

Members are unable to meet physical or emotional needs of members.

Parents do not demonstrate respect for each other's views on child rearing.

Family members are unable to express or accept wide range of feelings.

Members are unable to relate to each other for mutual growth and maturation.

Members are unable to accept help appropriately from other family members.

Members are unable to respect boundaries, individuality, and autonomy of other members.

Unhealthy decision-making process exists.

### Inneffective Family Coping: Compromised and Disabling

Compromised: insufficient, ineffective, or compromised support, comfort, assistance, or encouragement usually by a supportive primary person (family member or close friend). Client may need support to manage or master adaptive tasks related to his or her health challenge.

Disabling: behavior of significant person (family member or other primary person) that disables his or her own capacities and the client's capacities to effectively address tasks essential to either person's adaptation to the health challenge.

I. Compromised
   A. Subjective

Client expresses concern about family's response to his or her health problem.

Family describes preoccupation with personal reactions (e.g., fear, guilt, anticipatory grief, anxiety) to client's illness, disability, or situational or developmental crisis.

Family describes inadequate understanding of client's condition or treatment that interferes with effective assistive or supportive behavior.

   B. Objective

Family is unable to provide assistive or supportive behavior or with less than satisfactory results.

There is neglectful relationship with other family members as a result of client's illness

Family displays protective behavior disproportionate to the client's abilities or need for autonomy.

II. Disabling

Neglectful care of the client in regard to basic human needs or treatment of illness

Distortion of reality regarding the client's health problem, including extreme denial

Intolerance, rejection or abandonment

Client development of helpless, passive dependence on family

### Desired Outcomes

Family member attempting to describe growth impact of crisis on his or her own values, priorities, goals, or relationships

Family member moving in direction of health-promoting and enriching lifestyle

Family member successfully seeking contact with family unit

ensure that the family will be able to accomplish them and retain some sense of mastery and self-efficacy about the process. Taking little steps that are achievable is preferred to giant steps that misjudge what the family can realistically do and so never get accomplished.

The nursing role may vary depending on the setting and the skill and experience of the nurse. In most settings, the nurse focuses on facilitating and role modeling healthy family communication, helping the family solve problems, linking the family with other parts of the health care system, providing information, and supporting and strengthening family coping. More experienced nurses with specialized graduate training counsel families experiencing more intense problems in family dynamics. The nurse must be clear about his or her role and effectively communicate that role and its limitations to the family.

## Nursing Interventions with Families

Family communication theory provides the nurse with principles to use when offering nursing care, especially in assessing and intervening with families. Some of the ways nurses intervene with families include guiding family change, educating and problem solving during developmental crises, supporting family coping, enlisting the aid of family members in caring for family members, and helping family members coordinate resources.

The nurse enters the family system as a teacher, counselor, and advocate to help the family adjust itself to often dramatic change in life circumstances. The goal of nursing interventions is creation of a family system that allows for the growth of all members. The manner in which this care is implemented is determined not only by the needs of the family but also by the skill and experience the nurse brings to the situation. Nurses use communication principles to help families solve problems and attach to resources in ways that maintain their functioning during times of stress.

### Guiding Family Change

Change occurs more readily when at least one member of the system, often a person who is the most free from constraints and has some power in the family, changes his or her way of functioning within the family. In this way of thinking, interventions for families are not always directed at the member who is ill, injured, or at risk but at family members who are most able to engineer necessary change. Family change working through family strengths rather than focusing on its deficits is useful. Helping a family to become aware of information from the environment and to use what is available from outside itself often promotes family health. By showing interest in the coping strategies that have and have not worked, the nurse can help the family see how it has reorganized itself around the stressful situation.

### Educating and Problem Solving During Developmental Crises

Families traditionally care for their members during times of life transitions such as pregnancies, births, marriages, and deaths. Whereas most families come to the situation with an expectation of what they will be doing, they often need support or education when they are experiencing new developmental challenges. Everyone knows that an infant will demand that the family make some adjustments. However, it is not until the infant actually arrives that the family may realize it needs information or ideas about how to rearrange the activities of daily living. When more than one crisis occurs simultaneously, for example, the birth of a child with a congenital problem, the family who appeared to be prepared may need additional resources to cope with the pileup of demands.

A nurse who is aware of developmental family theory will attempt to locate the family within a stage in the life cycle and to assess the family's knowledge of the current developmental demands, the strategies it is using to meet these demands, and its success in meeting them. Some families need information about the "usual" course that can be expected. Others benefit from interventions that help them find balance between the developmental demands and situational stressors such as illness or job loss. Sometimes in families with an ill member, the needs of a healthy child become lost in the shuffle. The goal is to enable the family to accomplish its function for all its members, not just the ones who are ill or otherwise in the forefront. Strategies to help the family in stressful situations or crisis are described in Chapters 20 and 21.

## Enlisting the Aid of the Family for Care of an Ill Member

Other family members are often the identified caregivers for the ill members. The family member may be homebound, and family members may need to offer all the care or coordinate it with health professionals. In other situations, the ill member is more able to care for self but may need to enlist family support when changes are required in diet, activity, and so on. The nurse is the primary agent for coordinating and teaching this health care. Sometimes, however, the family members themselves need care. For example, many female caregivers themselves end up ill or resentful, having sacrificed satisfaction of personal needs to care for others in the family. The nurse needs to help the family recognize its limitations and hidden strengths and maintain a balance of health for all members.

## Supporting Family Coping

The family's perception of the event will greatly influence the outcome. For example, one family in which the father has lost his job may think of the loss as a challenge and an opportunity to move to a new location. Another family may be able to see only the negative consequences, such as the lost income and the anxiety that will result.

Starting with the family's information about itself, the nurse often is able to help members reframe a situation so that there is a healthier balance between self-needs and those created by the current stressors (Modricin & Robison, 1991). Each family has a different style of coping that may or may not be helpful in time of stress. If the coping style is adequate to meet the needs of the current situation, the nurse can encourage the family's methods even if others are available. Helping the family understand the implications of the pileup of demands that leads to crisis helps members think about their situation and realize that it is time limited.

Sometimes the family's style of coping is not useful. Suppose that the way one family copes is to look to the mother for all their support and the mother is the one who is ill. When the nurse and the family determine that the present style of coping is not working, then alternative solutions can be sought. The nurse can encourage the family to develop new ways of coping or can list alternatives and allow the family to choose coping styles that might be useful to them. Providing emotional support is crucial to helping families cope. Remaining aware of one's own values and staying calm and thoughtful can be very helpful to a family in crisis.

## Helping Families Coordinate Resources

Most families need some help coordinating resources. Sometimes family resources are limited or nonexistent. Other families may have plenty of financial and instrumental resources but need help finding their way through the maze of the health care system. Providing information and linking families to available resources is a frequent role of the nurse. This requires that the nurse have a working knowledge of community resources available to families and the best ways to access them. Encouraging families to use natural helping systems increases the network of emotional and economic support available to the family in time of crisis. Examples include contact with other relatives, neighbors, friends, and churches.

## Family as Focus of Care

Not only are families a resource to the health team during a client illness, but the family may also become the focus of care. As family members experience changes in family roles and family dynamics and begin to appreciate the loss a crisis or an illness can bring, they may need help in coping with the situation. The loss can involve a significant valued person, loss of a part of self, role-related losses, loss of personal property, and developmental loss such as loss of hearing or sight in old age. Robinson and McKenna (1998) suggested that one loss can precipitate multiple losses. For example, the Alzheimer's disease victim loses his memory. Accompanying this physical loss are additional psychological losses of role, communication, and independence, which occur simultaneously for both the client and the family. The nurse becomes a facilitator who can help the family strengthen its coping strategies. The nurse is in the position to offer emotional support and help the family solve problems during the crisis. Simply recognizing multiple losses inherent in a seemingly single loss is helpful.

Loos and Bell (1990) noted four explicit needs of families with critically ill clients: (1) relief of anxiety, (2) information, (3) to be with and helpful to the client, and (4) to alter and adjust to new roles. They suggested the use of circular questioning, shown in Box 13–9, as a way of helping clients develop the self-awareness needed to meet each of these needs.

## Evaluating Nurse–
## Family Interactions

Evaluation is the appraisal step of the nursing process in which judgments are made about the value of the care offered. Evaluation may include an estimation of the effectiveness of the nursing care, the quality of the nurse–family interactions, changes in the family's state that may require modification or termination of the care plan, and the family's response to the interventions.

Evaluation as a part of the nursing process does not start and stop at specific times but should begin during the planning stage when appropriate outcomes are established. Continuing simultaneously with implementation, evaluation provides the nurse and family with timely data to make decisions about the client's care.

More specifically, however, the nurse should be aware of the quality of the nurse–family interactions to be able to make judgments about the contributions of family members to the care outcomes. It is possible that a care plan could be formulated that looks promising and realistically is appropriate. Without the vehicle of an effective nurse–family relationship to implement the plan, however, the efforts have been wasted. With any family interaction, the nurse will want to ask the following:

Did I clarify my purpose and the boundaries of the meeting at the beginning?

Did the family understand why I was there and what we would attempt to do together?

After observing the way the family arrived at and started the interaction, what did family members tell me (nonverbally) about what they needed at that time?

Did it seem that I was engaged with each and every member of the family? Were there any members who were not involved or who were not made to feel important to the interaction?

How clearly could I see and describe the communication patterns within this family?

What did I observe that gave me feedback about the family's perception and emotional response to the interaction?

In what ways did I seek feedback to validate the accurate reception of my messages and my reception of the family's messages?

Was there any way I should have modified my verbal or nonverbal communication with this family?

## Communication Strategies

As they become more skilled and take on expanded roles, many nurses are finding themselves in the role of family therapist or coach. Nurses with advanced training and education are recognized increasingly as primary clinicians for many families. Families with disturbances in the way they operate should be referred to someone who is trained to counsel them. Changing family dynamics is not a quick or simple assignment, but it is one that many nurses are incorporating into their practices.

### Observation

The nurse using communications principles with families first examines the family's style of communication. Families have certain rules that govern the way they communicate. Their patterns of interaction repeat themselves and can be used as a source of information about family communication and members' relationships with one another. The nurse will want to observe what kinds of messages people in the family receive about themselves as people and about the problem at hand.

### Tailoring the Intervention to the Family Dynamics

As with individual relationships, the nurse begins with what the family knows and where the family unit is at the time in emotional understanding or need for knowledge. For example, if a family has a rule that all communication goes through the father, the nurse may initially choose to communicate with the family in this way. Different cultures have definite rules about the ways that

## ◆ Box 13–9. Sample Circular Questions for the Family of the Critically Ill

### Need for Relief of Anxiety

*Difference Questions:*

Who will be most relieved when father wakes up/gets better?

Who is most anxious/fearful about the illness?

What is the worst thing that could happen because of father's illness?

What is most helpful to mother to relieve her anxiety?

Is mother more anxious now or when she heard about son's accident?

*Behavioral Effect Questions:*

How does your mother show she is anxious?

What do you do when your mother cries?

*Triadic Questions:*

What does your brother do to help mother relieve her anxiety?

*Hypothetical Questions:*

If the children stayed with you, would you be more or less anxious?

If you went home, would you be more or less anxious?

### Need for Information

*Difference Questions:*

Who finds the information most helpful?

Who best understands what the doctors have explained to you?

When a new member of the family needs to be told about the patient, who explains best?

How do you understand what the doctors have told you?

How is your understanding different from your mother's?

*Hypothetical Questions:*

If you chose to ask for more information, who could you ask?

If you asked for more information, who would be most helpful?

### Need to Be with and Helpful to the Patient

*Difference Questions:*

Who finds most comfort in being near the patient?

Who is most uncomfortable at the bedside?

*Behavioral Effect Questions:*

How does your mother show she is uncomfortable?

What does your brother do to avoid going to the bedside?

How do you make sense of your brother not going to the bedside?

*Hypothetical Questions:*

If you could do one thing to help, what would it be?

*Triadic Questions:*

If mother wanted to help father while he is a patient, what do you think she could do?

### Need to Alter and Adjust to New Roles

*Difference Questions:*

Now that mother is ill, who is best at disciplining the children? Who is best taking care of the house? Who is closest to mother?

*Behavioral Effect Questions:*

How do they show they are close?

How does father/brother/sister help now that mother is in the hospital?

*Hypothetical Questions:*

If son/daughter were more helpful, what would they do?

From Loos F, Bell J. (1990). Circular questions: A family interviewing strategy. Dimensions of Critical Care Nursing 9(1):49. © Springhouse Corporation.

the nurse should approach the client, family members, and outside agencies. The nurse needs to respect differences in family dynamics as being the best way the family knows how to handle the problem at the time even if objectively this is not true. Exercise 13–6 presents a case study for reflection on family issues.

Taking steps to ensure that communication is direct, open, honest, and congruent sends information accurately to the family and increases the chance that the family will perceive it accurately. The nurse may sometimes intervene most effectively simply by being a role model of an effective communicator. Sometimes the nurse's ability to be outside the family and observe more accurately what goes on makes it easier to transmit information about family communication patterns that family members cannot observe. All family members deserve communication from the health care system that recognizes their importance and worth as individuals. How the nurse communicates to each member may be as important as what he or she chooses to say.

## Encouraging Self-Awareness

Helping each family member become more aware of self and of his or her impact on others in the family is a primary objective. Techniques for doing this include role-playing various positions or situations with some accompanying discussion of what that position feels like and about its continued use in the family.

## Clarification of Rules

The nurse is in the position as an outside observer to observe rules of which the family may not be aware. These rules may have to do with the expression of emotion, a family secret, avoidance of conflict, or maintenance of family equilibrium. However, the strongest rule that inhibits family growth is a rule that it is not all right to be different from the family. Helping the family become aware of its rules, clarifying what it wants the rules to be, and learning to replace implicit (embedded) with explicit (open and clear) communication help the family grow.

## Reframing

*Reframing* or relabeling is a way to look at both positive and negative aspects of a situation or communication. Usually this involves turning a negative perception into a positive one. The process helps people become aware of others' points of view and helps promote member self-esteem. It detours the blaming process and often shakes up the situation just enough for the family to begin trying something different. For example, a mother who criticizes her daughter's grades may be encouraged to reframe her statements to indicate her concern about how grades can affect her daughter's future.

## Giving Corrective Feedback

The nurse who takes the position of an informed observer uses corrective feedback in a neutral way. Role modeling appropriate communication is the first priority in corrective feedback, because even if you are not directly telling the family what you want, family members will be able to infer it from your behavior. Talking to all members, not responding to someone who speaks for another member but addressing that person directly, modeling clear and direct communication, demonstrating techniques for getting feedback, and taking risks to deal openly with negative feelings are all examples of ways the nurse can provide this feedback. Sometimes actual comments such as challenging generalizations ("always" and "never") or assumptions ("you assumed that he knew what you meant?") can be provided in ways that are nonthreatening and eventually perceived by the family as helpful information.

## Terminating with Families

All things come to an end, and so will the nurse's interaction with the family. Whether the interaction has been very brief or whether the nurse has seen the family for a long time, the nurse will want to work toward everyone leaving the encounter with a clear sense of what has happened and with hope that the family's progress will continue into the future.

For families, there are specific issues to consider. If nurses are committed to the value of improving communication skills, they will hope to leave the family with a better sense of how family members communicate and perhaps with more communication skill than they had before interaction with the nurse. The nurse might ask,

◆ Exercise 13-6. **Nursing Process Applied to Family Interactions**

**Purpose:** To practice skills needed with difficult family patterns

**Procedure:**

Read the case study and think of how you could interact appropriately with this family.

Mr. Z., aged 43, was chairing a board meeting of his large, successful manufacturing corporation when he developed shortness of breath, dizziness, and a crushing, viselike pain in his chest. An ambulance was called, and he was taken to the medical center. Subsequently, he was admitted to the coronary care unit with a diagnosis of impending myocardial infarction.

Mr. Z. is married, with three children: Steve, aged 14; Sean, aged 12; and Lisa, aged 8. He is the president and majority stockholder of his company. He had no history of cardiovascular problems, although his father died at the age of 38 of a massive coronary occlusion. His oldest brother died at the age of 42 from the same condition, and his other brother, still living, became a semiinvalid after suffering two heart attacks, one at the age of 44 and the other at 47.

Mr. Z. is tall, slim, suntanned, and very athletic. He swims daily, jogs every morning for 30 minutes, plays golf regularly, and is an avid sailor, having participated in every yacht regatta and usually winning. He is very health conscious and has had annual physical checkups, watches his diet, and quit smoking to avoid possible damage to his heart. He has been determined to avoid dying young or becoming an invalid like his brother.

When he was admitted to the coronary care unit, he was conscious. Although in a great deal of pain, he seemed determined to control his own fate. While in the unit, he was an exceedingly difficult patient, a trial to the nursing staff and his physician. He constantly watched and listened to everything going on around him and demanded complete explanations about any procedure, equipment, or medication he received. He would sleep in brief naps and only when he was totally exhausted. Despite his obvious tension and anxiety, his condition stabilized. The damage to his heart was considered minimal, and his prognosis was good. As the pain diminished, he began asking when he could go home and when he could go back to work. He was impatient to be moved to a private room so that he could conduct some of his business by telephone.

When Mrs. Z. visited, she approached the nursing staff with questions regarding Mr. Z.'s condition, usually asking the same question several times in different ways. She also asked why she was not being ''told everything.''

Interactions between Mr. Z. and Mrs. Z. were noted by the staff as Mr. Z. telling Mrs. Z. a list of things she needed to do. Very little intimate contact was noted.

Mr. Z. denied having any anxiety or concerns about his condition, although his behavior contradicted his denial. Mrs. Z. would agree with Mr. Z. when questioned in his company.

**Discussion:**

1. What questions would you ask the client and family to obtain data regarding their adaptation to crisis?

_____

_____

_____

2. What family nursing diagnosis would apply with this case study?

_____

_____

_____

◆ **Exercise 13-6. Nursing Process Applied to Family Interactions** *Continued*

3. What nursing interventions are appropriate to interact with this client and his family?

_____

_____

4. How would you plan to transmit the information to the family?

_____

_____

_____

Developed by Conrad J. (1993). University of Maryland School of Nursing.

"Did the family members become more aware of their communication styles during our interactions? Did they learn new, more effective ways of relating to each other?"

Leaving the family with a sense of what was accomplished is important and may help family members see progress that was obscure to them. Did we summarize the progress toward goals in such a way that all family members left the encounter with a sense of knowing what had happened and what was gained?"

Family needs may not have been met completely during the nursing encounter. Referrals, continuing the contact with another health professional, or family education about when to contact the health system may be needed. The nurse should ask, "What information needs to go to others about this family or for this family? Did we decide who would communicate this information and when?"

Finally, the nurse needs to assess the personal behaviors that influenced the relationship. Appraising self and using that information to adjust one's communication and interpersonal style can be growth producing for future contacts. The nurse will ask, "What feedback did family members give me about the way I communicated with them? In what ways did this interaction promote the growth and self-esteem of each member, including myself?"

Understanding the principles underlying family communication and learning to use them can be helpful in interactions with families. The nurse who can use open, honest, clear, direct, and congruent communication will be a better communicator, a better nurse, and probably a more effective and satisfied person. Exercise 13–7 provides experience with evaluating nurse–family interactions.

## SUMMARY

Chapter 13 provides an overview of family communication. Family is defined as "a self-identified group of two or more individuals whose association is characterized by special terms, who may or may not be related by bloodlines or law but who function in such a way that they consider themselves to be a family." Families have a structure, defined as the way in which members are organized. Family function refers to the roles people take in their families, and family process describes the communication that takes place within the family. Family frameworks identified in the chapter include Bowen's family systems theory, Duvall's developmental model, and Satir's interactional model. McCubbin's model of family coping is discussed.

The genogram is a primary assessment tool used to help families describe multigenerational transmission of family patterns. North American Nursing Diagnosis Association (NANDA) nursing diagnoses related to family communication and coping form the foundation for nursing interventions. Other assessment tools include a time line and ecomap. Nursing interventions are

---

◆ Exercise 13-7. **Evaluating Nurse–Family Communication**

**Purpose:** To help the nurse evaluate and improve his or her communication with families

**Procedure:**
Set up an interview with a family that has volunteered to help you with this assignment. Ask the family to discuss with you a real-life problem in the family. Be prepared for the session by writing down a goal and some questions to ask the family. Ask the family's cooperation in helping you improve your communication. After the session has been conducted, ask the family members to answer the following questions:

1. Did the interviewer clarify the purpose and time limits of the meeting at the beginning?
2. Did you understand the purpose and what you were supposed to do in the meeting?
3. How did the meeting begin? What was each person doing as the meeting started?
4. Did you feel involved in the discussion? Was anyone left out?
5. Did the interviewer make you feel that what you were saying was important and that he or she valued your opinion?
6. Can you identify any feelings or emotional reactions that occurred during the discussion? How did the interviewer respond to them?
7. Did the interviewer ever ask you to validate or clarify his or her ideas of what was happening?
8. Do you have any suggestions to help this person improve communication with a family group?

---

aimed at strengthening family functioning and may include guiding family change, educating and problem solving during developmental crises, supporting family coping, enlisting the aid of family members in caring for family members, and helping family members coordinate resources. Families with critically ill members need (1) relief of anxiety, (2) information, (3) to be with and helpful to the client, and (4) to alter and adjust to new roles. Circular questioning helps families develop the type of self-awareness they require to meet these four basic needs. Other strategies involve observation, role modeling communication, and support of the family's efforts to cope.

Evaluation may include an estimation of the effectiveness of the nursing care, the quality of the nurse–family interactions, changes in the family's state that may require modification or termination of the care plan, and the family's response to the interventions.

## REFERENCES

Barker P. (1998). Different approaches to family therapy. Nursing Times 94(14):60–62.

Bohlander J. (1995). Differentiation of self: An examination of the concept. Issues in Mental Health Nursing 16(2):165–184.

Bowen M. (1985). Family Therapy in Clinical Practice. Northvale, NJ, Jason Aronson.

Bruner J. (1990). Acts of Meaning. Cambridge, MA, Harvard University Press.

Dunst C, Trivette C, Deal A. (1988). Enabling and Empowering Families. Cambridge, MA, Brookline Books.

Duvall E. (1958). Marriage and Family Development. Philadelphia, JB Lippincott.

Framo JL. (1992). Family of Origin Therapy: An Intergenerational Approach. New York, Bruner/Mazel.

Glasscock F, Hales A. (1998). Bowen's family systems theory: A useful approach for a nurse administrator's practice. Journal of Nursing Administration 28(6):37–42.

Green R, Werner P. (1996). Intrusiveness and Closeness—Caregiving: Rethinking the Concept of Family Enmeshment. Family Process 35(2):115–131.

Hartman A. (1978). Diagrammatic assessment of family relationships. Social Casework 58:465–476.

Hawley D, DeHaan, L. (1996). Toward a definition of family resilience: Integrating life span and family perspectives. Family Process 35:283–298.

Hill R. (1949). Families Under Stress: Adjustment to the Crises of War, Separation and Reunion. New York, Harper & Brothers.

Innes M. (1996). Connecting Bowen theory with its human origins. Family Process 35(4):487–500.

Kerr M, Bowen M. (1988). Family Evaluations. New York, WW Norton.

Loos F, Bell J. (1990). Circular questions: A family interviewing strategy. Dimensions of Critical Care Nursing 9(1):46–53.

Mailick M, Vigilante F. (1997). The family assessment wheel: A social constructionist perspective. Families in Society 361–369.

McBride A. (1976). A Married Feminist. New York, Harper & Row.

McCubbin H, Cauble AE, Patterson J. (1982). Family Stress, Coping, and Social Support. Springfield, IL, Charles C Thomas.

McCubbin, HI, McCubbin MA, Thompson A. (1993). Resiliency in families: The role of family schema and appraisal in family adaptation to crisis. In Brubaker TH (ed.), Family Relations: Challenges for the Future (pp. 153–177). Newbury Park, CA, Sage.

McGoldrick M, Gerson R. (1985). Genogram in Family Assessment. New York, WW Norton.

Minuchin S. (1974). Families and Family Therapy. Boston, Harvard University Press.

Modricin MJ, Robison J. (1991). Parents of children with emotional disorders: Issues for consideration and practice. Community Mental Health Journal 27(4):281–292.

Otto H. (1963). Criteria for assessing family strength. Family Process 2:329–338.

Robinson D, McKenna H. (1998). Loss: An analysis of a concept of particular interest to nursing. Journal of Advanced Nursing 27:779–784.

Satir V. (1976). Making Contact. Millbrae, CA, Celestial Arts.

Satir V, Baumen J, Gerber J, Gomori M. (1991). The Satir Model: Family Therapy and Beyond. Palo Alto, CA: Science & Behavioral Books.

Von Bertalanffy L. (1968). General Systems Theory. New York, George Braziller.

Walsh F. (1996). The concept of family resilience: Crisis and challenge. Family Process 35(3):261–279.

Watzlawick P, Beavin JH, Jackson DD. (1967). Pragmatics of Human Communication. New York, WW Norton.

Whall A. (1990). The family as the unit of care in nursing: A historical review. In Ismeurt R, Arnold E, Carson V (eds.), Readings: Concepts Fundamental to Nursing. Springhouse, PA, Springhouse Corp.

Wright LM, Leahey M. (1984). Nurses and Families: A Guide to Family Assessment and Intervention. Philadelphia, FA Davis.

# 14

# Resolving Conflict Between Nurse and Client

Kathleen Underman Boggs

## OBJECTIVES

At the end of the chapter, the student will be able to

1. Define conflict, and contrast the functional with the dysfunctional role of conflict in a therapeutic relationship
2. Recognize and describe personal style of response to conflict situations
3. Discriminate among passive, assertive, and aggressive responses to conflict situations
4. Specify the characteristics of assertive communication
5. Identify four components of an assertive response and formulate sample assertive responses
6. Identify appropriate assertive responses and specific nursing strategies to promote conflict resolution in relationships

*Creative confrontation is a struggle between persons who are engaged in a dispute or controversy and who remain together, face to face, until acceptance, respect for differences, and love emerge; even though the persons may be at odds with the issue, they are no longer at odds with each other.*

Clark Moustakis (1974)

Conflict is a natural part of human relationships (Baker, 1995). There are times when we experience negative feelings about a situation or person. When this occurs in a nurse–client relationship, clear, direct communication is needed. This chapter emphasizes awareness of the dynamics associated with conflicts and the skills needed for successful resolution.

Knowing how to respond to emotions—personal emotions as well as those of others—allows the nurse to use them as a positive force rather than a negative one. Nurses frequently find themselves in dramatic situations in which a calm, collected response is required. To listen and to respond creatively to intense emotion when the nurse's first impulse is to withdraw or to retaliate demands a high level of skill. It requires self-knowledge, self-control, and empathy for what the client may be experiencing. It is difficult to remain cool under attack, and yet the nurse's willingness to stay with the angry client may mean more than any other response. Nurses need assertive skills to help them deal constructively with conflict (de Torynay, 1990).

## BASIC CONCEPTS
### Definition of Conflict

*Conflict* has been defined as tension arising from incompatible needs, in which the actions of one frustrate the ability of the other to achieve a goal (Valentine, 1995). Conflicts in any relationship are inevitable. They serve as warning that something in the relationship needs closer attention.

### Nature of Conflict

All conflicts have certain things in common: a concrete *content issue* and *process issues*, which involve our emotional response to the situation. It is immaterial whether the issue or associated feelings make realistic sense to the nurse. They feel real to the client and need to be addressed, or they will interfere with success in meeting goals. Most people experience conflict as uncomfortable, disquieting feelings about a person or situation. Previous experiences with conflict situations, the importance of the issue, and possible consequences for the client all play a role in the intensity of our reaction. For example, a client may have great difficulty asking appropriate questions of the physician regarding treatment or prognosis but experience no problem asking similar questions of the nurse or family. The reasons for the discrepancy in comfort level may relate to previous experiences with this physician or with authority figures. Alternatively, it may have little to do with the actual persons involved. Rather, the client may be responding to anticipated fears about the type of information the physician might give.

## Causes of Conflict

Psychological causes of conflict include misunderstanding, poor communication, differences in values or goals, personality clashes, and stress. Clashes occur between nurse and client or even between two clients.

---

◆ **Case Example**

Two women who gave birth this morning are moved to a semiprivate room on the postpartum floor. Ms. A. is 19, likes loud music, and is feeling fine. Her roommate, Mrs. B., is 36, has four children at home and wants to rest as much as possible (latent). The music and visitors to Ms. A. repeatedly wake up Mrs. B. (perceived), who yells at them (overt). The nurse arranges to transfer Mrs. B. to an unoccupied room (resolution).

---

A great deal of literature describes working situation conflicts, which deal with conflicts between nurse and others: managers, peers, physicians, and so on. In Chapter 22, we discuss the nurse's role communicating with other professionals.

## Understanding Personal Style of Response to Conflict

Conflicts do arise between nurse and client. Once identified, it becomes the nurse's responsibility to work to resolve the conflict, or the relationship process will become blocked. Energy is transferred to conflict issues instead of being used to build the relationship. To accomplish conflict resolution, nurses first need to have a clear understanding of their own personal response patterns to conflict. No one is equally effective in all situations.

Completing Exercise 14–1 may help you identify your personal responses.

Most interpersonal conflicts involve some threat to the nurse or client's sense of control or self-esteem. For example, no one likes to be criticized. Negative reactions might include anger, rationalization, or blaming others (Davidhizar, 1991). Examples of situations producing conflict between client and nurse are as follows:

- Being asked to do something you know would be unsafe
- Having the client try to shift responsibility for decision making to you
- Having your statements discounted
- Being asked to give more information than you feel comfortable sharing
- Having your feelings ridiculed
- Being pressured to give more time than you are able
- Encountering sexual harassment
- Being the target of a personal attack
- Wanting to do things the old way instead of trying something new
- Being asked to take on too much or too little responsibility

### Four Styles of Personal Conflict Management

Studies have repeatedly identified several distinct styles of response to conflict. Although not specifically addressing nurse–client conflict, the literature shows that in the past corporate managers felt that any conflict was destructive and needed to be suppressed. Current thinking holds that conflict can be healthy and can lead to growth. Concepts developed by Blake, Morton, Thomas, Rahim, and Bonoma can be applied to nursing (Baker, 1995; Feeney & Davidson, 1996; McElhaney, 1996; Valentine, 1995).

*Avoidance* is a common response to conflict. Sometimes an experience makes you so uncomfortable that you want to avoid the situation or person at all costs, so you withdraw. Studies have shown that females, nurses, people from Asian cultures, and people who tend to take the conflict very personally most often demonstrate this style of reaction to conflict. Many studies of nurses, including that by Cavanagh (1991), show that avoidance is the most often used strategy for managing conflict. This style is appropriate when the other individual is more powerful or the cost of addressing the conflict is higher than the benefit of resolution. Sometimes you just have to "pick your fights," focusing your energy on the most important issues. However, use of avoidance can just postpone the conflict, turning it into a lose-lose situation (McElhaney, 1996).

*Accommodation* is another common response, characterized by a desire to smooth over the conflict. The response is cooperative but nonassertive. Sometimes this involves a quick compromise or giving false reassurance. By giving in or obliging others, the person maintains peace but does not actually deal with the issue, so it will likely resurface in the future (Baker, 1995). It is appropriate when the issue is more important to the other person. "This lose-win situation promotes harmony and gains credits that can be used at a later date" (McElhaney, 1996, p. 49).

*Competition* is the response style characterized by domination. This is a contradictory style in which one party exercises power to gain their own personal goals regardless of the needs of the other. It is characterized by aggression and lack of compromise. Authority may be used to suppress the conflict in a dictatorial manner. This response style was frequently used in the past by corporate managers and leads to increased stress among subordinates (Dallinger & Hample, 1995). It is an effective style when there is a need for a quick decision.

*Collaboration* is a solution-oriented style of response. To manage the conflict, both parties commit to finding a mutually satisfying solution.

◆ Exercise 14–1. **Personal Responses to Conflict**

**Purpose:** To increase awareness of how you respond in conflict situations and the elements in situations—people, status, age, previous experience, lack of experience, place—that contribute to your sense of discomfort

**Procedure:**
Break up into small groups of two or three participants. Think of two conflict situations that you would feel comfortable sharing with the group: one you handled well and the other that you wished you had handled differently. (Variation: This exercise could be done as a homework assignment.)

**Part I:**
The following feelings are common correlates of interpersonal conflict situations that many people say they have experienced in conflict situations they have not handled well:

| | | | |
|---|---|---|---|
| Anger | Defensiveness | Exclusion | Manipulation |
| Annoyance | Deflation | Frustration | Obsequiousness |
| Antagonism | Devaluation | Hostility | Outmaneuvering |
| Anxiousness | Disappointment | Humiliation | Quarrelsomeness |
| Bitterness | Discountedness | Incompleteness | Resentment |
| Caught off guard | Embarrassment | Inferiority | Superiority |
| Competitiveness | Emptiness | Intimidation | Uneasiness |
| Criticism | Exasperation | Intrusion | Vengefulness |

Although these feelings generally are not ones we may be especially proud of, they are a part of the human experience. By acknowledging their existence within ourselves, we usually have more choice about how we will handle them.

Using words from the list to stimulate images of situations you actually have experienced, describe, as concretely as possible, the following:

1. The details of the situation: how did it develop? What were the content issues? Was the conflict expressed verbally or nonverbally? Who were the persons involved, and where did the interaction take place?

2. What you were feelings before experiencing the conflict. Did this situation stir up any images of previous conflictive situations? How would you describe the intensity of your feelings?

3. Why was the situation particularly uncomfortable for you?

1. _____

_____

2. _____

_____

3. _____

_____

**Part II:**
Now think of a conflict situation that you felt you handled well. Using Steps 1, 2, and 3 from Part I, apply the same process to this situation. Be very specific in describing the behaviors you used to cope with this situation.

1. _____

_____

◆ Exercise 14-1. **Personal Responses to Conflict** *Continued*

2. _____

_____

3. _____

_____

**Discussion:**
In what ways were these situations different? How were your responses different in this situation? What were the differences in outcome? What was your level of satisfaction? If you could redo your behaviors in the first interaction, what would you do differently?

Share your experiences with members of your dyad or triad. Note the commonalties of feeling experiences that prevent us from acting assertively when it clearly is in our best interests to do so. Identify behaviors that were different in the more successful conflict situation.

This involves directly confronting the issue, acknowledging the feelings, and using an integrative method to solve the problem. Jones and others (1990) suggested four steps for productive confrontation: (1) identify concerns of each party; (2) clarify assumptions; (3) identify the real issue; (4) work collaboratively to find a solution that satisfies both parties. This is considered to be the most effective style for genuine resolution. McElhaney called this a win-win situation.

## Factors that Influence Responses to Conflict

### Gender

Ample research demonstrates gender differences in managing conflict. Expression of emotion differs between genders (Brooks et al., 1996). Women have been socialized to react in ways that will assuage the other person's anger (Johnson & Arneson, 1991). Studies have shown that women tend to use more accommodative conflict management styles such as compromise and avoidance, whereas men tend to use collaboration more often and to prefer "competitive, unyielding and aggressive strategies" (Valentine, 1995, 144). However, the literature is inconclusive regarding the effects of gender and style on the outcome of conflict resolution.

### Culture

Many of a nurse's responses are determined by cultural socialization, which prescribes proper modes for behaviors. Personal style and past experiences influence the typical responses to conflict situations. Individuals from societies that emphasize group commitment and cooperation tend to use avoidance and less confrontation in their conflict resolution styles. People from cultures that value individualism more tend to more often use competing/dominating styles (Trubisky et al., 1991). Of course, nurses are individuals and have different attitudes toward the existence of conflict and respond to conflict differently, although the underlying feelings generated by conflict situations may be quite similar. Common emotional responses to conflict, listed in Exercise 14–1, include anger, embarrassment, and anxiety. Awareness of how we cope with conflict is the first step in learning assertiveness strategies. Fortunately, assertiveness and other skills essential to conflict resolution are learned behaviors that any nurse can master.

## Assessing the Presence of Conflict in the Nurse–Client Relationship

To foster resolution, the nurse must recognize the presence of conflict. Often awareness of our own feelings of discomfort are an initial clue. Box 14–1 lists the stages of conflict. Evidence of the presence of conflict may be *overt*, that is, observable in the client's behavior and expressed verbally. The conflict issues may be identified, expressed, and allowed to reach resolution so that constructive changes may take place. The relationship progresses and deepens. However, more often, conflict is *covert* and not so clear-cut. The conflict issues are hidden or buried among distracting feelings or tangential issues. The client talks about one issue, but talking does not seem to help, and the issue does not seem to get resolved. The client continues to be angry or anxious. Often the first clue to the existence of a conflict situation occurs when the client or the nurse becomes aware of a generalized sense of personal uneasiness. Frequently, the reasons for this feeling are not clear. In a covert conflict situation, the conflict acts as a hindrance to the progress of the relationship and the ultimate treatment goals. The conflict usually cannot be resolved until the issues can be revealed and explored.

Subtle behavioral manifestations of *covert conflict* might include the following: a reduced effort by the client to engage in the process of self-care; frequent misinterpretation of the nurse's words; behaviors that are out of character for the client; and excessive anger or undue praise for the nurse. For example, when the client seems unusually demanding, has a seemingly insatiable need for the nurse's attention, or is unable to tolerate reasonable delays in having needs met, the problem may be anxiety stemming from conflictive feelings.

It is important for the nurse to realize that intellectually clients may want to change, but emotionally the troublesome behavior may seem integral to the self. Clients must feel that it is in their best interests emotionally to change behaviors, and they must be able to feel that such change is also the goal of the nurse. As nurses, we affect the behavior of our clients in positive or negative ways through our actions. See Exercise 14–2 for practice in defining conflict issues.

Sometimes the feelings themselves become the major issue, so that valid parts of the original conflict issue are obscured. There is complete focus only on the feelings. The context issue is discounted or denied. These feelings can become a major obstacle and conflict can escalate. At best, confusing feelings with the issue clouds communication and makes it more difficult to respond appropriately. Usually conflictive feelings have to be put into words and related to the issue at hand before the client can understand the meaning of the conflict. Consider yourself as the nurse in the following situation.

### ◆ Case Example

Mr. J. is scheduled for surgery at 8 A.M. tomorrow. As the student nurse assigned to care for him, you have been told that he was admitted to the hospital 3 hours ago, and he has been examined by the house resident. The anesthesia department has been notified of the client's arrival. His blood work and urine have been sent to the laboratory. As you enter his room and introduce yourself, you notice that Mr. J. is sitting on the edge of his bed and appears tense and angry.

**Client:** I wish people would just leave me alone. Nobody has come in and told me about my surgery tomorrow. I don't know what I'm supposed to do, just lay around here and rot, I guess.

At this point, you probably can sense the presence of conflictive feelings, but it is unclear whether the emotions being expressed relate to anxiety over the surgery or to anger over some real or imagined invasion of privacy because of the necessary lab tests and physical exam. The client might also be annoyed by you or by a lack of information from his surgeon. He may feel

---

### ◆ Box 14-1. Stages of Conflict

1. Latent conflict, in which disparities exist
2. Perceived conflict, in which disparities are recognized
3. Felt conflict, in which feelings (such as anger) erupt
4. Overt conflict, in which feelings are acted out in observed behaviors
5. Resolution, in which the outcome is known to all participants

From Booth R. (1985). Conflict and conflict management. In Mason DJ, Talbot SW (eds.), Political Action Handbook for Nurses. Menlo Park, CA, Addison-Wesley. Used with permission.

◆ Exercise 14–2. **Defining Conflict Issues**

**Purpose:**　To help students begin to organize information and identify problem definitions in interpersonal conflict situations; in every conflict situation, it is important to look for the specific behaviors (including words, tone, posture, facial expression), feeling impressions (including words, tone, intensity, facial expression), and need (expressed verbally or through actions)

**Procedure:**
Three situations follow. Situation 1 is completed as a guide. In Situations 2 and 3, identify the behaviors, feeling impressions, and needs that the client is expressing and suggest a nursing action.

**Situation 1:**
Mrs. A., an Indian client, does not speak much English. Her baby was just delivered by cesarean section, and it is expected that Mrs. A. will remain in the hospital for at least 4 days. Her husband tells the nurse that Mrs. A. wants to breast-feed, but she has decided to wait until she goes home to begin because she will be more comfortable there and she wants privacy. The nurse knows that breast-feeding will be more successful if it is initiated soon after birth.

**Behaviors**
The client's husband states she wants to breast-feed but does not wish to start before going home. Mrs. A. is not initiating breast-feeding in the hospital.

**Nursing Inference:**
Assess meaning of behaviors: indirectly the client is expressing physical discomfort, possible insecurity, and awkwardness about breast-feeding. She may also be acting in accordance with cultural norms of her country or family.
　　Assess underlying needs: safety and security. Mrs. A. probably will not be motivated to attempt breast-feeding until she feels safe and secure in her home environment.
　　Suggested nursing action: Provide family support and guarantee total privacy for feeding.

**Situation 2:**
Mrs. S. is returned to the unit from surgery after a radical mastectomy. The doctor's orders call for her to ambulate, cough, and deep breathe and to use her arm as much as possible in self-care activities. Mrs. S. asks the nurse in a very annoyed tone, ''Why do I have to do this? You can see that it is difficult for me. Why can't you help me?''

Behaviors:

_____

_____

_____

Nursing inference:

Assess meaning of behavior.

_____

_____

_____

*Exercise continued on following page*

◆ **Exercise 14–2. Defining Conflict Issues** *Continued*

Assess underlying needs. _____

_____

_____

Suggested nursing action. _____

**Situation 3:**

Mr. C. is a 31-year-old client who was recently diagnosed with terminal cancer of the pancreas. He answers the nurse's questions with monosyllables and turns his head away. When the nurse questions him, he says in a low voice: ''There is no hope. They're going to keep me here until I die. Can't you give me my medication more often than every 3 hours? I'm going to die anyway.''

Behaviors:

_____

_____

_____

Nursing inference:

Assess meaning of behavior. _____

_____

_____

Assess underlying needs. _____

_____

_____

Suggested nursing action. _____

_____

the need to know that hospital personnel see him as a person and care about his feelings. Before the nurse can respond empathetically to the client's feelings, his feelings will have to be decoded.

---

**Nurse** (in a concerned tone of voice): You seem really upset. It's rough being in the hospital, isn't it?

---

Notice that the nurse's reply is nonevaluative and tentative. The nurse does not suggest specific feelings beyond those the client has shared. There is an implicit request for the client to

validate the nurse's perception of his feelings and to link the feelings with concrete issues. Verbal as well as nonverbal cues are included in the nurse's reply. Concern is expressed through the nurse's tone of voice and words. The content focus relates to the client's predominant feeling tone, because this is the part of the conflict the client has chosen to share with the nurse. It is important for the nurse to maintain a nonanxious presence. The nurse recognizes that client resistance can be a way to maintain personal stability, even though it may appear counterproductive to the relationship.

## Types of Conflict: Intrapersonal Versus Interpersonal

A conflict can be internal or intrapersonal; that is, it can represent opposing feelings within an individual. Alternatively, the conflict may be interpersonal, occurring between two or more people.

### Escalation of Intrapersonal and Interpersonal Conflict

Depending on the type of feedback received, an intrapersonal conflict can take on interpersonal dimensions. In the case presented next, the mother initially experiences an intrapersonal conflict. The wished-for perfect infant has not happened, and her personal ambivalence related to coping with her infant's defect is expressed indirectly through her partial noncompliant behavior. If the nurse interprets the client's behavior incorrectly as poor mothering and acts in a manner that reflects this attitude, the basically intrapersonal conflict can become interpersonal.

---

### ◆ Case Example

A mother with her first infant is informed soon after delivery that her child has a small cleft palate. The physician explains the infant's condition in detail and answers the mother's questions. The mother requests rooming in and seems genuinely interested in the infant. Each time the nurse enters the client's room, the mother complains that her child does not seem hungry and states how difficult it is to feed the baby. Although the nurse spends a great deal of time with them teaching the mother the special techniques necessary for feeding, and the mother seems interested at the time, she seems unable or unwilling to follow any of the nurse's suggestions when she is by herself. Later, the nurse finds out that the mother has been asking her roommate to feed her infant.

---

This client appears to be asking for guidance and to be resisting what is offered. Although she may simply need further instruction in technique, the presence of an underlying intrapersonal conflict is worth investigating. Before proceeding with teaching, the nurse needs to find out about the mother's perceptions. Does she feel competent in the mothering role? What does having a less than perfect child mean to her?

What are her fears about caring for an infant with this particular type of defect? Until the underlying feelings are identified, client teaching is likely to have limited success.

Seeking to understand the meaning of a conflict to a client from his or her perspective reframes the experience. In this situation, a client strength would be the mother's ability and willingness to express her uncomfortable feelings so that they can be addressed. Even though the mother may be unclear about the nature of her feelings, reframing the issues in this way builds on strengths instead of personal deficits. It is hoped that the client provides more specific input about her fears and the nurse provides acceptance of the client's right to have all types of feelings. Together they seek a solution.

### Interpersonal Sources of Conflict

When the source of conflict is interpersonal, the nurse needs to think through the possible causes of the conflict as well as his or her own feelings about it and respond appropriately, even if the response is a deliberate choice not to respond verbally. Interpersonal conflicts usually leave residual feelings that reappear unexpectedly and affect the nurse's ability to respond realistically and responsibly in future interactions.

## Functional Uses of Conflict

Traditionally, conflict was viewed as a destructive force to be eliminated (Booth, 1985). Current thinking holds that conflict can serve either a functional or a dysfunctional role in relationships. In fact, conflict is thought to be an inevitable part of today's changing health care environment (Jones et al., 1990; Porter, 1996). The critical factor is the willingness to explore and resolve it mutually. Appropriately handled, conflict can provide an important opportunity for growth. Box 14–2 gives helpful guidelines regarding your responsibilities when involved in a conflict, and Exercise 14–3 provides practice in using them.

## Dysfunctional Conflict

Several identifiable elements may occur in *dysfunctional conflict*: information is withheld; feelings are expressed too strongly; the conflict is obscured by a double message; feelings are de-

---

◆ Box 14-2. Personal Rights and Responsibilities in Conflict Situations

I have the right to respect from other people as a unique human being.

I have the responsibility to respect the human rights of others.

I have the right to make my own decisions.

I have the responsibility to allow others to make their own decisions.

I have the right to have feelings.

I have the responsibility to express those feelings in ways that do not violate the rights of others.

I have the right to make mistakes.

I have the responsibility to accept full accountability for my mistakes.

I have the right to decide how I will act.

I have the responsibility to act in ways that will not be harmful to myself or to others.

I have the right to my own opinions.

I have the responsibility to respect the rights of others to hold opinions different from mine.

---

distort the content issue. For example, some information is withheld so one of the participants must guess at what is truly going on in the mind of the other participant in the interaction.

In other dysfunctional conflicts, the feelings are stated accurately, but they are expressed so strongly that the listener feels attacked. The listener then tends to respond in a defensive manner. Consequently, the relationship is damaged. In dysfunctional communication, the outcomes provide little sense of satisfaction or accomplishment.

## Behavioral Responses Used to Resolve Conflict

The importance of knowing your own personal responses to conflict has been discussed. The next step in conflict resolution is to clearly identify the conflict issues. Then separate out the emotional feelings associated with the conflict. Of the four conflict management responses described earlier, the most satisfactory is collaboration using integrative problem-solving skills. This process is mutually entered into by both parties with the expectation of a win-win outcome. The issues of each are identified and their feelings acknowledged. Solutions are discussed, and the best one is used to resolve the conflict (Feeney & Davidson, 1996). Skills needed to participate in this problem-solving process are confrontation, active listening, and appropriate *assertive behavior*.

nied or projected onto others; conflicts are not resolved, so issues build up.

Nonproductive conflicts are characterized by feelings that are misperceived or stated too intensely. The problem occurs when the emotions

---

◆ Exercise 14-3. **Behavioral Responses to Interpersonal Conflict**

**Purpose:**  To help students experience the feelings associated with responses to conflict

**Situation:**
A newly employed staff nurse is routinely assigned to care for the most critically ill clients, yet her workload is the same as that of other nurses on the floor. In her 2-month evaluation conference with her manager, the nurse receives less than satisfactory ratings on ''ability to complete work on time.''

**Procedure:**
Choose a partner. Using the behaviors suggested in Box 14-2, take turns role-playing a response. Pause between response positions to reflect on the feelings generated by being in that position. After each person has had a turn, the class should discuss the common feelings: what your body felt like, which communication position felt most comfortable, and why.

**Discussion:**  Take 5 minutes to share results with the class.

## Nature of Assertive Behavior

*Assertive behavior* is defined as setting goals, acting on those goals in a clear and consistent manner, and taking responsibility for the consequences of those actions. The assertive nurse is able to stand up for the rights of others as well as for his or her own rights. Box 14–3 lists the characteristics of assertive behaviors. Four components identified by Lazarus are the ability to (1) say no, (2) ask for favors, (3) appropriately express both positive and negative thoughts and feelings, and (4) initiate, continue, and terminate the interaction. This honest expression of yourself does not violate the needs of others but does demonstrate self-respect rather than deference to the demands of others.

According to Angel and Petronko (1987), the two goals of assertiveness are to (1) stand up for your personal rights without infringing on the rights of others and (2) reduce anxiety, which often prevents us from behaving assertively. Assertive behaviors range from making a simple, direct, and honest statement about one's beliefs to taking a very strong, confrontational stand about what will and will not be tolerated in the relationship. Assertive responses contain *"I"*

*statements* that take responsibility. This behavior is in contrast to *aggressive behavior*, which has a goal of dominating while suppressing the other person's rights. Aggressive responses often consist of "you" statements that fix blame and undue responsibility on the other person.

Assertiveness is a learned behavior. Many nurses, especially women, have been socialized to act passively. Passive behavior is defined as a response that denies our own rights to avoid conflict. An example is remaining silent and not responding to a client's demands for narcotics every 4 hours when he displays no signs of pain out of fear that he might report you to his physician. Passivity can be evidenced by the acceptance of a negative, unfair comment without any further discussion of the impact the comment had on you.

Assertiveness needs to be practiced to be learned (Exercises 14–4 to 14–8). Effective nursing encompasses the mastery of assertive behavior (see Box 14–3). Studies show that nonassertive behavior in a professional nurse is related to lower levels of autonomy (Schutzenhofer, 1992). Continued patterns of nonassertive responses have adverse psychological effects on the nurse and a negative influence on the standard of care the nurse delivers (McCanton & Hargie, 1990). Evaluate your own assertiveness with Exercises 14–6 and 14–7.

## APPLICATIONS

## Nursing Strategies to Enhance Conflict Resolution

Strategies that have been found to be useful in conflict resolution are described here. Successful use of these strategies varies with the skill level of the participants and the nature of the situation. Mastery takes practice.

### Prepare for the Encounter

Careful preparation often makes the difference between being successful and failing to assert yourself when necessary. In discussing assertive communication, Flanagan (1990, p. 49) noted that for communication to be effective it must be carefully thought out in terms of certain basic questions:

- Purpose: what is the purpose or objective of

---

> ◆ Box 14–3. Characteristics Associated with the Development of Assertive Behaviors

- Use strategies that respect the rights of self and others.
- Express your own position, using "I" statements.
- Make clear statements.
- Speak in a firm tone, using moderate pitch.
- Assume responsibility for personal feelings and wants.
- Make sure verbal and nonverbal messages are congruent.
- Address only issues related to the present conflict.
- Structure responses to be tactful and show awareness of the client's frame of reference.
- Understand that undesired behaviors, not feelings, attitudes, and motivations, are the focus for change.

◆ Exercise 14–4. **Responding Assertively**

**Purpose:** To help you define your position in a conflict situation in an assertive manner

**Procedure:**
Think of three interpersonal situations in which you wished you had acted more assertively. What behaviors would you alter? For each of these situations, specify how you would relate in an assertive manner. (Example: Your employer schedules you to work overtime or your teacher incorrectly gives you a lower grade than you believe you earned. Sample response: I would tell my boss that I had exams at school and I wasn't going to be able to continue to work every weekend.)

1. _____

2. _____

3. _____

If you are like most people, you find it difficult to express yourself clearly about your position in conflict situations. Sometimes you may not recognize that you are involved in a conflict situation until the situation is well under way.

**Discussion:**
1. What were some of the variables that made it difficult for you to express yourself assertively?
2. As you listen to other students' responses, what common themes emerge?
3. How could you use this information in your professional responses to conflict?

this information? What is the central idea, the one most important statement to be made?
- Organization: what are the major points to be shared and in what order?
- Content: is the information to be shared complete? Does it convey who, what, where, when, why, and how?

- Word choice: has careful consideration been given to the choice of words?

If you wish to be successful, you must consider not only what is important to you in the discussion but also what is important to the other person. Bear in mind the other person's frame of

◆ Exercise 14–5. **Pitching the Assertive Message**

**Procedure:**
List the five vocal pitches commonly used in conversation: whisper, soft tone with hesitant delivery, moderate tone and firm delivery, loud tone with agitated delivery, screaming. Place enough individual slips of paper in a hat so that every student in class can draw one. Divide into groups, and have each student take a turn drawing and demonstrating the tone while the others in the group try to identify correctly which person is giving the assertive message.

**Discussion:** How does tone affect perceptions of a message's content? (This exercise was contributed by Saretha Boggs.)

◆ Exercise 14–6. **Assertiveness Self-Assessment Quiz**

**Purpose:** To help students gain insight into own responses

**Procedure:**
Read and answer *yes, no,* or *sometimes.* A score of 10 or more items without a *no* answer suggests the need to practice assertiveness.

Do you

1. Feel self-conscious if someone watches you work with a client?
2. Feel confident in your nursing judgment?
3. Hesitate to express your feelings?
4. Avoid problems rather than try to solve them?
5. Hesitate to call a physician about a client problem?
6. Avoid questioning people in authority?
7. Swear at others?
8. Feel uncomfortable speaking up in class?
9. Ever say ``I hate to bother you . . .''?
10. Feel people take advantage of you at work?
11. Ever turn down a classmate who asks you to do his or her work?
12. Complain to your friends rather than to the person with whom you have a problem?
13. Avoid protesting an unfair grade or evaluation?
14. Have trouble starting a conversation?

◆ Exercise 14–7. **Assertive Responses**

**Purpose:** To increase awareness of assertiveness

**Procedure:**
Have four students volunteer to read each answer to the following scenario:
   You are working full time, raising a family, and taking 12 credits of nursing classes. The teacher asks you to be a student representative on a faculty committee. You say

a. I don't think I'm the best one. Why don't you ask Karen? If she can't, I guess I can.
b. Gee, I'd like to but I don't know. I probably could if it doesn't take too much time.
c. I do want students to have some input to this committee, but I am not sure I have enough time. Let me think about it and let you know in class tomorrow.
d. I have worked myself to death for this school. Everyone always expects me to do everything. Let someone else work for a change!

**Discussion:**
Ask students to choose the most assertive answer and comment about how other options could be altered.

---

◆ Exercise 14–8. **Staff-Focused Consultation**

**Purpose:** To pool ideas for resolving conflict and providing consistent care

**Procedure:**
Read the case study about Mr. P. (page 343) and identify four strategies based on this staff-focused consultation.

1. _____

2. _____

3. _____

4. _____

**Analysis of Effective Staff-Level Interventions:**
In this case study, once the manager became aware of the difficulty the staff was having coping with Mr. P., strategies to help staff included the following:

Arranging a group meeting of caregivers who were responsible for the client

Using a consultant

Ventilating feelings, with a focus on their own reactions and feelings, not on complaints about the client's behavior

Elevating awareness of their own feelings of anger and other emotions, showing that these are common reactions exhibited by several nurses in the group

Developing increased awareness among staff of the cause of the client's unacceptable behavior

Developing a plan for handling the client's unacceptable behavior, perhaps behavior modification strategies

Obtaining consensus (for all shifts to use)

Committing the plan to writing

---

reference when acting assertively. The following clinical example illustrates this idea.

◆ **Case Example**

Mr. R. is an 80-year-old bachelor who lives alone. He has always been considered a proud and stately gentleman. He has a sister, 84 years old, who lives in Florida. His only other living relatives, a nephew and his wife, also live in another state. He recently changed his will, excluding his relatives, and he refuses to eat. When his neighbor brings in food he eats it, but he won't fix anything for himself. He tells his neighbor that he wants to die and that he read in the paper about a man who was able to die in 60 days by not eating. As the visiting nurse assigned to his area, you have been asked to make a home visit and assess the situation.

The issue in this case example is not one of food intake alone. The nurse's attempts to talk about why it is important for the client to eat or to express a point of view in this conflict immediately on arriving is not likely to be successful. The client's behavior suggests that he feels there is little to be gained by living any longer. His actions suggest further that he feels lonely and may be angry with his relatives. Once you correctly ascertain his needs and identify the specific issues, you may be able to help Mr. R. resolve his intrapersonal conflict. His wish to die may not be absolute or final because he eats when food is prepared by his neighbor, and he has not yet taken a deliberate, aggressive move to end his life. Each of these factors needs to be assessed and validated with the client before an accurate nursing diagnosis can be made.

### Organize Information

Organizing your information and validating the appropriateness of your intervention with another knowledgeable person who is not directly

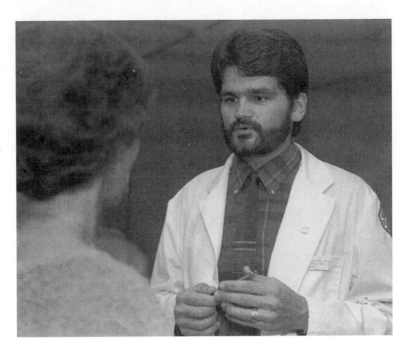

Reaching a common understanding of the problem in a direct, tactful manner is the first step in conflict resolution. (Courtesy University of North Carolina at Charlotte College of Nursing)

involved in the process is useful. Sometimes it is wise to rehearse out loud what you are going to say.

## Manage Own Anxiety

If you experience stage fright before engaging in a conflict situation that calls for an assertive response, know that you are in good company. Most people experience some variation of a physical response when taking interpersonal risks. Before you actually enter the client's room, take a few deep breaths. Inhale deeply and count 1–2–3 to yourself. Hold your breath for a count of two and exhale, counting again to four slowly. Fortify yourself with positive statements (e.g., "I have a right to respect"). Usually anticipation is far worse than the reality.

## Time the Encounter

Timing can be critical in responding assertively to a conflict situation. Conflictive situations lead to varying degrees of energy depletion. Once fatigue sets in, the value of any assertive behavior on your part may be diminished. Select a time when the client or colleague is most likely to be receptive.

You might accompany your assertive state-

ment with comfort measures, such as arranging the table attractively. Nonverbal support of verbal statements adds strength to the meaning of the communication.

Timing is also important if an individual is very angry. The key to assertive behavior is choice. Sometimes it is better to allow ventilation of some "emotional steam" before engaging in conversation. In this case, the assertive thing to do is to choose silence accompanied by a calm, relaxed body posture and eye contact. These nonverbal actions convey acceptance of feeling and a desire to understand. Validating the anger and reframing the emotion as adaptive is useful. Comments such as "I'm sorry you are feeling so upset" recognize the significance of the emotion being expressed without enlarging the frame of reference beyond what is being expressed.

## Use Clear, Congruent Communication

Choose direct declarative sentences. Use objective words, directly state your wants, and honestly convey your emotions. Make sure verbal and nonverbal communication is congruent. Avoid mixed messages. For example, Larry is a staff nurse who works the 11–7 shift, and he needs to get home to make sure his children get on the bus to school. The day shift nurse is consistently late receiving his report. He uses a soft voice and smiles as he tells her he would like to begin the report. Another example is Mr. C., the 29-year-old client in room 122 who constantly makes sexual comments to a young student nurse. She laughs as she tells him to cut it out.

## Take One Issue at a Time

It is best to start by focusing on the original issue, although Fritchie (1995) and others suggested that you may need to first focus on the feelings associated with the conflict, because it is these that generally escalate conflict. It is always best to start with one issue at a time. Focus on the present issue, because the past cannot be changed. Limiting your discussion to one topic issue at a time enhances the chance of success. It usually is impossible to resolve a conflict that is multidimensional in nature with one solution. By breaking the problem down into simple steps, automatic responses are avoided, and enough time is allowed for a clear understanding. In the case example just given, the nurse might paraphrase the client's words, reflecting the meaning back to the client to validate accuracy. Once the issues have been delineated clearly, the steps needed for resolution may appear quite simple. As one issue is resolved, others may disappear of their own accord or assume a different perspective. At the very least, a sense of mutuality develops because both parties become actively involved in the process of resolving the conflict, and the client is assured of the nurse's interest. At times, however, the conflict is such that a behavioral change is needed before the conflict can be fully resolved.

## Make a Request for a Behavior Change

Asking someone for a needed behavior change is handled best when the request takes into consideration the person's developmental stage, cultural and value orientation, and other life factors likely to be affected by the change. The person's level of readiness to explore alternative options also needs to be considered. Additionally, for an ill client, level of self-care as well as outside support systems are factors. To approach the task without this information is risky and haphazard.

There obviously will be situations in which such a thorough assessment is not possible, but each of these variables affects the success of the confrontation. For example, a client with dementia who makes a pass at a nurse may simply be expressing a need for affection in much the same way that a small child does; this behavior needs a loving touch rather than a reprimand. A 30-year-old client with all his cognitive faculties who makes a similar pass needs a more confrontational response.

Often what appears to be an inappropriate response in our culture is a highly acceptable way of interacting in a different culture. For example, some clients experience conflict related to taking pain medication. In the cultures of these clients, pain is supposed to be endured with a stoicism that is incompatible with reality. It is often necessary to help such clients express their discomfort when it occurs and to give them guidelines as well as explicit permission to develop a different behavior. It is easier for the client to take such medication when he can assure the family that the nurse said he needed to take it. By focusing on the behavior required to meet the client's physical needs, the nurse bypasses placing a value on the rightness or wrongness of the behavior. Refer to other chapters for a more detailed discussion of cultural differences that can create conflict.

Client readiness is vital. The behavior may need to be confronted, but the manner in which the confrontation is approached and the amount of preparation or groundwork that has been done beforehand is a determinant of success. Know specifically the behavior you wish to have the client change. Make sure that the client is capable physically and emotionally of changing the behavior.

## Evaluate the Conflict Resolution

Evaluation of the degree to which an interpersonal conflict has been resolved depends somewhat on the nature of the conflict. Sometimes a conflict cannot be resolved in a short period of time, but the willingness to persevere is a good indicator of a potentially successful outcome. Accepting small goals is useful when large goal attainment is not possible. The ideal interactive process is one in which a climate of openness and trust leads to an increase in communication in the form of feedback and increased problem solving (Jones et al., 1990).

For a client, perhaps the strongest indicator of conflict resolution is the degree to which he or she is actively engaged in activities aimed at accomplishing tasks associated with treatment goals. Two questions you as the nurse might want to address if modifications are necessary are

1. What is the best way to establish an environment that is conducive to conflict resolution? What else needs to be considered?
2. What self-care behaviors can be expected of the client if these changes are made? They need to be stated in ways that are measurable.

Both the nurse and the client benefit from conflict resolution. The nurse gains because successful resolution permits movement toward treatment goals and increases confidence and self-esteem. The client achieves a clearer understanding of the actions needed to resolve conflicts as well as an opportunity to explore alternative solutions for coping with difficult situations.

## Defusing Intrapersonal Conflict

Intrapersonal conflicts develop out of ambivalent or opposing feelings within an individual. The client with a myocardial infarction who insists on conducting business from the bedside probably feels conflicted about the restraints placed on his or her activities, as does the diabetic client who sneaks off to the food vending machine for a hamburger.

There are times when the conflictive feelings also begin intrapersonally within the nurse (e.g., in working with parents of an abused child or treating a foul-mouthed alcoholic client in the emergency room). Such situations often stir up strong feelings of anger or resentment. When the conflict is judged to be intrapersonal in nature, nurses may need to help themselves defuse destructive emotions before proceeding further. The following are interventions the nurse can use to defuse interpersonal conflict in a potentially destructive interaction:

1. Identify the presence of an emotionally tense situation.

2. Talk the situation through with someone.
3. Provide a neutral, accepting environment.
4. Take appropriate action to reduce tension.
5. Evaluate the effectiveness of the strategies.
6. Generalize behavioral approaches to other situations.

For the nurse, the first step in coping with difficult emotional responses is to recognize their presence and to assess the appropriateness of expressing emotion in the situation. If expressing the emotion does not fit the circumstances, one must deliberately remain unruffled when every natural instinct argues against it. Ambivalence, described as two opposing ideas or feelings related to any life situation or relationship coexisting within the same individual, is a relatively common phenomenon.

It is not the responsibility of the nurse to help a client resolve all intrapersonal conflict. Deal only with those that occur within the context of the immediate clinical situation and threaten to sabotage the goals of the therapeutic relationship. Long-standing conflicts require more expertise to resolve. In such cases, the nurse identifies the presence of possible conflict, refers the client to the appropriate resource, communicates with the personnel chosen, and supports the client's participation.

### Identify Potential Conflict Situations

The initial interpersonal strategy used to help clients reduce strong emotion to a workable level is to provide a neutral, accepting interpersonal environment. Within this context, the nurse can acknowledge the client's emotion as a necessary component of adaptation to life. The nurse conveys acceptance of the individual's legitimate right to have any feeling. Telling a client "I'm not surprised that you are angry about . . ." or simply stating "I'm sorry you are hurting so much" acknowledges the presence of an uncomfortable emotion in the client, conveys an attitude of acceptance, and encourages the client to express the feeling and the circumstances generating the emotion. Once a feeling can be put into words, it becomes manageable because it has concrete boundaries.

### Talk About It

The second step in defusing the strength of an emotion is to talk the emotion through with someone. For the client, this someone is often the nurse. For the nurse, this might be a nursing supervisor or a trusted colleague. Unlike complaining, the purpose of talking the emotion through is to help the person connect with all of his or her personal feelings surrounding the incident. If one client seems to produce certain negative emotional reactions on a nursing unit, the emotional responses may need the direct attention of all staff on the unit.

### Use Tension-Reducing Actions

The third phase is to take action. The specific needs expressed by the emotion suggest actions that might help the client come to terms with the consequences of the emotion. This responsibility might take the form of obtaining more information or of taking some concrete risks to change behaviors that sabotage the goals of the relationship. Convey mutual respect, and avoid any "putdown" type of comment about yourself or the client.

Sometimes the most effective action is simply to listen. Active listening in a conflict situation involves concentrating on what the other person is upset about. Listening can be so powerful that it alone may reduce the client's feelings of anxiety and frustration (Shearer & Davidson, 1997).

In psychiatric settings, taking a walk, going to the gym to use the punching bag, taking a warm bath, and writing are neutralizing interventions the nurse can suggest to control a client's initial anxiety behaviors. Stepping in before the client's behaviors escalate to the point at which they are no longer under the client's conscious control can defuse an emotionally tense situation. If the client is so consumed by emotion that he or she constitutes a danger to himself or others and talking is futile, the nurse should allow a significant amount of physical space and face the client but avoid backing the client into a corner. The nurse should speak in a low, calm tone to the client and move slowly to the nurses' station. Many hospitals and psychiatric units have a "code blue" that is used to summon trained help.

### Evaluate

The final step in the process is to evaluate the effectiveness of responses to emotions and to generalize the experience of confronting difficult emotions to other situations. Each step in the process may need to be taken more than once and refined or revised as circumstances dictate.

## Developing Assertive Skills

### Demonstrate Respect

Responsible assertive statements are made in ways that do not violate the rights of others or diminish their standing. They are conveyed by a relaxed, attentive posture and a calm, friendly tone of voice. Statements should be accompanied by the use of appropriate eye contact.

### Use "I" Statements

Assertive or self-expressive statements that begin with "I" suggest that the person making the statement accepts full personal responsibility for his or her own feelings and position in relation to the presence of conflict. It is not necessary to justify your position unless the added message clarifies or adds essential information (Smythe, 1990).

Statements that begin with "You" sound accusatory and always represent an assumption because it is impossible to know exactly, without validation, why someone acts in a certain way. Because such statements usually point a finger and imply a judgment, most people respond defensively to them.

"We" statements should be used only when you actually mean to look at an issue collaboratively. Thus, the statement "Perhaps we both need to look at this issue a little closer" may be appropriate in certain situations. However, the statement "Perhaps we shouldn't get so angry when things don't work out the way we think they should" is a condescending statement, thinly disguised as a collaborative statement. What is actually being expressed is the expectation that both parties should handle the conflict in one way: my way.

### Make Clear Statements

Statements, rather than questions, set the stage for assertive responses to conflict. When questions are used, "how" questions are best because they are neutral in nature, they seek more information, and they imply a collaborative effort. "Why" questions ask for an explanation or an evaluation of behavior and often put the other person on the defensive. It is always important to state the situation clearly, describe events or expectations objectively, and use a strong, firm, yet tactful manner. The following case example shows how a nurse can use the three levels of assertive behaviors to meet the client's needs in a hospital situation without compromising his or her own needs for respect and dignity.

### ◆ Case Example

Mr. G. is a 35-year-old executive who has been hospitalized with a myocardial infarction. He has been acting seductively toward some of the young nurses, but he seems to be giving Miss O. an especially hard time.

**Client:** Come on in, honey, I've been waiting for you.

**Nurse** (using appropriate facial expression and eye contact and replying in a firm, clear voice): Mr. G., I would rather you called me Miss O'Hara.

**Client:** Aw, come on now, honey. I don't get to have much fun around here. What's the difference what I call you?

**Nurse:** I feel that it does make a difference, and I would like you to call me Miss O'Hara.

**Client:** Oh, you're no fun at all. Why do you have to be so serious?

**Nurse:** Mr. G., you're right. I am serious about some things, and being called by my name and title is one of them. I would prefer that you call me Miss O'Hara. I would like to work with you, however, and it might be important to explore the ways in which this hospitalization is hampering your natural desire to have fun.

In this interaction, the nurse's position is defined several times using successively stronger statements before the shift can be made to refocus on underlying client needs. Notice that even in the final encounter, however, the nurse labels the behavior, not the client, as unacceptable. Persistence is an essential feature when first attempts at assertiveness appear too limited. After a careful appraisal of an interpersonal encounter, if you find that a client's behavior is infringing on your rights as a human being, it is not only desirable but also essential that the issues be addressed directly in a tactful manner. If you do not, it is quite likely that the undesirable behavior will continue until you are no longer willing to tolerate it.

### Use Proper Pitch and Tone

The amount of force used in delivery of an assertive statement depends on the nature of the conflict situation as well as on the amount of confrontation needed to resolve the conflict successfully. Starting with the least amount of assertiveness required to meet the demands of the situation conserves energy and does not place the nurse into the bind of overkill. It is not necessary to use all of one's resources at one time or to express ideas strongly when this type of response is not needed. You can sometimes lose your effectiveness by becoming long winded in your explanation when only a simple statement of rights or intent is needed. Long explanations detract from the true impact of the spoken message. Getting to the main point quickly and saying what is necessary in the simplest, most concrete way cuts down on the possibility of misinterpretation. This approach increases the probability that the communication will be constructively received.

Pitch and tone of voice contribute to another person's interpretation of the meaning of your assertive message. A soft, hesitant, passive presentation can undermine an assertive message as much as vocalizing the message in a harsh, hostile, and aggressive tone. A firm but moderate presentation often is as effective as content in conveying the message (see Exercise 14–6).

### Analyze Personal Feelings

At the other end of the spectrum are behaviors that cause conflictive feelings. For example, clients may have opinions about such issues as abortion, parenting techniques, and homosexuality that differ markedly from those of the nurse. The client has the right to hold such opinions, even if the nurse cannot agree with them philosophically.

Part of an initial assessment of the nature of an interpersonal conflict situation includes a differentiation of the nurse's intrapersonal contribution to the conflict from that of the client's. It is not wrong for nurses to have ambivalent feelings about taking care of clients with different lifestyles and values. However, the nurse needs to acknowledge this. In the prior case example, if the nurse seemed unsure in her choice of words, it is almost predictable that Mr. G. would have continued to show disrespect to the nurse, and the conflict would not have been addressed.

### Focus on the Present

The focus of assertive responses should always be on the present. Because it is impossible to do anything about the past except learn from it, and the future is never completely predictable, the present is the only reality in which we have much decision-making power as to how we shall act.

To be classified as assertive, the behavior must reflect deliberate choice. It is not always necessary to use words to be assertive. Sometimes it is better to listen quietly to what someone has to say, to think carefully about the message, and to plan to come back later when the person is in a more receptive frame of mind. Assertive communication is open, direct, honest, and appropriate to the interpersonal demands of the situation.

To be assertive in the face of an emotionally charged situation demands thought, energy, and commitment. Assertiveness also requires the use of common sense, self-awareness, knowledge, tact, humor, respect, and a sense of perspective. Although there is no guarantee that the use of assertive behaviors will produce desired interpersonal goals, the chances of a successful outcome are increased because the information flow is optimally honest, direct, and firm. Often the use of assertiveness brings about changes in ways that could not have been anticipated. Changes occur because the nurse offers a new resource in the form of objective feedback with no strings attached. Within a nurse–client relationship, the nurse's definition of self, in relation to conflict issues, leaves room for the client to experience the conflict directly, to exercise the right of making a personal judgment based on an accurate appraisal of individual needs, and to determine the best possible action in line with those needs.

**Structure Your Response.** In mastering assertive responses, it may be helpful initially to use the four steps of an assertive response first presented by Angel and Petronko (1983, p. 27), who also provided the following example:

1. Express empathy: "I understand that _____"; "I hear you saying _____ ."

2. Describe your feelings or the situation: "I feel that _____"; "This situation seems to me to be _____ ."
3. State expectations: "I want _____"; "What is required by the situation is _____ ."
4. List consequences: "If you do this then _____ will happen" (state positive outcome); "If you don't do this, then _____ will happen" (state negative outcome).

For example, the nurse might

1. Express empathy: "I understand that things are difficult at home."
2. Describe feelings or the situation: "But your 8-year-old daughter has expressed a lot of anxiety, saying, 'I can't learn to give my own insulin shots.'"
3. State expectations: "It is necessary for you to be here tomorrow when the diabetic teaching nurse comes so you can learn how to give injections and your daughter can too with your support."
4. List consequences: "If you get here on time, we can be finished and get her discharged in time for her birthday on Friday."

## Clinical Encounters with Angry or Difficult Clients

Every nurse encounters clients who refuse to comply with the treatment plan, who exhibit hostile behaviors toward the staff, perhaps eventually withdrawing from any positive interaction with the nurse. As Maynard (personal communication, 1998, based on Maynard & Chitty, 1971) noted, there are numerous nonverbal clues to anger, including clenched jaws or fists, turning away, "forgetting" or being late for appointments, and refusing to maintain eye contact. Verbal cues by a client may, of course, include use of an angry tone of voice, but they may also be disguised as witty sarcasm and condescending or insulting remarks. To become comfortable in dealing with client anger, the nurse must first become aware of his or her own reactions to anger so that the nurse does not threaten or reject the individual expressing anger. Successful interventions include the following:

1. Identify anger. Help the client recognize his or her own anger by pointing out cues and

attempting to validate them with the client (e.g., "I notice you are clenching your fists and talking more loudly than usual. These are some things people do when they are feeling angry. Are you feeling angry now?"; Maynard, personal communication, 1998, developed from Maynard & Chitty, 1971).

2. Give permission for anger (e.g., "Everyone gets angry at this" and "It's natural to be angry in these circumstances").

3. Help the client own the angry feelings by getting the client to verbalize things that make him or her angry. Perhaps suggest a hypothetical situation.

4. Realistically analyze the current situation that is disturbing the client.

5. Assist the client in developing a plan to deal with the situation (e.g., the nurse could use techniques such as role-playing to help the client express anger appropriately, use "I" statements such as "I feel angry" rather than "You make me angry"). Bringing behavior up to a verbal level should help alleviate the need for other acting out/destructive behaviors.

Box 14–4 lists some useful strategies for coping with difficult clients. An additional strategy available for helping nurse–client problem inter-

actions is the staff-focused consultation, illustrated in the following situation.

---

### ◆ Case Example

Mr. P., aged 29, has been employed for 6 years as a construction worker. Four weeks ago, while operating a forklift, he was struck by a train, leaving him a paraplegic. After 2 weeks in intensive care, he was transferred to a neurological unit. When staff members attempt to provide physical care, such as changing his position or getting him up in a chair, Mr. P. throws things, curses angrily, and sometimes spits at the nurses. Staff members become very upset; several nurses have requested assignment changes. Some staff members try bribing him with food to encourage good behavior; others threaten to apply restraints. The manager schedules a behavioral consultation meeting with a psychiatric nurse or clinical specialist. The immediate goal of this staff conference is to bring staff feelings out into the open and to facilitate increased awareness of the staff's behavioral responses when confronted with this client's behavior.

---

The outcome goal is to use a problem-solving approach to develop a behavioral care plan, so that all staff members respond to Mr. P. in a consistent manner.

Students are particularly prone to feel rebuffed when they first encounter negative feedback from a client. Support from staff, instructor, and peers, coupled with efforts to understand the underlying reasons and the client's feelings, help the student resist the trap of avoiding the relationship (Lerner & Byrne, 1991). To develop these ideas further, practice Exercise 14–7.

## SUMMARY

Conflict represents a hostile encounter or a mental struggle between two opposing thoughts, feelings, or needs. It can be intrapersonal in nature, deriving from within a particular individual, or interpersonal, when it represents a clash between two or more people.

All conflicts have certain things in common: a concrete content issue and a process of expression. Expressions of passionate feelings about the issue may occur. Generally, intrapersonal conflicts stimulate feelings of emotional discomfort. A neutral, supportive interpersonal environment

---

> ### ◆ Box 14–4. Potential Approaches for Dealing with Anxious or Difficult Clients
>
> 1. Provide education. Explain all options, with outcomes.
> 2. Develop a nursing care plan: involve patient in care and set goals; review and re-evaluate whether nurse and client have same goals; focus on mutual goals and progress.
> 3. Use incentives and withdrawal of privileges to modify unacceptable behavior.
> 4. Use medical and nonmedical interventions to decrease anxiety (medicine, touch, relaxation, guided imagery).
> 5. Set limits, give family permission to rest, to leave, and so on.
> 6. Promote trust by providing immediate feedback.

helps reduce emotions to a workable level. Other strategies to defuse strong emotion include talking the emotion through with someone and temporarily reducing stress through the use of distraction or additional information.

Most interpersonal conflicts involve some threat to one's sense of power to control an interpersonal situation or to ways of thinking about the self. Giving up ineffective behavior patterns in conflict situations is difficult; such patterns are generally perceived to be safer because they are familiar.

Conflictive feelings usually have to be put into words and related to the issue at hand before the meaning of the conflict becomes understandable. When the source of conflict is interpersonal in nature, before making a response the nurse needs to think through the possible causes of the conflict as well as his or her own feelings about it.

Behavioral responses to conflict situations fall into one of four categories. A number of strategies have been successfully used by nurses to manage client–nurse conflicts, including assertion. Assertive behaviors range from making a simple statement, directly and honestly, about one's beliefs to taking a very strong, confrontational stand about what will and will not be tolerated.

## REFERENCES

Anderson MA, Helms LB. (1998). Comparison of continuing care communication. Image 30(3):255–260.

Angel G, Petronko DK. (1987). Developing the New Assertive Nurse: Essentials for Advancement (2nd ed.). New York, Springer.

Baggs JG, Schmitt MH. (1997). Nurses' and resident physicians perceptions of the process of collaboration in an MICU. Research in Nursing & Health 20(1):71–80.

Baker KM. (1995). Improving staff nurse conflict resolution skills. Nursing Economics 13(5):295–298.

Balzer-Riley JW. (1996). Communications in Nursing. St. Louis, CV Mosby.

Booth R. (1985). Conflict and conflict management. In Mason DJ, Talbot SW (eds.), Political Action Handbook for Nurses. Menlo Park, CA, Addison-Wesley.

Brooks A, Thomas S, Droppleman P. (1996). From frustration to red fury: A description of work-related anger in male registered nurses. Nursing Forum 31(3):4–15.

Dallinger JM, Hample D. (1995). Personalizing and managing conflict. International Journal of Conflict Management 6(3):273–289.

Davidhizar R. (1991). Impressing the boss who criticizes you. Advances in Clinical Care Nursing 6(2):39–41.

de Torynay R. (1990). Helping students deal with controversy. Journal of Nursing Education 29(4):149.

Droppleman PG, Thomas SP. (1996). Anger in Nurses. American Journal of Nursing 96(4):26–31.

Feeney MC, Davidson JA. (1996). Bridging the gap between the practical and the theoretical: An evaluation of a conflict resolution model. Peace and Conflict: Journal of Peace Psychology 2(3):255–269.

Ferrucci P. (1982). What We May Be. Los Angeles, Jeremy P. Tarcher.

Flanagan L. (1990). Survival Skills in the Workplace: What Every Nurse Should Know. Kansas City, MO, American Nurses Association.

Fritchie R. (1995). Conflict and its management. British Journal of Hospital Medicine 53(9):471–473.

Johnson J, Arneson P. (1991). Women expressing anger to women in the workplace. Women's Studies in Communication 14(2):24–41.

Jones MA, Bushardt SC, Cadenhead G. (1990). A paradigm for effective resolution of interpersonal conflict. Nursing Management 21(2):64B, 64F–64K.

Lerner H, Byrne MW. (1991). Helping nursing students communicate with high-risk families. Nursing and Health Care 12(2):98–101.

Levis AJ. (1996). Shifting our attention from content to process. Journal of Psychotherapy Integration 6(2):127–134.

Maynard C. (1998). Personal communication.

Maynard C, Chitty L. (1971). Dealing with anger: Guidelines for nursing intervention. Journal of Psychiatric Nursing and Mental Health Services 17(36):June.

McCanton PJ, Hargie O. (1990). Assessing assertive behavior in student nurses: A comparison of assertive measures. Journal of Advanced Nursing 15(12):1370–1376.

McElhaney R. (1996). Conflict management in nursing administration. Nursing Management 27(3):49–50.

Moustakis C. (1974). Finding Yourself, Finding Others. Englewood Cliffs, NJ, Prentice Hall.

Peterson LW, Halsey J, Albrecht TL, McGough K. (1995). Communicating with staff nurses: Support or hostility? Nursing Management 26(6):36–38.

Porter L. (1996). Conflict. Seminars in Perioperative Nursing 5(3):119–126.

Schutzenhofer KK. (1992). Nursing education and professional autonomy. Reflections 18:7.

Shearer R, Davidson R. (1997). When a co-worker complains. Canadian Nurse 93(1):47–48.

Smythe E. (1990). Surviving Nursing. Menlo Park, CA, Addison-Wesley.

Trubisky P, Ting-Toomey S, Lin, S. (1991). The influence of individualism-collectivism and self-monitoring on conflict styles. International Journal of Intercultural Relations 15:65–84.

Valentine PEB. (1995). Management of conflict: Do nurses/women handle it differently? Journal of Advanced Nursing 22:142–149.

## Electronic References

http://www.cios.org

## Suggested Readings

Bower S, Bower G. (1991). Asserting Yourself: A Practical Guide for Positive Change. Reading, MA, Addison-Wesley.

Chenevert M. (1988). Special Techniques in Assertiveness Training for Women in the Health Professions. St. Louis, CV Mosby.

Hamilton J, Kiefer M. (1986). Survival Skills for the New Nurse. Philadelphia, JB Lippincott.

Kramer M. (1974). Reality Shock: Why Nurses Leave Nursing. St. Louis, CV Mosby.

Raudsepp E. (1991). Six ways to becoming more assertive. Nursing 91 21(3):112–116.

# 15

# Health Promotion and Client Learning Needs

Elizabeth Arnold

**OBJECTIVES**

At the end of the chapter, the student will be able to

1. Define health promotion
2. Contrast motivational frameworks in health promotion
3. Identify factors related to a client's readiness to learn
4. Describe factors related to a client's ability to learn
5. Discuss the role of self-awareness in health promotion

---

*You cannot teach a man anything, you can only help him discover it within himself.*

Galileo

---

Chapter 15 introduces health promotion and motivational frameworks as the basis for health teaching and outlines communication strategies the nurse can use to help clients promote their health and well-being. As we enter the 21st century, health promotion has become a potent force in health care (Fraser, 1998). The current focus of health care in the United States is on helping all health care consumers achieve optimal health and well-being through self-re-

sponsibility for healthy lifestyles and active cooperation in health maintenance. A health promotion–disease prevention focus views the client as an informed consumer and valued partner in a vertical health care delivery system. Political and social initiatives identified in *Healthy People 2000* (U.S. DHHS, 1991) and subsequent documents reinforce the concept of community-based health care delivery and preventive care. The goals of health promotion and prevention include understanding health-related threats to vulnerable populations, ensuring equity in health care, and preserving and enhancing quality of life for all health care consumers.

Health is viewed as a resource. Clients invest in their health when they collaborate with the nurse in a problem-solving process to improve and maintain maximum health and well-being. A wellness focus emphasizes health promotion and protection factors. A health maintenance emphasis stresses health prevention activities to strengthen and restore the health of individuals. Clients are expected to assume much greater responsibility for their personal health care, and nurses are an invaluable resource in helping them through health teaching across the full continuum of care. Many treatments, such as intravenous chemotherapy, parenteral nutrition, and that involved in the care of ventilator-dependent clients, are carried out in the home rather than in hospitals.

The extent to which people engage with health service providers to promote, maintain, and restore their health and well-being is important in determining the content and process of appropriate health teaching. Factors related to the client's readiness and ability to learn help the nurse understand the client's perspective. Individualized health teaching plans recognize and respect client preferences and learning needs. Understanding and responding appropriately to client learner needs are critical in today's managed care health care environment.

## BASIC CONCEPTS
### Definition

*Health promotion* is defined in clinical practice as "organized actions or efforts that enhance, support, or promote the well-being or health of individuals, families, groups, communities or societies" (Kulbok et al., 1997, p. 17). The concept of *well-being* consists of attitudes supporting a lifestyle of balance and well-being in six personal dimensions: intellectual, physical, emotional, social, occupational, and spiritual (Chandler et al., 1992; Omizo et al., 1992). Well-being is a subjective experience, always defined by the client, with its meaning validated by the nurse. Health promotion strategies aim at helping people modify their lifestyles and make personal choices to improve their health prospects and quality of life (Maltby & Robinson, 1998). Through increased self-understanding and improved self-care, people are able to actualize their health potential. Box 15–1 lists priority

---

### ◆ Box 15–1. Healthy People 2000: Priority Areas

**Health Promotion**

1. Physical activity and fitness
2. Nutrition
3. Tobacco
4. Alcohol and other drugs
5. Family planning
6. Mental health and mental disorders
7. Violent and abusive behavior
8. Educational and community-based programs

**Health Protection**

9. Unintentional injuries
10. Occupational safety and health
11. Environmental health
12. Food and drug safety
13. Oral health

**Preventive Services**

14. Maternal and infant health
15. Heart disease and stroke
16. Cancer
17. Diabetes and chronic disabling conditions
18. Human immunodeficiency virus infection
19. Sexually transmitted diseases
20. Immunization and infectious diseases

**Strategies to Meet Objectives**

21. Professional and access issues in clinical preventive services
22. Development of surveillance and data systems to track progress

areas for healthy people as identified by the U.S. Department of Health and Human Services (DHHS).

To help clients achieve the goal of optimal well-being, the nurse uses one-to-one counseling and group education formats to meet educational health care objectives related to maintenance of health, prevention of illness, restoration of health, coping with impaired functioning, and rehabilitation. Health promotion activities are available to all clients regardless of health status and include primary prevention strategies such as parenting classes as well as wellness promotion activities not directly related to any specific disease (e.g., stress management and exercise).

Nursing interventions for health promotion support client autonomy in selecting health care options that fit the person as well as the situation. Jones and Meleis (1993) characterized health as empowerment, a contextual definition of health in which the nurse helps clients use a critical thinking process to resolve their health problems and acts as an advocate in facilitating access to those resources most likely to support their health and well-being. Guidelines proposed by the U.S. Preventive Services Task Force for health education and counseling are presented in Table 15–1.

## Table 15-1. Recommendations of the U.S. Preventive Services Task Force: Strategies in Health Education and Counseling

1. Frame the teaching to match the client's perceptions.
2. Fully inform clients of the purposes and expected effects of interventions and when to expect these effects.
3. Suggest small changes rather than large ones.
4. Be specific.
5. Add new behaviors rather eliminating established behaviors whenever possible.
6. Link new behaviors to old behaviors.
7. Obtain explicit commitments from the client regarding action.
8. Refer clients to community resources.
9. Use a combination of strategies.
10. Monitor progress through follow-up contact.

Adapted from U.S. Preventive Services Task Force. (1996). Guide to Clinical Preventive Services (2nd ed). Baltimore, MD, Williams & Wilkins. Used with permission.

## Health Promotion and Disease Prevention

The combination of health promotion and disease prevention is essential to helping clients achieve their goal of optimal health and well-being. In the document *Healthy People 2000*, **prevention** is defined broadly as "a culture, or a way of thinking and being, that actively promotes responsible behavior and the adoption of lifestyles that are maximally conducive to good health" (U.S. DHHS, 1991, p. v).

Nursing considers three aspects of prevention—primary, secondary, and tertiary prevention—in a seamless continuum of health care delivery.

- *Primary prevention*, defined as actions taken to preclude illness or to prevent the natural course of illness from occurring, focuses on teaching people how to establish and maintain lifestyles conducive to optimal health. The nurse teaches clients how to avoid health-related problems in their particular age, cultural, or social group. Examples include prenatal clinics, parenting courses, stress management programs, genetic screening, and most forms of health education.
- *Secondary prevention* involves interventions designed to promote early diagnosis of symptoms or timely treatment after the onset of the disease. The purpose of secondary preventive teaching programs is to catch health problems early, thus minimizing their effects on a person's life. Examples include screening surveys, mammograms, purified protein derivatives (PPDs), and glaucoma, diabetes, respiratory, and blood pressure screenings.
- *Tertiary prevention* describes rehabilitation strategies designed to minimize the handicapping effects of a disease. The goal of tertiary prevention is the same as those of primary and secondary prevention: to help clients achieve the highest level of wellness possible, at this level through restoration of function to whatever extent is possible. Education can play as critical a healing role as medication or surgery in tertiary prevention. Examples include teaching a cancer victim about chemotherapy, helping a stroke victim with bladder retraining to avoid infection, and teaching a client to cope effectively with the necessary adjustments a serious physical, social, or emotional illness imposes.

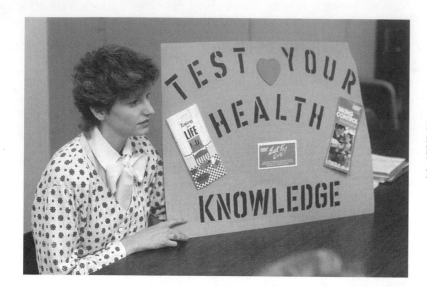

Primary prevention strategies include community education at health fairs. (Courtesy of the University of Maryland School of Nursing)

As clients take increasing responsibility for their health care, they must be knowledgeable about medication dosage and side effects, therapeutic protocols, signs and symptoms of illness, diet, and self-monitoring strategies. Health promotion activities involve proactive decision making at all levels of prevention related to identifying and treating the multideterminants of health for the purpose of maintaining and improving the general health and well-being of individuals, families, and communities (Edelman & Mandel, 1998).

## APPLICATIONS

Characteristics of the helping relationship are important in health teaching for health promotion and parallel those found in Carl Rogers' (1969) client-centered teaching process. He insisted that the teacher must start where the learner is, structuring the learning process to support the learner's natural desire to learn and mindful of learner characteristics that enable or impede the process. Rogers proposed that "if the teacher could be congruent—that is honest and open to the point of transparency—with her student, if she could show acceptance and regard for her student in spite of the latter's failures and mistakes, and if she could demonstrate a genuine understanding of the student's point of view, the student would be likely to learn" (Hallett, 1997).

Learners differ in their abilities, intellectual curiosity, motivation for learning, learning styles, and rate of learning. Learner variables important in the teaching-learning process generally fall into two categories: readiness to learn and ability to learn. These factors may exist in combination or as isolated characteristics. Whereas the nurse can readily help people who want to learn, less is achieved in a learning situation when the learner is unwilling or unable to learn. Unconditional acceptance of the client as he or she is now enhances trust and cooperation in a mutual process of learning.

Finding ways to engage clients in the learning process is the first step in planning effective teaching interventions. Hoff (1987) told the story of a stranger who asked him for directions to a certain street. In response, he pointed to the street and gave the stranger very explicit instructions on how to get there. Shortly thereafter, he noticed the stranger going in the opposite direction. When he told him he was going in the wrong direction, the stranger told him: "Yes, I know, I'm not quite ready yet."

So it is with client engagement with health care. Teaching cannot begin until the client is ready. The teachable moment takes place when the learner feels that there is a need to know the information and has the capacity to learn it. Factors affecting learning readiness are identified in Box 15–2.

┌─────────────────────────────────────────────────────────────────────────────┐
◆ Box 15-2. Factors that Influence Learning Readiness

| | |
|---|---|
| Physical | Pain, fatigue, disability, sensory deprivation |
| Psychological | Motivation, altitude, belief about health and illness, emotional response to illness |
| Intellectual | Literacy, ability to comprehend |
| Socioeconomic/cultural | Ethnicity, religious beliefs, health values, family roles and relationships, support structures, financial concerns, home environment |

From Ruzicki D. (1989). Realistically meeting the educational needs of hospitalized acute and short-stay patients. Nursing Clinics of North America. 24(3):631. Reprinted with the permission of WB Saunders Company, Philadelphia.
└─────────────────────────────────────────────────────────────────────────────┘

## Motivation

*Motivation* is the force that activates behavior and directs it toward a goal. It is a fundamental component of learner readiness. Without it, the learner and teacher have an almost insurmountable task. It is like trying to start a car with no gas. The driver can push the car, but it will not move on its own. Without client motivation, the nurse can "push," but the learner, like the car, will make very little movement. Before implementing teaching strategies related to content, the nurse must help the client see a need to learn the required information (Vitousek, Watson & Wilson, 1998). Two theories that have application for increasing motivation are Pender's health promotion model and Proschaska and DiClemente's stage model of change.

## Frameworks for Assessing Learner Readiness

### Health Promotion Model

Pender's (1996) health promotion model expands on an earlier health belief model developed by Rosenstock and his associates in the 1950s. This model proposes that a person's willingness to engage in health promotion behaviors is best understood through examining a person's beliefs about the seriousness of a health condition and his or her ability to influence personal health and well-being (Fig. 15–1). Unless people believe that (1) they are susceptible to the disease, (2) they are likely to have serious life changes should they contract the disease, (3) they are capable of taking direct action to avoid or reduce the severity of the disease, (4) the action they would have to take is less threatening than the

threat of the disease, they are unlikely to take a health action.

Pender's health promotion model emphasizes movement toward a positive valuing of health and well-being. It highlights self-actualization by collaborating with clients to acknowledge and take responsibility for achieving the highest level of well-being possible. Cognitive perceptual factors, which include a person's definition of health, perceptions of health status, benefits, and barriers to health-promoting behaviors, strengthen or weaken interest in engaging in health-promoting behaviors. Pender called them "the primary motivational mechanisms for acquisition and maintenance of health-promoting behaviors" (p. 60). Modifying factors are external inputs that serve as "cues to action" in a person's decision to seek health care or to engage in health-promoting activities. Examples of modifying factors are schools that require immunizations, family experiences with a disorder or preventive measures, and interpersonal reminders, such as a family member's experience with the health care system, the mass media, and ethnic approval. Figure 15–2 presents Pender's health promotion model.

### ◆ Case Example

Mary Nolan knows that walking will help diminish her potential for developing osteoporosis, but the threat of having this disorder in her 60s is not sufficient to motivate her to take action in her 40s. Mary does not feel any signs or symptoms of the disorder, and it is easier to maintain a sedentary life. The nurse will have to understand the client's internal value system and other factors that influence readiness to learn to create the most appropriate learning conditions and types of

**Belief About Health Threat**

•*Health Values*
I am concerned about my health.
•*Beliefs About Vulnerability*
I am at risk because my mother
had breast cancer.
•*Beliefs About the Severity of the Disorder*
Breast cancer is a leading cause
of death in women.

**Belief That Preventive Health Behaviors
Can Decrease Health Threat**

•*Beliefs That Specific Health Behaviors
Can Minimize Health Threat*
Mammograms can detect early cancers.
•*Beliefs That Benefits of Preventive Health
Behaviors Outweigh Costs*
Even though it seems inconvenient and
costly, yearly mammograms can minimize
my risk of dying from breast cancer.

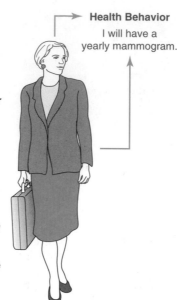

**Health Behavior**
I will have a
yearly mammogram.

Figure 15–1. Example of health-belief model applied to the health behavior of yearly mammograms.

teaching strategies Mary will need to effect positive change in health habits. The nurse might show Mary a video of the changes osteoporosis creates in spinal structure or ask an older adult with this disease to share her experience.

An example of the health promotion model applied to breast cancer prevention is presented in Figure 15–1. Exercise 15–1 provides practice with applying the health promotion model to common health problems.

## Transtheoretical Model of Change

Prochaska and DiClemente (1992) describe motivation to change as a state of readiness that fluctuates and can be influenced by external encouragement. Their change model identifies six stages through which people pass in coping with a health problem, and describes motivational strategies the nurse can use to encourage compliance. Motivational strategies match the stages of change and are designed to increase the likelihood that the client will follow the recommended course of action toward change. The transtheoretical model is particularly effective for use with clients who are resistant to standard teaching strategies. Old patterns are hard to break. The fear of destroying old familiar patterns may be particularly strong when the new patterns designed to take its place are unknown or uncertain. Most people will go through the stages of change more than once before effecting a stable change. Box 15–3 presents stages of change with suggested approaches and sample statements.

When using this model, the nurse's comments start where the client is in the process and expand the learning field to include more and relevant information that the client may not have considered. If the client is a rational agent and capable of decision making, the decision about treatment remains with the client (Gauthier, 1993). For example, the nurse might use the following format if the client is in the contemplation stage.

### ◆ Case Example

**Nurse:** I know that you think you can manage yourself at home. But most people really need some rehabilitation after a stroke to help them regain their strength. If you go home now without the rehabilitation, you may be shortchanging yourself by not taking the time to develop the skills you need to be independent at home.

In the maintenance phase, the nurse may need to help the client renew resolve by pointing out behaviors that indicate a temporary setback.

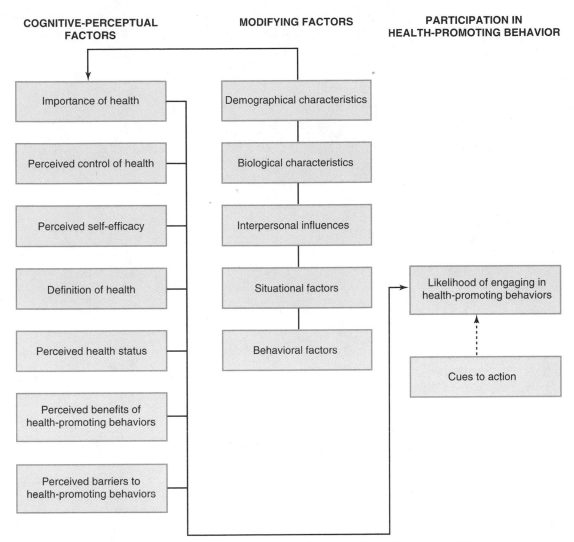

**COGNITIVE-PERCEPTUAL FACTORS**

- Importance of health
- Perceived control of health
- Perceived self-efficacy
- Definition of health
- Perceived health status
- Perceived benefits of health-promoting behaviors
- Perceived barriers to health-promoting behaviors

**MODIFYING FACTORS**

- Demographical characteristics
- Biological characteristics
- Interpersonal influences
- Situational factors
- Behavioral factors

**PARTICIPATION IN HEALTH-PROMOTING BEHAVIOR**

- Likelihood of engaging in health-promoting behaviors
- Cues to action

Figure 15–2. Health-promotion model. (From Pender N. [1996]. Health Promotion in Nursing Practice. Norwalk, CT, Appleton & Lange, p. 58.)

◆ **Case Example**

**Nurse:** I notice that we don't seem to be making much headway in applying what you are learning about dietary changes required by your high cholesterol. I wonder if there are some issues that we have not addressed that may be getting in the way.

Stated in a proactive, positive way, this dialogue can motivate the client to consider possible barriers to behavioral change or actions in need of modification. The nurse makes a direct statement without judging the client and asks the client to participate with the nurse in problem solving as to why this has occurred. The simple process of talking through concerns with the nurse and then with significant others unmasks fears and negative energy that can get in the way of effective learning.

---

◆ Exercise 15-1. **The Health Belief Model and Common Health Problems**

**Purpose:** To help students gain experience with use of the health belief model

**Procedure:**
1. Using the health care model as a guide, interview a person with a health care problem.
2. Record the person's answers and develop a diagram of the health care model using the person's answers.
3. Comment on the individual perceptions, modifying factors, and cues to action you found in the client data to determine the likelihood of taking recommended preventive health actions.

**Discussion:**
1. Were you surprised at the client's knowledge about the target health problem or interpretation of the meaning of it?
2. As you compare your client's answers with those of your classmates, do any common themes emerge?
3. How could you use the information you gained from your client and from doing this exercise in future practice?

---

## Social Learning Theory

Bandura (1987) considered learning to be a social process. He identified three sets of motivating factors: physical motivators, social incentives, and cognitive motivators that promote learning. Exercise 15–2 explores significant learning experiences. Physical motivators can be internal such as a memory of previous discomfort or a symptom that the client cannot ignore.

### Case Example

Francis Edison agrees wholeheartedly with his nurse that smoking is bad and is likely to cause an earlier death from emphysema. However, in his mind, it is impossible for him even to contemplate giving up smoking. His mindset precludes learning until he can see the connection between giving up cigarettes and avoiding painful symptoms. A severe bronchitis creating air hunger and a hacking cough finally convinces Francis to give up cigarettes.

---

Unfortunately, waiting until this happens may prove lethal. Knowing that many clients find it difficult to appreciate the need to give up old habits or to try new behaviors without a personally valid reason, the nurse might deliberately use Bandura's theory to help Francis. In the following statement, the nurse makes the connection between Francis's actions and his physical symptoms. The nurse combines the concept of a physical motivator with a social incentive related to something the client values to help Francis recognize how changes in his health behavior can improve his health and well-being.

### Case Example

**Nurse:** I'm a little worried that you are continuing to smoke because it does affect your breathing. There is nothing you can do about the damage to your lungs that is already there, but if you stop smoking it can help preserve the healthy tissue you still have [physical motivator] and you won't have as much trouble breathing. I bet your grandson would appreciate it if you could breathe better and be able to play with him [social incentive].

---

The second set of motivators identified by Bandura (1987) is social incentives. Approval and disapproval of others who potentially have the power to reward or punish have significant motivating power for many people. Social incentives such as praise and encouragement increase self-esteem and give the client reason to continue learning. The social incentive in the prior case example is the opportunity to enjoy his grandson.

#### ◆ Box 15-3. Stages of Change and Suggested Approaches

| Client Stage | Characteristic Behaviors | Suggested Approach | Example |
|---|---|---|---|
| Precontemplation | Does not think there is a problem, is not considering the possibility of change | Raise doubt, give information feedback to raise awareness of a problem and health risks | "Your lab tests show some liver damage. These tests can be predictive of serious health problems and premature death." |
| Contemplation | Thinks there may be a problem; thinking about change; goes back and forth between concern and nonconcern | Tip the balance, allowing open discussion of pros and cons of changing behavior, build motivation for change, help the client justify a positive commitment | "It sounds as though you think you have a problem with drinking, but you are not sure that you are an alcoholic. What would your life be like if you gave up alcohol completely?" |
| Determination | Decides there is a problem and is willing to make a change: "I guess I do need to reduce my drinking" | Help the client choose the best course of action to take in coping with the problem | "What kinds of changes will you have to make in order to stop drinking?" |
| Action | Engages in actions to effect change | Help the client take active steps to action, reviews progress, gives feedback | "I like the fact that you are committed to saying no when someone offers you a drink." |
| Maintenance | Perseveres with positive behavioral change | Help client identify and use strategies to sustain progress; point out positive changes; accept temporary setbacks | "It's hard to let go of old habits, but you have been abstinent for 3 months now and your liver tests are significantly improved." |

Bandura (1987) referred to the third set of motivators as cognitive motivators described as internal thought processes associated with change. Changes in health status frequently dictate permanent changes in the client's lifestyle and self-perceptions. Clients with newly diagnosed chronic conditions have to change their attitudes and develop a new set of behaviors to cope with their illness. This is a difficult process for many clients, who secretly entertain the fantasy that they will be able to resume their former lives and that their functional ability will be the same. Both clients and family caregivers may have reservations about their competence to carry out treatments in the home or make changes in lifestyle without ongoing support (Exercise 15-3).

## Factors Affecting Readiness to Learn

Typically, health teaching is done with clients who are trying to adjust to recent and problematic life events, often accompanied by personal rejection, compromised body function, loss of a job, or end of an intimate relationship. They must make major life decisions at the worst possible time and under the worst possible conditions. The emotional fallout from these situations has a significant bearing on the learning process.

Nurses need to remember that learning is never smooth or linear in its development. Rather than challenge the client's learning pattern, the nurse needs to understand it and incorporate it into new opportunities for learning

---

◆ Exercise 15–2. **Significant Learning Experiences**

**Purpose:** To identify elements that make for successful learning experiences

**Procedure:**
Write a short paragraph about a significant learning situation in which you

1. Identify the most significant learning situation you have experienced. Use the situation that comes to mind first.
2. Describe the learning outcomes you achieved (e.g., developed a skill, gained insight, changed behavior, learned some new information, learned something about yourself).
3. Describe the activities and circumstances that contributed to making this learning situation so significant.

**Discussion:**
Use a chalkboard or flip chart to record student themes and activities in the significant learning situation.

1. Were you surprised at the situation that you chose for this exercise? In what ways?
2. In what ways were the activities and circumstances contributing to the memorability of this learning situation similar or different from those of others in your group?
3. What previously held assumptions/values were challenged or reaffirmed by this learning situation?
4. What did you learn from this exercise that you could use in your nursing practice?

---

(Blackie, Gregg & Freeth, 1998). This is the art of health teaching. Psychosocial and physical factors that can affect the learner's ability to learn include previous knowledge and experience about the illness as well as its personal and cultural meaning.

### Previous Knowledge and Experience

Closely linked to culture and often intertwined with it are culturally relevant knowledge and experiences of the client that make the client less able to engage in a traditional learning process. Each learning situation has a past as well as a present reality. Past experience, perceptual associations, and talking with others about their symptoms have provided the client with a set of assumptions and knowledge that must be factored into the teaching process. Previous knowledge, although often an asset, can present barriers and confusion for the client in learning new information.

For example, in a study of low-income, inner-city pregnant women, most of who had no prenatal care, the women were receiving ongoing teaching from friends and relatives. Some of the information was valid, but other information (such as the belief that a pregnant woman should not have intercourse or take a bath because she will drown the fetus) was wrong. Even more critical, cultural understandings related to inducing labor if the infant is overdue by taking large doses of laxatives or jumping off stairs are potentially unsafe health practices (St. Claire & Anderson, 1989). The nurse needs to know not only what information the client has received but also whom the client looks to and respects for health teaching purposes. Focusing on accurate information without destroying the credibility of well-meaning and influential informal health teachers in the client's life is part of the art of health teaching. Nothing is gained by injuring the reputation of the person who gave the client the information. Instead, the nurse might say, "There have been some new findings that I think you might be interested in. The most current thinking suggests that (give example) works well in situations like this." With this statement, the nurse can introduce a different way of thinking without challenging the person identified in the client's mind as expert.

◆ Exercise 15-3. **Facilitating Readiness to Confront Medical Events**

**Purpose:** To identify elements in teaching that can promote readiness

**Procedure:**
Identify as many specific answers as possible to the following questions.

1. Patrick drinks four to six beers every evening. Last year he lost his job. He has a troubled marriage and few friends. Patrick does not consider himself an alcoholic and blames his chaotic marriage for his need to drink. There is a strong family history of alcoholism.

What kinds of information might help Patrick want to learn more about his condition? _____

_____

2. Lily has just learned she has breast cancer. Although there is a good chance that surgery and chemotherapy will help her, she is scared to commit to the process and has even talked about taking her life.

What kinds of health teaching strategies and information might help Lily become ready to learn about her condition? _____

_____

3. Shawn has just been diagnosed as having epilepsy. He is ashamed to tell his friends and teachers about his condition. Shawn is considering breaking up with his girlfriend because of his newly diagnosed illness.

How would you use health teaching to help Shawn cope more effectively with his illness? ___

_____

4. Marilyn, a 14-year-old, has been admitted to the hospital with a bleeding ulcer. She has never been seriously ill before and has never been in the hospital before, even to visit a friend. She is scared and refuses to cooperate with her nurses.

What kinds of information and support might help Marilyn cope more effectively with her current circumstances? _____

_____

Assessment and inclusion of previous learning continue throughout the teaching process. This allows the nurse to make the teaching meaningful to the client and relevant to changes in the client's condition. As the client's condition worsens or becomes stable, the teaching content and strategies necessarily change. For example, one family facing an unexpected diagnosis of cancer or stroke may need information about the condition and the care and treatment involved. Another family in the same situation may need to deal with their grief and the normal reactions of shock, disbelief, denial, and anger before they are ready to hear about the condition and the different treatment options. Some families are overwhelmed by a sense of loss. Unexpected threats to health or life force individuals and their families to consider their own vulnerability and to acknowledge the possible loss of vital family members.

## Changes in Social Support

Changes in social support or the health status of significant others can affect the client's willing-

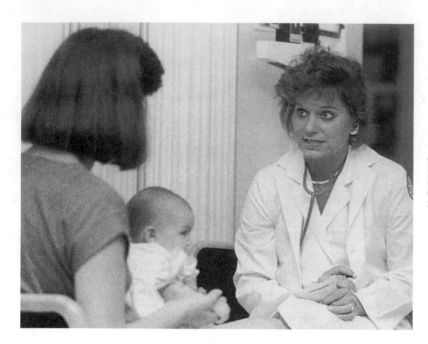

Assessing the client's readiness to learn is the first step in effective health promotion activities. (Courtesy University of Maryland School of Nursing)

ness or ability to learn. Many elderly clients have depended on others for direction and for overseeing treatment. When these supports are no longer available, through death or incapacity, the client may lack not only motivation but also the skills to know how to learn or to know what is expected.

### ◆ Case Example

Edward Flanigan, an 82-year-old man who was recently widowed, has diabetes. There is no evidence of memory problems, but there are some significant emotional components to his current health care needs. All his life, his wife pampered him. Although Edward administered his insulin daily, his wife reminded him to take it and make certain that he followed his diabetic diet. Now that his wife is dead, Edward takes no interest in controlling his diabetes. The home care nurse who visits him on a regular basis is discouraged because, despite careful instruction and seeming comprehension, Edward appears unwilling to follow the prescribed diabetic diet and is not consistent in taking his medication. Predictably, he goes into diabetic crisis. His family worries about him, but he is unwilling to consider leaving his home of 42 years.

In this case, the nurse learned that his wife assumed all responsibility for Edward. She paid the bills, monitored his diet, and prepared all his meals. Edward did not know how to cook, and he had never grocery shopped in his 45 years of marriage. Emotional issues of loss and change complicate the learning needs of this client. Edward could function and maintain his health as long as he could rely on his wife for support. This support is no longer available.

Although it may difficult for the nurse to understand how a grown, educated man might not know how to grocery stop or prepare his own food, dependency on others happens, and it affects how a client responds to health teaching about diet. Teaching objectives might incorporate helping Edward to understand and accept the normal process of grieving and include referral to supportive resources in his crisis situation. Helping him expand his social support system and consider alternative ways to meet his health and dependency needs would be a critical component of his teaching care plan. He might need instruction about grocery shopping, cooking, or Meals on Wheels to implement a diet teaching plan. Considering Edward's unique learning needs from a holistic, caring, as well as educational, perspective might make a difference in Edward's ability to learn and in his readiness to take responsibility for self-care.

A simple way to find out the client's perceptions and attitudes is simply to ask the client and family what they already know about the topic or what they associate with it. This is important information about personal fears, expectations, and what is important to the client. The more obvious the links between previous experiences and the new knowledge, the deeper is the learning (Glover & Bruning, 1990).

There are other questions the nurse might ask. For example, is the client able, without the consistent support of a significant other, to learn and take responsibility for self-care? Will the nurse have to help the client cope with changes in self-image and identity before or concurrently with providing concrete information? The sensitivity of the nurse in accurately perceiving the unique and immediate learning needs, so strongly intertwined with the emotional meaning of the health need, will facilitate the learning process.

## Active Involvement of the Learner

Active involvement of the learner enhances learning. Think about the differences between classes in which you are passive and those in which you are expected to be actively involved. Instructors who provide practical examples and invite participation from the class generally hold student interest more than do those who simply lecture.

Most people learn best when they engage more than one sense in the learning process. Practical learning takes place through doing. People feel a sense of pride and accomplishment from having successfully mastered active hands-on involvement with something they were not quite sure they could accomplish (Fig. 15–3). The same thing happens in health promotion. A highly participatory learning format with the opportunity to try out new behaviors is far more effective than giving simple instructions to a client or family or doing it for them because it is easier and faster to do so. Health promotion strategies require a sensitive appraisal and choice of strategy, unique in every case, and matched to the relevant needs of the individual, family, or group. Exercise 15–4 explores learning readiness further.

◆ **Case Example**

Soon Mrs. Hixon began learning how to dress herself. At first she took an hour to complete this task. But with guidance and practice, she eventually dressed herself in 25 minutes. Even so, I practically had to sit on my hands as I watched her struggle. I could have done it so much faster for her, but she had to learn, and I had to let her (Collier, 1992, p. 63).

## Inclusion of Family Members

Active learning also requires critical decisions to determine the extent to which family members are to be involved either in a supportive role or as the primary recipients of the teaching process. For example, the family or caregiver would be involved as a primary unit in certain cultures, with children, and with clients who have sensory or cognitive deficits. Content presentations to these family members would be the same as that given to the client if the client were able to assume full responsibility for self-care.

On the other hand, family members take supportive roles in cases involving teenagers, clients in crisis, elderly clients with intact cognitive abilities, and those with a depressive disorder that compromises concentration. The difference in content and strategies for these family members would center on what they needed to know to support the learner. They may or may not need detailed content given to the client; they do need information about strategies to enable their loved one to take responsibility for self-care management.

Strategies to encourage active involvement of the client might include self-monitoring strategies, such as recording eating patterns or thoughts and feelings surrounding anxiety attacks. Information and anticipatory guidance about what to expect when the client goes home and early warning signs of complications or potential problems are given to family members as well as clients. Return demonstrations are essential components of any psychomotor learning because performance errors can be corrected instantly.

## Physical Barriers to Learning

Sometimes the client's condition precludes teaching. A client in pain cannot focus on any-

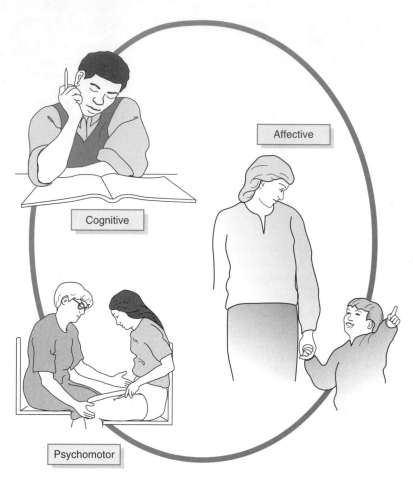

**Figure 15–3.** People learn best when more than one sense is involved.

Cognitive

Affective

Psychomotor

◆ **Exercise 15-4. Applying Maslow's Theory to Learning Readiness**

**Purpose:** To develop skill in facilitating learning readiness

**Procedure:**
Students will break up into four groups and receive a case scenario that depicts a client learning need. Using Maslow's hierarchy of needs, determine where the client is and plan your teaching approach based on their current level. Include in your plan the supportive measures that would be necessary to foster readiness to learn.

**Discussion:**
Each group will present their case and plan. Discuss how the use of Maslow's hierarchy can be effective in addressing learning needs and nursing approach. Discuss factors that contribute to resistance to learning and noncompliance. Discuss the supportive measures that nurses must include as part of the learning process with clients.

thing else. A client emerging from the shock of a difficult diagnosis may require teaching in small segments or postponement of serious teaching sessions until the physical problems are under greater control.

## Ability to Learn

Many clients are ready to learn, but they are not able to learn with traditional learning formats (Hemmings, 1998). Assessment of the client's ability to learn and accommodating the learning format to the learner's unique characteristics makes a difference. If the client cannot understand what is being taught, learning does not take place. Clients give up or "tune out," not because they do not want to know the information but because they lack the skills to obtain and assimilate it. Many psychological, physiological, intellectual, and emotional factors affect a client's capacity to learn new information and ways of behaving.

For example, certain physical conditions make health teaching difficult. Nausea, weakness, or speech or motor impairments may make it difficult for the client to maintain concentration. Medications or the period of disorientation after a diagnostic test or surgical procedure can influence the level of the client's ability to participate in learning. Careful assessment will usually reveal when the client's physical or emotional condition is a barrier to learning. The client with significant thought disorders may need very concrete instructions and frequent prompts to perform adequately.

Concurrent health care problems that could interfere with the goals or process of teaching are important pieces of data that influence what can and should be taught. For example, an exercise program might be useful for an overweight person, but if the client also has a cardiac condition or other problem that would limit activity, this information has a direct impact on the goals and strategies of the intervention.

Some situations favor learning. The anxiety associated with crisis can be used productively, provided it is not extreme. Mezirow (1990) noted that crisis and life transitions provide a format for the most significant adult learning. Attention is likely to be at its peak during these times. Crisis learning is particularly effective with many homeless and Medicaid clients, who frequently do not voluntarily seek health care at any other time. Health teaching for these clients should be immediate, practical, designed to resolve the crisis situation, and carefully organized to maximize client attention.

People learn material differently. Some people learn better with short segments, whereas others prefer to learn all of the material and break it down later. Scheduling shorter sessions with time in between to process information helps prevent sensory overload (Demuth, 1989). This is particularly true in health teaching of the elderly. Too much information in too short a time breeds frustration for the elderly client who needs extra time to process and integrate information.

To appreciate the significance of allowing processing time to prevent sensory overload, compare your own level of interest, attention, and learning during the last hour of class on a heavy lecture day with that during the first hours. Chances are your attention has diminished by the last hour of class. A simple strategy that helps break up learning segments is to change the pace by inserting an activity, visual aid, or discussion point.

## Low Literacy

Low literacy is not the same as low intelligence, although frequently people confuse the two. There is an assumption that educationally disadvantaged or functionally illiterate people are less responsible learners. However, just because a person is educated does not mean he or she will be more ready to assume responsibility for changing difficult behaviors than a less educated individual. Nor does it mean that an illiterate person cannot learn.

A persistent stigma about low literacy and learning disabilities exists even though it is unfounded. For this reason, many people try to hide the fact that they cannot read or do not know the meaning of complex words. They fake their inability to understand by appearing to agree with the educator and by not asking questions. Using symbols and images with which the client is familiar helps overcome the barriers of low literacy. Simple, concrete words convey the same message as more sophisticated language. For example, one client referred to testing his urine for diabetes as "testing for sugar in the piss." This language had meaning for him. Describing diabetes in abstract terms would have little relevance for this client, who would have difficulty following and participating in the learning process. Taking the time to understand the client's use of words and phrases provides the nurse with words and ideas that can be used as building blocks in helping the client understand difficult health-related concepts. Otherwise the client may misunderstand what the nurse is saying.

### ◆ Case Example

The discharge nurse said to a new mother, "Now you know to watch the baby's stools to be sure they're normal. You do know what normal stools look like, don't you?" The mother replied, "Oh, yeah, sure . . . I've got four of them in my kitchen" (Doak et al., 1985).

The nurse should keep instructions as simple as possible, presenting ideas in an uncomplicated, step-by-step format. Familiar words supplemented by common pictures provide an extrasensory input for the client and improve retention. Drawings and photographs provide additional cues, allowing the client to understand meanings he or she would be unable to grasp through words alone (Fig. 15–4).

Use the literal meanings of words rather than nonliteral terminology. "Call the doctor if you

run into trouble" may not mean that the client will call the physician if symptoms develop unless the precise reasons for calling the doctor are described and understood. A better direction is "Call the doctor on Monday if you still have pain or swelling in your knee." These same instructions, written exactly as they were spoken, act as a reminder once the person leaves the actual teaching situation. In addition to using simple words and literal interpretations, the nurse should use the same words to describe the same thing. For example, if you use "insulin" in one instance and "medicine" or "drug" later to describe the same medication, the client may become confused.

Logical sequencing of content is particularly important in teaching the low-literacy client. Doak et al. (1985) suggested thinking about the order of a teaching session from the client's perspective and advocated the following series of questions as a framework for instruction about medication:

- What do I take?
- How much do I take?
- When do I take it?
- What will it do for me?
- What do I do if I get a side effect?

By selecting small, related pieces of data and structuring them into informational chunks, the client can remember the information better through association even if one fact is forgotten. Whenever possible, link new tasks and information with what the client already knows. This strategy, important with all clients, is particularly advantageous with the low-literacy client. It takes advantage of previous learning and helps reinforce self-esteem by reminding the client of competencies learned in the process of instruction.

When technical words are necessary for clients to communicate about their condition with other health professionals, clients need direct instruction about appropriate words to use. As with culturally diverse clients, keeping sentences short and precise and using active verbs help clients understand what is being taught. Box 15–4 provides guidelines for the nurse in teaching low-literacy clients.

### The Learning-Disabled Client

The learning-disabled client, whether because of mental illness, learning disability, or attention

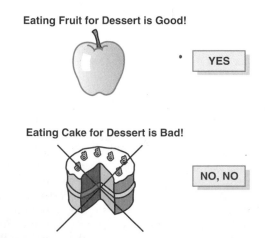

**Eating Fruit for Dessert is Good!**

YES

**Eating Cake for Dessert is Bad!**

NO, NO

**Figure 15–4.** Diabetic teaching for low-literacy clients: example of teaching aids.

> ### ◆ Box 15–4. Guidelines for Teaching Low-Literacy Clients
>
> 1. Teach the smallest amount possible to do the job.
> 2. Make your point as vividly as you can. (Use visual aids and examples for emphasis.)
> 3. Incorporate as many senses as possible in the learning process.
> 4. Have the client restate and demonstrate the information.
> 5. Review repeatedly.
>
> ---
>
> Adapted from Doak CC, Doak LG, Root JH. (1985). Tips on teaching patients. In Doak CC, Doak LG, Root JH (eds.), Teaching Patients with Low Literacy Skills. Philadelphia, JB Lippincott, p. 4. Reprinted with the permission of JB Lippincott Company, Philadelphia.

deficit disorder (ADD), may require adaptation of normal teaching strategies to learn new material. Learning disability is defined as "impairment in one or more aspects of a broad range of functional areas comprising such processes as attention, memory, visual perception, receptive language, expressive language, motor output and higher order conceptualization" (Levine, 1980, p. 312). The concept of learning disability covers a wide range of learning handicaps, ranging from severe impairment of learning potential in many functional areas to mild disability in one area and marked excellence in others.

Nurses should be aware that a learning-disabled client possibly has a history of feelings of failure or frustration. As in any other teaching situation, communication skills such as empathy and sincere interest are used to establish a sense of rapport. Data about the type of learning disability help the nurse avoid the kind of content the client has difficulty processing. For example, the client may have difficulty with numbers but not with word concepts. Concrete concepts may present little difficulty, but abstract or symbolic material may require great effort to process. Some clients have trouble reproducing a word or picture from memory but experience little difficulty recognizing written words and symbols in picture format. Other clients have problems with written materials but have normal auditory processing skills for the words they hear. Fine motor

deficits can present as eye–hand coordination problems that can hamper learning psychomotor skills. Poor retention of multiple-step instructions, confusion about time relationships, and sequencing difficulties can be problems for some learning-disabled clients. In each case, the nurse's approach should convey understanding of the client's deficits. Supporting the client's strengths, using a mode of delivery the client can understand, and providing additional time for processing are key to successful instruction of the learning-disabled client.

Many learning-disabled clients have above average intelligence but need additional time to process information (Freed, 1998). Learning disabilities are amplified in high-stimuli environments and anxiety-provoking situations. Learning-disabled clients respond best to very small group or one-to-one teaching formats. The environment in which information is presented can be structured to limit distractions. New information is best presented in small units, using easily understood vocabulary and visual aids to make concepts "concrete." Choosing learning materials to compensate for client deficiencies and reinforce strengths, frequent positive reinforcement, and a strong, informed advocacy for the learning-disabled client help make the learning situation manageable. Many of these strategies are also useful with clients suffering from ADD.

### Developmental Level

Developmental level affects both teaching strategies and subject content, and the nurse will find that clients are at all levels of the learning spectrum with regard to their social, emotional, and cognitive development. However, developmental learning capacity is not always age related and is easily influenced by culture and stress. Parents can provide useful information about the child's immediate life experiences and use of words in relating to them.

Teaching strategies for young children should be simple, concrete, and directly linked with the child's immediate life experience. For example, in teaching preschoolers to swim, one instructor used an example of blowing up a balloon to help them understand how to breathe under water. One child did this easily because it was a part of her experience at home. The other preschooler seemed at a loss. In the next class, a substitute teacher taught the same concept using the example of blowing out a candle. This time the situation was reversed for the two children: The child who could not grasp the idea the first time was able to use the example of the candle and perform the teaching task. The other child experienced difficulty because she did not have a similar experience with blowing out candles. Other health personnel can record vocabulary words of importance on the chart as well for use.

School-age children struggling with Erikson's stage of industry have an interest in building competencies. Focusing teaching on the development of competency, whether physical, psychological, or cognitive, takes advantage of the child's natural stage of development. Children of this age are eager to learn about better ways of taking care of themselves. Box 15–5 presents an application of a teaching sequence for school-age children.

*Androgogy* refers to the "art and science of helping adults learn" (Knowles, 1980). According to Knowles, adult learners favor a problem-focused approach to learning. They are interested in learning skills and knowledge that will help them master life problems. Self-directedness is a key component of the adult teaching-learning process. Adults like to be in control of their learning process. They appreciate structure and advance organizers, but only as structures within which they can create their own sense of how the learning will apply in their lives. To facilitate the process, the nurse might use the following overview: "Today, I am going to give

---

### Box 15–6. Learning as a Natural Process

We cannot teach another person directly; we can only facilitate his learning.

A person learns significantly only those things which he perceives as being involved in the maintenance of, or enhancement of, the structure of self.

Experience that is perceived as inconsistent with self can only be assimilated if the current organization of self is relaxed and expanded to include it.

The educational situation that most effectively promotes significant learning is one in which the threat to the self of the learner is reduced to a minimum.

From Knowles M. (1990). The Adult Learner: A Neglected Species, pp. 3233. Copyright @ 1990 by Gulf Publishing Company, Houston, TX. Used with permission. All rights reserved.

---

you some information about food groups and specific quantities you will need to know about in controlling your diabetes. Then we can see how you might be able to incorporate this information into menu planning, given your work schedule and family eating habits." It is up to the adult client to help the nurse determine how these necessary changes in diet will be integrated into the client's current lifestyle.

Individual responsibility through taking action and reflecting on the consequences ensures ownership and stimulates learning in the adult client. The adult's orientation to learning is "life centered." Adult learners need to be able to see the practicality of what they are learning. Experience is a rich resource that can be used wisely in planning nursing interventions. They can discriminate between essential information and irrelevant data. Many adult learners are insulted when the nurse does not seem to know the difference. The adult client expects the nurse to inquire about previous life experience and to incorporate this knowledge into the teaching plan. Box 15–6 describes the natural learning process elements required for adult learners.

Elderly clients learn as well as younger clients if the material is presented in ways that acknowledge their different developmental learning

---

### Box 15–5. Application: Nutrition Class for Fifth Graders

1. Ask children to identify their favorite foods.
2. Present factual information about the pyramid.
3. Ask the children to tell their peers about the foods they eat and to identify the food groups to which they belong.
4. Give each child a diet worksheet to record his or her food intake for the next week; encourage the children to select foods from each food level.

needs. They respond best to learning formats that integrate knowledge from the past, involve the use of more than one sense, and are practical. Most elderly clients appreciate recognition of their long years of experience in choosing content. The elderly learner responds best in a learning milieu in which the nurse faces the client when talking and speaks clearly and slowly in a low-pitched voice.

The nurse needs to allow for the additional reaction time that elderly clients need (Kick, 1989; Kim, 1986). Sufficient time to practice and frequent praise encourage elderly clients to take an active role in their learning process. Frequent, shorter learning sessions are better than long formats.

The elderly client may have difficulty with some psychomotor tasks (e.g., removing bottle caps or filling syringes) because of dexterity loss. Pride may prevent the client from revealing this to the nurse. Assuming that elderly clients lack the capacity to understand the instructions is a common error. Health care providers often direct instruction to the elderly client's younger companion even when the client has no cognitive impairment. This action disconfirms the elderly client and diminishes self-worth. The sensitive nurse observes the client before implementing teaching and gears teaching strategies to meet the individual learning needs of each elderly client. Box 15–7 presents teaching strategies for use with clients at different developmental levels.

## Culture

Culture adds to the complexity of the teaching-learning process in health care. Culturally, learners come from many different value systems with different beliefs, interaction styles, and language backgrounds. Language barriers can make learning virtually impossible for a client. Pictures, the use of dictionaries, and the help of translators may be necessary supports to the learning process.

Incorporating the client's cultural beliefs about health into teaching promotes better acceptance. Such beliefs include assumptions about health and illness, the causes of and treatments for different types of illnesses, and traditionally accepted health actions or practices to prevent or treat illness.

Appropriate client education for culturally diverse clients should include both the client and the client's social support system (Tripp-Reimer & Afifi, 1989). In many cultures, the family assumes a primary role in the care of the client even when the client is physically and emotionally capable of self-care. All parties needing information, especially those expected to support the learning process of the client, should be included from the outset in developing a realistic teaching plan as well as implementing and evaluating the plan. Otherwise, the teaching plan may be sabotaged when the client goes home.

Client motivation and participation increase with the use of indigenous teachers and cultural recognition of learning needs. The culturally sensitive nurse develops knowledge of the preferred communication style of different cultural groups and uses this knowledge in choosing teaching strategies. For example, Native Americans like stories. Their tradition of telling stories orally is a primary means of teaching that the nurse can use as a teaching methodology. Box 15–8 presents guidelines for teaching the culturally diverse client.

## Self-Awareness

The nurse has an ethical and legal responsibility in health teaching to maintain the appropriate expertise and interpersonal sensitivity to client needs required for effective learning. Equally important is the need to understand the complexity of the teaching process in health care and to appreciate one's role as health educator. There are as many perceptual realities as there are persons. The nature of those realities makes each learning experience and the resources the client has to commit to the process different (Rogers, 1969).

It is easy enough to remain engaged and to provide interesting teaching formats for the self-directed, highly motivated learner. However, it takes energy and imagination to impart hope to clients and to stimulate their emotions and interest when they see little reason to participate in learning about self-care management. It is discouraging for the nurse when the client feels helpless and does not want to change, or participates with little change in outcome. There is a tendency to feel rejected when a client does not

---

**◆ Box 15–7. Recommended Teaching Strategies at Different Developmental Levels**

| Developmental Level | Recommended Teaching Strategies |
| --- | --- |
| Preschool | Allow child to touch and play with safe equipment. Relate teaching to child's immediate experience. Use child's vocabulary whenever possible. Involve parents in teaching. |
| School-age | Give factual information in simple, concrete terms. Focus teaching on developing competency. Use simple drawings, models to emphasize points. Answer questions honestly and factually. |
| Adolescent | Can use metaphors and analogies in teaching. Give choices and multiple perspectives. Incorporate the client's norm group values, personal identity issues in teaching strategies. |
| Adult | Involve client as an active partner in learning process. Encourage self-directed learning. Keep content and strategies relevant and practical. Incorporate previous life experience into teaching. |
| Elderly | Incorporate previous life experience into teaching. Accommodate for sensory and dexterity deficits. Use short, frequent learning sessions. Use praise liberally. |

---

**◆ Box 15–8. Suggested Strategies for Teaching the Culturally Diverse Client**

1. Speak slowly (plan the teaching session to last at least twice as long as a typical session).
2. Make the sentence structure simple (use active, not passive, voice; use a straightforward subject-verb pattern).
3. Avoid technical terms (for example, use "heart" rather than "cardiac"), professional jargon, and American idioms ("red tape").
4. Provide instructional material in the same sequence in which the patient should carry out the plan.
5. Do not assume you have been understood. Ask the patient to explain the protocol; optimally, if appropriate, obtain a return demonstration.

From Tripp-Reimer T, Afifi LA. (1989). Cross cultural perspectives on patient teaching. Nursing Clinics of North America 24(3):615. Reprinted with the permission of WB Saunders Company, Philadelphia.

value our information and betrayed when the outcomes do not match the effort the nurse has put into teaching the client. When these feelings occur, it is important to detach one's ego from achieving perfect success and to reflect on one's own motivations and investment in the process.

Health promotion is a mutual interpersonal process. The nurse is responsible for the health teaching. The client assumes responsibility for the outcome. At all times, the nurse respects the client's autonomy. Some clients want symptom relief, whereas others want more in-depth teaching. The desired level of change ultimately is up to the client. At the same time, the nurse has an ethical responsibility to provide appropriate health teaching, and the right to hope that if the information is not used now, perhaps later it will be.

## SUMMARY

Teaching for health promotion is a more concentrated form of therapeutic communication. Two theoretical frameworks, the health belief model and the health promotion model, are important in understanding the readiness of the client to participate in health-enhancing activities. Preventive health education is designed to teach people how to promote and maintain their highest level of wellness. Three types of health prevention—primary, secondary, and tertiary—are described. Effective preventive education starts where the client is and builds on the client's knowledge base and perceptual understandings. Learning takes place in three distinct yet often highly interrelated areas: cognitive, affective, and psychomotor. Learner variables, important as the foundation of client education, generally fall into two categories: client's readiness to learn and client's capacity to learn. Personal and community factors such as physical condition, literacy, culture, emotional context, interpersonal dynamics, and previous experience influence learning. Self-awareness and critical reflection of experiences, important in other aspects of the nurse–client relationship, continue to be significant elements for the nurse in teaching conversations with clients. Nurses participate routinely in community health promotion and disease prevention activities. They are a major resource in helping clients understand their illnesses and represent a primary intervention in assisting clients to develop effective ways of coping with illness. Helping clients achieve optimal wellness is the primary goal of all health teaching?

## REFERENCES

Bandura A. (1987). Human agency in social cognitive theory. American Psychologist 44:1175–1184.

Blackie C, Gregg R, Freeth D. (1998). Promoting health in young people. Nursing Standard 12(36):39–46.

Chandler C, Holden J, Kolander C. (1992). Counseling for spiritual wellness: Theory and practice. Journal of Counseling and Development 71:168–175.

Collier S. (1992). Mrs. Hixon was more than the C.V.A. in 251. RN '92 22(11):62–64.

Demuth J. (1989). Patient teaching in the ambulatory setting. Nursing Clinics of North America 24(3):645–654.

Doak CC, Doak LG, Root JH. (1985). Teaching Patients with Low Literacy Skills. Philadelphia, JB Lippincott.

Edelman C, Mandel C. (1998). Health Promotion Throughout the Lifespan. (4th ed.) St. Louis, Mosby–Year Book.

Fraser A. (1998). Health promotion for everyone. Nursing Standard 12(25):19.

Freed P. (1998). Perseverance: The meaning of patient education in psychiatric nursing. Archives of Psychiatric Nursing 12(2):107–113.

Gauthier C. (1993). Philosophical foundations of respect for autonomy. Kennedy Institute of Ethics Journal 3(1):21–37.

Glover J, Bruning R. (1990). Educational Psychology: Principles and Applications (3rd ed.). Glenview, IL, Scott, Foresman.

Hallett C. (1997). The helping relationship in the community setting: The relevance of Rogerian theory to the supervision of Project 2000 students. International Journal of Nursing Studies 34(6):415–419.

Hemmings D. (1998). Health promotion for people with learning disabilities in the community. Nursing Times 94(24):58–59.

Hoff B. (1987). The Tao of Pooh. New York, Penguin Books.

Jones P, Meleis A. (1993). Health is empowerment. Advances in Nursing Science 15(3):114.

Kick E. (1989). Patient teaching for elders. Nursing Clinics of North America 24(3):681–686.

Kim KK. (1986). Response time and health care learning of elderly patients. Research in Nursing and Health Care 9:233–236.

Knowles M. (1980). The Adult Learner: A Neglected Species (2nd ed.). Palo Alto, CA, Mayfield.

Kulbok P, Baldwin J, Cox C, Duffy R. (1997). Advancing discourse on health promotion: Beyond mainstream thinking. Advances in Nursing Science 20(1):12–20.

Levine M. (1980). The child with learning disabilities. In Scheiner A, Abroms I (eds.), The Practical Management of the Developmentally Disabled Child. St. Louis, MO, CV Mosby.

Maltby H, Robinson S. (1998). The role of baccalaureate nursing students in the matrix of health promotion. Journal of Community Health Nursing 15(3):135–142.

Manning S. (1992). The nurses I'll never forget. RN '92 22(8):47.

Mezirow J. (1990). Fostering Critical Reflection in Adulthood: A Guide to Transformative and Emancipatory Learning. San Francisco, Jossey-Bass.

Omizo M, Omizo S, d'Andrea M. (1992). Promoting wellness among elementary school children. Journal of Counseling and Development 71(3):194–198.

Pender N. (1996). Health Promotion in Nursing Practice (3rd ed.). Norwalk, CT, Appleton & Lange.

Prochaska J, DiClemente C, Norcross J. (1992). In search of how people change: Applications to addictive behaviors. American Psychologist 47(9):1102–1114.

Rogers C. (1969). Freedom to Learn: A View of What Education Might Become. Columbus, OH, Merrill.

Ruzicki D. (1989). Realistically meeting the educational needs of hospitalized acute and shortstay patients. Nursing Clinics of North America 24(3):629.

St. Claire P, Anderson N. (1989). Social network advice during pregnancy: Myths, misinformation and sound counsel. Birth 16(3):103–107.

Tripp-Reimer T, Afifi LA. (1989). Cross-cultural perspectives on patient teaching. Nursing Clinics of North America 24(3):613–619.

U.S. Department of Health and Human Services. (1991). Healthy People 2000. Washington, DC, U.S. Government Printing Office.

Vitousek K, Watson S, Wilson G. (1998). Enhancing motivation for change in treatment-resistant eating disorders. Clinical Psychology Review 18(4):391–420.

# 16

# Health Teaching in the Nurse–Client Relationship

Elizabeth Arnold

## OBJECTIVES

At the end of the chapter, the student will be able to

1. Define health teaching and describe the role of the nurse
2. Contrast selected theoretical frameworks used in health teaching
3. Identify different types of formats found in health teaching
4. Use the nursing process to develop, implement, and evaluate a teaching care plan
5. Specify teaching strategies relevant to health teaching
6. Describe applications in different care settings

---

*When adults teach and learn in one another's company, they find themselves engaging in a challenging, passionate, and creative activity. The acts of teaching and learning—and the creation and alteration of our beliefs, values, actions, relationships, and social forms that result from this—are ways in which we realize our humanity.*

Brookfield (1986)

---

368

❖❖ This chapter examines relevant health teaching principles in the nurse–client relationship and outlines strategies that the nurse can use to enhance the health and well-being of clients, families, and communities. Health teaching has always been an integral part of relationship but even more so in a managed-care health care delivery system with mandated limitations on time and resources (Greiner & Valiga, 1998). Nurses carry much larger caseloads and generally have much less time to spend with their clients. They must help their clients achieve favorable health outcomes with fewer visits and rely on creative teaching strategies to achieve this goal.

A radical shift in health care delivery from an illness-focused, hospital-based approach to a community-based, wellness-oriented care emphasis creates new learning conditions and a broader base of health teaching content that includes primary prevention and quality of life issues (Ragland, 1997).

## IMPORTANCE OF HEALTH TEACHING

The importance of health teaching as a fundamental nursing function is indisputable. The Joint Commission on Accreditation of Hospital Organizations (JCAHO) has established educational standards requiring health care agencies to provide systematic health education

- *Standard PF 1* specifies that the client and family must be provided with appropriate education to increase their knowledge of their diagnosis, illness and treatment needs, and the skills and behaviors needed to promote their recovery and rehabilitation.
- *Standard PF 2* specifies that the client and family receive education in line with their assessed learning needs, abilities, and readiness to learn and appropriate to their length of stay. Implicit in this standard is the need to use individualized teaching strategies.
- *Standard PF 3* specifies that discharge instructions given to the client and family are also provided to the care provider who will be responsible for the client's continuing care.
- *Standard PF 4* specifies that the health care agency must have an identifiable education plan demonstrating coordinated learning activities

and resources based on client and family needs. Implicit in this standard is ongoing health care team involvement in the educational process (Miller & Capps, 1997).

Professional nursing standards, developed by the American Nurses Association (ANA), also reinforce the importance of health teaching as an essential nursing intervention in the standard "the nurse assists clients, families, and groups to achieve satisfying and productive patterns of living through health teaching" (ANA, 1982). Most state Nurse Practice Acts mandate health teaching as an independent professional nursing function; third-party reimbursement for Medicare defines health teaching as a skilled nursing intervention.

Educating clients about their condition and treatment options is a legal and ethical responsibility of the nurse related to informed consent, as identified in Chapter 2. The nurse frequently is the health professional in the best position to judge the necessary amount of disclosure and individualized health teaching clients need to understand their health condition and the information required for informed consent.

Informed consent is designed to protect client rights. It must be voluntarily given for a specific act, and an adult with sound mind and no coercion must give it. Health teaching requirements include (1) explanation of the procedure, test, treatment; (2) description of possible risks and adverse effects; (3) description of potential benefits; and (4) disclosure of possible alternative procedures or treatments (Usher & Arthur, 1998). Opportunity to ask questions and to receive knowledgeable answers is an essential part of the health teaching process.

## BASIC CONCEPTS
### Definition

*Health teaching* is defined as a specialized creative interpersonal nursing intervention whereby the nurse provides information, emotional support, and health-related skill training to clients for the purpose of helping individuals and their families cope effectively with health problems and achieve maximum well-being.

Although health teaching is a term with many definitions, most do not address the complexity of the teaching process in health care (Wellard, Turner & Bethune, 1998). They fail to include the multiple communication factors required of the nurse, who must find creative ways to teach highly complex information that is practical, applicable, and appropriate to highly diverse learners. For example, the "learner" in a health care setting can be a client, the client's family, a caregiver, or a community. Whereas most teaching situations require that the students enter with a similar level of education and knowledge, health teaching must be designed to meet the diverse learning needs of individuals from markedly different socioeconomic, educational, and experiential backgrounds. In health care, a highly educated client, a noncompliant client, and a low-literacy client may have the same medical condition with similar needs for health teaching. Specific teaching strategies, type of involvement of others, and level of content will need to reflect these unique learning needs.

The process of health teaching involves assessing client learner needs, selecting the appropriate knowledge a client needs, planning and implementing the health teaching, and evaluating whether the desired behavioral or attitudinal change has occurred. Written documentation of all phases of the teaching learning process is necessary. Included in the documentation is the client's response to the health teaching.

## Health Teaching Domains

The scope of health teaching involve three domains: cognitive (understanding content), affective (changing attitudes and promoting acceptance), and psychomotor (hands-on skill development). The three domains are interrelated. Cognitive knowledge is a prerequisite to skill development and attitude change. When people practice a skill, they also develop "cognitive knowledge" about the factors that contribute to success and the actions that need to be avoided. Attitude changes always include cognitive information the person lacked previously about a situation or person.

*Cognitive learning* is most appropriate when a person lacks knowledge related to his or her illness and treatment (e.g., a client with a nursing diagnosis of knowledge deficit related to a recent diagnosis of diabetes). Key learning objectives for a diabetic client in the cognitive domain will involve an understanding of diabetes, the role of diet, exercise and insulin in diabetic control, and trouble signs that require immediate attention. The client obtains pertinent cognitive knowledge from hearing instructions, watching others, reading, and listening to experts. Cognitive outcomes include having a basic understanding of the disease process and treatment protocols and being able to apply new information to meet personal health needs. A teaching outcome in the cognitive domain might read "The client will be able 'to translate instructions on a medicine bottle into action'" (Redman, 1997, p. 39). Information clients and families need related to informed consent falls into the cognitive domain.

*Affective learning* refers to emotional learning with the goal of changing attitudes that inform and direct behavior related to compliance and acceptance of lifestyle modifications for optimal health and well-being. Behavioral change in the affective domain usually takes longer than increasing knowledge in the cognitive domain (Leahy & Kizilay, 1998) because people do not always accept their condition even though they "know" everything there is to know about it. It is a more personalized form of learning with desired outcomes of acceptance, compliance, and self-responsibility for health care.

---

◆   **Case Example**

Jack cognitively understands that adhering to his diabetic diet is essential to control of his diabetes. He can tell you everything there is to know about the relationship of diet to diabetic control. Although he follows his diet at home because his wife does the cooking, he eats snack foods at work and insists on extra helpings at dinner. Jack has an affective learning need to cope with treatment protocols successfully. Desired outcomes for Jack's learning in the affective domain include his accepting responsibility for treatment compliance and demonstrating an interest in learning more about self-care.

---

The nurse can use the motivational strategies presented in Chapter 15 to engage this client in taking the responsibility needed for self-care. Other teaching strategies include role-playing and discussions in a safe supportive atmosphere in which clients can explore their experiences openly.

*Psychomotor learning* refers to learning a skill through "hands-on practice." It is a critical prerequisite for self-care management of health because a person can learn only so much from reading about skill or through observation. "Doing it," receiving feedback, and practicing is the best way to master a psychomotor skill" (see Fig. 15–4). The nurse can demonstrate the skill followed by a return demonstration by the client with coaching from the nurse (e.g., teaching a diabetic client to titrate the dosage, fill the syringe, and self-inject). Performing the skill over and over again with constructive feedback allows the learner to become proficient as the skill becomes a natural part of the person's life. Outcomes relate to (1) being able to perform the motor skill, (2) developing confidence and proficiency in performing health care skills, and (3) being able to adjust the performance of the skill when challenged with new situations.

## Theoretical Frameworks

### PRECEDE Model

The PRECEDE (*P*redisposing, *R*einforcing, *E*nabling *C*auses in *E*ducational *D*iagnosis and *E*valuation) is a health education model that examines the components of behavioral intention that can influence an individual's willingness to learn new health-related behaviors. Developed by Greene and colleagues in 1980, this community-based health education model proposes that the learning needs of individuals must be assessed within the context of their community and social structures, rather than in isolation, for teaching success. This model examines the interaction of predisposing, enabling, and reinforcing factors as relevant to help ensure a successful teaching program (Table 16–1).

### Client-Centered Health Teaching

The process of health teaching is a client-centered process that integrates knowledge of the content area, self-awareness, and a good understanding of teaching-learning principles with knowledge of the client's learning needs and provision of emotional support. The same critical conditions for successful relationship—empathy, genuineness, respect—apply to health teaching. The nurse acts as a guide, information provider. As a *guide*, the nurse coaches clients on actions they can take to improve their health and offers suggestions on modifications needed as their condition changes. As information providers, the nurse helps clients become more aware of why, what, and how they can learn to take better care of themselves. The nurse acts as a knowledgeable resource to help the client think through choices and develop different perspectives (Rankin & Duffy-Stallings, 1996). As a *partner in learning*, the nurse collaborates with the client to understand barriers to treatment and to foster those that maintain or enhance optimal well-being. Through the nurse–client teaching relationship, clients begin to challenge old, unworkable ideas and habits, transform unproductive understandings and actions, and act on new perspectives.

Rogers (1983) described learning as a natural, human process in which people want to engage and viewed a client-centered interpersonal relationship as the ideal format in which learning takes place. The best teaching takes place when the learner has a positive relationship with the teacher. When most people think of their own learning, they typically find that their most satisfying learning experiences took place in a learning environment in which they felt accepted and valued. Their remembering of content almost

---

Table 16–1. **Behavioral Factors in the PRECEDE Model**

| | |
|---|---|
| Predisposing Factors: | Previous experience, knowledge, beliefs and values that can affect the teaching process—examples: culture, prior learning |
| Enabling Factors: | Environmental factors that facilitate or present obstacles to change—examples: transportation, scheduling, availability of follow-up |
| Reinforcing Factors: | Perceived positive or negative effects of adopting the new learned behaviors including social support—examples: family support, risk of recurrence, avoidance of a health risk |

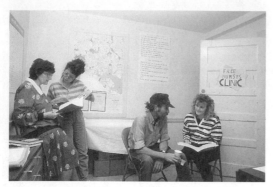

Health teaching can be done in one-to-one formats as well as in group formats. (Courtesy of the University of Maryland School of Nursing)

always contains recall of interactions with a teacher or mentor who believed in them, supported their self-integrity, and enhanced their self-worth. Conversely, memories of negative learning experiences often include having felt disconfirmed as a person. The following case example speaks to health teaching that confirms the learner.

### ◆ Case Example

"There was Nadine, who was an excellent preoperative teacher. She was the first person who clearly explained what a bladder augmentation entailed. She described different tubes I'd have and the purpose of each. When I returned from surgery, she helped me cope with my body image by teaching me how to use my bladder and by being a compassionate listener" (Manning, 1992, p. 47).

A client-centered teaching approach involves engaging clients as active partners in the learning process and helping them take responsibility for their own learning. There is no single correct way to teach. Teaching methodologies vary from situation to situation as the nurse strives to make new content comprehensible and interesting to the clients. Self-disclosure appropriate to the situation and the relationship adds to the human quality of the teaching experience.

### Concepts of Empowerment

The concept of empowerment is important in helping individuals and their families take charge of their health through teaching strategies emphasizing self-management. No single element or strategy ensures success, and the nurse does not motivate the client directly. Empowerment principles place the learner in charge of his or her learning and build on personal strengths to achieve learning objectives. A highly participative learning environment in which the nurse functions as a teaching instrument and the learner assumes primary responsibility for the learning process encourages empowerment (Post-White, 1998). Empowerment factors include motivation of the client to learn new behaviors, support of others (family, friends, others with the same condition, counselors, and clergy), models of appropriate behavior, goal setting, and relevant health information.

Empowerment strategies *enable* clients to take as much responsibility as possible for learning about their health alteration by letting them take the lead and encouraging them to be as creative as possible in devising health management strategies that has personal meaning. Spending time with the client initially to find out what is relevant from the client's perspective and building the teaching plan from the perspective of the client's need to know empowers the client.

In an empowering learning environment, nurses assume the role of providing enough information and emotional support—but no more than is required—to allow the client free access to unique ways of coping with health needs. The nurse, as teacher, provides content messages that describe health information in unambiguous, concrete, objective terms using the client's terminology and allows the client to respond in his or her unique way. Another principle the nurse can incorporate in the learning process includes giving instructions that are specific in meaning so that the client knows exactly what is expected.

Setting mutual goals with clients and following up with periodic reviews help clients become proactive in planning specific ways to achieve learning goals. The goals provide a benchmark for evaluating success. Clients who have specific and challenging goals coupled with ongoing support and reinforcement from the nurse do best. Reinforcement for successful performance encourages clients to continue learning because it offers immediate positive feedback and builds the client's confidence and self-esteem.

## Concepts of Critical Thinking

Helping clients achieve a sense of mastery includes the development of **critical thinking** strategies. These strategies provide a learning framework for problem solving through which persons can identify and analyze the assumptions underlying the actions, decisions, values, and judgments of themselves and others. These strategies help (1) guide actions, (2) decipher the meaning of unknown and uncertain reality, and (3) reassess the justification for what is already known.

The nurse can provide the client with adapting-teaching strategies that match the client's motivational stage and enhance the teaching process by giving examples and using analogies. Analogies may be used, such as "Think about how difficult it was for you to learn to ride a bicycle. Now that you know how to ride it, you don't worry about it because it is an automatic skill. The anxiety you are experiencing in learning how to give yourself insulin is similar. It will decrease with practice, and it will become an automatic part of your life." By using a reflective process, clients are able to generalize the problem-solving process beyond a specific situation.

Critical thinking facilitates learning by helping clients to restructure a problem so that it is amenable to change. Critical thinking is a creative, flexible process. The critical thinker develops the capacity to imagine entirely different and creative ways of thinking about and acting in a wide variety of life situations. Exercise 16–1 will enable the student to chart development of his or her own thinking skills. Imagination in critical thinking processes differs from intuitive thinking in that it is a disciplined cognitive process combined with analysis and synthesis of real data. The critical thinker considers other stake-holder positions such as those of the caregiver at home. An application of critical thinking to the teaching process requires that the nurse be as aware of potential pitfalls and limitations in thinking as of real possibilities in the situation.

## Behavioral Models

Many people look at behavioral models of learning with suspicion. The reality is that we all learn behaviors as the result of behavioral cues. Paychecks, performance appraisals, and disciplinary actions, for example, "reinforce" desired behavior and discourage unwanted behavior.

Behavioral approaches use a structured learning format in which learning occurs by linking a desired behavior with reinforcement for performing the behavior. Although sometimes viewed as a mechanistic learning strategy, behavioral approaches prove effective with individuals who are unable to process needed instruction cognitively and with clients who are unmotivated. Children, adolescents, and seriously mentally ill clients require skills training for very different reasons and respond best to behavioral learning strategies (Curran & Monti, 1986).

## Behavioral Concepts

### Reinforcement

**Reinforcement** refers to the situational consequences of performing specified behaviors. Behaviorists believe that reinforcement strengthens or weakens learner responses.

Skinner (1971) defined positive reinforcers as "any event that increases the probability of a response" and negative reinforcers as "any event that decreases the probability of a response." The different types of reinforcers used with behavioral approaches are found in Box 16–1.

To be effective, reinforcers should have meaning to the client. Referred to as the Premack principle, nurses need to choose activities and rewards that the client values. Reinforcement immediately after successful performance is more effective. Once the behavior is learned, the nurse can introduce new content and distribute rewards less frequently. Progressive learning challenges with appropriate support stimulate the client's interest and desire to continue learning.

### Modeling

**Modeling** is a behavioral strategy that refers to learning by observing another person performing a behavior. Nurses "model" behaviors both unconsciously and consciously in their normal conduct of nursing activities as well as in actual teaching situations. Bathing an infant, feeding an older person, and talking to a scared child in front of significant caregivers provide opportunities for informal teaching through modeling desired behaviors.

◆ Exercise 16–1. **Guidelines for Reflective Journals**

This exercise may be completed as a one-time experiential learning exercise, or it may be used over a semester.

**Definition:**
Reflection is ''the process of reviewing one's repertoire of clinical experience and knowledge to invent novel approaches to complex clinical problems. Reflection also provides data for self-examination and increases learning from experience'' (Saylor, 1990, p. 8.).

**Purpose:**
The capacity to examine one's actions, thoughts, and feelings about professional practice is of particular significance in the development of professional attitudes. Reflective journals allow students to raise important questions, reflect on activities and progress, and consider new approaches and resources.

**Procedure:**
Your *first* journal entry should be a short narrative reflecting on the persons, circumstances, situations, and values that drew you to consider nursing as a profession.

In *subsequent* weeks, or as a one-time learning experience, your journal entry should focus on your educational experience and address the following questions:

What was the most significant experience I had this week? (The experience can be an incident, an encounter, or a discovery about self, client, nursing professor, nursing profession.)
In what ways was it important?
What questions did it raise for me personally? Professionally?
How could I use what I learned from this experience in my nursing practice?

**Discussion:**
1. what makes an incident significant for a person?
2. How do people learn from critical incidents in their lives?
3. In what ways did you use critical thinking to develop the meaning of this incident?
4. In what ways can you use this exercise in future nursing practice?

---

◆ Box 16–1. Types of Reinforcement

| Concept | Purpose | Example |
|---|---|---|
| Positive reinforcer | Increases probability of behavior through reward | Stars on a board, smiling, verbal praise, candy, tokens to purchase items |
| Negative reinforcer | Increases probability of behavior by removing aversive consequence | Restoring privileges when client performs desired behavior |
| Punishment | Decreases behavior by presenting a negative consequence or removing a positive one | Time outs, denial of privileges |
| Extinguishing | Decreases behavior by ignoring it | Disregards undesired behavior and ignores the person when behavior is performed |

## Shaping

*Shaping* is the term used to describe specific behavioral steps that result in the desired behavior. Shaping as a behavioral strategy to increase learning is a common occurrence in our lives. The grades students receive in this course, the approval or disapproval of an instructor, and written comments on care plans and papers all help "shape" student behaviors by providing positive or negative reinforcement of their learning. In health care, providing constructive feedback and verbally encouraging client efforts reinforce learning and shapes future attempts. Simple building steps also move the learner from the familiar to the unfamiliar.

## Implementing a Behavioral Approach

The nurse starts the teaching process using a behavioral approach with a careful description of the behavior requiring change. Each behavior is described as a single behavior unit (e.g., failing to take a medication, cheating on a diet, participating in unit activities). Numerical unit assignment allows the nurse and the client to monitor progress and to chart setbacks.

The next step in the process is to define the problem in behavioral terms and to validate the problem statement with the client (e.g., "The client does not take his medication as prescribed" or "The client does not attend any unit activities"). A behavioral approach requires the cooperation of the client and a mutual understanding of the problem on the part of the nurse and the client. Active listening skills will alert the nurse to any concerns or barriers to implementation.

Next the nurse and client reframe the problem as a solution statement (e.g., the client the client will attend all scheduled unit activities). If the problem and solution are complex, the nurse breaks them down into simpler definitions, beginning with the simplest and most likely behavior to stimulate client interest. The nurse identifies the tasks in sequential order, defines specific consequences, positive and negative, for behavioral responses, and solicits the client's cooperation.

Once these steps are complete, the nurse establishes a learning contract with the client that serves as a formal commitment to the learning process. This contract describes

- Behavioral changes that are to occur
- Conditions under which they are to occur
- Reinforcement schedule
- Time frame

Contracts spell out the responsibilities of each party and the consequences if behaviors are implemented or, in the case of undesired behaviors, persist. The nurse rewards the client for each instance of expected behavior. If the client is noncompliant or needs to pay more attention to a particular aspect of behavior, the nurse can say, "This (name the behavior or skill) needs a little more work." One advantage of a behavioral approach is that it never considers the client as bad or unworthy.

◆ **Case Example**

Peggy Braddock, a student nurse, was working with a seriously mentally ill client with diabetes. All types of strategies were used to help the client take responsibility for collecting and testing her urine. Regardless of whether she was punished or pushed into performing these activities, the client remained resistant. To avoid taking her insulin injections, the client would take urine from the toilets or would simply refuse to produce a urine sample. Peggy decided to use a behavioral approach with her. She observed that the client liked sweets. Consequently, the reward she chose was artificially sweetened Jell-O cubes. To earn a Jell-O cube, the client had to bring her urine to Peggy. After some initial testing of Peggy's resolve to give the cubes only for appropriate behavior, the client began bringing her urine on a regular basis. Once this behavior was firmly established, Peggy began to teach the client how to give her own insulin. The reward remained the same. Peggy also used the time she spent with the client to build trust and acceptance. She wrote her plan in the Kardex, and other nurses used the same systematic approach with the client. Over time, the client took full responsibility for testing her urine and for administering her own insulin.

Exercise 16–2 is designed to provide experience working with some of the common elements of a behavioral learning approach.

## APPLICATIONS
## Constructing a Teaching Plan
### *Assessment*

For health teaching to be effective, the nurse and client must have a clear understanding of actual

◆ Exercise 16–2. **Using a Behavioral Approach**

**Purpose:** To help students gain an appreciation of the behavioral approach in the learning process

**Procedure:**
Think about a relationship you have with one or more people that you would like to improve. The person you choose may be a friend, teacher, supervisor, peer worker, parent, or sibling.

1. Set a goal for improving that relationship.
2. Develop a problem statement as the basis for establishing your goal.
3. Identify the behaviors that will indicate you have achieved your goal.
4. Identify the specific behaviors you will have to perform to accomplish your goal.
5. Identify the personal strengths you will use to accomplish your goal.
6. Identify potential barriers to achieving your goal.
7. In groups of four or five students, present your goal-setting agenda, and solicit feedback.

**Discussion:**
1. Do any of your peers have ideas or information that might help you reach your goals?
2. Are there any common themes, strengths, or behaviors related to goal setting that are found across student groups?
3. What did you learn about yourself that might be useful in helping clients develop goals using a behavioral approach?

and potential health problems. Nurses use a variety of sources to gather and validate data with special attention paid to the factors presented in Chapter 15 related to client readiness and ability to learn. From the start, the nurse actively engages the client in the teaching process. Assessment focuses on *predisposing factors* within the client as well as on informational aspects needed by the client.

• What specific information does the client need to enhance self-management?
• What attitudes does the client hold that potentially could enable or hinder the learning process?
• What specific skills does this client need for self-management?

Checking out how much the client already knows aids the nurse in knowing the appropriate level and amount of knowledge the client needs to have for self-care management. The nurse gives the client permission to ask questions, and by introducing the idea that most people do have questions, the client feels freer to question data or ask for more explanation.

Probing the learner's beliefs about his or her illness and proposed treatment is an essential aspect of the assessment process. Beliefs and values influence learning. For example, the client who believes that any drugs taken into the body are harmful will have a hard time learning about the insulin injection he needs to take every day. The client who thinks that if one tablet to relieve pain is good and thus two must be better may not understand the need to take only one pill every 4 hours.

Preliminary questions in a teaching assessment can include "Can you tell me what this illness has been like for you," and "Can you tell me what your doctor has told you about your treatment?" Types of follow-up questions the nurse can use to assess client learning needs are found in Box 16–2. Through the client's responses to key questions, the goals of a teaching plan begin to emerge. The nurse will want to explore potential *enabling factors* such as limited health insurance, transportation difficulties, lack of follow-up facilities, and cultural dietary considerations so that these factors will not be barriers to the client's implementation of the teaching plan.

If other family members will be involved in

> ◆ Box 16–2. Questions to Assess
> Learning Needs

> What does the client already know about his or her condition and treatment?
>
> In what ways is the client affected by it?
>
> In what ways are those intimately involved with the client affected by the client's condition or treatment?
>
> To what extent is the client willing to take personal responsibility for seeking solutions?
>
> What goals would the client like to achieve?
>
> What will the client need to do to achieve those goals?
>
> What resources are available to the client and family that might affect the learning process?
>
> What barriers to learning exist?

the care of the client, the nurse will need to assess the family's general patterns of health care behaviors, expectations for the client, and knowledge of the client's condition is significant assessment data. Many well-planned teaching interventions do not produce the desired outcomes because the family fails to understand or fully support the client's efforts to implement new behaviors (*reinforcing factors*). At the conclusion of the assessment interview, the nurse needs to summarize important points. This strategy helps to validate any misinformation the nurse may have about the assessment data that has been collected. Exercise 16–3 provides practice with collecting assessment data as a basis for establishing nursing diagnoses in health teaching.

## Planning

Health teaching addresses specific health care needs. Sample nursing diagnoses that respond to teaching interventions are found in Box 16–3. The nursing diagnosis clarifies the specific nature of the learning need. For example, a knowledge deficit related to a lack of knowledge about signs and symptoms of hyper- and hypoglycemia requires different content and strategies from a nursing diagnosis of "knowledge deficit related to how to prefill syringes and administer insulin."

Teaching plans should focus on what the client *needs* to know. Smith (1987) noted that nurses often teach too much detail about the fine medical or scientific points of a condition and too

little about the side effects of medication, self-care management, and coping strategies. This situation occurs when the nature of the knowledge deficit is assumed rather than developed with the client. To forestall this happening, the nurse might give a broad opening. For example, the nurse could say "There is some information I'd like to give you that will be useful for you to know before you go home, but first I'd like to ask you a few questions that will help me better understand your needs. Is that okay with you?"

Although it is important to keep health teaching concise, incomplete information can be dangerous. For example, a nurse on the evening shift instructed an 85-year-old man to keep his arm in an upright position after a treatment procedure. The nurse neglected to tell him that he could release his arm once the needle was securely in place. The man called his wife at 5 A.M. the next day to tell her he did not think he could hold his arm in that position any longer. The man had been awake all night, his arm felt numb, and he was at his wits' end because of incomplete health teaching. Too much information puts the learner into informational overload so that critical content is not learned; not enough direction can also prove harmful.

### Developing Learning Goals

Setting clear learning goals that the client is interested in meeting and has the necessary resources to achieve is essential to success. Questions that help the client take an active role in setting goals include "How would you like for things to be different?" and "Let's take one step at a time. What do you think would be a good first step?" The answers to these questions give the client autonomy in choosing goals and the nurse important information as to whether the client's goals are realistic.

In developing relevant goals, the nurse focuses on what the client and family *want* to know about a topic as well as what they need to know. Client interest is a good place to start, whenever possible. Health teaching goals should be comprehensive enough to provide needed information and yet narrow enough to be achievable. Included in the development of outcome goals is a broad statement about what the client needs to achieve maximum health potential (e.g., "Following health teaching, the client will maintain dietary

◆ **Exercise 16-3. Role-Play of an Assessment Interview**

**Purpose:** To develop an appreciation for the many aspects of an assessment interview

**Procedure:**
1. Recall an experience that you, a member of your family, a friend, or an acquaintance had with an illness requiring health treatment that you would be willing to share with your class group. You should have enough information about the person to assume the general characteristics of the situation.
2. Using the factors identified in Chapter 15, role-play the person you chose.
3. Select a partner, and role-play the part of the person as though you were a client.
4. Your partner should take on the role of the interviewer and use the questioning guidelines in the assessment interview to develop an appropriate assessment from the role-play. (20 minutes)
5. Reverse the process with your partner so that each participant has an opportunity to experience each role. (20 minutes)

**Discussion:**
1. Which was the harder role to take: client or interviewer?
2. Were you surprised at any of the information that emerged?
3. After doing this exercise, what pieces of information do you think are most relevant?
4. What kinds of nursing diagnoses could you develop from this assessment information?
5. What implications for future nursing practice do you see from doing this exercise?

control of his diabetes"). An interim goal might be "Following health teaching, the client will develop a ADA diet plan for 1 week." Setting realistic goals prevents disappointment on the part of both nurse and client. Achieving small goals stimulates success and encourages the client to take charge. Box 16-4 summarizes guidelines to use in the development of effective health teaching goals and objectives.

Exercise 16-4 provides experience with developing relevant behavioral goals.

### Establishing Priorities

In today's health care environment, time is an issue. Teaching goals often need to be modest, and the content can cover only essential content. Here the nurse needs to structure the learning session to include the key elements: "What is the minimum information the client needs to know?" and "What kinds of activities are abso-

---

◆ **Box 16-3. Sample Nursing Diagnoses Amenable to Health Teaching**

| | |
|---|---|
| Potential for injury or violence | Anxiety |
| Ineffective coping | Noncompliance |
| Alterations in parenting or family process | Impaired home maintenance management |
| Self-care deficits | Knowledge deficit |

---

◆ **Box 16-4. Guidelines for Developing Effective Goals and Objectives**

- Link them to the nursing diagnosis.
- Make them action oriented.
- Make them specific and measurable.
- Define objectives as behavioral outcomes.
- Design objectives with a specific time frame for achievement.
- Show a logical progression with established priorities.
- Review periodically and modify as needed.

---

◆ Exercise 16-4. **Developing Behavioral Goals**

**Purpose:** To provide practical experience with developing teaching goals

**Procedure:**
Establish a nursing diagnosis related to health teaching and a teaching goal that supports the diagnosis in each of the following situations:

1. Jimmy is a 15-year-old adolescent who has been admitted to a mental health unit with disorders associated with impulse control and conduct. He wants to lie on his bed and read Steven King novels. He refuses to attend unit therapy activities.
2. Maria, a 19-year-old single woman, is in the clinic for the first time because of cramping. She is 7 months pregnant and has had no prenatal care.
3. Jennifer is overweight and desperately wants to lose weight. However, she cannot walk past the refrigerator without stopping, and she finds it difficult to resist the snack machines at work. She wants a plan to help her lose weight and resist her impulses to eat.

**Discussion:**
1. What factors did you have to consider in developing the most appropriate diagnosis and teaching goals for each client?
2. In considering the diagnosis and teaching goals for each situation, what common themes did you find?
3. What differences in each situation contributed to variations in diagnosis and teaching goals? What contributed to these differences?
4. In what ways can you use the information in this exercise in your future nursing practice?

---

lutely essential for the client and family to have knowledge of in meeting client health care needs?" Focusing on a specific topic is better than trying to cover a global subject. Everything else should be treated as extraneous data to be saved for a different time or referred elsewhere.

Health teaching can never be eliminated because the nurse lacks time, but it can be streamlined. Even in the most limited situation, scheduling a definite block of time for teaching to occur is essential. Otherwise, other duties will always receive higher priority.

Matching teaching strategies with client need is important. For example, children should be given general information without going into too much detail, whereas adults usually need details. Clients with English as a second language may require additional learning time. Clients experiencing a procedure for the first time need to have more detailed information than clients who require only follow-up information.

### Developing Measurable Objectives

Health teaching objectives describe the tasks needed to accomplish identified goals. They should be achievable, measurable, and related to specific health outcomes. To determine whether an objective is achievable, consider the client's level of experience, educational level, resources, and motivation. Then define the specific learning objectives needed to achieve the health goal. The objectives, like the terminal health goal, should relate to the nursing diagnosis. For example, the nursing diagnosis might read "Knowledge deficit related to diabetic diet." The expected outcome might be "Dietary control of diabetes by time of discharge in 60 days." Each related learning objective should describe a single learning task. Including the time frame by which each objective should be achieved reinforces commitment. Examples of progressive learning objectives related to diabetic control might include the following:

• The client will identify the purpose of a diabetic

diet and appropriate foods by the end of the first teaching session.

- The client will identify appropriate foods and serving sizes allowed on a diabetic diet by the end of the second teaching session.
- The client will demonstrate actions for urine testing for sugar at home by the third teaching session.
- The client will identify foods to avoid on the diabetic diet and the rationale for compliance by the fourth teaching session.
- The client will describe symptoms and actions to take for hyperglycemia and hypoglycemia by the end of the fifth teaching session.
- The client will develop a food plan for one week by discharge in two weeks.

## Structuring the Environment

The type of teaching format determines the most appropriate setting. Teaching sessions conducted in a quiet, well-lighted area stress the importance of the learning endeavor. If health teaching is done in the home, all of those involved in the health care of the client should be included. Small children need to be cared for elsewhere, and the telephone should not become a distraction. Stating these conditions before the teaching session begins prevents misunderstandings and unnecessary disturbances. In hospital situations, the client frequently is in bed or sitting in a chair. The learning environment is relatively informal, but having enough space for equipment and demonstration is critical.

## Timing

Timing is essential because learning takes place only when the learner is ready. The client's condition, energy level, and emotional attitudes may temporarily preclude teaching. If possible, the client should choose the best time for health teaching. When this is not possible, the nurse needs to make every attempt to pick times when energy levels are high, the client is not distracted by other things, it is not visiting time, and the client is out of pain. Some people learn better in the morning; others are more alert in early evening. Careful observation of the client will help determine the most appropriate times for learning. Consider when the client is more talkative and interested in what is going on.

Allowing the client enough time to process a difficult diagnosis or change in condition may be critical before health teaching can begin. It is futile to engage in a serious teaching process when the client is unreceptive. This does not mean that the nurse abandons the teaching project, but simply that the "stage" must be set before the "play" can begin.

Timing is a significant issue in planning the duration of teaching sessions. The nurse needs to consider how much time is needed to learn this particular skill or body of knowledge. Complicated and essential skills need blocks of time and repeated practice with feedback. Some clients can absorb only a small amount of information at a time. Some information can be provided as written back-up material.

Not all health teaching is formal. Simple, spontaneous health teaching takes minutes, yet it can be as effective as more formal teaching sessions. For example, in *Heartsounds*, the wife of a heart patient noted that

---

A nurse came in while he was eating dinner. "Dr. Lear," she said, "after angiography the patients always seem to have the same complaints, and I thought you might want to know about them. It might help." (This was a good nurse. I didn't know it then, because I didn't know how scared he was. But later I understood that this was a damned good nurse.) "Thanks, it would help," he said. "It's mostly two things. The first is, they say that during the test, they feel a tremendous rush. It's very sudden and it can be scary."

. . . Now he told the nurse, "Okay, the flush. And what's the other thing?"

"It's . . . well, they say that at a certain point, they feel as though they are about to die. But that feeling passes quickly." He thanked her again. He was very grateful.

(Lear, 1980)

---

Later, during the actual procedure, Dr. Lear remembers the nurse's words and finds comfort:

---

Easy. Easy. You're supposed to feel this way. This is precisely what the nurse described. The moment you feel you are dying.

(Lear, 1980)

---

This teaching intervention probably took less than 2 minutes, yet its effect was long lasting and healing. There are countless opportunities for this type of health teaching in clinical practice if the nurse consciously looks for them.

Timing and length of sessions are important issues for learners handicapped by memory deficits, lack of insight, poor judgment, and limited problem-solving abilities. These learners respond best to a learning environment in which the content is presented in a consistent, concrete, and patient manner, *with clear and frequent cues to action.* Providing sufficient time to practice and offering frequent encouragement help elderly clients who have difficulty learning in sophisticated, fast-paced environments (Brillhart & Stewart, 1989; Check & Wurzbach, 1984). Box 16–5 covers important aspects of timing in health teaching.

**Selecting Appropriate Content**

Essential content in most teaching plans includes information about the health care problem, risk factors, treatment, and self-care skills the client will need to manage at home (Lee et al., 1998). Attitudes that will affect the client's adjustment and compliance with treatment also require attention.

---

◆ Box 16–5. Factors Involved in Timing

Client readiness
Time needed to learn skill or body of knowledge
Possible need for attitude change by client
Time constraints of nurse
Client priorities about information or skill
Client's energy level
Atmosphere of trust

---

The nurse should consider the client's perception of the acceptability of the content. Some topics are more acceptable and more easily learned than others. Is the content complicated or likely to make the client uncomfortable? If so, the nurse must be able to organize it in such a way that the client can relate to it. Clients learn more effectively when they understand the goals of the learning session and when the content helps them connect new knowledge to what they already know.

To make content comprehensible to the client is an art. Content that builds on the person's experiences, abilities, interests, motivation, and skills is more likely to engage the learner's attention. Attention to the reading level of clients helps ensure that the pamphlet can be read. Clients with perceptual difficulty or an inability to speak can sometimes respond to picture boards and line drawings. Large print pamphlets and audiotapes are learning aids for those with sight problems (Smith, 1987).

**Selecting Appropriate Teaching Methods**

No one teaching strategy can meet the needs of all clients. Recognizing distinctive differences in client learning needs is critical in choosing the most appropriate teaching strategies.

Additionally, in health care the nurse needs to adjust teaching strategies to meet client needs as their medical condition changes. Preoperation teaching strategies should differ from those used immediately after the operation. The amount of information given, the pace of the teaching, and the level of learner involvement necessarily reflect the client's physical condition and learning needs in each time frame (Fig. 16–1).

Planning to use a variety of teaching strategies is most effective. For example, mothers respond positively to posters showing normal infant features and development because they can see as well as hear that head molding and skin rashes are typical. The nurse might provide one-to-one instruction for the client related to diabetic teaching, with additional sessions scheduled to include the family caregiver in open discussion of dietary modifications if this person prepares the meals. Another factor to consider is how people learn best. Box 16–6 displays characteristics of different learning styles.

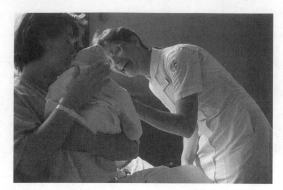

Figure 16–1. Affective learning can include role modeling. (Courtesy of the University of Maryland School of Nursing)

## Implementation

A key element in successful health teaching is an enthusiastic presentation that demonstrates a thorough knowledge of the subject matter, a keen understanding of the client's learning needs, and a genuine interest in the client. The client must be actively involved in the process. Effective teaching involves not only a healthy exchange of information but plenty of opportunities to ask questions and to receive feedback.

### Sequencing the Learning Experience

Presentations in which ideas logically relate to one another are more effective than those that are poorly organized. People learn best when there is a logical flow and building of information from simple to complex. Information that builds on previous knowledge and experience is even

better. The nurse sets the stage for the learning process by presenting a simple overview of what will be taught and why the information will be important to them. The overview is followed by the main points the nurse needs to cover with opportunity for client feedback. If the material is complex, it can be broken down into smaller learning segments. For example, diabetic teaching could include

• Introduction, including what does the client know
• Basic pathophysiology of diabetes
• Diet and exercise
• Demonstration of insulin injection with return demonstration
• Recognizing signs and symptoms of hyper- and hypoglycemia
• Care of skin and feet
• How to talk to the doctor

It is important to allow enough time for questions. A strong closing summarizing major points reinforces the learning process. Exercise 16–5 provides practice with developing a miniteaching plan.

### Using Clear Language

Using clear and precise language is critical to understanding because many words have several meanings even in English. For example, the word "cold" can refer to temperature, an illness, an emotional tone, or a missed opportunity. Providing information with abstract and vague language leaves the learner wondering what the nurse actually meant. For example, "Call the doctor if you

---

### ◆ Box 16–6. Characteristics of Different Learning Styles

| Visual | Auditory | Kinesic |
|---|---|---|
| Learns best by seeing | Learns best with verbal instructions | Learns best by doing |
| Likes to watch demonstrations | | Hands-on involvement |
| Organizes thoughts by writing them down | Likes to walk things through | Needs action and likes to touch, feel |
| Needs detail | Detail not as important | Loses interest with detailed instructions |
| Looks around; examines situation | Talks about situation: pros, cons | Tries things out |

◆ **Exercise 16–5. Developing Teaching Plans**

**Purpose:** To provide practice with developing teaching plans

**Procedure:**
1. Develop a miniteaching plan for one of the client situations listed below.
2. Use guidelines presented in Chapters 15 and 16 in the development of your teaching plan.
3. Include the following data: a brief statement of client learning needs and a list of related nursing diagnoses in order of priority. For one nursing diagnosis, develop a long-term goal, short-term learning objectives, a teaching time frame, content to be covered, teaching strategies, and methods of evaluation.

**Situations:**
1. Jim Dolan feels stressed and is requesting health teaching on stress management and relaxation techniques.
2. Adrienne Parker is a newly diagnosed diabetic. Her grandfather had diabetes.
3. Vera Carter is scheduled to have an appendectory in the morning.
4. Marion Hill just gave birth to her first child. She wants to breast-feed her infant, but she does not think she has enough milk.
5. Barbara Scott wants to lose weight.

have any problems" can mean many different things. "Problems" can refer to side effects of the medication, a return of symptoms, problems with family acceptance, changed relationships, and even alterations in self-concept. The best way to provide information and instructions is to use clear behavioral descriptions that include

• Who needs to be involved
• Identification of specific behaviors
• What needs to happen
• Under what specific circumstances

An example of a clear statement the nurse might use is "If you should develop a headache or feel dizzy in the next 24 hours, call the emergency room doctor right away."

### Using Visual Aids

Visual aids are useful tools to supplement the words of the nurse because they help reinforce a message and provide concrete visual images. Simple images and few words work better than complex visual aids (Huntsman & Binger, 1981). Visual aids are particularly relevant in explaining complex anatomy or displaying external symp-

toms such as a rash or mole changes. For example, the nurse might show a client a skeleton model to explain a collapsed disc. A chart or model showing the heart might help another client understand the anatomy and physiology of a heart disorder.

Films and videotapes are especially useful in teaching clients with limited reading skills, and they have the advantage of allowing clients to

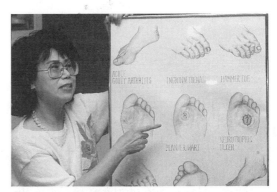

Visual aids provide concrete images that help clients remember essential information. (Courtesy University of Maryland School of Nursing)

◆ Exercise 16-6. **Using Advance Organizers as a Teaching Strategy**

**Purpose:** To help students understand the value of verbal cues (advance organizers) in health teaching

**Procedure:**
1. Identify a segment of course content you need to know or a skill you need to learn, and develop a mnemonic to organize and help you remember it.
2. Write down the verbal cue and explicitly what it stands for in helping you remember important information.
3. Share your results with your classmates in the group.

**Discussion:**
1. In what ways was it easy or difficult for you to develop your mnemonic?
2. What benefits or difficulties do you envision in using it?
3. Do mnemonics work better for some types of information than others?
4. In what ways can you use the insights you gained in your future nursing practice?

watch them at their convenience. Later discussion with the nurse helps to correct misinterpretations and emphasize pertinent points.

## Using Advance Organizers

Advance organizers, consisting of cue words related to more complex data, help clients anticipate and respond to more complex information in their own minds. Using a *mnemonic*, defined as a key letter, word, or phrase, helps clients organize important ideas. For example, the nurse might use the word "diabetes" to help a client remember key concepts about diabetes.

D = diet
I = infections
A = administering medications
B = basic pathophysiology
E = eating schedules
T = treatment for hyper/hypoglycemia
E = exercise
S = symptom recognition

Each letter stands for one of the concepts needed for comprehensive diabetic education. Taken together, the client has a useful tool for remembering *all* of the important concepts. A mnemonic can be letters of the alphabet, places, or words, in fact any associations that have personal or group meanings for the persons developing them. Nursing students can use mnenomics to help them remember key points. The word

association fosters identification in much the same way that linking new information to previously learned information does. For example, the four Fs (fat, forty, female, family history) can help students remember risk factors for gallbladder disorder. Developing mnemonics can be fun and creative. Exercise 16–6 provides an opportunity to see the value of mnemonics in learning content.

## Providing Transitional Cues

Sometimes people do not understand an instruction because the nurse fails to make the necessary transitions that link one idea to another. Johnson noted that "being complete and specific seems so obvious, but often people do not communicate the frame of reference they are using, the assumptions they are making, the intentions they have in communicating or the leaps in thinking they are making" (quoted in Flanagan, 1990). Directions may seem simple and obvious to the nurse, but clients may have difficulty with elementary material simply because the information is new to them. Transition statements can help the client see how the ideas fit together.

### ◆ Case Example

Statement A

**Nurse:** The doctor wants you to take a half a pill for the first week and increase the dose to a full pill after the first week. You should call him if you experience any side effects such as nausea or headaches.

Statement B

**Nurse:** This medication works well for most people, but some people tolerate it better than others. The doctor would like you to take a half a pill for the first week so that your system has a chance to adapt to it, and the doctor can see how you are responding before you take the full dose. If you have no side effects, he would like you to increase the dose to a full pill after the first week. The most common side effects are nausea or headaches. They don't occur with most people, but each person's response to medication is a little different. He would like you to call him if you notice these side effects.

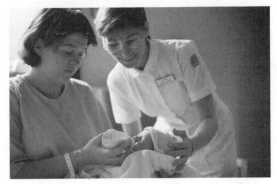

Giving immediate feedback is important with learning psychomotor tasks. (Courtesy University of Maryland School of Nursing)

Although the second statement takes a little longer, it includes clear transitions between ideas that will make it easier for the client to remember the instructions. Including transitional cues helps the client to see the rationale for the change in dosage, and because it seems logical, there is a greater probability of compliance.

## Repeating Key Concepts

Most learners need more than one exposure to new content or skill development. Review new information frequently. If possible, have more than one session for each learning segment. Although it may feel redundant, repeating yourself and restating key elements help the client process material by going over it mentally. Having the opportunity to practice self-care skills that the client can apply immediately enhances the teaching process (Bohny, 1997). Allowing extra time for the client to talk about and do return demonstrations of tasks reinforces learning.

## Giving and Seeking Feedback

In a research study of factors considered necessary to a successful patient teaching program on medications, clients identified feedback as an essential element (Mullen & Green, 1985). To appreciate its significance, consider your performance if you did not receive feedback from your instructor. Feedback about how the client is accomplishing teaching goals should be descriptive, not evaluative, and should include both posi-

tive and negative elements. One way of doing this is to describe all of the behaviors that contributed to an outcome rather than selectively choosing only those in need of alteration.

Effective feedback is honest and based on concrete data. It is important to differentiate between observational data and personal interpretations or conclusions, and to focus on the "what" needs to change, not the "why" of behaviors. Determining motivation is a guessing game, because most of the time noncompliance is multifactorial.

Many clients respond better to teaching feedback that allows them to explore alternatives rather than a direct solution. The nurse's solution, brilliant though it may be, may not work for a client because the problem, as the client perceives it, is different. Other times, the client and nurse view a problem similarly, but the client is aware of flaws in the nurse's proposal that would make it difficult for the client to implement it. Feedback usually should be designed to stimulate further discussion.

Feedback given as soon as possible after observation is more likely to be accurately reported and hence more readily accepted by the client. Behavioral statements on a continuum (i.e., "You need a little more practice" or "You are able to draw up the medication okay, but you need a little more work with selecting sites") are more effective than absolute statements such as "You still are not doing this correctly." Exercise 16–7 provides practice with giving feedback in health teaching.

---

◆ Exercise 16-7. **Giving Teaching Feedback**

**Purpose:** To give students perspective and experience in giving usable feedback

**Procedure:**
Divide the class into working groups of three or four students.

1. Give a 3-minute sketch of some aspect of your current learning situation that you find difficult (e.g., writing a paper, speaking in class, coordinating study schedules, or studying certain material).
2. Each person in turn offers one piece of usable, informative feedback to the presenter. In making suggestions, use the guidelines on feedback given in this chapter.
3. Feedback suggestions are placed on a flip chart or chalkboard.

**Discussion:**
1. What were your thoughts and feelings about the feedback you heard in relation to resolving the problem you presented to the group?
2. What were your thoughts and feelings in giving feedback to each presenter?
3. Was it harder to give feedback in some cases than in others? In what ways?
4. What common themes emerged in your group?
5. In what ways can you use the self-exploration about feedback in this exercise in teaching conversations with clients?

---

Indirect feedback given through nodding, smiling, and sharing information about the process and experiences of others reinforces learning. Acknowledging the contributions of participants in group learning provides encouragement for active participation, and repeating questions or answers emphasize key concepts.

Another strategy is to ask the client to repeat the instructions in his or her own words and to describe for the nurse the actions that need to be taken if the instructions cannot be followed exactly or fail to produce the desired effect. Asking the client to repeat as you go along reinforces each piece of information and eliminates the problem of delivering a comprehensive teaching plan only to discover that the client lost your train of thought after the first few sentences.

### Coaching the Client

*Webster's Ninth New Collegiate Dictionary* defines coaching as "instructing or training, for example, of a player in fundamental rules and strategies of a game." Clients may need coaching through unfamiliar and often painful procedures, and it is a particularly effective strategy to use when the client needs to gain control (Lewis & Zahlis,

1997). In most cases, the nurse will teach self-management problem-solving skills in primary prevention through "coaching" the client.

Coaching involves a number of skills presented in this and other chapter, which are displayed in Figure 16–2. It is a teaching strategy that fully respects the client's autonomy in developing appropriate solutions because the client is always in charge of the pace and direction of the learning. In addition to giving appropriate information, coaching involves taking the client step by step through the procedure or activities in a mutual dialogue in which the client makes suggestions about care.

To coach a client successfully, the nurse must know and appreciate the client as an individual. This helps the nurse to know what information the client needs and how best to guide a particular client in taking charge of a situation. Sometimes the coaching a client needs relates to negotiating a complex health care system or developing better ways to have personal needs met.

The secret of successful coaching is to provide enough information to help the client take the next step without taking over. Exercise 16–8 provides practice with coaching as a teaching strategy.

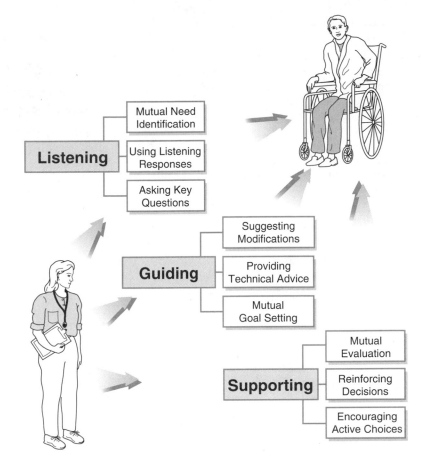

**Figure 16–2.** The nurse's role in coaching clients.

---

◆ **Exercise 16-8. Coaching Exercise**

Identify the steps you would use to coach clients in each of the following situations. Use Figure 16-2 as a guide to develop your plan.

1. A client returning from surgery with pain medication, ordered as needed
2. A client newly admitted to a cardiac care unit
3. A client with a newly inserted intravenous catheter for antibiotic medications
4. A child and his parents coming for a preoperative visit to the hospital before surgery

Share your suggestions with your classmates.

**Discussion:**
1. What were some of the different coaching strategies you used with each of these clients?
2. In what ways were your coaching strategies similar to or unlike those of your classmates?
3. How could you use the information you gained from this exercise to improve the quality of your helping?

## Evaluation of Client Teaching

The Joint Commission of Health Care Organizations (JCHCO) requires documentation of client teaching. Notes about the initial assessment should be detailed, comprehensive, and objective. Included in the documentation are the teaching actions and the client response directly linked to nursing diagnosis. For example, the nursing documentation for ongoing home health teaching about diabetic control would start with client assessment data and might be written as follows.

---

*4/8/98 Blood glucose check normal. Vital signs stable. Client on insulin for 10 years; has difficulty prefilling syringes. Lives with son who works. Nursing diagnosis: knowledge deficit related to prefilling syringes and ineffective coping in self-medication related to poor eyesight. Nurse prefilled syringes, wrote out med schedule, and discussed in detail with client. Client receptive to medication instruction, but may have difficulty with insulin prefill secondary to poor vision. Instructed client on medications, signs and symptoms to report to MD, diet and safety measures. Client able to repeat instructions. Spoke with son regarding medication supervision.*

M. Haggerty, RN

---

Accurate documentation serves another critical purpose in health teaching. It helps ensure continuity and prevents duplication of teaching efforts. The client's record becomes a secondary vehicle of communication, informing other health care workers of what has been taught and what areas need to be addressed in future teaching sessions. This is important for two reasons. First, the client can lose interest or become confused when the same information is repeated or is given in such a different way that the client is unsure which is "the correct information." Second, because many insurance carriers will not pay for parallel teaching, nurses need to share their teaching with other members of the inter-disciplinary health team. This helps to avoid additional costs for the client and prevent complicating the client's life with insurance company questions about claim information.

## Teaching Applications in Different Settings

Health teaching takes place in a variety of settings—informal one-to-one relationships, formal structured group sessions, and family conferences. The nurse may conduct scheduled teaching groups related to health care issues (e.g., in medication and rehabilitation discharge groups). Family conferences incorporate formal and informal teaching strategies for providing families with information they will need to help the client recover and for answering the many questions families have about their loved ones in the clinical setting. The media provide mass health teaching, particularly in primary prevention, such as safe sex and drug abuse prevention commercials. Written instructions, videotapes, and informational pamphlets provide supplemental health teaching. Health teaching in the home help clients and their family in a variety of traditional and nontraditional ways. Most recently, telehealth has emerged as a technical means of providing information to clients in their home by telecasting health information through video or interactive teaching formats using telephone and television. This type of health teaching is important in rural areas, where distance precludes ongoing nursing support.

### Group Presentations

Group presentations offer the advantage of being able to teach a number of people at one time, and the format allows people to learn from each other as well as from the teacher. Health teaching topics that lend themselves to a group format include care of the newborn, diabetes, oncology, and pre- and postnatal care (Redman, 1993).

Formal group teaching should be structured in a space large enough to accommodate all participants. Temperature is important. A hot, stuffy room causes people to become drowsy. Learners tend to focus on the coldness of the room rather than what the instructor is saying when this is a factor. The learner should be able to hear and see the instructor, all of the equipment, and visual aids without strain. Space to practice and equipment to take notes give people a sense of purpose.

The nurse needs to make sure that the room is available and should plan to arrive a little early for setup. If the teaching plan calls for use of equipment or flip charts for visual aids, they need to be available and in working order. Nothing is more disconcerting than to be unable to integrate teaching aids and props into the discussion. Consistency and planning help provide a structured environmental framework for the teaching process and decrease instructor anxiety. Should the equipment not work, it is better to eliminate the planned teaching aid completely than to spend a portion of the teaching session trying to fix it.

Preparation and practice can ensure that your presentation is clear, concise, and well spoken. Practice giving the information in a natural manner, particularly if the information is emotionally laden for you, the client, or both. If your teaching includes visual aids or equipment, developing an ease with incorporating them into your teaching process will make it easier, and you will appear more confident. In a group presentation, you also will need to establish rapport with your audience. This means being receptive to the learner's style, making courteous observations, and initiating discussion appropriately. Use simple gestures such as smiling, nodding, and responding.

A quote at the beginning that captures the meaning of the presentation or a humorous opening grabs the audience's attention. Make eye contact immediately, and continue to do so throughout the teaching session. Extension of eye contact to all participants communicates acceptance and inclusion. Strengthen content statements with careful use of specific examples. Citing a specific problem and the ways another person dealt with it gives general statements credibility. Repeating key points and summarizing them again at the conclusion of the session helps reinforce learning.

If you plan to use overhead transparencies, use a font that is large enough to see from a distance (32 point is recommended) and include no more than four to five items per transparency. Gauge the number of overheads that you will need, and remember that the anticipated time for teaching may appear longer than it actually will be because of questions from the audience.

To be a good teacher, one must also be a good listener. Asking questions confidently and thoughtfully as they relate to your understanding of participant circumstances conveys interest in the client's learning needs. Giving answers that are direct and clear reinforces the presentation. It is important for the nurse to anticipate questions and be on the alert for blank looks.

No matter how good a teacher you are, you will from time to time experience the "blank look." When this occurs, it is appropriate to ask, "Does anyone have any questions about what I just said?" or "This content is difficult to grasp; I wonder if you have any questions or concerns about what I have said so far?"

If you do not know the answer to a question, do not bluff it. It is appropriate to say, "That is a good question. I don't have an answer at this moment, but I will get back to you with it." Sometimes in a group presentation, another person will have the required information and with encouragement will share it. Group members provide a rich learning resource that often is overlooked.

Handouts and other materials provide additional reinforcement. Make sure that the information is accurate and complete, easy to understand, and logical. Sometimes it is useful to have a nonprofessional who is unfamiliar with the topic review written instructions for clarity and logic before using them with clients. Asking clients for feedback also helps. Exercise 16–9 provides an opportunity to practice health teaching in a group setting.

## Discharge Teaching

Discharge health teaching become extremely important when the client is in a health care facility for a restricted period of time or when the number of home visits to clients in the community are limited. When the client is ready for discharge, the nurse asks a set of questions focused on the discharge process and what is likely to happen when the client returns home. Appropriate questions are found in Box 16–7.

Family conferences are used as teaching sessions during discharge planning. Topics commonly covered in discharge planning include information about the nature of the illness or injury, a summary of individual progress in meeting treatment goals, and information about care

---

◆ Exercise 16-9. **Group Health Teaching**

**Purpose:** To provide practice with presenting a health topic in a group setting

1. Plan a 15- to 20-minute health presentation on a health topic of interest to you, including teaching aids and methods for evaluation.

**Suggested Topics:**

| | |
|---|---|
| Nutrition | Weight control |
| Drinking and driving | Mammograms |
| High blood pressure | Safe sex |
| Dental care | |

2. Present your topic to your class group.

---

of the client once the client leaves the hospital. Reinforcement of teaching about medications and referrals to community health and support groups are also a part of the teaching session. For example, there may have to be some modifications in medication schedules to fit individual and family lifestyles. The family should have ample opportunity to ask questions and to have them answered completely and honestly. Written instructions and a postdischarge telephone number support learning and provide necessary transitional support for client and family (Cagan & Meier, 1983).

### Health Teaching in the Home

As health care moves to community-based care, with a case mix of unstable, acutely ill home care clients and constrained funding for community home-based care, skilled health teaching becomes an increasingly important component of health care delivery. In home care, the nurse is a guest in the client's home. Part of the teaching assessment includes appraisal of the home environment, family supports, and resources as well as client needs.

Although the principles of health teaching remain the same, regardless of setting, the nurse implements them differently in home care settings because there is more time available and the teaching can be adapted to the client's individual situation. Teaching aids and structured teaching strategies available in the hospital setting may not be available. However, in many ways the home offers a teaching laboratory unparalleled in the hospital. The nurse can actually "see" the improvisations in equipment and technique that are possible in the home environment. Family members may have ideas that the nurse would not have thought of, which can make care easier. It is more natural for the client to reproduce teaching outcomes in the home environment where they initially learned a procedure.

The nurse should call before going to the client's home. This is common courtesy, and it protects the nurse's time if the client is going to be out. The tools of the trade are housed in a bag the nurse carries into the home. Before setting the bag down on a table, the nurse should spread a clean paper to protect both the client's table and the bag. It is important for the nurse to talk the client through procedures and dressing changes in much the same way as was done in

---

◆ Box 16-7. Assessing Learning Needs at Discharge

1. What potential problems are likely to prevent a safe discharge?
2. What potential problems are likely to cause complications or readmission?
3. What prior knowledge or experience does the patient and family have with this problem?
4. What skills and equipment are needed to manage the problem at home?
5. Who (what agency) will assume responsibility for continuing care?

the hospital. The nurse models appropriate behaviors (e.g., washing hands in the bathroom sink before touching the client). Simple strategies, such as not washing one's hands in the kitchen sink where food is prepared, encourage the client to do likewise.

Caregivers often do not recognize that there is a teaching need or what to ask. There are certain basic pieces of information that all clients and caregivers need. Conley and Burman (1997) suggested that caregivers need information related to the client's disease "including its progression, symptoms and side effects, treatment options, and what to expect in the future" (p. 812).

Teaching outcomes for clients in their homes relate to (1) increased knowledge, (2) optimal functioning, and (3) better self-care management. They are not mutually exclusive. In addition to content knowledge about the client's condition and treatment interventions, the nurse must have a working knowledge of community resources. Helping clients access supportive services, particularly when working with clients who are not by nature assertive, can be extremely helpful to families who would not otherwise do so even with the appropriate written information. The nurse must be able to select from a number of existing resources and create new ones through novel uses of family and community support systems. An understanding of Medicare, Medicaid, and other insurance, including regulations, required documentation, and reimbursement schedules, is factored into the management of health care teaching in home health care.

The community health–home care nurse works alone. Consequently, there is a need for creativity as well as competence in providing health teaching. Teaching in home care settings is rewarding. Frequently, the nurse is the client's only visitor. Other family members often display a curiosity and willingness to be a part of the learning group, particularly if the nurse actively uses knowledge of the home environment to make suggestions about needed modifications.

Teaching in home care has to be short term and comprehensive because most insurance companies will provide third-party reimbursement only for intermittent, episodic care. Nurses need to plan teaching sessions realistically so that they can be delivered in the shortest time possible.

Content needs to reflect specific information the client and family need to provide immediate effective care for the client, *nothing more and nothing less*. Sometimes it is tempting to include everything the learner needs to know. Because there are so many regulations regarding the length and scope of skilled nursing interventions imposed by third-party reimbursement guidelines, the nurse needs to pay careful attention to health teaching content and formats.

### Telehealth

Telehealth is a new means of providing ongoing client education and tracking client compliance. As an adjunct to home visiting, telecommunicated nursing directives that can be listened to or viewed repeatedly is helpful to many clients with chronic diseases such as acquired immunodeficiency syndrome, diabetes, and congestive heart failure (Kinsella, 1997).

## SUMMARY

Chapter 16 describes the nurse's role in health teaching. Theoretical frameworks, client-centered teaching, critical thinking, and behavioral approaches guide the nurse in implementing health teaching. The PRECEDE model helps nurses look at the learner in his or her social context, and the nursing process provides an organizing structure for health teaching. Teaching is designed to access one or more of the three domains of learning: cognitive, affective, and psychomotor. Assessment for purposes of constructing a teaching plan centers on three areas: What does the client already know? What is important for the client to know? What is the client ready to know? Essential content in all teaching plans includes information about the health care problem, risk factors, and self-care skills needed to manage at home. No one teaching strategy can meet the needs of all individual clients. The learning needs of the client will help define relevant teaching strategies. Several teaching strategies, such as coaching, use of mnemonics, and visual aids, are described. Repetition of key concepts and frequent feedback make the difference between simple instruction and teaching that informs. Documentation of the learning process is essential. The client's record becomes a vehicle of communication, informing other health care workers what has been taught and what areas need to be addressed in future teaching sessions.

## REFERENCES

American Nurses Association. (1982). Professional Nursing Standards. New York, National League for Nursing.

Bohny B. (1997). A time for self-care: Role of the home health nurse. Home Health Nurse 15(4):281–286.

Brillhart B, Stewart A. (1989). Education as the key to rehabilitation. Nursing Clinics of North America 24(3):675.

Brookfield S. (1986). Understanding and Facilitating Adult Learning. San Francisco, Jossey-Bass.

Cagan J, Meier P. (1983). Evaluation of a discharge planning tool for use with families of high risk infants. Journal of Obstetrical, Gynecological and Neonatal Nursing 12:275–281.

Check JF, Wurzbach ME. (1984). How elders view learning. Geriatric Nursing 1:37–39.

Conley V, Burman M. (1997). Informational needs of caregivers of terminal patients in a rural state. Home Health Care Nurse 15(11):808–817.

Curran J, Monti P (ed.). (1986). Social Skills Training. Washington Square, NY, New York University Press.

Flanagan L. (1990). Survival Skills in the Workplace: What Every Nurse Should Know. Kansas City, MO, American Nurses Association.

Greiner P, Vagiga T. (1998). Creative educational strategies for health promotion. Holistic Nursing Practice 12(2):73–83.

Huntsman A, Binger J. (1981). Communicating Effectively. Wakefield, MA, Nursing Resources.

Kinsella A. (1997). Telehealth and home care nursing. Home Health Care Nurse 15(11):796–797.

Leahy J, Kizilay P. (1998). Fundamentals of Nursing Practice: A Nursing Process Approach. Philadelphia, WB Saunders.

Lear MW. (1980). Heartsounds. New York, Pocket Books (Simon & Schuster), pp. 120–121.

Lee N, Wasson D, Anderson M, et al. (1998). A survey of patient education post discharge. Journal of Nursing Care Quality 13(1):63–70.

Lewis F, Zahlis E. (1997). The nurse as coach: A conceptual framework for clinical practice. Oncology Nursing Forum 24(10):1695–1702.

Manning S. (1992). The nurse I'll never forget. RN 92 22(8):47.

Miller B, Capp SE. (1997). Meeting JCAHO patient education standards. Nursing Management 28(5):55–58.

Mullen P, Green L. (1985). Meta-analysis points the way toward more effective teaching. Promotion of Health 6:68.

Post-White J. (1998). Wind behind the sails: Empowering our patients and ourselves. Oncology Nursing Forum 25(6):1011–1017.

Ragland G. (1997). Instant Teaching Treasures for Patient Education. St. Louis, MO, CV Mosby.

Rankin SH, Duffy-Stallings K. (1996). Patient Education: Issues, Principles and Guidelines (3rd ed.). Philadelphia, JB Lippincott.

Redman BK. (1993). The Process of Patient Education (7th ed.). St. Louis MO, CV Mosby.

Redman BK. (1997). The Practice of Patient Education (8th ed.). St. Louis, MO, CV Mosby.

Rogers C. (1983). Freedom to Learn for the 80's. Columbus, OH, Merrill.

Saylor CR. (1990). Reflection and professional education: Art, science and competency. Nurse Educator 15(2):811.

Skinner BF. (1971). Beyond Freedom and Dignity. New York, Knopf.

Smith CE. (1987). Patient Education: Nurses in Partnership with Other Health Professionals. Orlando, FL, Grune & Stratton.

Webster's Ninth New Collegiate Dictionary. (1985). Springfield, MA, Merriam Webster.

Wellard S, Turner D, Bethune E. (1998). Nurses as patient-teachers: Exploring current expressions of the role. Contemporary Nurse 7(1):12–14.

Usher K, Arthur D. (1998). Process consent: A model for enhancing informed consent in mental health nursing. Journal of Advanced Nursing 27:692–697.

## PART IV

## Responding to Special Needs

# 17

# Communicating with Clients Experiencing Communication Deficits

### Kathleen Underman Boggs

**OBJECTIVES**

At the end of the chapter, the student will be able to

1. Identify common communication deficits

2. Describe nursing strategies for communicating with clients experiencing communication deficits

*As Hubert Humphrey was fond of saying, the moral test of a society is how well it treats people in the dawn of life (children), people in the twilight of life (the elderly), and people in the shadows of life (the poor, the sick, the handicapped). We in the field of communication still have far to go in our contribution to these groups.*

Thompson (1984)

❖ This chapter presents an overview of common communication deficits and suggests communication strategies to use when working with clients experiencing them. Communication deficits may occur as a result of more permanent physical handicaps such as hearing loss, blindness, aphasia, or mental illness. Alternatively, communication deficits can arise from sensory deprivation related to temporary mobility and environmental limitations in an intensive care unit (ICU) (Fig. 17–1).

A primary nursing goal is to maximize the client's independence. When working with some clients who have sensory deficits, the nurse may need to modify the general therapeutic communication strategies presented earlier in this book. Multiple deficits may coexist. For example, children with motor dysfunction related to cerebral palsy have shown to have significant sensory deficits (Cooper et al., 1995). It is important for the nurse to remember that two individuals can be equally impaired but not equally disabled. People compensate for their impairment in different ways. The social, psychological, and behavioral context in which a communication handicap develops accounts for some of the differences in the ways people handle their disability.

## BASIC CONCEPTS
### Types of Deficits
#### *Hearing Loss*

People's sense of hearing alerts them to changes in the environment so they can respond effectively. The listener hears not only sounds and words but also a speaker's vocal pitch, loudness, and intricate inflections accompanying the ver-

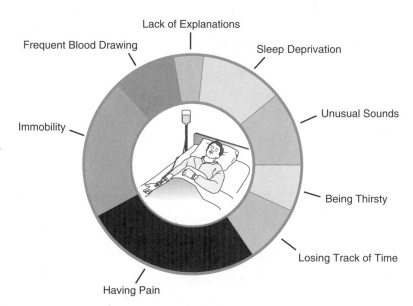

Figure 17–1. Situational factors affecting client responses to critical care units.

Lack of Explanations

Frequent Blood Drawing

Sleep Deprivation

Unusual Sounds

Immobility

Being Thirsty

Losing Track of Time

Having Pain

balization. Subtle variations can completely change the sense of the communication. Combined with the sounds, intensity, and organization of the verbal symbols, they allow the client to perceive and interpret the meaning of the sender's message. When this channel of communication is compromised through injury, illness, or the aging process, the client is at an enormous disadvantage in relationships with others. The extent of the loss is not always appreciated because the person looks normal, and the effects of partial hearing loss are not always readily apparent. Deprived of a primary means of receiving signals from the environment, the client with a hearing loss frequently withdraws from relationships.

### Blindness

Vision is used by clients to decode the meaning of messages. They watch the sender's facial expression and gestures for clues about interpreting the meaning of the message. All of the nonverbal cues that accompany speech communication, such as facial expression, nodding, and leaning toward the client, are lost to blind clients. Because clients cannot see nurses' faces or observe their nonverbal signals, nurses need to use words to express what the client cannot see in the message.

### Speech and Language Deficits

Clients who have speech and language deficits resulting from neurological trauma present a different type of communication problem. Normal communication allows people to perceive and interact with the world in an organized and systematic manner. People use language to express self-needs and to control environmental events. Language is the system people rely on to represent what they know about the world. When the ability to process and express language is disrupted, many areas of functioning are assaulted simultaneously. Aphasia, defined as a neurological linguistic deficit, produces a sudden alteration of communication that invariably has an impact on the sense of self. The person is intimately affected by feelings of loss and social isolation imposed by the communication impairment. Some of the reactions of self and others occur not as reactions to the disabling condition

itself but as responses to the meaning of the deficit. For example, it is not uncommon for employers and family members to wonder whether the client with a stroke has intellectual impairment as well as language impairment. Although this may be the case for some clients, others with mild neurological disruptions may simply need more time for cognitive processing.

*Aphasia* represents a speech-language disorder that is most frequently associated with neurological trauma to the brain. Aphasia can present as primarily an expressive or receptive disorder. The client with expressive aphasia can understand what is being said but cannot express thoughts or feelings in words. Receptive aphasia creates difficulties in receiving and processing written and oral messages. With *global aphasia*, the client has difficulty with both expressive language and reception of messages.

### Serious Mental Illness

Clients with serious mental disorders have a different type of communication deficit resulting from a malfunctioning of the neurotransmitters that normally transmit and make sense out of messages in the brain. Social isolation, impaired coping, and low self-esteem accompany the client's inability to receive or express language signals from the milieu. The emotional impact of these disabilities reflects the degree of severity of the deficits and the coping skills of the client.

The communication deficits found in clients with serious mental dysfunctions are related to their psychiatric disorders. Psychotic clients have intact sensory channels, but they cannot process and respond appropriately to what they hear, see, smell, or touch. The most serious communication difficulties are found in clients with autism (a childhood disorder characterized by a profound inability to communicate) and schizophrenia. Alterations in the biochemical neurotransmitters in the brain that normally conduct messages between nerve cells and help orchestrate the person's response to the external environment tangle messages and distort meanings. It is beyond the scope of this text to discuss in detail the psychotic client's communication deficits or the most appropriate strategies to use in communicating with this client. Such coverage is found in the many excellent psychiatric nursing texts available to the student. It is appropriate here, however, to appreciate the profound thought disintegration and communication problems psychotic clients face and to suggest basic guidelines for interacting with them.

The psychotic client usually presents with a poverty of speech and limited content. Speech appears blocked, reflecting disturbed patterns of perception, thought, emotions, and motivation. The client demonstrates a lack of vocal inflection and unchanging facial expression, which makes it difficult for anyone to truly understand the underlying message. Many clients display illogical thinking processes in the form of illusions, hallucinations, and delusions. Common words assume new meanings known only to the person experiencing them. The client thinks concretely and is unable to make abstract connections between ideas. Words and ideas are loosely connected and difficult to follow. Spontaneous movement is decreased, and the schizophrenic client exhibits inappropriate affect or appears nonresponsive to conversation. What the client hears may be overshadowed by the client's mental disorder, resulting in pervasive distorted perceptions.

### Environmental Deprivation

Communication is particularly important in nursing situations characterized by sensory deprivation, physical immobility, and limited environmental stimuli. In the emergency room as well as the ICU, perceptions and dialogue are limited by the nature of the unit and by the unstable nature of the conditions precipitating admission. Yet even in the most high-tech setting, the potential for caring remains an underlying theme (Ray, 1987).

For the most part, the client is kept physically immobile, so that by default the relationship with the critical care nurse often becomes the most important one to the client. Nurses who show concern for the client as a person and who have a sensitive awareness of what the client may be experiencing in a strange environment help the client maintain a sense of self in a bewildering situation. A nurse who is with the client psychologically as well as physically helps the client develop meaning from the current situation.

Temporary, reversible changes in cognitive equilibrium occur because there are few organizing structures to anchor the client. Such clients, surrounded by high-tech equipment, usually find themselves in settings in which there are no gender distinctions, privacy is at a minimum, and there is not even a window from which to view the outside world. The immediate environment is unfamiliar, circumscribed, upsetting, and punctuated with strange sounds. Medical emergencies are the rule rather than the exception, and the client's usual support system is excluded except for brief visits. It is often difficult for the client to differentiate noises and equipment as important or insignificant. Everything seems equal and strange. As Cooper (1993) pointed out, the ICU "is not the ordinary world of human experience." The lack of familiar landmarks and varied stimuli in a hospital special care unit (the ICU, labor room, or emergency room, for instance) limit a person's ability to use environmental cues to direct behavior. Moreover, clients usually are frightened, in pain, and unable to communicate easily with others. Barriers to communication can also include the client's inability to respond in a conversation, usually because of intubation or sedation.

Research indicates that the subsequent gradual decline of cognitive abilities and the absence of interpersonal stimulation are related. Clients with normal intellectual capacity can appear dull, uninterested, and lacking in problem-solving abilities if they do not have frequent interpersonal stimulation.

## APPLICATIONS
## Communications Strategies
### Hearing Loss

Assessment of the effects of auditory sensory loss should include the age of onset and the severity. Hearing loss that occurs after the development of speech means that the client has access to word symbols and language skills. Deafness in children can cause developmental delays, which may need to be taken into account in planning the most appropriate communication strategies (Jaffe & Luterman, 1980). Hearing deficits have been shown to be associated with depression (Kalayam et al., 1995). Box 17–1 lists some strategies for improving communication with the hearing impaired.

---

◆ **Box 17–1. Specific Strategies to Maximize the Quality of the Communication Process**

1. Stand or sit so that you face the client and the client can see your facial expression and mouthing of words. Communicate in a well-lighted room.
2. Use facial expressions and gestures that reinforce the verbal content.
3. Use gestures and speak distinctly without exaggerating words. Partially deaf clients respond best to well-articulated words spoken in a moderate, even tone.
4. Write important ideas and allow the client the same option to increase the chances of communication.
5. Help elderly clients adjust hearing aids. Lacking fine motor dexterity, the elderly client may not be able to insert aids to amplify hearing.
6. Allow more time to communicate information.
7. Become familiar with the client's communication pattern, likes, and dislikes.
8. Use an intermediary, such as a family member who knows sign language, to facilitate communication.

---

Clues to hearing loss occur when clients appear unresponsive to sound or respond only when the speaker is directly facing them. The nurse should ask clients whether they use a hearing aid and whether it is working properly. Auditory amplifiers such as assisted listening devices, hearing aids, and telephone attachments counterbalance certain types of hearing loss. Frequently, clients have hearing aids but fail to use them because they do not fit well or are hard to insert. Other people complain that the hearing aid amplifies all sounds indiscriminately, not just the voices of people in conversation, and they find this distracting. Exercises 17–1 and 17–2 will help you understand what it is like to have a hearing deficit.

◆ **Case Example**

Two student nurses were assigned to care for 9-year-old Timmy, who is a deaf mute. When they went into his room for assessment, he was alone and appeared anxious. No information was available as to his ability to read lips, the nurses were not sure what reading skills he had, and they did not know sign language. So, instead of using a pad and paper for communication, they decided to role-play taking vital signs by using some funny facial expressions and demonstrating on a doll.

---

## Blind Clients

The blind person experiences the world as full of shadows and lacking in detail. Visual impairment has been shown to be associated with a higher occurrence of paranoia (Blazer et al., 1996). It is important to use words as you approach the blind client so as not to startle him or her. It also is helpful to mention your name as you enter the client's room. Even people who are partially blind appreciate hearing the name of the person to whom they are speaking, because otherwise they may have to guess.

The nurse needs to use words to supply additional information to counterbalance the missing visual cues. For example, a blind elderly client commented to the student nurse that she felt the student was uncomfortable talking with her and perhaps did not like her. Not being able to see the student, the client interpreted the hesitant uneasiness in the student's voice as evidence that the student did not wish to be with her. The student agreed with the client that she was quite uncomfortable but did not explain further. Had the client been able to see the apprehensive body posture of the student, she would have realized that the student was quite shy and might have been ill at ease with *any* interpersonal relationship. It was a serious but not necessarily a fatal error in communication. In such a situation, the student might have clarified the reasons for her discomfort, and the relationship could have moved forward. Unfortunately, she did not do this, and the client was left feeling that her emotions were inconsequential, inappropriate, or misunderstood.

The social isolation experienced by blind clients can be profound, and the need for human contact is important. Touching the client lightly *as* you speak alerts the client to your presence. Voice tones and pauses that reinforce the verbal content are helpful. The client needs to be informed when the nurse is leaving the room.

◆ Exercise 17–1. **Loss of Sensory Function in Geriatric Clients**

**Purpose:** To assist you to get in touch with the feelings often experienced by older adults as they lose sensory function. If the younger individual is able to ''walk in the older person's shoes,'' he or she will be more sensitive to the losses and needs created by those losses in the older person.

**Procedure:**
1. Students separate into three groups.
2. Group A: place cotton balls in your ears. Group B: cover your eyes with a plastic bag. Group C: place cotton balls in your ears and cover your eyes with a plastic bag.
3. A student from Group B should be approached by a student from Group A. The student from Group B is to talk to the student from Group A, using a whispered voice. The Group A student is to verify the message heard with the student who spoke. The student from Group B is then to identify the student from Group A.
4. The students in Group C are expected to identify at least one person in the group and describe to that person what he or she is wearing. Each student who does not do the description is to make a statement to the other person and have that individual reveal what he or she was told.
5. Having identified and conversed with each other, hold hands or remain next to each other and remove the plastic bags and cotton balls (to facilitate verification of what was heard and described).

**Discussion:**
1. How did the loss you experienced make you feel?
2. Were you comfortable performing the function expected of you with your limitation?
3. What do you think could have been done to make you feel less handicapped?
4. How did you feel when your ''normal'' level of functioning was restored?
5. How would you feel if you knew the loss you just stimulated was to be permanent?
6. What impact can you project this experience might have on your future interactions with older individuals with such sensory losses.

From Glenn BJ, former member, State Health Coordinating Council—Acute Care Committee, 1993, 1998.

Compensatory interventions for the blind include a plentiful assortment of auditory and tactile stimuli such as books on tape and in Braille and music.

When a blind client is being introduced to a new environmental setting, the nurse should orient the client by describing the size of the room and the position of the furniture and equipment. If other people are present, the nurse should name each person. A good communication strategy is to ask the other people in the room to introduce themselves to the client. In this way, the client gains an appreciation for their voice configurations. The nurse should avoid any tendency to speak with a blind client in a louder voice than usual or to enunciate words in an exaggerated manner. This may be perceived by some clients as condescending or insensitive to the nature of the handicap. Voice tones should be kept natural. Exercise 17–3 will give you a sense of what it is like to be visually impaired.

The blind client needs guidance in moving around in unfamiliar surroundings. One way of preserving the client's autonomy is to offer your arm to the client instead of taking the client's arm. Mention steps and changes in movement as they are about to occur to help the client navigate new places and differences in terrain. The client will be less socially isolated if the nurse helps him or her maintain contact and involve-

◆ Exercise 17–2. **Hearing Loss Exercise**

**Purpose:** To help raise consciousness regarding hearing as a channel of communication and experience the loss of hearing function

**Procedure:**
1. Watch the first 5 minutes of a television show with the sound turned off. All students should watch the same show (e.g., the 6 o'clock news report or a rerun of a situation comedy). Write down what you think was said during this time period. Your instructor will either tape or listen to the broadcast.
2. Share your observations of the television show and describe for each other in turn what went on.
3. After completion of the exercise, the instructor will summarize what actually happened in the broadcast or show the videotape

**Discussion:**
1. Were perceptual differences noted in how each student interpreted the show? If so, what implications do you think these differences have in working with deaf clients?
2. How frustrating was it for you to watch the show without sound? How did it make you feel?
3. What could the characters in the show have done to make it easier for you to receive information without sound?
4. What did you learn about yourself from this exercise?

◆ Exercise 17–3. **Experiencing What It Is Like to Be Blind**

**Purpose:** To help students understand what it is like to be blind

**Procedure:**
1. Have students pair up. One student should be blindfolded.
2. The other student should guide the ''blind'' student on a walk around the campus.
3. During the walk, the student guide should converse with the ''blind'' student about the route they are taking.
4. The students should return to the classroom after 15 minutes and reverse roles for a second 15-minute walk.

**Discussion:**
1. What did it feel like to be temporarily blind?
2. In what ways was the student guide helpful and considerate of your handicap?
3. What actions did you wish your student guide had taken that would have made the walk easier?
4. What trust issues arose for you as a result of being dependent on another person?
5. In what ways can you use the learning from this exercise in your nursing practice?

ment with as much of the environment as the client's capabilities will allow.

### Deaf-Blind Clients

The deaf-blind client presents a special communication challenge to the nurse, but many of the strategies described previously can be used in combination to facilitate communication. Methods of communication used by these clients include reading and writing in Braille and use of American Sign Language. Although these skills are not common among nurses, several other techniques can be used by any nurse to communicate with the deaf-blind client. Capital letters can be printed in the client's palm. Touch becomes very important. The nurse can help the client touch and feel the position of different items in a room. Walking deaf-blind clients around their environment allows for sensory knowledge that otherwise would be inaccessible to them. Other suggestions are listed in Box 17–2.

The **Optacon** is a reading device that converts printed letters into a vibration that can be felt by the deaf-blind client. The **Tellatouch** is a portable machine into which the nurse types a message that emerges in Braille.

### Clients with Speech and Language Deficits

Assessment of the type of aphasia aids the nurse in selecting the most appropriate intervention. Expressive language problems are evidenced in an inability to find words or to associate ideas with accurate word symbols. In some instances, clients can find the correct word if given enough time and support. Other clients have difficulty organizing their words into meaningful sentences or describing the sequence of events. Clients with receptive communication deficits have trouble following directions, reading information, and writing. They hear the words but have difficulty classifying data or relating data to previous knowledge. Common properties of familiar items are not connected. This inability limits short-term memory and is sometimes misinterpreted as a short-term memory deficit associated with dementia. These clients appreciate the nurse who helps them supply the missing connections. Clients who lose both expressive and receptive communication abilities have global aphasia. Even though they appear not to understand, the nurse should explain in very simple terms what is happening. Using touch, gestures, eye movements, squeezing of the hand can improve chances of communication and should be attempted.

Clients with speech and language deficits become frustrated when they are not understood and may refuse to repeat themselves. The level of concentration required by the nurse to capture every word and its meaning is tiring. Clients fatigue easily and need short, positive sessions to reinforce their efforts. Otherwise, they may become nonverbal as a way of regaining energy and composure. Changes in self-image occasioned by physical changes, the uncertain recovery course and outcome of strokes, shifts in family roles, and the disruption of free-flowing verbal interaction among family members make the loss of functional communication particularly agonizing for clients. The inability to talk about these profound changes increases the client's feelings of social

---

#### ◆ Box 17–2. Suggestions for Helping the Deaf-Blind Client

1. Let the person know when you approach by a simple touch, and always indicate when you are leaving.
2. Make positive use of any means of communication available.
3. Develop and use your own special sign to identify yourself to the client.
4. Encourage the client to verbalize speech, even if the person uses only a few words or the words are difficult to understand at first.
5. Keep the client informed.
6. Use touch and close physical proximity while you are with the client; give the person something substantial to touch in your absence.
7. Do not lead or hold the client's arm when walking; instead, allow the person to take your arm.
8. Develop and use signals to indicate changes in pace or direction while walking.

Data from Armstrong NT. (1991). Nursing care of the deaf-blind client. Insight 16(3):21. Used with permission.

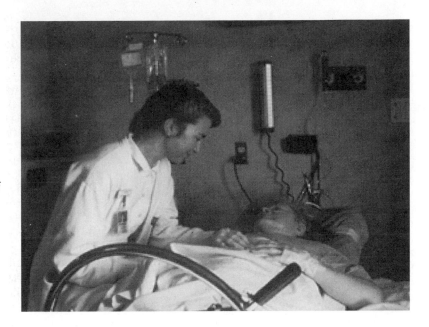

Touch, eye movements, and sounds can be used to communicate with clients experiencing aphasia. (Courtesy University of Maryland School of Nursing)

isolation and fear. Even more important than verbal interaction with the aphasic client is the attitude the nurse brings to the interaction. When the nurse is sensitive to these concerns and is able to express them, clients report feeling supported and reassured.

When the capacity to communicate through words is lost through illness or injury, the client must learn different ways to compensate for normal speech production skills. Any language skills that are preserved should be exploited. Other means of communication can be used, such as pointing, gesturing, using pictures, and repeating phrases. Sounds and eye movements can develop into unique communication systems between nurse and client.

Flexibility and accurate assessment of learning needs are keys to developing the most effective teaching strategies with aphasic clients. For example, Collier (1992, p. 63) described an aphasic client's initial reluctance to participate in self-care teaching and the strategies the nurses used to engage the client.

If the client is able to use short phrases and simple sentences, this should be encouraged. It does not matter if the sentence does not make complete grammatical sense or is expressed in a halting way. The important thing is that the cli-

ent is communicating and the communication is understandable. Anything the nurse can do to encourage and support verbal expressive abilities is useful (Box 17–3). If the client is in speech therapy, the nurse can be an important source of

---

### Box 17–3. Strategies to Assist the Client with Speech and Language Difficulties

1. Avoid prolonged, continuous conversations; instead, use frequent, short talks.
2. When clients falter in written or oral expression, supply needed compensatory support.
3. Praise efforts to communicate, and make learning new ways to communicate a creative game.
4. Provide regular mental stimulation in a nontaxing way.
5. Help clients focus on the faculties still available to them for communication.
6. Allow extra time for delays in cognitive processing of information.
7. Encourage the client to practice what is learned in speech therapy.

support. Exposure to varied social environments without the pressure to talk helps the client with a communication deficit remain connected. The nurse can point out familiar objects as they tour the immediate environment on foot or with the client in a wheelchair.

### Clients with Serious Mental Illness

The nurse faces a formidable challenge in trying to establish a relationship with the psychotic client in a community setting. The most important modifications needed in communicating with psychotic clients center on taking a more proactive approach. Research by Blazer and associates (1996) found that 1 of every 10 older adults in a community sample displayed symptoms of paranoia. Other studies suggest about a 2% incidence of more severe undiagnosed mental illness in community elders.

Rarely will the psychotic client approach the nurse directly. It is the nurse who must reach out and try different communication strategies. Patience and respect for the client are essential. The client generally responds to questions, but the answers are likely to be brief, and the client does not elaborate without further probes. Knowing this is the most common form of response helps the nurse depersonalize the impact of a response that conveys little information. Although the client appears to rebuff any social interaction, it is important to keep trying to connect (Box 17–4). People with

mental illnesses like schizophrenia are easily overwhelmed by the external environment (information may be obtained electronically via www.schizophrenia.com).

Keeping in mind that the client's unresponsiveness to words, failure to make eye contact, unchanging facial expression, and monotonic voice are patterns of the disorder and not a commentary on the nurse's communication skills helps the nurse continue to engage with the client.

If the client is hallucinating or using delusions as a primary form of communication, the nurse should not challenge their validity directly. Nor should there be prolonged discussions of illogical thinking. Instead, the nurse might say "I know that your sense that God is going to destroy the world tomorrow seems very real to you, but I don't see it that way."

Often the nurse can identify the underlying theme the client is trying to convey with the delusional statement. For example, the nurse might say to the client making the previous statement, "It sounds as though you feel powerless and afraid at this moment." The technique of listening to the client carefully, using alert posture, nodding to demonstrate active listening, and trying to make sense out of the underlying feelings models effective communication for the client and helps the nurse to decode nonsensical messages. If the nurse expects the client to talk crazy, the client will oblige. However, if the nurse is willing to look beyond the misleading exterior to the way the individual experiences reality and wishes to be seen by others, a different picture can emerge. A mark of the growing trust in a relationship with a psychotic client is expanded rational conversation and a willingness to remain with the nurse for increasing periods of time.

### Clients Experiencing Environmental Deprivation

It is not that the client actually is forgotten, but nurses in the high-tech ICU environment often forget the client is still a psychosocial being. The human concerns of the client assume a secondary priority, receiving less attention than the more immediate physical needs. In the rush to stabilize the client physically, communication is of poor quality; nurses verbalize less often or are

---

> ◆ **Box 17–4. Strategies to Assist with the Schizophrenic Client**
>
> 1. Keep contact short; avoid longer interactions.
> 2. Use simple, concrete sentences.
> 3. Use props and actions, such as games, magazines, going for walks, discussing simple topics, curling a client's hair, or manicuring the client's nails.
> 4. Avoid crowding the client's personal space.
> 5. Maintain eye contact while speaking in a calm voice.
> 6. Express positive feelings by saying "I like it when you do. . . . "
> 7. Express negative feeling by saying "I get uncomfortable when you. . . . "

less sensitive to the client's behavioral cues (Turnock, 1991).

When a client is not fully alert, it is not uncommon for nurses to speak in the client's presence in ways they would not if they thought the client could fully understand what is being said. Such situations are unfortunate for two reasons: first, because hearing is the last sense to go, and clients have been able to repeat whole conversations; second, because the client may hear only parts of what is said and misinterpret it. A rule of thumb is *never to say anything you would not want the client to hear.*

In addition to conveying a caring, compassionate attitude, the nurse may use several of the strategies for communicating listed in Box 17–5.

An example of orienting cues would be the labeling of meals as breakfast, lunch, or dinner. Linking events to routines, for example, saying, "The x-ray technician will take your chest x-ray right after lunch" helps secure the client in time and space. When the client is unable or unwilling to engage in a dialogue, the nurse should continue to initiate communication in a one-way mode (Turnock, 1991).

### ◆ Case Example

**Nurse:**  I am going to give you your bath now. The water will feel a little warm to you. After your bath, your wife will be in to see you. She stayed in the waiting room last night because she wanted to be with you. (No answer is necessary if the client is unable to talk, but the sound of a

human voice and attention to the client's unspoken concerns can be very healing.)

The client should be called by name. Nurses need to identify themselves and explain procedures in simple language even if the client does not appear particularly alert. Clients who are awake or even semialert should not be allowed to stare at a blank ceiling for extended periods of time. Changing the client's position frequently benefits the person physiologically and offers an opportunity for episodic dialogue with the nurse. The nurse is frequently in a position to create a more stimulating environment. For example, a simple animated conversation that taps into the client's world of knowledge can provide a source of ongoing emotional support because of the indirect recognition of the client's intellectual and perceptual qualities.

If the client in the ICU becomes temporarily delusional or experiences hallucinations, the nurse can use strategies similar to those used with the psychotic client. The client is reassured if the nurse does not appear bothered by the symptoms and is able to confirm to the client that experiencing strange sensations, thoughts, and feelings is a common occurrence in the ICU.

## SUMMARY

This chapter discusses the specialized communication needs of clients with communication deficits. Basic issues and applications for communicating with clients experiencing sensory loss of hearing and sight are outlined. Sensory stimulation and compensatory channels of communication are needed for clients with sensory deprivation. The mentally ill client has intact senses, but information processing and language are affected by the disorder. It is important for the nurse to develop a proactive communication approach with psychotic clients. The aphasic client has trouble expressing or receiving communication, or both. Nurses can develop alternative methods of communicating with these clients. Clients in the ICU can experience a temporary distortion of reality. Such clients need frequent cues that orient them to time and place as well as sensory stimulation.

## REFERENCES

Armstrong NT. (1991). Nursing care of the deaf-blind client. Insight 16(3):20–21.

---

### ◆ Box 17–5. Strategies for Communicating with Clients in the ICU

1. Encourage the client to display pictures or a simple object from home.
2. Orient the client to the environment.
3. Frequently provide information about the client's condition and progress.
4. Reassure the client that cognitive and psychological disturbances are common.
5. Give explanations before procedures by providing information about the sounds, sights, and feelings the client is experiencing.
6. Provide the client with frequent orienting cues to time and place.

Blazer D, Hays J, Salive ME. (1996). Factors associated with paranoid symptoms in a community sample of older adults. The Gerontologist 36(1):70–75.

Collier S. (1992). Mrs. Hixon was more than the CVA in 251. Nursing 22(11):62–64.

Cooper J, Majnemer A, Rosenblatt B, Birnbaum R. (1995). The determination of sensory deficits in children with hemiplegic cerebral palsy. Journal of Child Neurology 10(4):300–309.

Cooper M. (1993). The intersection of technology and care in the ICU. Advances in Nursing Science 15(3):23–32.

Elvins R. (1991). Attitudes to people with mental handicaps. Nursing Standard 5(34):29–32.

Jaffe B, Luterman D. (1980). The child with a hearing loss. In Scheiner A, Abroms I (eds.), The Practical Management of the Developmentally Disabled Child. St. Louis, MO, CV Mosby.

Kalayam B, Meyers BS, Kakuma T, et al. (1995). Age at onset of geriatric depression and sensorineural hearing deficits. Biological Psychiatry 38(10):649–658.

McCann K, McKenna HP. (1993). An examination of touch between nurses and elderly patients in a continuing care setting in N. Ireland. Journal of Advanced Nursing 18(5):838–846.

Peters S. (1998). Responding to pediatric pain. Advanced Practice Nurse 6(2):79–80, 96.

Ray M. (1987). Technological caring: A new model in critical care. Dimensions of Critical Care Nursing 6(3):169–173.

Robinson BE, Bacon JG. (1996). The "if only I were thin. . . ." treatment program: Decreasing the stigmatizing effects of fatness. Professional Psychology: Research & Practice 27(2):175–183.

Turnock C. (1991). Communicating with patients in ICU. Nursing Standard 9(5):38–40.

Wood D. (1991). Communication and cognition. American Annals of the Deaf 136(3):247–251.

## Electronic

http://www.deaflibrary.org/

http://www.schizophrenia.com/family/communicationskills.html

## Suggested Readings

Niewenhuis R. (1989). Breaking the speech barrier. Nursing Times 85(15):34–36.

Vaccari C, Marschark M. (1997). Communication between parents and deaf children: Implications for social-emotional development. Journal of Child Psychology and Psychiatry 38(7):793–801.

Velligan DI, Mahurin RK, Eckert SL, et al. (1997). Relationship between specific types of communication deviance and attentional performance in patients with schizophrenia. Psychiatry Research 70(1):9–20

# 18

# Communicating with Children

## Kathleen Underman Boggs

**OBJECTIVES**

At the end of the chapter, the student will be able to

1. Identify how developmental levels impact the child's ability to participate in interpersonal relationships with caregivers
2. Describe modifications in communication strategies to meet the specialized needs of children

3. Describe interpersonal techniques needed to interact with concerned parents of ill children

*A revolution is occurring in the world of pediatric medicine which will have profound effects on the way we practice and in the venue in which patients are encountered . . . with unique opportunities to actively prevent future illness by altering life habits at an early stage.*

Bernstein & Shelov (1996)

❖❖ This chapter is designed to help the nurse recognize and apply communication concepts related to the nurse–client relationship in pediatric clinical situations. Each nursing situation represents a unique application of communication strategies. Tools needed by caregivers to provide effective and ethical care are cognitive, interpersonal, and attitudinal. For each of these domains, the child's and family's socioeconomic status and cultural background must be considered (Bernstein & Shelov, 1996). As the prior quotation reveals, major changes in society are impacting on the health care of children. Some research suggests that societal changes have also increased the communication initiatives taken by children with health care providers (Meeuwesen & Kaptein, 1996).

Communicating with children at different age levels requires modifications of the skills learned in previous chapters. By understanding the child's cognitive, developmental, and functional level, the nurse is able to select the most appropriate communication strategies. Children undergo significant age-related changes in the ability to process cognitive information and in the capacity to interact effectively with the environment. To have an effective therapeutic relationship with a child, the nurse needs an understanding of feelings and thought processes from the child's perspective. Developing rapport requires that the nurse know about the interpersonal world as the child perceives it and convey honesty, respect, and acceptance of feelings.

## BASIC CONCEPTS

Childhood is very different from adulthood. The child has fewer life experiences from which to draw and is still in the process of developing skills needed for reasoning and communicating. All children's concepts of health and illness must be considered within the developmental framework (Burns et al., 1996). Erikson's concepts of ego development and Piaget's description of the progressive development of the child's cognitive thought processes form a theoretical basis for the child-centered nursing interventions described in this chapter. Both theorists say that the child's thought processes, ways of perceiving the world, judgments, and emotional responses to life situations are qualitatively different from those of the adult. Cognitive and psychosocial development unfold according to an ordered hierarchical scheme, increasing in depth and complexity as the child matures.

## Child's Developmental Environment

Jean Piaget's (1972) descriptions of stages of cognitive development provide a valuable contribution toward understanding the dimensions of a child's perceptions. Cognitive development and early language development are integrally related, as evidenced by the mutual nonverbal communication that occurs between infant and caretaker. Although current developmental theorists expand on Piaget's theoretical model by recognizing the effects of the parent–child relationship and a stimulating environment on developing communication abilities, his work forms the foundation for the understanding of childhood cognitive development. Piaget observed cognitive development occurring in sequential stages (Box 18–1). The ages are only approximated since Piaget himself was not specific.

### Piaget's Stages

In the first stage of cognitive maturation, the *sensorimotor period,* the infant explores its own body as a source of information, gradually modifying reflexive responses to include more purposeful interactions with the environment. As the infant gains more motor control, cognitive behaviors become more intentional, and the infant begins to differentiate between objects in the environment. At about 8 months of age, the infant clearly is able to distinguish the primary caregiver in the environment from less familiar persons. The infant may begin to vocalize some awareness that objects may be dissimilar in nature and function. By the end of this stage, the infant is developing an understanding of symbolic thinking and thus begins to use language to communicate.

The second stage of cognitive development emerges around the age of 2. In this stage, known as the *preoperational period,* the toddler is markedly egocentric, unable to see another's viewpoint, and for this reason unable to engage productively in interactive, cooperative play. However, there is a genuine interest in being

---

### ◆ Box 18–1. Stages of Cognitive Development

| Age | Piaget's Stages | Characteristics | Language Development |
|---|---|---|---|
| Birth–2 years | Sensorimotor | Infant learns by manipulating objects. At birth, reflexive communication, then moves through six stages to reach actual thinking. | Communication largely nonverbal; vocabulary of more than four words by 12 months, increases to >200 words and use of short sentences before age 2. |
| 2–6 years | Preoperational | Beginning use of symbolic thinking. Imaginative play. Masters reversibility. | Actual use of structured grammar and language to communicate. Uses pronouns. Average vocabulary >10,000 words by age 6. |
| 7–11+ years | Concrete operations | Logical thinking. Masters use of numbers and other concrete ideas, classification, conservation, etc. | Mastery of passive tense by age 7 and complex grammatical skills by age 10. |
| >12+ years | Formal operations | Abstract thinking. Futuristic, takes a broader, more theoretical perspective. | Near adultlike skills. |

Adapted from Piaget J. (1972). The Child's Conception of the World. Savage, MD, Littlefield, Adams and Co.

---

with other children, playing alongside them in parallel play. In the preoperational stage of cognitive development, children are not able to make cognitive connections between past events and a given end result.

The preschool child is still unable to distinguish fantasy from reality, to consider another's viewpoint, and to accept the possibility of alternative options. Images are developed through concrete devices. Verbal explanations should be accompanied by opportunities for the child to use concrete, touchable objects and to play in a cooperative take-turns fashion with other children. As the child makes the transition to the concrete operational stage, there is a growing ability to categorize information and to internalize more structures into thinking about things. At the end of the preoperational period in the early elementary school years, the child begins to notice the cause-and-effect relationships in situations and is able to describe differences in objects having some similarities (Crain, 1992; Piaget, 1972).

The third stage of cognitive development, referred to as the **concrete operations period,** extends from approximately 7 to 11 years of age and beyond. The child now is capable of structural cooperative play with complex rules. Children can comprehend concepts presented in graphic detail and are beginning to appreciate the possibility of developing alternative solutions to problems. The child is able to distinguish between concrete, disparate groups of objects. Health teaching with children in this stage of cognitive development should be closely aligned with reality and presented with concrete images.

The final stage of cognitive development described by Piaget is the **formal operations period.** Starting at about 12 years of age in some children and continuing through adulthood, abstract reality and logical thought processes emerge. Cooperation, collaboration, and social conscience are noted. The formal operational thinker is able to consider several alternative options at the same time and to set long-term goals. Adolescents who have developed formal operational thinking abilities are capable of making health-related judgments about their care. Whenever possible, they should be given the opportunity to exercise this right.

Wide individual differences exist in the intellectual functioning of same-age children. Variations also occur across situations, so that the child under stress or in a different environment may process information at a lower level than he or she would under normal conditions. Because two children of the same chronological age may have quite different skills as information processors, the nurse needs to assess level of functioning. Language alternatives familiar to one child because of certain life experiences may not be useful in providing health care and teaching with another. Application of nursing care to children draws heavily from Erikson's model of psychosocial development. Integrating cognitive and psychosocial developmental approaches into communication with children at different ages enhances its effectiveness.

## Understanding the Ill Child's Needs

Difficulties arise in adult–child communications in part because of the child's cognitive level in an early developmental stage. Children have limited social experience in interpreting subtle nuances of facial expression, inflection, and word meanings. When illness and physical or developmental disabilities occur during formative years, situational stressors are added that affect the way children perceive themselves and the environment. Illness may lead to significant alterations in role relationships with family and peers. The nurse needs to assess not only the physical care needs of the child but also the impact of the illness on the child's self-esteem and on his or her relationships with family and friends. Factors affecting the child's response may include the chronicity of illness, its impact on lifestyle, the child's cognitive understanding of the disease process, and the family's ability to cope with care demands.

If the child needs to be hospitalized, this is a situational crisis for the child and the entire family. Hospitalization is always stressful. Hospitalized children have to contend not only with physical changes but also possibly separation from family and friends as well as living in a strange, frightening, and probably hurtful environment. The family needs to learn new interactional patterns and coping strategies that take into consideration the meaning of an illness and disability in family life. Because personal disappointments and frustrations are feelings many families are reluctant to share freely when a child is ill, important behavioral responses frequently are stifled in fathers as well as in mothers.

## APPLICATIONS

## Assessment

Assessing a child's reaction to illness requires knowing the child's normal patterns of communication. Interactions are observed between parent and child. The child's behavioral responses to the entire interpersonal environment (including nurse and peers) are assessed. Are the child's interactions age appropriate? Are behaviors organized, or is the child unable to complete activities? Does the child act out an entire play sequence, or is such play fragmented and disorganized? Do the child's interactions with others suggest imagination and a broad repertoire of relating behaviors, or is communication devoid of possibilities? Once baseline data have been collected, the nurse plans specific communication strategies to meet the specialized needs of the child client (Fig. 18–1). An overview of nursing adaptations needed to communicate effectively with children are summarized in Box 18–2.

### Regression as a Form of Childhood Communication

A severe illness can cause a child to show behaviors that are reminiscent of an earlier stage of development. A certain amount of regression is normal. Common behaviors include whining, teasing other children, demanding undue attention, withdrawal, or having "toileting accidents." In most cases, the underlying dynamic is the powerlessness and inadequacy the child feels in attempting to cope with a potentially overwhelming, frightening environment. Reassuring the parent that this is a common response to the stress of illness can be reassuring.

Because children have limited life experience to draw from, they exhibit a narrower range of

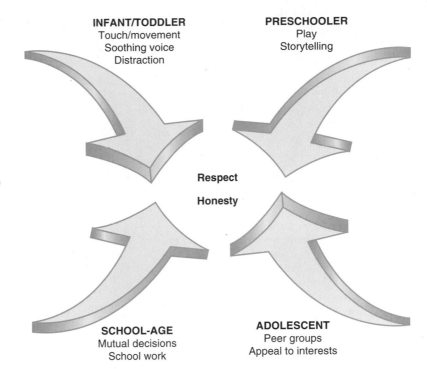

**INFANT/TODDLER**
Touch/movement
Soothing voice
Distraction

**PRESCHOOLER**
Play
Storytelling

**Respect**

**Honesty**

**SCHOOL-AGE**
Mutual decisions
School work

**ADOLESCENT**
Peer groups
Appeal to interests

Figure 18–1. Nursing strategies must be geared toward the developmental level of the child.

behaviors in coping with threat. The quiet, overly compliant child who does not complain may be more frightened than the child who screams or cries. This should alert you to the child's emotional distress. The nurse needs to obtain detailed information regarding the usual behavioral responses of the family and child. Some behaviors that look regressive may be a typical behavioral response for the child (e.g., the 2-year-old who wants a bedtime bottle). A complete baseline history offers a good counterpoint for assessing the meaning of current behaviors.

## Age-Appropriate Communication

Whenever possible, the nurse should communicate with language familiar to the child. Elicit specific words used for toileting, pain, and so on. Parents are valuable resources in understanding the child and interpreting behavioral data. If possible, they should be part of the nurse's interpersonal relationship with the child. An assessment of vocabulary and understanding is essential in fostering communications. The nurse can assist a child who is having difficulty finding the right words by reframing what the child has said and repeating it in a slightly different way. Another strategy is to ask the parent what words the child uses to express specific health-related concerns.

The afflicted child's peers often have difficulty accepting individual differences created by health deviations. They lack the knowledge and sensitivity to deal with physical changes that they do not understand, as evidenced by "bald" jokes about the child receiving chemotherapy. Children with hidden disorders such as diabetes, some forms of epilepsy, or minimal brain dysfunction are particularly susceptible to interpersonal distress. For example, it may be difficult for juvenile diabetics to regulate their intake of fast foods when all of their friends are able to eat what they want. When peer pressure is at its peak in adolescence, a teenager with a newly diagnosed convulsive seizure disorder may find it difficult to tell peers he no longer can ride his bicycle or drive a car. Unless appropriate interpersonal support is provided by the family and nurse, such children have to cope with an indistinct assault to their self-concept all by themselves. A summary of age-appropriate strategies are provided in Box 18–3.

## Communicating with Ill Children in the Hospital and Ambulatory Clinic

Overestimating a child's understanding of information about illness results in confusion, increased anxiety, anger, or sadness (Marcus, 1988). Beyond physiological care, ill children of all ages need the support they would receive from parents, including stimulation to talk, listen, and play. They have major difficulties verbalizing their true feelings about the treatment experience. The nurse can be a primary resource in adapting interventions to meet the ill child's needs.

### Infants

Cues to assessment of the preverbal infant include tone of the cry, facial appearance, and body movements. Because the infant uses the senses to receive information, nonverbal communication such as touch are important tools for the pediatric nurse. Tone of voice, rocking motion, use of distraction, and a soothing touch can be used in addition to or in conjunction with verbal explanations. Face-to-face position, bending or moving to the child's eye level, maintaining eye contact, and making a reassuring facial expression further help the nurse to interact with infants.

Nurse should anticipate developmental behaviors such as "stranger anxiety" in infants between 9 and 18 months of age. Rather than reaching to pick a child up immediately, the nurse might smile and extend a hand toward the child or stroke the child's arm before attempting to hold the child. In this way, the nurse acknowledges the infant's inability to generalize to unfamiliar caregivers. If the child is able to talk, asking the child his or her name and pointing out a notable pleasant physical characteristic conveys the impression that the nurse sees the child client as a unique person. To a tiny child, this treatment can be synonymous with caring.

### Toddlers

Almost all small children receiving invasive treatment feel some threat to their safety and security, one of Maslow's hierarchy of human needs. This need is exaggerated in toddlers and young children, who cannot articulate their needs or understand why they are ill. To help the child's comprehension, nurses use phrases rather than long sentences and repeat words for emphasis. Because the toddler has a limited vocabulary, the caretaker may need to "put into words" the feelings that the ill child is conveying nonverbally.

Evaluate the agency environment: Is it safe? Does it allow for some independence and auton-

**◆ Box 18-3. Key Points in Communicating with Children According to Age Group**

## Infants

Nonverbal communication is a primary mode.

Use stroking, soft touching, holding; soothe with crooning voice tone.

*Kinesthetic Communication*

Use motion (e.g., rocking) to reassure. Allow freedom of movement, and avoid restraining when possible.

Infants are bonded to primary caregivers only. Those older than 8 months may display anxiety when approached by strangers.

Use parents to give care. Arrange for one or both parents to remain nearby.

Establish rapport with the caregiver (parent) and at first keep at least 2 feet between nurse and infant. Talk to and touch the infant and initially smile often.

Learn specifically how the primary caregiver provides care in terms of sleeping, bathing, and feeding, and attempt to mimic these approaches.

Always allow the mother to be within sight of her child, and vice versa.

*Vision: 20/200–20/300 at Birth*

Encourage the infant's caregivers (parents) to use a lot of intimate space interaction (8–18 inches). Mimic the same when trust is established.

*Minimal Receptive Language Skills*

Use a soft, slow voice tone; smile often; sit down as often as possible or stoop down so as to look less imposing.

Talk out loud in an active listening manner. Say such things as "Mommy is here and she loves you"; "Mommy will keep you safe."

*Separation Anxiety When Primary Caregiver Is Absent*

Provide for kinesthetic approaches; offer self while infant is protesting (e.g., stay with the child; pick the child up and rock or walk; talk to the child about Mommy and how much the child cares for Mommy and Daddy).

*Short Stature*

Sit down on chair, stool, or carpet to decrease posture superiority.

## Toddlers

*Limited Vocabulary and Verbal Skills*

Make explanations brief and clear. Use the child's own vocabulary words for basic care activities. Assess (e.g., use the child's words for defecate [poop, gooies] and urinate [pee-pee, tinkle]). Learn and use self-name of the child.

*Speaks in Phrases*

Rephrase the child's message in a simple, complete sentence; avoid baby talk.

*Limited Vocabulary*

Use vocabulary skills to get to know the primary caregiver *first* before approaching the child. For example, allow the child to see that the nurse can be a friend of Mommy.

*Kinesthetic Communication*

Allow ambulation where possible (toddler chairs, walkers). Pull the child in a wagon often if child cannot achieve mobility.

*Struggling with Issues of Autonomy and Control*

Allow the child some control (e.g., say "Do you want a half a glass or a whole glass of milk?")

Reassure the child if he or she displays some regressive behavior (e.g., if child wets pants, say "We will get a dry pair of pants and let you find something fun to do").

*Box continued on following page*

◆ **Box 18–3. Key Points in Communicating with Children According to Age Group** *Continued*

## Toddlers

Allow the child to express anger and to protest about his or her care (e.g., say "It's okay to cry when you are angry or hurt").

Allow the child to sit up or walk as often as possible and as soon as possible after intrusive or hurtful procedures. Say "It's all over and we can do something more fun."

Use nondirective modes, such as reflecting an aspect of appearance or temperament (e.g., "You smile so often") or playing with a toy and slowly coming closer to and including the child in play.

*Fear of Bodily Injury*

Show hands (free of hurtful items) and say "There is nothing to hurt you. I came to play/talk."

*Egocentrism*

Allow child to be self-oriented and accepted. Use distraction if another child wants the same item or toy rather than expect the child to share.

*Direct Questions*

Use a nondirective approach. Sit down and join the parallel play of the child. Reflect messages sent by toddler (nonverbally) in a verbal and nonverbal manner. For example, say "Yes, that toy does lots of interesting and fun things."

*Separation Anxiety*

Accept protesting when parent(s) leave. Hug, rock the child, and say "You miss Mommy and Daddy! They miss you too." Play peek-a-boo games with child. Make a big deal about saying "Now I am here."

Show an interest in one of the child's favorite toys. Say "I wonder what it does" or the like. If the child responds with actions, reflect them back.

## Preschoolers

*Speaks in Sentences but Is Unable to Comprehend*
*Abstract Ideas*

Use simple vocabulary; avoid lengthy explanations. Focus on the present, not the distant future; use concrete, meaningful references. For example, say "Mommy will be back after you eat your lunch" (instead of "at 1 o'clock"). Use play therapy, drawings.

*Unable to Tolerate Direct Eye-to-Eye Contact (Some Preschoolers)*

Use some eye contact and attending posture. Sit or stoop, and use a slow, soft tone of voice.

*May React Negatively and with Increased Anxiety If a Long Explanation Is Given Regarding a Painful Procedure*

Complete the procedure as quickly as possible; give explanations about its purpose afterward. For example, say "Jimmy, I'm going to give you a shot" (quickly administer the injection). "There. All done. It's okay to cry when you hurt. I'd complain, too. This medicine will make your tummy feel better."

*Short Attention Span and Imaginative Stage*

Explain, using imagination (puppetry, drama with dress-ups); use music.

Use play therapy: allow the child to play with safe equipment used in treatment. Talk about the needed procedure happening to a doll or teddy bear, and state simply how it will occur and be experienced. Use sensory data: say, for example, "The teddy bear will hear a buzzing sound."

*Concrete Sense of Humor Beginning*

Tell corny jokes and laugh with the child.

*Continuing Need to Have Control*

Provide for many choices (e.g., "Do you want to get dressed now or after breakfast?")

◆ Box 18-3. Key Points in Communicating with Children According to Age Group *Continued*

## School Age

*Developing Ability to Comprehend*

Include the child in concrete explanations about condition, treatment, protocols.

Use draw-a-person to identify basic knowledge the child has, and build on it.

Use some of the same words the child uses in giving explanations.

Use sensory information in giving explanations (e.g., "You will smell alcohol in the cast room.")

*Assuming Increased Responsibility for Health Care Practices*

Reinforce basic care activities in teaching.

*Increased Need for Privacy*

Respect privacy: Knock on the door before entering; tell the client when and for what reasons you will need to return to his or her room.

## Early Adolescence

*Increased Comprehension About Possible Negative Threats to Life or Body Integrity, Yet Some Difficulty in Adhering to Long-Term Goals*

Verbalize issues about treatment protocols that require giving up immediate gratifications for long-term gain. Explore alternative options (e.g., tell a diabetic adolescent who must give up after-school fries with friends that he or she could save two breads and four fats exchanges to have a milkshake).

*Confidentiality May Be an Issue*

Reassure the adolescent about the confidentiality of your discussion, but clearly state the limits of this confidentiality. If, for example, the child should talk of killing himself, this information needs to be shared with parents and staff.

*Struggling to Establish Identity and Be Independent*

Allow participation in decision making, wearing own clothes. Avoid an authoritarian approach when possible. Avoid a judgmental approach. Use a clarifying and qualifying approach. Actively listen. Accept regression.

*Beginning to Demonstrate Abstract Thinking*

Use abstract thinking, but look for nonverbal cues (puzzled face) that may indicate lack of understanding. Then clarify in more concrete terms.

*Uses Colloquial Language or Street Slang*

Couch your dialogue with the use of some of the client's words.

*Sexual Awareness and Maturation*

Offer self and a willingness to listen. Provide value-free, accurate information.

From Joyce Ruth, MSN, University of North Carolina College of Nursing at Charlotte, 1998.

omy? Care in the ambulatory setting is facilitated if a parent or caregiver is present. Care in the hospital is enhanced by agency policies that promote parent–child contact, such as unlimited visiting hours, rooming-in, or use of audiocassettes of a parent's voice. Familiar objects make the environment safer. According to Wincott (1971), transitional objects such as a teddy bear, blanket, or favorite toy remind the alone or frightened child that the security of the parent is still available even when he or she is not physically present. Some hospitals have a prehospital orientation in which they present small children with a familiar transitional object to bring with them when they return for the actual hospitalization. Box 18–4 presents a representative nursing care problem.

Distraction is a successful strategy with tod-

---

◆ **Box 18–4. Representative Nursing Problem: Dealing with an Irritable Toddler**

### Situation

Tommy, age 2 years, is hospitalized for a minor surgical procedure. Ms. K. is a single parent and unable to room-in because of family responsibilities. The father is unavailable. The toddler is very fussy and irritable when his mother is not around, crying frequently and demonstrating aggressive behaviors during caretaking activities.

### Nursing Diagnosis

Ineffective coping related to separation anxiety and stress of hospitalization

### Nursing Goals

Reduce stress of hospitalization related to separation anxiety and loss of consistent mothering; provide warm, secure environment.

### Interventions

1. Assign consistent substitute self-care agent who will provide warm, nurturing care.
2. Accept the child's behavior (crying, screaming) as healthy manifestations of separation anxiety; do not attempt to suppress the child's expression of anger or nonverbally communicate to the child that he is "bad" for acting this way.
3. Position self near the child while he or she is crying or angry and provide nonverbal support (touch, tactile stimulation) to demonstrate acceptance of the child's behavior.
4. Provide a transitional object or familiar objects from home that will comfort and soothe the child.
5. Allow liberal visiting hours so the mother may visit at her convenience.
6. Adhere to the child's home routines as much as possible during hospitalization to create a secure environment for the child.
7. Allow the child the opportunity to express anger at being "deserted" through such play activities as pounding a board with pegs, playing with large wooden spoons and nonbreakable pots, or drawing with thick crayons on paper.
8. If limits must be set to reduce aggressive behavior, make sure the limits are few in number and are consistently followed by all health care personnel.

From M. Michaels, University of Maryland School of Nursing, 1987.

---

dlers in ambulatory settings. Use of stuffed animals, wind-up toys, "magic" exam lights that blow out can turn fright into delight. One advanced practice nurse recommended the use of a musical watch during otoscopic exams, telling the child that "children who sit very still can hear a song when I look into their ears" (Flarity, 1997).

### Preschoolers

Throughout the preoperational period, young children tend to interpret language in a literal way. For example, the child who is told that he will be "put to sleep" during the operation tomorrow may think it means the same as the action recently taken for a pet dog who was too ill to live. Children do not ask for clarification, so messages can be misunderstood quite easily.

Preschool children have limited auditory recall and are unable to process auditory information quickly. They have a short attention span. Verbal communication with the preschool child should be clear, succinct, and easy to understand (Enlow & Swisher, 1986).

Before the age of 7, most children cannot make a clear distinction between fantasy and reality. Everything is "real," and anything strange is perceived as potentially harmful. Anything the nurse can do to make the child's environment stable, real, and manageable will be helpful to the preschool client.

In the hospital, young children need frequent

concrete reminders to reinforce reality. Assigning the same caregiver reduces insecurity. Visiting the preschooler at the same time each day and posting family pictures are simple strategies to reduce the child's fears of abandonment (Petrillo & Sanger, 1980). The nurse can link information to activities of daily living. For example, saying, "Your mother will come after you take your nap" rather than "at 2 o'clock" is much more understandable to the preschool client.

Assessment of the preschooler's ability to communicate involves a careful evaluation of the actual child's level of understanding. Children need to be assessed for misconceptions and troubling problems, preferably using free play and fantasy storytelling exercises. Egocentrism can be a normal developmental process that may prevent children from understanding why they cannot have a drink when they are fasting before a scheduled test. Explanations given long beforehand may not be remembered. If something is going to hurt, the nurse should be forthright about it, while at the same time reassuring the child that he or she will have the appropriate support. Simple explanations reduce the child's anxiety. No child should ever be left to figure out what is happening without some type of simple explanation. Box 18–2 can help you focus on specific communication strategies with the hospitalized preschooler.

### Play as a Communication Strategy

The preschooler lacks a suitable vocabulary to express complex thoughts and feelings. Small children cannot picture what they have never experienced. Play is an effective means by which a puzzling and sometimes painful real world can be approached. Play allows the child to create a concrete experience of something unknown and potentially frightening. By constructing a situation in play, the child is able to put together the components of the situation in ways that promote recognition and make it a concrete reality. When the child can deal with things that are small or inanimate, the child masters situations that to him or her might otherwise be overwhelming. Cartoons, pictures, or puppets can be used to demonstrate actions and terminology. Dolls with removable cloth organs help children understand scheduled operations.

Preschoolers tend to think of their disabilities or illnesses, their separation from parents, and any painful treatments as punishment. Play can be used to help children express their feelings about an illness and to role-play coping strategies. Allowing the young child to manipulate syringes, give "shots" to a doll, or put a bandage or restraint on a teddy bear's arm allows the child to act out his or her feelings. The child becomes "the aggressor." Play can be a major channel for communication in the nurse–client relationship involving a young child. Preschool children develop communication themes through their play and work through conflict situations in their own good time; the process cannot be rushed. As the child develops trust in the interpersonal environment, themes are clarified and goals can be accomplished.

Play materials vary with the age and developmental status of the child. Simple, large toys are used with young children; more intricate playthings are used with older preschoolers. Clay, crayons, and paper become modes of expression for important feelings and thoughts about problems.

Play can be the pediatric health care professional's primary tool for assessing preschool children's perceptions about their hospital experience, their anxieties and fears, and their coping ability (Parish, 1986). Preschoolers love jokes, puns, and riddles; the cornier, the better. Using jokes during the physical assessment, such as "Let me hear your lunch" or "Golly, could that be a potato in your ear?" helps form the bonds needed for successful relationship with the preschool client. Box 18–5 presents a typical nursing care problem.

### Storytelling as a Communication Strategy

A communication strategy often used with young children is the use of story plots. Gardner (1986) described a mutual storytelling technique in which the caregiver asks the child whether he would like to help make up a story. If the child is a little reluctant, the nurse may begin as described in Exercise 18–1. At the end of the story, the child is asked to indicate what lesson might be learned from the story. If the child seems a little reluctant to give a moral to the story, the nurse might suggest that all stories have something that can be learned from them. The nurse

---

### ◆ Box 18–5. Representative Nursing Problem: Dealing with a Fearful Preschooler

#### Situation

While climbing a tree in his backyard, John A., 4 1/2 years, falls and breaks his left femur. He is hospitalized for 2 weeks of traction before application of a hip spica cast. During routine morning care, John tells you he was a naughty boy for climbing the tree and now he's being punished. He goes on to say, "If I don't do everything the nurses tell me to do, then this big hairy monster will sneak in during the night and break my other leg."

#### Nursing Diagnosis

Ineffective coping related to hospitalization and threats to body integrity due to immature cognitive structures and simplistic, "magical" view of morality

#### Nursing Goals

Reduce the stress of hospitalization and increase the child's sense of control; reduce threats to body integrity.

#### Intervention

1. Maintain mutual respect while talking to the child by not ridiculing or belittling his fears or perceptions.
2. Use reflection to determine what he has been told about the accident, what his parents' reactions were, and so forth.
3. Respond to the feeling tone of what the child is saying rather than content; help him understand what he is feeling (fear, anger, helplessness) rather than why he is feeling that way.
4. Talk slowly and casually; do not overwhelm or frighten him with lengthy explanations; when appropriate, reassure him that no one is to blame.
5. Assign a primary nurse or consistent caregiver to ensure continuity of care and to provide a sense of security for the child.
6. Encourage the parents to visit frequently and even become involved in the child's care; such involvement will tell the child his parents are concerned and care about him.
7. Using the concept of storytelling, have the child make up a story about a particular event or show him a picture of an event and have him describe what is happening.
8. Because 4 1/2-year-olds enjoy manipulative or constructive play, provide toys that require being put together or even "fixed"; provide materials for making a cast and have the child "fix" a doll's broken leg; have the child tell you how the doll's leg was broken.
9. Provide a nightlight in his room and discuss all the different things that scare monsters (e.g., lights).

From M. Michaels, University of Maryland School of Nursing, 1987.

---

analyzes the themes presented by the child, which usually reveal important feelings. Is the story fearful? Are the characters scary or pleasing? The child should be praised for telling the story. The next step in the process is for nurses to ask themselves, "What would be a healthier resolution or a more mature adaptation than the one used by the child?" The nurse could suggest an alternative ending or plot. In the nurse's version of the story, the characters and other details remain the same initially, but the story contains a more positive solution or suggests alternative answers to problems. The object of mutual storytelling is to offer the child an opportunity to explore different alternatives in a neutral communication process with a helping person. Exercise 18–1 provides an opportunity to experiment with a mutual storytelling strategy.

◆ Exercise 18–1. **Using a Mutual Storytelling Technique**

**Purpose:**  To give practical experience with the mutual storytelling technique

**Procedure:**

1. Use the mutual storytelling process described in the text with a 5- to 8-year-old child in your neighborhood.
2. Write down the story the child told and suggest alternate endings.
3. Share your stories with each other in turn during the next class period.

**Discussion:**

1. How difficult was it for you to engage the child? If you had trouble, what alternate actions would you incorporate in using the technique again?
2. Were you surprised at the story the child produced? If so, in what ways?
3. What did you learn about the child when using this technique?
4. What conclusions might you draw from hearing the other students relate their experiences about the use of this technique? In what situations was it most effective? Least effective?
5. What did you learn about yourself as a helping person in using this technique?

**Sample Answer:**

*Nurse*: Once upon a time in a land far away, there lived a . . .
*Child*: dragon
*Nurse*: a dragon who ate . . .
*Child*: carrots.
*Nurse*: The dragon ate carrots and slept . . .
*Child*: in a cave.
*Nurse*: One day he left the cave to go out and find many sweet carrots to eat, but as he walked along he ran into a . . .
*Child*: bike.
*Nurse*: He was afraid of the bike and so he . . .
*Child*: kicked it and ran away.
*Nurse*: After he ran away, is there any more to the story?
*Child* (upset): He got hit with a stick.
*Nurse*: What is the message to this story? What does it tell us? . . .
*Child*: about running away not to be punished.

## School-Age Children

As children move into concrete operational thinking, they begin to internalize the reasons for illness: illness is caused by germs, or you have cavities because you ate too much candy or did not brush your teeth. In later childhood, most children become better able to work verbally with the nurse. It still is important to prepare responses carefully and to anticipate problems, but the child is capable of expressing feelings and ventilating frustration more directly through words. Use Exercise 18–2 to reformulate medical technology into age-appropriate expressions.

Assessment of the child's cognitive level of understanding continues to be essential; the nurse searches for concrete examples to which the child can relate rather than giving abstract examples. If children are to learn from a model, they must see the model performing the skill to

◆ Exercise 18-2. **Age-Appropriate Medical Terminology**

**Purpose:** To help you think of terminology appropriate to use with young clients

**Procedure:**
Reformulate the following expressions using words a child can understand.

Cardiac catheterization
NPO
Sedation
Nausea
Urine specimen
Vital signs
Anesthesia
Enema
Dressings
Infection
Injection
Disease
Inflammation
Operating room
Isolation
Intake and output
IV needle

**Discussion:**
Think of any experiences you might have had as a child client or may have observed. What were some of the troublesome words you found in these experiences?

be learned. School-age children thrive on explanations of how their bodies work and enjoy understanding the scientific rationales for their treatment. School-age children and adolescents should themselves become the primary source of information needed by the nurse (Enlow & Swisher, 1986). The parent may be consulted for validation.

### Using Audiovisual Aids as a Communication Strategy

Audiovisual aids and reading material geared to the child's level of understanding may supplement verbal explanations. Details about what the child will hear, see, smell, and feel are important. Diagrams can be used to help provide simple, accurate scientific information. For the younger school-age child, expressive art can be a useful method to convey feelings and to open up communication (Parish, 1986). The older school-age child or adolescent might best convey feelings by writing a poem, a short story, or a letter. This written material can assist the nurse in understanding hidden thoughts or emotions. Williams (1987) suggested that self-photographs are an innovative short cut to developing meaningful talk sessions with emotionally disturbed children.

### Mutuality in Decision Making

Children of this age need to be involved in discussions of their illness and in planning for their care. Explanations giving the rationale for care are useful. Involving the child in decision making may decrease fears about the illness, the treatment, or the effect on family life. Videotapes and written materials may be useful in involving the child in the management phase of care. Lewis, Pantell, and Sharp (1991) noted that, although children often are included in data gathering, there is a tendency to exclude them from management and diagnostic information. In this study, when children were included in discussions of medical recommendations, the children were more satisfied with their care and recalled more information.

## Adolescents

An understanding of adolescence and the intensity of the search for identity is essential for the nurse working with teenagers. Even teens enjoying good health are forced to deal with new health issues such as acne, menstrual problems, and sexual activity (Tindall et al., 1994). The adolescent vacillates between childhood and adulthood and is emotionally vulnerable. The ambivalence of the adolescent period may be expressed through withdrawal, rebellion, lost motivation, and rapid mood changes. All of these behaviors are normal in varying degrees as teenagers examine values and standards. However, identity issues become more difficult to resolve when the normal opportunities for physical independence, privacy, and social contacts are compromised by illness or handicaps. Sick, well, or disabled, all adolescents have questions about their developing body and sexuality. They have the same longings and desires. Problems may be greater for ill teens because the natural outlets for their expression with peers are curtailed by the disorder or by hospitalization. Use of peer groups, adolescent lounges (separate from the small children's playroom), and a telephone in the rooms, as well as provisions for wearing one's own clothes, "fixing up" hair, or attending hospital school may help teenagers adjust to hospitalization. When the developmental identity crisis becomes too uncomfortable, adolescents may project their fury and frustration onto family or staff. Identifying rage as a normal response to a difficult situation can be very reassuring.

Assessment of the adolescent should occur in a private setting. Attention to the client's interpersonal comfort and space will have a tremendous impact on the quality of the interaction. To the teenager, the nurse represents an authority figure. The need for compassion, concern, and respect is perhaps greater during adolescence than at other times in the life span. Often lacking the verbal skills of adults, yet wishing to appear in control, adolescents do well with direct questions. Innocuous questions are used first to allow the teenager enough space to check the validity of his or her reactions to the nurse. In caring for a teen in an ambulatory office or clinic, I always conduct part of the history interview without the parent present. If the parent will not leave the exam room, this can be done while walking the teen down to the laboratory. Questions about substance use, sexual activity, and so on demand confidentiality.

To assess a teen's cognitive level, find out about his or her ability to make long-term plans. An easy way to do this is the "3 wishes question." Ask the teen to name three things he or she would expect to have in 5 years. Answers can be analyzed for concreteness, realism, goal-directness, and so on. Questions for psychosocial assessment are provided in Box 18–6.

### Using Hobbies as a Communication Strategy

Adolescents still rely primarily on feedback from adults and from friends to judge their own competency. A teen may not yet have developed proficiency and comfort in carrying on verbal conversations with adults. The teen may respond best if the nurse uses several modalities to communicate. Using empathy, conveying acceptance, and using open-ended questions are three useful strategies (Tindall et al., 1994). Sometimes more innovative communication strategies are needed. In the following case example, the teen

---

◆ Box 18–6. Psychosocial Assessment of Adolescents

1. Level of self-care responsibility
2. Quality of relationships with significant others, including health practices such as safe sex for those who are sexually active
3. Self-concept, body image, and personal identity
4. Threats to developmental integration of body functions, such as may occur with an ostomy
5. Age-appropriate interpersonal and cognitive functioning

has a difficult time talking, so the use of another modality is appropriate.

◆ **Case Example**

Ashley, a first-year student nurse, becomes frustrated during the course of her conversation with her assigned client, 17-year-old Cary, admitted 5 days ago to the psychiatric unit. Despite a genuine desire to engage him in a therapeutic alliance, the client would not talk. Attempts to get to know him on a verbal level seemed to increase rather than decrease his anxiety. The nurse correctly inferred that, despite his age, this adolescent needed a more tangible approach. Knowing that the client likes cars, Ashley brought in an automotive magazine. Together they looked at the magazine; the publication soon became their special vehicle for communication, bridging the gap between the client's inner reality and his ability to express himself verbally in a meaningful way. Feelings about cars gradually generalized to verbal expressions about other situations, and Cary quickly began describing his life dreams, disappointments, and attitudes about himself. When Ashley left the unit, he asked to keep the magazine and frequently spoke of her with fondness. This simple recognition of his awkwardness in verbal communication and use of another tool to facilitate the relationship had a positive effect.

## Dealing with Care Problems

### Pain

The literature has identified a lack of understanding about pain in children as a barrier to giving optimal nursing care (Craig et al., 1996). For years, children's ability to feel pain has been underrated by adult caregivers. This may in part be due to the child's limited capacity to communicate the nature of their discomfort. Infants indicate pain with physiological changes, including diaphoresis, pallor, increased heart rate, increased respirations, and decreased oxygen saturation. Effective nonpharmacological interventions for pain include pacifiers, rocking, physical contact, and sometimes even swaddling (Page & Halvorson, 1991). Nurses now are educated to use age-specific pain assessment instruments with toddlers and preschoolers. Exercise 18–3 will stimulate discussion about care for children in pain.

### Anxiety

Illness is often an unanticipated event. Uncertainty and even anxiety should be expected when both treatment and outcome are unknown. Young children react to unexpected stimuli, to painful procedures, and even to the presence of strangers with fear. Older children fear separation from parents, but also may fear injury, loss of body function, or even just being perceived by friends as "different" because of their illness. Exercise 18–4 helps develop age-appropriate explanations that may reduce anxiety.

### Acting-Out Behaviors

Behavior problems in adolescents present a special challenge to the nurse. Clear communication of expectations, treatment protocols, and hospital rules is of value. As much as possible, adolescents should be allowed to act on their own behalf in making choices and judgments about their functioning. At the same time, adolescents still need

---

◆ **Exercise 18–3. Pediatric Nursing Procedures**

**Purpose:** To give practice in preparing young clients for painful procedures

**Procedure:**
Timmy, age 4 years, is going to have a bone marrow aspiration. (The insertion of a large needle into the hip is a painful procedure.)

**Discussion:**
Answer the following questions:

1. What essential information does Timmy need?
2. If this is a frequently repeated procedure, how can you make him feel safe before and after the procedure?
3. How soon in advance should you prepare him?

◆ Exercise 18-4. **Preparing Children for Treatment Procedures**

**Purpose:** To help students apply developmental concepts to age-appropriate nursing interventions

**Procedure:**
Students divide into four small groups and design an age-appropriate intervention for the following situation. As a large group, each small group spokesperson writes the intervention on the board in the age labels column.

**Situation:**
Jamie is scheduled to go to the surgical suite later today to have a central infusion catheter inserted for hyperalimentation. This is Jamie's first procedure on the first day of this first hospitalization experience.

**Discussion:**
Group focuses on comparing interventions across the age spans.

1. How does each intervention differ according to the age of the child? (Make age-appropriate interventions for preschooler, school-age child, and adolescent.)
2. What concept themes are common across the age spans? (Education components: assessing initial level of knowledge; assessing ability to comprehend information, readiness to receive information; adapting information to cognitive level of child.)
3. What formats might be best used for each age group? (Role-play with dolls, pictures, comic books, educational pamphlets, peer group session, etc.)

limits on behavior. Limit setting assumes special importance in adolescence, when, of necessity, it becomes a more collaborative experience.

Limits define the boundaries of acceptable behaviors in a relationship. Initially determined by the parents or the nurse, limits can be developed mutually as an important part of the relationship as the child matures. Determining consequences has a positive value in that it provides the child with a model for handling frustrating situations in a more adult manner.

Once the conflict is resolved and the child has accepted the consequences of his or her behavior, the child should be given an opportunity to discuss attitudes and feelings that led up to the need for limits as well as his or her reaction to the limits set.

Although communication about limits is necessary for the survival of the relationship, it needs to be balanced with time for interaction that is pleasant and positive. Sometimes with children who need limits frequently, discussion of the restrictions is the only conversation that takes place between nurse and client. When this is noted, nurses might ask themselves what feelings the child might be expressing through his or her actions. Putting into words the feelings that are being acted out helps children trust the nurse's competence and concern. Usually it is necessary for the entire staff to share this responsibility. Box 18–7 and Box 18–8 present a step-by-step proposal for setting limits within the context of the nurse–client relationship.

## More Helpful Strategies for Communicating with Children

Adapting general communications strategies studied earlier in this book to interactions with children requires some imagination and creativity. Exercise 18–5 should provoke some light-hearted activities that may strengthen pediatric care skills.

### Active Listening

Knowing what a child truly needs and values is the heart of successful interpersonal relationships in health care settings. The process of active listening takes form initially from watching the be-

From Felker D. (1974). Building Positive Self-Concepts. Minneapolis, MN, Burgess Publishing. Reprinted with permission.

---

### ◆ Box 18–7. Guidelines for Developing Workable Consequences for Unacceptable Behavior

**Effective consequences are**

- Logical and fit the situation
- Applied in a matter-of-fact manner without lengthy discussion
- Situation centered rather than person centered
- Applied immediately after the transgression

---

haviors of children as they play and interact with their environments. As a child's vocabulary increases and the capacity to engage with others develops, listening begins to approximate the communication process that occurs between adults, with one important difference. Because the perceptual world of the child is concrete,

the nurse's feedback and informational messages should coincide with the child's developmental level. Buscaglia (1986) described the type of listening needed in a poem by an anonymous writer.

---

*When I ask you to listen and you start giving me advice, you have not done what I asked.*

*When I ask you to listen to me and you feel you have to do something to solve my problem, you have failed me, strange as that may seem.*

*Listen! All that I asked was that you listen, not talk or do—just hear me.*

*When you do something for me that I can or*

---

### ◆ Box 18–8. Outline of a Limit-Setting Plan

1. Have the child describe his or her behavior.

*Key:* Evaluate realistically.

2. Encourage the child to assess behavior. Is it helpful for others and himself?

*Key:* Evaluate realistically.

3. Encourage the child to develop an alternative plan for governing behavior.

*Key:* Set reasonable goals.

4. Have the child sign a statement about his or her plan.

*Key:* Commit to goals.

5. At the end of the appropriate time period, have the child assess his performance.

*Key:* Evaluate realistically.

6. Provide positive reinforcement for those aspects of performance that were successful.*

*Key:* Evaluate realistically.

7. Encourage the child to make a positive statement about his performance.

*Key:* Teach self-praise.

*If the child's performance does not meet the criteria set in the plan, return to Step 3 and assist the child in modifying the plan so that success is more possible. If, on the other hand, the child's performance is successful, help him or her to develop a more ambitious plan (e.g., for a longer time period or for a larger set of behaviors).

From Felker D. (1974). Building Positive Self-Concepts. Minneapolis, MN, Burgess Publishing. Reprinted with permission.

◆ **Exercise 18-5. Strategies for Conducting an Assessment on the Toddler and the Preschooler**

**Purpose:** To help students adapt assessment skills to younger children

**Procedure:**
Each student will state one technique he or she has seen successfully used by a health care worker attempting to auscultate heart sounds in a toddler. Change this scenario to examining the child's ear with an otoscope. Change the context from hospital to ambulatory care or outpatient clinic. Then change the age to preschooler.

---

*need to do for myself, you contribute to my fear and inadequacy.*

*But when you accept as a simple fact I do feel what I feel, no matter how irrational, then I can quit trying to convince you and get about this business of understanding what is behind this irrational feeling.*

*And when that's clear, the answers are obvious and I don't need advice.*

*Irrational feelings make sense when we understand what's behind them.*

*So, please listen and just hear me.*

*And if you want to talk, wait a minute for your turn—and I'll listen to you.*

---

Working with children is rewarding, hard work that sometimes must be evaluated indirectly. For instance, George was the primary care nurse who had worked very hard with a 13-year-old girl over a 6-month period while the girl was on a bone marrow transplant unit. He felt bad when, at discharge, the girl stated, "I never want to see any of you people again." However, just before leaving, the nurse found her sobbing on her bed. No words were spoken, but the child threw her arms around George and clung to him for comfort. For this nurse, the child's expression of grief was an acknowledgment of the meaning of the relationship. Children, even those who

are verbal, often communicate through behavior rather than verbally when under stress.

### Authenticity

Life crises are an inevitable part of life. Many parents and health professionals ignore children's feeling or deceive them about procedures, illness, or hospitalization in the mistaken belief that they will be overwhelmed by the truth. Just the opposite is true. Children, like adults, can cope with most stressors as long as they are presented in a manner they can understand and given enough time and support from the environment to cope. In fact, very ill children often are a source of inspiration to the adults working with them because of their courage in facing the truth about themselves and dealing with it constructively. Completing Exercise 18–6 may stimulate some discussion.

A nurse should never allow any individual, even a parent, to threaten a child. For example, many a parent has been heard to say, "You be good or I'll have the nurse give you a shot." It is appropriate to interrupt this parent. Children respect honest expression of emotions in adults. Being real with children is a crucial factor in the development of a therapeutic relationship.

◆ **Case Example**

In a community setting, an older student nurse, with a family of her own, was monitoring a family in which the mother had terminal cancer. There were three children in the family, and the identified client of the student was a 13-year-old boy. He was abnormally quiet, and it was difficult to draw him out. Halfway through the semester, the boy's father died unexpectedly of a heart attack. When the boy and student nurse next met, the nurse asked the boy whether there was

---

◆ **Exercise 18-6. Working with the Newly Diagnosed Human Immunodeficiency Virus-Positive Teenager**

**Purpose:** To stimulate class discussion about how to deal with the adolescent who is difficult to communicate with. Questions can be done out of class, with class time used only for discussion.

**Procedure:**
Read the case situation and answer the questions that follow.

**Situation:**
Bill, age 17 years, seeks treatment for gonorrhea. He is hospitalized for further testing after his initial workup reveals he is seropositive for human immunodeficiency virus (HIV) type 1. For 2 days on the unit he has cried, cursed, and been uncooperative. Staff tends to avoid him when possible. A team of residents begins a bone marrow aspiration procedure in the treatment room after obtaining his absent parents' permission. (They have expressed condemnation and have not yet been to visit.) A technician walks in and out of the room to obtain supplies while the doctors concentrate on completing the procedure. A student nurse is asked to come in to help restrain Bill, who is alternately screaming, crying, and being very quiet.

1. What communication strategies could this student use as he squeezes into this small room? (Clue: verbal and nonverbal directed to the client and to the doctors)
2. What assessment might the nurse want to make? (Clue: what are Bill's feelings about his diagnosis?)
3. What can be inferred about Bill's current behavior?
4. What interventions would you suggest for initiating interaction with his parents?
5. What additional data are needed before attempting any teaching about acquired immunodeficiency syndrome?

---

anything special that had happened between father and son that the boy would remember about his father. The boy replied that the day before his father's death he had received a letter of acceptance to the same school his father had attended, and he had shared this with his father. He said his father was very proud that he had been accepted. The student nurse could feel her eyes fill as the boy revealed himself to her in this special way. Her sharing of honest emotion was a significant turning point in what became a very important relationship for both participants. It was a moment of shared meaning for both of them and, from that time on, the needed common ground for communication existed.

Being real does not mean being overly familiar. Trying to interact with older children and adolescents as though the nurse is a buddy is confusing to the client. What the child wants is an emotionally available, calm, caring, competent resource who can protect, care about, and, above all, listen to him or her.

## Conveying Respect

It is easy for adults to impose their own wishes on a child. Respecting a child's right to feel and to express his or her feelings appropriately is important. Providing truthful answers is a hallmark of respect. When interacting with the older child, using the concept of mutuality will promote respect and should foster more positive and lasting health care outcomes (Henson, 1997). Confidentiality needs to be maintained unless the nurse judges that revealing information is necessary to prevent harm to the child or adolescent. In such cases, the child needs to be advised of the disclosure.

## Providing Anticipatory Guidance to the Child

The American Academy of Pediatrics has published guidelines for health care providers working with well children in the community. These suggestions focus on health promotion information to be given to caretakers at appropriate ages. Managed care has brought an increased focus on the role a child can assume in being responsible for his or her own health care. It is never too early to begin. For example, McCarthy and Hobbie (1997) provided very clear written handouts for incorporating violence prevention into well-child visits made to nurse practitioners. This shift in placing responsibility for good health practices onto the individual is in line with recommendations in *Healthy People 2010 AD*.

## Interacting with Parents of Ill Children

According to some estimates, up to 20 or 30 percent of all children have some form of chronic illness (Sterling et al., 1997). Having an ill child is stressful for parents. Many research studies have shown that loss of the ability to act as the child's parent, to alleviate the child's pain, and to comfort the child is more stressful than factors connected with the illness, including coping with uncertainty over the outcome. Other stressors include financial and marital strains. Stress may vary across cultures (Rei & Fong, 1996; Sterling et al., 1997). For example, Hispanic parents in the Rei and Fong study cited coping with strange sights, sounds, and equipment as being highly stressful. Other studies pointed to a lack of needed information and support from professionals as being a top stressor, exacerbating already existing family problems and resulting in feelings of fear and helplessness. Exercise 18–7 may increase student awareness of family conflict situations.

Parents frequently have questions about discussing their child's illness or disability with

---

◆ **Exercise 18–7. Conflicts Experienced by Care Providers of HIV-Positive Children**

**Purpose:** To stimulate student discussion of role conflict

**Procedure:**
Students break into small groups to read and discuss the following case. In class compare responses.

**Situation:**
Janet is a 24-year-old nurse who graduated 2 years ago. She is transferred to a new unit exclusively admitting children with acquired immunodeficiency syndrome (AIDS). She enjoys her work, finding the children's physical, social, and psychological needs challenging. She also enjoys the collegial attitudes of her coworkers. However, her parents, with whom she still lives, are pressuring her to quit. Also she has recently become involved with a man with whom she is discussing marriage. He shares her parents' concerns about her work. Janet doesn't want to give up this job she loves and feels to leave would be akin to deserting clients who need her skills and with whom she has established therapeutic relationships. However, she doesn't want to live in conflict with her loved ones.

**Discussion:**

1. This is a long-standing conflict. What successful coping strategies has Janet used?

2. What factors are operating to increase her conflict? Consider your own family's feeling about your contact with AIDS clients.

3. What options would you suggest for Janet? There are no wrong answers, and many nurses do resolve this type of conflict by withdrawing from the situation. Suggest other more adaptive responses.

Contributed by Gail Tumulty, RN, PhD, Saudi Arabia.

others. Telling siblings and friends the truth is important. For one thing, it provides a role model for the siblings to follow in answering the curious questions of their friends. Issues such as overprotectiveness, discipline, time out for parents to replenish commitment and energy, and the quality and quantity of interactions with the hospitalized child have a powerful impact on the child's growth and development.

More frustrating to nurses are parents who are critical of the nurse's interventions, displacing the anger they feel about their own powerlessness onto the nurse (Box 18–9). The nurse may be tempted to become defensive or sarcastic or simply to dismiss the comments of the parent as irrational. However, a more helpful response would be to place oneself in the parents' shoes and to consider the possible issues. Asking the parents what information they have or might need, simply listening in a nondefensive way, and allowing the parents to vent some of their frustrations facilitate the possibility of dialogue about the underlying feelings. The listening strategies given in Chapter 10 are helpful. Sometimes a listening response that acknowledges the legitimacy of the parent's feeling is helpful: "I'm sorry that you feel so bad" or "It must be difficult for you to see your child in such pain." These simple comments acknowledge the very real anguish parents experience in health care situations having few palatable options. If possible, parental venting of feeling should occur in a private setting out of hearing range from the child. It is very upsetting to children to experience splitting in the parent–nurse relationship.

Rei and Fong (1996) suggested that nurses can reduce parental stress by educating them about their child's condition. When the child has a chronic illness, the family is called on to continually adjust the family system to adapt to changing demands in the child's health. More than 10 percent of the population has a chronically ill or disabled child to care for (Clawson, 1996). Because nursing care is largely moving to care in the home, nurses will have an increasing need to help families cope with seriously, chronically ill children. At times, the nurse will be called on to act as the child's advocate in giving parents helpful information, anticipatory guidance, and complex technical assistance in caring for the health and developmental needs of their child (Dixon & Stein, 1987). Guidelines for communicating with parents are presented in Box 18–10.

### Anticipatory Guidance in the Community

Every parent is entitled to a full explanation of the child's disability and treatment. Because the parents usually assume responsibility for the child's care after they leave the hospital, it is essential to encourage active involvement from the very beginning of treatment. Many parents look to the nurse for guidance and support in this process. In ambulatory well-child clinics, parents of well children need facts about normal development, milestones to expect, as well as prevention of illness.

## Community, Family, and Nurse Partnerships

According to Hoeman (1997), forming a partnership with the family can be the best method a nurse has to address the complex health care needs of children with chronic illnesses. Parents' participation in the care of their child and active involvement in decision making regarding the youngster's treatment ensure a more stable environment for the child. The focus of care is shifting to community partnership movements across the world. Parents are the central figures in care planning, with significant input as to which community social formal and friend networks and which professionals will be mobilized to provide care to their child. Successful collaboration requires active commitment to meet client needs by all parties involved (Paavilainen & Astedt-Kurki, 1997).

## SUMMARY

Working with children requires patience, imagination, and creative applications of therapeutic communication strategies. Children's ability to understand and communicate with nurses is largely influenced by their cognitive developmental level and by limited life experiences. Nurses need to develop an understanding of feelings and thought processes from the child's perspective, and communication strategies with children should reflect these understandings.

◆ Box 18-9. Representative Nursing Problem: Dealing with a Frightened Parent

### Situation

During report, the night nurse relates an incident that occurred between Mrs. Smith, the mother of an 8-year-old admitted for possible acute lymphocytic leukemia, and the night supervisor. Mrs. Smith told the supervisor that her son was receiving poor care from the nurses and that they frequently ignored her and refused to answer her questions. While you are making rounds following the report, Mrs. Smith corners you outside her son's room and begins to tell you about all the things that went wrong during the night. She goes on to say, "If you people think I'm going to stand around and allow my son to be treated this way, you are sadly mistaken."

### Problem

Frustration and anger caused by a sense of powerlessness and fear related to the son's possible diagnosis

### Nursing Diagnosis

Ineffective coping related to hospitalization of son and possible diagnosis of leukemia

### Nursing Goals

Increase the mother's sense of control and problem-solving capabilities; help the mother develop adaptive coping behaviors.

### Method of Assistance

Guiding; supporting; providing developmental environment

### Interventions

1. Actively listen to the client's concerns with as much objectivity as possible; maintain eye contact with the client; use minimal verbal activity, allowing the client the opportunity to express her concerns and fears freely.
2. Use reflective questioning to determine the client's level of understanding and the extent of information obtained from health team members.
3. Listen for repetitive words or phrases that may serve to identify problem areas or provide insight into fears and concerns.
4. Reassure the mother when appropriate that her child's hospitalization is indeed frightening and it is all right to be scared; remember to demonstrate interest in the client as a person; use listening responses (e.g., "It must be hard not knowing the results of all these tests") to create an atmosphere of concern.
5. Avoid communication blocks, such as giving false reassurance, telling the client what to do, or ignoring the concerns. Such behavior effectively cuts off therapeutic communication.
6. Keep the client continually informed regarding her child's progress.
7. Involve the client in her son's care; do not overwhelm her or make her feel she has to do this; watch for cues that tell you she is ready "to do more."
8. Acknowledge the impact this illness may have on the family; involve the health team in identifying ways to reduce the client's fears and provide for continuity in the type of information presented to her and other family members.
9. Assign a primary nurse to care for the client's son and serve as a resource to the client. Identify support systems in the community that might provide help and support to the client.

From M. Michaels, University of Maryland School of Nursing, 1987.

---

◆ **Box 18–10. Guidelines for Communicating with Parents**

Present complex information in informational chunks.

Repeat information and allow plenty of time for questions.

Keep parents continually informed of progress and changes in condition

Involve parents in determining goals; anticipate possible reactions and difficulties.

Discuss problems with parents directly and honestly.

Explore all alternative options with parents.

Share knowledge of community supports; help parents role-play responses to others.

Acknowledge the impact of the illness on finances, on emotions, and especially on the family, including siblings.

Use other staff for support in personally coping with the emotional drain created by working with very ill children and their parents.

---

Various strategies for communicating with children of different ages are suggested, as are strategies for communicating with their parents. A marvelous characteristic of children is how well they respond to caregivers who make an effort to understand their needs and take the time to relate to them.

## REFERENCES

Bernstein D, Shelov SP. (1996). Pediatrics. Baltimore, Williams & Wilkins.

Burns CE, Barber N, Brady MA, Dunn AM. (1996). Pediatric Primary Care: A Handbook for Nurse Practitioners. Philadelphia, WB Saunders.

Buscaglia L. (1986). Loving Each Other: The Challenge of Human Relationships. Thorofare, NJ, Charles B. Slack.

Clawson JA. (1996). A child with chronic illness and the process of family adaptation. Journal of Pediatric Nursing 11(1):52–61.

Craig KD, Lilley CM, Gilbert CA. (1996). Social barriers to optimal pain management in infants and children. Clinical Journal of Pain 12(3):232–242.

Crain W. (1992). Theories of Development: Concepts and Application (3rd ed.). Englewood Cliffs, NJ, Prentice Hall.

Dixon S, Stein M. (1987). Encounters with Children. Chicago, Year Book Publishers.

Enlow A, Swisher S. (1986). Interviewing and Patient Care (3rd ed.). New York, Oxford.

Erikson EH. (1963). Childhood and Society. New York, Norton.

Flarity K. (1997). Practice Pointers. The Nurse Practitioner 22(11):106.

Gardner R. (1986). Therapeutic Communication with Children (2nd ed.). New York, Science Books.

Hensen RH. (1997). Analysis of the concept of mutuality. Image 29(1):77–81.

Hoeman SP. (1997). Primary care for children with spina bifida. Nurse Practitioner 22(9):60–72.

Kaplan DW, Calonge N, Guernsey BP, Hanrahan MB. (1998). Managed care and school based health centers. Archives of Pediatric and Adolescent Medicine 152(1): 25–33.

Lewis CC, Pantell RH, Sharp L. (1991). Increasing patient knowledge, satisfaction, and involvement: Randomized trial of a communication intervention. Pediatrics 88(2): 351–358.

Marcus DM. (1988). Manifestations of the therapeutic alliance in children and adolescents. Child and Adolescent Social Work 5(2):71–83.

McCarthy V, Hobbie C. (1997). Incorporating violence prevention into anticipatory guidance for well child visits. Journal of Pediatric Helath Care 11(5):222–226.

McMahon L. (1995). Developing skills in therapeutic communication in daily living with emotionally disturbed children and young people. Journal of Social Work Practice 9(2):199–216.

Meeuwesen L, Kaptein M. (1996). Changing interactions in doctor-parent-child communication. Psychology & Health 11(6):787–795.

Paavilainen E, Astedt-Kurki P. (1997). The client-nurse relationship as experienced by public health nurses: Toward better communication. Public Health Nursing 14(3): 137–142.

Page GG, Halvorson M. (1991). Pediatric nurses: The assessment and control of pain in preverbal infants. Journal of Pediatric Nursing 6(2):99–106.

Parish L. (1986). Communicating with hospitalized children. Canadian Nurse 82(1):21–24.

Petrillo M, Sanger S. (1980). Emotional Care of Hospitalized Children (2nd ed.). Philadelphia, JB Lippincott.

Piaget J. (1972). The Child's Conception of the World. Savage, MD, Littlefield, Adams.

Rei RM, Fong C. (1996). The Spanish version of the Parental Stressor Scale: Pediatric intensive care unit. Journal of Pediatric Nursing 11(1):3–9.

Reichert E. (1994). Play and animal assisted therapy. Family Therapy 21(1):55–62.

Santrock JW. (1997). Life-span Development. Madison, Brown & Benchmark.

Spees CM. (1991). Knowledge of medical terminology among clients and families. Image 23(4):225–229.

Sterling YM, Peterson J, Weekes DP. (1997). African-American families with chronically ill children. Journal of Pediatric Nursing 12(5):292–300.

Tindall WN, Beardsley RS, Kimberlin CL. (1994). Communication Skills in Pharmacy Practice. Philadelphia, Lea & Febiger.

Williams BE. (1987). Reaching adolescents through portraiture photography. Child and Youth Care Quarterly 16(4):241–245.

Wincott D. (1971). Playing and Reality. London, Tavistock.

## Electronic References

*http://www.aap.org/.*

Healthy People 2010. (1999). *http://web.health.gov/healthypeople/*

## Suggested Readings

Brammer L. (1988). The Helping Relationship: Process and Skills (4th ed.). Englewood Cliffs, NJ, Prentice Hall.

Eland JM. (1990). Pain in children. Nursing Clinics of North America 25(4):871–884.

Giger JN, Davidhizar R. (1990). Transcultural nursing assessment: A method for advancing nursing practice. International Nursing Review 37(1): 199–202.

Hansen B, Evans M. (1981). Preparing a child for procedures. Maternal Child Nursing 6:392.

# 19

# Communicating with Older Adults

## Judith W. Ryan

**OBJECTIVES**

At the end of the chapter, the student will be able to

1. Identify age-related physical, cognitive, and psychosocial-environmental changes that can affect communication
2. Identify two theoretical frameworks used with the older adult client
3. Discuss appropriate assessment strategies and related nursing interventions

4. Describe blocks to communication with the older adult
5. Specify communication strategies for use in long-term care of the older adult
6. Describe communication strategies to use with clients demonstrating cognitive impairment

*Perhaps above all I am proud of a straightforward clearness of vision, in part a gift of the gods, but also to no little degree due to the scientific training and inner discipline. By means of this I have met life face to face. I have loved a fight, and I have realized that Love is God and Work is his prophet; that his ministers are Age and Death.*

Dubois (1975)

◆ Chapter 19 focuses on communication strategies used in the nurse–client relationship with the older adult. The term "older adult" encompasses persons 65 years of age and older. By the year 2030, projections are that this age group will encompass 22 percent of the U.S. population (U.S. Department of Health and Human Services, 1991). The older adult population represents the most diverse of the age groups. Their life exposures and experiences contribute to the status and quality of life that exists for them.

Understanding the principles of communication as they relate to relationships with older adults requires a clear understanding of the uniqueness of older persons. Unfortunately, the stereotypical image of the older adult is that of a homogeneous, somewhat frail, not very mentally competent person. Older adults vary greatly in capabilities, interests, and capacities for relationships. Whereas some are frail and have reduced intellectual function as a result of disease, others retain a high level of physical and intellectual function until their death.

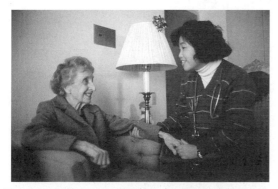

To whatever extent possible, the older client needs to take responsibility for choices and goal setting in health care.

In the past and currently in some cultures, the older adult was revered and acknowledged as the keeper of wisdom. The transmission of knowledge and tradition from generation to generation was primarily through word of mouth. The older generation served a valuable function in teaching the younger generation the ways of life. Because fewer people lived to advanced years, their unique contribution to society was considered special. As society has evolved and the printed word has become the primary transmitter of knowledge, the need for, and value of, the older adult has diminished. In addition, with more people living to advanced years, the novelty of their existence is gone. Advances in technology and medicine have also increased the numbers of older persons who survive with significant disease and limitation, thereby placing a strain on society and the health care system.

As direct providers of care to older adults in their homes, in long-term care settings, and in hospitals, nurses are held accountable for defining standards of care for the older adult and, increasingly, for delivering appropriate psychosocial care to this segment of our population. Older adults experience a gradual deterioration of their functional abilities, making them more in need of the services of professional nurses. The usual social supports dwindle as a result of death or illness. Communication becomes a major determinant of success in health promotion, health teaching, and compliance health care issues (Burke & Sherman, 1993).

## BASIC CONCEPTS

Communication problems that many nurses experience with older adults arise from both the societal discrimination and stereotyping that occurs as well as a lack of understanding about the physical changes that take place in older adults. The sensory losses that occur with normal aging, especially the hearing and vision changes, contribute to alterations in developing therapeutic relationships. About one third of adults older than 65 years have enough hearing impairment so that their social interactions are adversely affected (Mills, 1985). The third dimension of communication difficulties flows from psychosocial changes in the older adult's environment, which limit availability of social support and normal interpersonal stimuli.

## Physical Changes in Normal Aging

As a person ages, a number of physical changes occur, all of which can affect self-concept, self-esteem, and communication ability. Although in many instances the impact of these physical changes can be modified with diet, exercise, and a positive attitude, they nevertheless occur with regularity in everyone. The diminishment of vision and hearing acuity is fairly universal, and the general physical deterioration, which everyone experiences to a greater or lesser degree, increases vulnerability to illnesses such as cancer, cardiovascular and respiratory disorders, and degenerative bone loss. Many of these factors narrow previous physical functional ability, can affect body image, and lead to a re-evaluation of the self-concept depending on the significance of these changes to the individual.

## Age-Related Changes in Cognition

Age-related changes in cognition for healthy adults are minimal. Without the ravages of disease, the older adult has no loss of intelligence at all but may require more time for completing verbal tasks or retrieving information from long-term memory (Byrd, 1986; McIntyre & Craik, 1987; Petros et al., 1983). In addition, older adults are less likely to make guesses when they are presented with ambiguous testing items in mental status exams or respond less well if they are under time pressure to perform. Therefore, communication with healthy older adults does not require special modification based on changes in their cognition. Allowing a little extra time for processing may be all that is required for successful communication.

For approximately 5 percent of the population older than age 65 and 20 percent of those who reach the age of 80, however, there are abnormal cognitive changes. These abnormal age-related changes are profound and progressive and are referred to as Alzheimer's disease and related dementias. Dementia is characterized by memory loss, personality changes, and a deterioration in intellectual functioning that affects every aspect of the victim's life. A small percentage of dementias are caused by organic problems, such as drug toxicity, metabolic disorders, and depression, and may be reversed with treatment. Therefore, the nurse can play a vital role in helping clients and their families seek appropriate diagnosis and treatment.

## Psychosocial and Environmental Changes

Communication is affected by the environment. As people age, they are more likely to suffer multiple losses of people, activities, and functions that were very important to them. Occupational changes in the form of retirement can have the dual impact of significantly changing a person's lifestyle, both financially and as a source of meaning. A decrease in income can be difficult for many people because it limits a person's options. Emotional energy that used to find expression in work, friendships, and creative activities may lose its earlier intensity as the familiar landmarks in a life tapestry are altered by age. For people who have placed a high value on their achievement in a job, there can be a perceived loss of status and self-esteem. Losses of people significant to the older adult occur with increasing regularity, through death of friends and family and adult children moving away.

The client may express a decreased capacity for mastery in many areas of his or her life, feelings of helplessness, and a loss of self-esteem. In its more severe forms, there is a loss of purpose and sense of identity. Whenever the nurse senses from the client that there is a loss of emotional energy in life and feelings of desolation about his or her situation, the nurse needs to obtain more information. A life without purpose is a life without meaning, and everyone needs to feel that their lives have meaning. Statements indicating a need for further exploration include

"What good am I anymore?"
"I just need a friend or someone who cares about me."
"I can't do any of the things I used to do."
"I wish I were dead."

Depression is a common finding in the older adult, and age is one of the strongest risk factors for suicide among white males (Waters & Goodman, 1990). Somatization of vague physical complaints also is cause for concern. Because age is such an important risk factor for suicide, statements reflecting helplessness and hopelessness should never be taken lightly.

Older clients face many negative situational stressors, but they also carry a lifetime of strengths that can be temporarily forgotten. Whereas deficits are real and must be acknowledged, it is the client strengths that form the basis for planning and interventions. Generally, people who have demonstrated resiliency in tackling life's difficult issues during earlier stages of

their lives will continue to do so as they face the tasks of aging. Exercise 19–1 can help you understand the value of resiliency as an adaptive mechanism in promoting well-being.

## Theoretical Frameworks

### Erik Erikson

Erikson's (1982) model of psychosocial development can be used in the assessment of the older adult's health care needs. Erikson portrayed the psychosocial maturational crisis of old age as that of ego integrity versus ego despair. Ego integrity relates to the capacity of older clients to look back on their lives with a deep sense of satisfaction and their willingness to let the next generation carry on their legacy. Threads from all of life's previous psychosocial crises, trust, autonomy, purpose, competence, identity, intimacy, and generativity will resurface during this period. The extent to which these crises were successfully resolved in the past influence their impact in the present.

Ego despair is defined as the failure of a person to accept his or her life as appropriate and mean-

---

◆ Exercise 19–1. **Psychosocial Strengths and Resiliency**

**Purpose:**   To promote an understanding of psychosocial strengths in life accomplishment

**Procedure:**
1. Interview an older adult (75 years or older) who, in your opinion, has had a fulfilling life. Ask the person to describe a few of his or her most satisfying achievements, and what he or she did to accomplish them. Do the same for a few of the person's most challenging moments. The interview should be taped or written immediately after the interview.
2. In a written format, reflect on this person's comments and your ideas of what strengths this person had that allowed him or her to achieve a sense of well-being and to value his or her accomplishments.

**Discussion:**
1. On a blackboard or flip chart, identify the accomplishments that people have identified. Classify them as work related or people related.
2. Were you surprised at any of the older adult's responses to the question about most satisfying experiences? Most challenging experiences?
3. What common themes emerged in the overall class responses that speak to the lived experience of an adult?
4. Using the information from Discussion Step 1 and your written notes on the strengths this person possesses, identify the strengths the older adult identified on the same blackboard or flip chart. Follow the directions for Discussion Steps 2 and 3.
5. How can you apply what you learned from doing this exercise in your future nursing practice?

ingful. It can be temporary, lifted by a more realistic appraisal of one's life, or permanent, leading to feelings of emotional desolation, bitterness, and hostility. Empowerment is a particularly useful concept to use as the basis for intervention. Sometimes in the throes of reverses of life, the older adult loses sight of a proven track record of coping skills. The nurse can help clients get in touch with their ability to create their own path in old age, as they have done in other situations.

### Abraham Maslow

Another theoretical framework used in assessing the needs of the older adult and directing appropriate interventions is that of Maslow. The needs of the older adult are superimposed on Maslow's hierarchy of needs, as identified in Figure 19–1.

## APPLICATIONS

The assessment of older adults should focus on their level of functioning rather than on chronological age, especially because the span of old age covers 30 plus years. Functional level is a far more accurate indicator of the client's issues and relationship needs. Functional abilities in the older adult can range from vigorous, active, and independent to frail and highly dependent, with serious physical, cognitive, psychological, and sensory deficits (Waters & Goodman, 1990).

## Assessing Sensory Deficits

Sensory deficits can have a direct and significant impact on communication. Understanding the normal changes that occur with aging as well as the common diseases that affect hearing and vision will guide the nurse in devising interventions. Hearing deficits have been associated with perceived poor health and depression in the older adult (Wallhagen et al., 1996).

### Hearing

Hearing loss associated with normal aging begins after age 50 and is due to loss of hair cells (which are not replaced) in the organ of Corti in the inner ear. This change leads initially to a loss in the ability to hear high-frequency sounds (e.g., *f, s, th, sh, ch*) and is called *presbycusis*. Later the loss includes the sounds of the explosive conso-

nants (*b, t, p, k, d*), whereas the lower frequency sounds of vowels are preserved longer. Older adults also have difficulty perceiving sounds, especially against background noises, and in understanding fast-paced speech. The most understandable speech for older adults is about 125 words per minute (McCroskey & Kasten, 1982).

### Therapeutic Strategies to Use with Hearing Changes

In addition to the strategies suggested in Chapter 17 for the hearing impaired, several strategies can be used to improve communication with an older adult who has age-related partial hearing loss. It is important to remember that the older adult who does not hear well is not cognitively deficient. With a little planning in modifying communication with the hearing-impaired older adult, the relationship should not be any different from one with a client who does not have this disability. Nurses should do the following:

Determine whether hearing is better in one ear, and then direct speech to that side.

Help elderly clients adjust hearing aids. Lacking fine motor dexterity, the elderly client may not be able to insert aids to amplify hearing. Check the batteries.

Speak distinctly but in a normal voice.

Address the person by name before beginning to speak. It focuses attention.

Do not speak rapidly; about 125 words a minute is best.

If your voice is high pitched, lower it.

If the older adult does not understand, use different words when repeating the message.

Face the older adult so he or she can use facial expression and/or lip reading to enhance comprehension. For example, humor is often communicated by subtle facial expressions.

Use gestures and facial expression to expand the meaning of the message.

Do not talk with your hands in front of your mouth or with food or gum in the mouth.

Keep background noises to a minimum (e.g., turn down the radio or television when talking).

Obtain feedback periodically to monitor what the person hears.

### Vision

Vision decreases as people grow older. Colors lose their vividness, and images can be blurred.

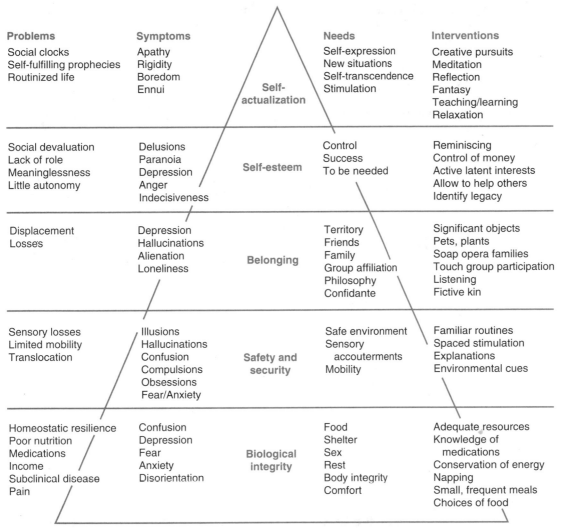

**Figure 19–1.** Maslow's hierarchy of needs applied to the assessment of older adult clients. From Ebersole P, Hess P. (1990). Toward Healthy Aging. St. Louis, CV Mosby. Used with permission.

Loss of vision can affect a person's ability to perform everyday activities, including dressing, preparing meals, taking medication, driving or using other transportation, handling the checkbook, and using the telephone. It also affects functional ability to engage in many hobbies or leisure activities, such as reading, doing handiwork, and watching television. In short, a significant decrease in visual function almost invariably affects an individual's ability to function autonomously. The nurse can play a vital role in supporting the independence of the visually impaired client by taking a few simple actions.

### Strategies to Use with the Visually Impaired

Have eyeglasses in place if they are worn.

Identify yourself by name when you enter the room or initiate conversation.

Stand in front of the client and use head movements.

Verbally explain every written piece of information, allowing time for the client to ask questions. Do not assume that because the person appears to be reading a document that it has been read accurately. Ask questions to determine the level of comprehension.

Appropriate lighting and other visual aids can enhance vision.

Remove any hazards, such as obstructed pathways or glares from lighting.

Use words to describe landmarks and where you are taking the client.

Exercise 19–2 is designed to help you understand the impact of sensory impairments on communication.

## Assessing and Responding to Psychosocial Needs

### Beginning with the Client's Story

Assessment of the older adult always begins with the client's story. It is important to see and hear what is happening from the older person's perspective (Waters & Goodman, 1990). In this way, value-laden psychosocial issues, such as independence, fears about being a burden, role changes, and vulnerability, can be brought to the surface.

---

◆ **Case Example**

**Nurse:**  You seem concerned that your stroke will have a major impact on your life.

**Client:**  Yes, I am. I'm an old woman now, and I don't want to be a burden to my family.

**Nurse:**  In what ways do you think you might be a burden?

**Client:**  Well, I obviously can't move around as I did. I can't go back to doing what I used to do, but that doesn't mean I'm ready for a nursing home.

**Nurse:**  What were some of the things you used to do?

**Client:**  Well, I raised three children, and they're all married now with good jobs. That's hard to do in this day and age. I did a lot for the church. I held a job as a secretary for 32 years, and I got several awards for my work.

**Nurse:**  It sounds as though you were very productive and were able to cope with a lot of things. You are right that this time in your life is different. It isn't possible to do the things you did previously, but you have a proven track record of coping with life. What you have given to your family is important, but it also is important to allow them to give some things to you. It can be very meaningful to them and to you. Let's think about some ways you can make your life more satisfying and as rewarding as it has been in the past.

---

In this dialogue, the nurse listens carefully to what the older adult is expressing and uses this information to help the client reframe problems as challenges to be addressed in the present. Suc-

---

◆ Exercise 19-2. **What Is It Like to Experience Sensory Decline?**

**Purpose:**  To promote an understanding of the effects of sensory decline on the activities of daily living

**Procedure:**
1. Put cotton in your ears and gloves on your hands, and smear a pair of glasses with a very thin coat of petroleum jelly.
2. With a partner take a short walk and carry on a conversation about what you are experiencing. Now try to find some change in your wallet as though you were making a purchase.

**Discussion:**
1. What does it feel like to have diminished functional ability?
2. In what ways did your feelings about yourself change?
3. How do you think your experience will affect your appreciation and response to the older adult?

cessful past achievements can be used as tools to help the client face necessary transitions and take control of his or her life. Helping the client identify sources of social support, personal resources, and coping strategies can alter the impact of physical and emotional stressors associated with age-related transitions. Exercise 19–3 provides a glimpse into the life stories of the older adult.

### Using a Proactive Approach

For many reasons, the older adult needs the nurse to assume initial responsibility for directing the interview in the initial stages of the relationship. At first, new situations can cause transitory confusion for many older adults. Knowing what to expect helps decrease anxiety and build trust. Many clients are aware of the stereotypes associated with aging and are reluctant to expose themselves as inadequate in any way.

When the nurse has concern about the cognitive capability of the older adult, it is prudent to perform a mental status assessment early in the interview to avoid obtaining questionable data. A variety of mental status exams are available for use with the older adult and any of them can be much more productive if the nurse takes the time to modify the process and approach as presented in Box 19–1.

The older adult appreciates having the nurse provide structure to the history-taking interview by explaining the reasons for it and the outline of what it will involve. The I–thou position stressed in earlier chapters is used to enhance connectedness. Questions that the older adult perceives as relevant and that follow a logical sequence are likely to hold the client's interest. Having an opportunity to talk about oneself can be extremely beneficial.

Of equal importance is the sensitivity of the nurse to the unexpressed fears of the older adult. Often the client has a strong concern that in accepting external or professional services, there is a loss of independence. In the client's mind, accepting help is the first step toward the nursing home. Consequently, the older adult may minimize difficulties. The nurse may need to assess environmental supports directly and should always bear in mind the possible association in the older adult's mind between accepting any help and independent living. For example, an older adult in cardiac rehabilitation told his nurse that he had a bedside commode and no stairs in his home. When the nurse visited the home, there was no commode, and the client's home had a significant number of stairs. He told the nurse that he was afraid she would take steps to change his living arrangements if these facts were known.

### Promoting Client Autonomy

The nurse plays a critical role in helping older adults maintain their autonomy. For many cli-

---

◆ **Exercise 19–3. Hearing the Story of the Older Adults in One's Family**

**Purpose:**  To promote an understanding of the older adult

**Procedure:**
1. Interview an older adult in your family (minimum age 75). If there are no older adults in your family, interview a family friend whose lifestyle is similar to that of your family.
2. Ask this person to describe what growing up was like for him or her, what is different today from the way it was when he or she was your age, what are the important values that he or she has held, and whether there have been any changes. Ask this person what advice he or she would give you, based on experience, about how to achieve satisfaction in life.

**Discussion:**
1. Were you surprised at any of the answers the older adult gave you?
2. What are some common themes you and your classmates found related to values and the type of advice the older adult gave each of you?
3. What implications do the findings from this exercise have for your future nursing practice?

## ◆ Box 19-1. Mental Status Exam for the Older Adult

1. Establish rapport with client and gain client's trust and acceptance before mental status examination.

2. Rule out possibility of sensory deficits (especially hearing and visual losses) before mental status examination.

3. Rule out possibility of toxic effects accruing from medication and drug dependencies before mental status examination.

4. Assess the presence, if any, of agitation, acute anxiety, and depression resulting from recent stressful events before mental status examination.

5. Assess client's retention and recall by using information, experiences, and events that have been known to have registered.

6. Test client's memory for events by selecting events that are of considerable interest and significance to the elderly client.

7. Memory of recent events should be tested by asking client to recall events that occurred in the past 8 to 24 hours (e.g., name of visitors; important event of the day).

8. Memory of more remote events may be evaluated by asking client to recall dates of important past events (birthday, anniversary date, age) and names of persons who had considerable significance for the client.

9. An independent assessment should be obtained from the client's family of the extent of the client's motivation and interest in the surroundings before the mental status examination.

10. Assessment of client's capacity for basic self-care tasks should be done before the mental status examination.

11. The nature of cognitive tasks expected of the client in the mental status examination must make allowance for the limited educational attainment of some clients and also for the impoverished nature of the client's current environment.

12. Questions of understanding, recall, and integration of materials in the mental status examination must definitely take into account the lifestyle, cultural bias, and previous interests of the elderly client.

13. Elderly clients should not be expected to engage in psychological tests that involve prolonged capacity for memory and attention.

14. Mental status tests should be supplemented by the use of other psychological tests involving observation of behavioral symptoms of the elderly client.

15. Careful assessment of mental status should be conducted over a longer time to preclude the possibility of off days or client's distress on a given testing day.

From Fry PS. (1986). Depression, Stress and Adaptations in the Elderly: Psychological Assessment and Intervention. Rockville, MD, Aspen, p. 62. Used with permission.

ents, being independent means that they are still in charge of their lives. It is easy for the nurse to confuse the fact that an older adult appears frail, with an inability to function. As the nurse assists the client to clarify values, make choices, and take action, a stronger understanding of the unique needs and strengths of the client emerges. An open-ended approach to understanding the client as a person is helpful to both nurse and client. Often in relating their life story and exploring options relevant to the current situation with the nurse, older clients are able to step back and look at the present in a more positive way.

## ◆ Case Example

**Nurse:** Mr. Matturo, it sounds as if being in charge of your life is very important to you.

**Client:** Yes, it is. I grew up on a farm and was always taught that I should pull my own weight. You have to on a farm. I've lived my entire life that way. I've never asked anyone for anything.

**Nurse:** I can hear how important that is to you. What else has been important?

**Client:** Well, I was a marine sergeant in World War II, and I led many a platoon into battle. My men depended on me, and I never let them down. My wife says I've been a good provider, and I've always taught my children to value honor and the simple way of life.

**Nurse:** It sounds as though you have led a very interesting and productive life. Tell me more about what you mean by honor and the simple way of life.

As the client expresses important information about values and life experiences, previous coping strategies can be identified. At the end of the dialogue, the nurse might summarize what the client has expressed and say to the client, "Do you think you might be able to use any of these life skills now?" It is easier for the client to imagine possible coping skills when they are linked to principles of coping in the past. The precise actions may be quite different, but the problem-solving process may be quite similar. With this line of open-ended questioning, the nurse uses the client's story as the baseline for planning and implementing nursing care. That care is individualized and sensitive to the older adult's needs and values.

### Acting as the Client's Advocate

The nurse plays an important role as advocate with the older adult client. When there is a breakdown in the client's ability to meet essential needs, sometimes they can be addressed with some very simple environmental modifications and referrals. It is important to engage the client in actively exploring appropriate environmental support (e.g., homemaker services, leisure activities, and home nursing support). Introducing the need for external supports, however, without first building rapport and helping the client establish a sense of his or her personal strengths is likely to be counterproductive. Framing suggestions for external supports in terms of helping the older adult maintain independent living as long as possible often works with clients who are reluctant to use them.

Advocating for the client with the family also is important. Seen from the client's eyes in this essay, the dilemma of allowing the older adult both enough freedom and enough protection is eloquently described:

*My children are coming today. They mean well. But they worry.*

*They think I should have a railing in the hall. A telephone in the kitchen. They want someone to come in when I take a bath. They really don't like my living alone.*

*Help me to be grateful for their concern. And help them to understand that I have to do what I can as long as I can.*

*They're right when they say there are risks. I might fall. I might leave the stove on. But there is no real challenge, no possibility of triumph, no real aliveness without risk.*

*When they were young and climbed trees and rode bicycles and went away to camp, I was terrified, but I let them go.*

*Because to hold them would have hurt them.*

*Now our roles are reversed. Help them see.*

*Keep me from being grim or stubborn about it. But don't let them smother me.*

From *Green Winter* by Elise Maclay.

Groups are an important source of social support for the older active adult. They help restore hope and re-establish a sense of personal worth. The model of empowerment, described in Chapter 5, and the wide variety of groups available for the older adult, described in Chapter 12, offer hope to clients by helping them receive needed emotional support and providing guidance to select the most appropriate tools. It becomes easier with support to mobilize resources in the environment that will assist an individual in developing a different productive way of being in old age.

### Blocks to Communication

A few special considerations or cautions are relevant when communicating with older adults.

Whereas these can be problems across the life span, they seem more prevalent in interactions with older persons. It is very easy to impede communication with any of the following:

## Offering Cliché Reassurances

For example, an older man says "I just got back from burying my wife; she was sick with cancer a long time." Communication-blocking responses might be "Well, at least her suffering is over" or "In time your grief will lessen." These are not particularly helpful comments, and they certainly do not promote a response from the client. In addition, they do not contribute to an assessment of the impact of this situation on the client. A better option might be "How are you doing?" or "I have some time. Would you like to talk?"

## Giving Advice

Telling an older adult what to do in a given situation rather than exploring the options available is a common block to communication (e.g., "With your bad arthritis you really do need to start a walking program or you will start to lose function"). A better response is "With your bad arthritis, I worry about your losing your mobility. What kinds of things do you do to stay physically active?"

## Answering Your Own Questions

Sometimes older adults require more time to hear and understand the communication, so that their responses are not as rapidly forthcoming as with younger persons. For example, "Which do you want: tomato, orange, or apple juice?" may be quickly followed by "I guess you would like apple juice" if a response from the older adult did not come fast enough. Another example of not waiting for an answer is "How would you describe your chest pain?", followed too quickly by "Is it sharp, dull, pricking, or aching?" The older adult should be allowed the additional few seconds to determine an answer ("It's burning") before the question is made "multiple choice." This provides a much better data-gathering approach when the cognitively intact older adult is allowed to use his or her own words to describe a problem or concern rather than having the caregiver provide the terminology.

## Giving Excessive Praise or Reprimands

Often giving effusive praise can be detrimental because it blocks most responses except "thank you." For example, "You have done a wonderfully fantastic job in organizing your medications" does not readily allow the older adult to ask questions or raise a concern about some aspect of what has been done. A better response might be to recognize the accomplishment and ask whether there are any remaining concerns about the medications. Also, reprimanding or scolding the older adult can be demeaning as well as a block to communication. For example, "Haven't you finished your lunch yet? You are the slowest one on the unit. What am I going to do with you?" could be more appropriately managed by identifying that this person eats slowly and perhaps could benefit from getting meals first.

## Defending Against a Complaint

Many older adults have no difficulty in criticizing their environment or treatment by others, and it is often to the nurse that this criticism is verbalized. For example, "No one answered my call light last night, and I almost fell going to the bathroom by myself" may elicit a defensive response, such as "The unit was really busy last night. We had two admissions." A better approach is to determine what underlies the comment. Is the older adult afraid of being alone, of falling, or of something else? A better response is "What was happening with you last night?"

## Using Parenting Approaches or Behaviors

When nurses use such approaches, older adults may be embarrassed or feel demeaned. It is treating them like children, using terms such as "honey," "sweetie," or "doll" rather than asking them the names by which they would like to be addressed. Additionally, the nurse may answer for the older adult when someone asks the person a question. For example, the chaplain asks an older woman, "How are you doing today?" and the nurse answers for her, "Oh, she is just fine." There is a simple rule to follow when communicating with older adults: the older adult *is* an adult and should be acknowledged as such and related to in an adult manner.

## Communication Strategies in Long-Term Care Settings

The rigid lifestyle imposed by many long-term care facilities reinforces clients' awareness of their diminished capacity to care for themselves independently and to choose voluntary activities that have meaning to them. It is difficult to avoid feeling like an object of care rather than a person in such situations. The nurse plays a central role in helping clients preserve their sense of person-hood by creating a nursing environment that is supportive of clients' independence and that pro-motes quality of life for older adult clients.

Liukkonen (1993) reported that many older adults in long-term facilities suffer from loneli-ness and long for someone simply to listen to them. Older adults who are institutionalized in hospitals or nursing homes often appreciate short, frequent conversations. Like everyone else, the need to be acknowledged is paramount to the older client's sense of self-esteem. Con-tinuity of care with one primary caregiver, when possible, helps foster the development of a com-fortable nurse–client relationship.

### Dealing with Memories and Reminiscences

It is not uncommon for healthy older persons to share the memories from youth or earlier days with those who are around. Whereas this is a meaningful way in which older adults review their life in an attempt to establish meaning and reconcile conflicts and disappointments (Butler, 1963), it can also be frustrating for the people who have heard the stories 100 times and so turn off or avoid interacting with the persons. Rather than responding with, "Oh my, here he goes again with that Model T story," it is better to respond to the story and enter it with the older adult to learn more about why it has special rele-vance or meaning. It is an opportunity to gain insight into the person, who he or she was, what aspirations and dreams were fulfilled or unful-filled, what contributions are valued, and what goals are yet to be attained. Reminiscing also has been demonstrated to increase self-esteem, mood, morale, and socialization (Lappe, 1987).

Several suggestions have been made by Cox and Waller (1987) in connection with responding to the reminiscences of the older person:

1. *Ask exploring questions.* In the Model T story, one might ask "What made you buy that car?" or "How did you get the money to buy it?"
2. *Use the memory as a bridge to other information.* "What other types of cars did you have after that?" "Were you usually the one in your social group who had the car. Where would you go?"
3. *Find a cue for a question within frequently heard stories.* "Cars seem very important to you. What was it like for you when you had to give up driving last year?"
4. *Practice ways to tell the person that you have heard the story before.* (This should be done only if the repetition occurs within the same conver-sation, or close to it.) "Oh yes, I remember the Model T episode when you drove the car into the Madison County reservoir. What other unusual or amusing things happened to you during your life?"

### Role Modeling

Role modeling is an aspect of care that indirectly affects the interpersonal relationships older adults have with their caregivers. Because ancil-lary personnel often constitute the largest group of primary caregivers in long-term care settings, it is particularly important for professional nurses, who frequently supervise them, to serve as positive role models. This means that the pro-fessional nurse needs to be actively involved with older adult clients and willing to share observa-tions with other personnel. People learn not only what is taught but also what is "caught," in the form of attitudes toward the older adult. Al-though as students you may not think that ancil-lary personnel are paying attention to you, they are very much aware of how you interact with clients. If professional attitudes are positive and supportive, they influence positively the care a nurse's aide gives to clients.

## Communication Strategies with the Cognitively Impaired Adult

Assessment of cognitive function should occur early in the communication process with older adults. Some older adults with moderately severe communication deficits retain all of their intellectual abilities. Other older adults retain enough of their sensory functions to communicate effectively, but the means of processing information, learning, and responding become dysfunctional. Most communication deficits associated with memory loss are cumulative and progressive. Unfortunately, in the early stages, environmental conflicts may be heightened because of the older adult's seemingly normal superficial verbal behaviors. Only when one tries to engage the older adult in a deeper conversation does the degree of communication deficit become apparent. For example, the client may say "I'm feeling great; Martha and I visited the grandchildren, and we had a great time." However, when asked what he actually did on the visit, he may be unable to answer with any real detail.

In a more advanced loss of cognition, the older adult is unable to express complete thoughts. He or she has difficulty finding the words to use, and sentences are unfinished. The dementia victim, unable to continue, stops in midsentence or continues with phrases that have little to do with the intended meaning. In such cases, the nurse can help by filling in the missing words, smiling, supplying the logical meaning, and then asking the client whether this is what he or she meant. Another strategy is to almost finish a sentence and have the client supply the last word. In fact, anything to help reduce the client's anxiety about groping for thoughts that do not come helps the person continue.

Another communication difficulty is *apraxia,* defined as the loss of the ability to take purposeful action even when the muscles, senses, and vocabulary seem intact. This condition causes a person to appear to register on a command, but then to act in ways that suggest he or she has little understanding of what transpired verbally. When the cognitively impaired adult fails to follow through on the agreed-on action, the nurse may interpret the behavior as uncooperative or obstinate. Talking the client through a procedure, step by step, providing additional cues, and allowing additional time for processing information reduce the person's anxiety and improve performance.

## Reminiscence

Relationships with older adults with mild to moderate cognitive disability can take advantage of the simple fact that remote memory (recall of past events) is retained longer than memory for recent events. Asking older adults about their past life experiences often serves as a way to connect verbally with those who might have difficulty telling you what they had for breakfast 2 hours ago. A memory is a gift to the nurse from someone who is sharing part of him- or herself and who might have little or nothing else to give (Ebersole & Hess, 1998). For some reason, once older adults with mild memory deficits begin to reminisce about their past, communication flows more freely and retention of messages is stronger. Mentally impaired persons become more verbal and will even assist others in remembering events when in a reminiscence group (Baker, 1985). The nurse can act as an advocate in learning about the dementia victim's needs, expressed as past occurrences, and can translate them into current requirements for care.

## Repetition and Instructions

The nurse should have additional means of communicating with older adults experiencing memory loss. It is very appropriate to address the older adult by his or her name several times before beginning the communication. This approach can be useful in focusing the older adult's attention on what is coming next. By selecting a simple, relevant thought from a stream of loosely connected ideas, the nurse permits the conversation to continue, often to the visible relief of the impaired dementia victim. Restating ideas, using the same words and sequence, are simple communication strategies that allow a conversation to continue.

By speaking in simple sentences, repeating phrases, and giving directions one at a time, the nurse enables the older adult to use his or her remaining capabilities. For example, asking the older adult to make a cup of coffee might be beyond his comprehension. However, breaking the request down into smaller steps—"Open the cupboard," "Open the drawer," "Take out a spoon," "Close the drawer," "Open the jar of instant coffee," and so on—may make the activity possible and thus reinforce self-esteem.

## Use of Touch

Gaining eye contact and using touch are also helpful to maintain focus. The use of appropriate touch with the cognitively impaired can be a helpful tool, but its applicability must be determined on an individual basis. For some people, being touched increases their agitation and confusion, whereas for others being touched is a calming and welcome action.

Nurses should be sensitive to their own style of touching: how it is done, to whom, when, and why. The older adults who are least likely to experience touch from nurses are men and those who have severe cognitive impairment (Watson, 1975).

There is also a hierarchy of places on the body that are appropriate to touch: the hands, shoulders, back, and arms. Although the thigh and face are relatively personal parts of the body, they are frequently selected when touching older adults. These areas should not be chosen as sites for touching until rapport has been established.

## Use of Multiple Modalities

Using more than one sense in communication facilitates the process. For example, touching the hand with the hairbrush in it and saying "Now use the brush to fix your hair" provides an additional focus for the older adult. When helping a dementia victim groom and dress, knowing that stiffening can occur because of an automatic neurological response and that this manifestation is not due to a resistive and rejecting person enables the nurse to be more sensitive to the older adult. Sometimes waiting 15 minutes and trying again can be a productive option.

## Use of Distraction for Disruptive Behaviors

Because older adults with memory loss lack the cognitive ability to develop alternatives, they can have what appears to be temper tantrums in response to real or perceived frustration. These tantrums are called ***catastrophic reactions*** and represent a completely disorganized set of responses. They are often difficult for the nurse to comprehend or manage. Usually there is something in the immediate environment that precipitates the reaction, but fatigue, overstimulation, misinterpretations, and inability to meet expectations may also be contributing factors. The emotion may be appropriate even if its behavioral manifestation is not. In these situations, the nurse can use distraction to move the older adult away from the offending stimuli in the environment or to diffuse the troublesome feeling through postponement. For example, the nurse might say to the older adult, "We will do that later; right now, let us go out on the porch," while gently leading the person away. Direct confrontation and an appeal for more civilized behavior usually serve to escalate rather than diminish the episode.

Often there are warning signs of an impending catastrophic reaction, such as restlessness, refusals, or general uncooperativeness; by redirecting the dementia victim, the outburst may be avoided. It is important for the nurse to model the appropriate responses to this behavior and to explain to the family members and staff what is happening and what to do to prevent or address it.

### Sample Clinical Situation

Problem: an 86-year-old woman exhibits disturbed attention and confusion.

Nursing diagnosis: inadequate coping related to organic memory loss

Nursing goals: minimize factors that contribute to inattentiveness.

Nursing approach: compensatory and supportive

Method of assistance: guiding, supporting, providing an understanding environment

Nursing interventions

1. Look directly at the client when talking.
2. Call the client by name several times.
3. Position self in the client's line of vision.
4. Rest hands on the client's hands.
5. Give clear, simple directions in a step-by-step manner.
6. Direct conversation toward concrete, familiar objects.
7. If attention lapses, let the client rest a few minutes before trying to regain his or her attention.
8. Provide simple activities that will encourage purposeful action.
9. Repeat messages slowly, calmly, and patiently until client shows some sign of comprehension.
10. Vary the words to fit the client's ability to comprehend.
11. Modify the environmental stimuli that affect attention.
12. Assist the family to understand that inatten-

tion and failure to respond is due to her inability to process information cognitively.

The evaluation of the effectiveness, appropriateness, and efficiency of the nursing actions with the dementia victim does not occur through words, as it does with other nurse–client relationships. Behaviors of the client in which agitation is reduced, cooperation is obtained, and the client responds positively to the caregiver are indicators of effective nursing interventions and successful outcomes.

## SUMMARY

Chapter 19 emphasizes the use of therapeutic communication skills with older clients. Understanding the principles of communication as they relate to relationships with older adults requires a clear understanding of the uniqueness of older persons.

Older adults vary greatly in capabilities, interests, and capacities for relationships. Whereas some are frail, with reduction of intellectual function as a result of disease, others retain a high level of physical and intellectual functioning until their death. Technological advances and better nutrition have reduced mortality rates, increased the life span, and correspondingly increased the number of older adults who now require health care. Communication difficulties can occur because of changes in sensory and cognitive functioning in the older adult as well as significant changes in social support systems. The nurse can provide the older client with a therapeutic environment that supports the client's independence and that helps the client compensate for failing physical, cognitive, and emotional functioning. Strategies such as reminiscing, encouraging spousal support, and treating the older client with dignity are proposed. A care plan for the cognitively impaired client is presented. As a primary provider of long-term care, the nurse is in a unique role to support and meet the communication needs of the older client.

## REFERENCES

Baker N. (1985). Reminiscing in group therapy for self-worth. Journal of Gerontological Nursing 11:21.

Burke M, Sherman S (eds.). (1993). Gerontological Nursing: Issues and Opportunities for the Twenty First Century. New York, National League for Nursing Press.

Butler R. (1963). Life review: An interpretation of reminiscences in the aged. Psychiatry 26:65.

Byrd M. (1986). The effects of previously acquired knowledge on memory for textual information. International Journal of Aging and Human Development 24(3):231.

Cox BJ, Waller L. (1987). Communicating with the Older Adult. St. Louis, MO, Catholic Health Association of the United States.

Ebersole P, Hess P. (1998). Toward Healthy Aging: Human Needs and Nursing Response (5th ed.). St. Louis, MO, CV Mosby.

Erikson E. (1982). The Life Cycle Completed. New York, Norton.

Fry PS. (1986). Depression, Stress and Adaptations in the Elderly: Psychological Assessment and Intervention. Rockville, MD, Aspen.

Lappe J. (1987). Reminiscing: The life review therapy. Journal of Gerontological Nursing 13:12.

Liukkonen A. (1993). The content of nurses' oral shift reports in homes for older adult people. Journal of Advanced Nursing 1095–1100.

Maclay E. (1977). Green Winter: Celebrations of Old Age. New York, Reader's Digest Press.

McCroskey RL, Kasten RN. (1982). Temporal factors and the aging auditory system. Ear Hear 3:124–127.

McIntyre J, Craik F. (1987). Age differences in memory for item and source information. Canadian Journal of Psychology 41:175.

Miles R. (1985). The auditory system. In Pathy MSJ (ed.), Principles and Practice of Geriatric Medicine (6th ed.). London, Wiley, 841–854.

Petros TV, Zehr HD, Chabot RJ. (1983). Adult age differences in accessing and retrieving information from long-term memory. Journal of Gerontology 38:589.

Wallhagen MI, Strawbridge WJ, Kaplan GA. (1996). Six-year impact of hearing impairment on psychosocial and physiologic functioning. The Nurse Practitioner 21:11.

Waters E, Goodman J. (1990). Empowering Older Adults: Practical Strategies for Counselors. San Francisco, Jossey-Bass.

Watson W. (1975). The meaning of touch: Gerontological nursing. Journal of Communication 25:104–112.

U.S. Department of Health and Human Services. (1991). Healthy People 2000. Washington, DC, Public Health Service.

# 20

# Communicating with Clients in Stressful Situations

Elizabeth Arnold

## OBJECTIVES

At the end of the chapter, the student will be able to

1. Define stress and sources of stress
2. Identify selected theoretical frameworks of stress and coping
3. Identify factors influencing the impact of stress
4. Specify the relationship between stress and disease
5. Identify expressions of grief
6. Identify basic concepts of coping
7. Apply the nursing process to the care of clients in stressful situations
8. Identify strategies for burnout prevention

*I knew I was being childish; still I acted terribly. I insulted nurses and doctors, repeatedly questioned their judgment . . . basically acted like a jerk. If only someone could have realized what was happening to me.*

Bluhm (1987)

◆◆ Chapter 20 provides a framework for understanding basic concepts of stress and coping in the nurse–client relationship. Stress is a normal part of life, an inevitability that no human being can escape. Factors that create stress can be external or internal. People feel stressed when there is (1) a threat to the person's self-integrity or well-being, (2) a loss of something important to the person's well-being and self-esteem, or (3) a challenge to be overcome. Most people struggling with health care issues are stressed. Making difficult decisions under less than ideal circumstances creates stress and is the rule rather than the exception.

Some stressors in health care can be modified with problem solving. Others cannot be changed. Terminal illness, chronic pain, death of a person, end of a relationship, and serious injury may require acceptance, a constructive outlook, and strategies to maintain self-esteem in the face of overwhelming, often unfair, and irreversible circumstances. Helping a person explore new directions and develop a different perspective can be just as important as the more traditional problem-solving strategies used to cope with stress (Michalenko, 1998).

Incorporating coping and stress management principles in the nurse–client relationship enables the nurse to communicate effectively with clients in stressful health care situations ranging from health promotion to care of the terminally ill. By learning to care for others experiencing stress, nurses can apply similar concepts in their own lives. One cannot give from an empty cupboard!

## BASIC CONCEPTS
### Definition

*Stress* is defined as a physiological, psychological, and spiritual response to the presence of a stressor. A *stressor* is defined as any demand, situation, internal stimulus, or circumstance that threatens a person's personal security and balance. Whether or not the stressor is objectively dangerous is immaterial; it is a personal experience that affects the whole person. Stress disrupts normal functioning and causes people to act in ways they ordinarily would not. People respond to stress as an integrated mind–body experience. Unrelieved stress leads to physiological changes.

Physical illness can produce emotional strain, tension, and anxiety. When a person perceives threat to self or loses a close and supportive relationship with a significant other, there is an immediate emotional arousal that can lead to clinical depression or anxiety disorders. Psychological stress arouses powerful emotional reactions ranging from exhilaration, anxiety, anger, frustration, and disbelief to sadness and functional immobilization (Emmons, 1991; Epstein & Katz, 1992). Pain and suffering challenge spiritual beliefs.

### Sources of Stress

Common sources of personal stress are described in Table 20–1. Men and women experience and respond to stress differently (Gadzella et al., 1991). Men are more likely to respond with anger or denial, whereas women internalize stress and may experience depression. A person's language, ethnic background, religion, social support, cultural and economic levels, and education affect their unique behavioral response to stress (Leininger, 1991).

Although not intended to do so, the experience of hospitalization creates stress. Individual identity is minimized with the donning of the short hospital gown and a wrist band. Physical discomfort, strange noises and lights, unfamiliar people asking personal questions, and strange equipment heighten the stress most clients already feel coping with their health needs. With experience, *the nurse can anticipate stress reactions and inquire about important client feelings.*

The stress of hospitalization is not limited to the client. Parents witnessing the children of other parents die cannot help but project that experience onto their own situation and experience grieving of their own (Johnson, 1997). The nurse is a valuable resource in providing emotional support and health-related information to clients and their families that help reduce the sense of insecurity associated with not knowing what to expect or how to respond in an unfamiliar, stressful health care situation.

### Special Issues for Children

Children experience stress but frequently lack the voice to tell others about it. Stress in a child can present as withdrawal or acting-out behavior (Greene & Walker, 1997). Frequently, adults as-

Table 20-1. **Personal Sources of Stress**

| PHYSICAL STRESSORS | PSYCHOLOGICAL STRESSORS | SPIRITUAL STRESSORS |
|---|---|---|
| Aging process | Loss of a job | Loss of role |
| Illness | Death of a significant person | Loss of meaning |
| Injury | Getting married or divorced | Questioning of values |
| Pain | Becoming a single parent | Change in religious affiliation |
| Mental disorder | Moving from a familiar place | |
| | Role overload, conflict, change | |

Data from McCaffery M, Beebe A. (1989). Pain: Clinical Manual for Nursing Practice. St. Louis, Mosby.

sume the child's stress is less or that they should be spared the full knowledge of what has happened. Most children know something is dreadfully wrong even if they do not voice their concerns.

Dying children often are aware that they are terminal, but feel so socially isolated that they are unable to express their grief and depression (Stephenson, 1985). They do not want to upset their parents or siblings. When they have been given false information or reassurance, they do not know what to believe because their intuition and body symptoms do not compute with the information they are receiving from people they trust. This can compound their stress.

Children who have a parent suffering from cancer or other serious illness face special challenges that may go unrecognized by their overstressed parents. Nurses can play the dual role of helping children cope with a seriously ill parent and their parents cope with altered parenting skills and helping their children understand and accept what is happening (Lewandowski, 1996). In a study of stress and coping of parents of children in a pediatric intensive care unit, the most common stressors identified were loss of parenting role, uncertainty about outcome, and information need, all of which are amenable to stress reduction through empathetic, problem-focused nursing intervention (LaMontagne & Pawlak, 1990).

Children express their stress according to their stage of development and established family patterns. Although it is particularly difficult to tell a child what is going on, all children need to have their questions answered simply and honestly. Because parents often are so consumed with their own stress, the nurse must help the child identify important feelings and make sure that they are addressed. Asking children what they know about their illness and how they think they are doing prompts them to voice significant fears and concerns. To obtain more detail, the nurse might ask the child how other people—parents, grandparents, and siblings—think they are doing. Small children can be encouraged to express their feelings through drawings and manipulating puppets.

### Special Issues for the Frail Elderly

Grieving as a stress response at the other end of the life span can be different. For the frail elderly who have lost hope, particularly those without a consistent social support system, grief is experienced as a prolonged, meaningless existence in a body that no longer responds to their commands and with the loss of almost all that matters—friends, family, and work. The frail elderly frequently mourn the social death they experience, and instead of fearing physical death, they long for it. Theirs is a chronic stress, unrelieved by the presence of a social support system that their younger counterparts have at their disposal. The nurse is in a unique position to help frail elderly clients fill this gap.

### Hidden Stressors

Practical, social, and financial considerations can create significant stress for a client, but they often are missed because the focus is on the diagnosed physical or psychological disorder. Nurses who are reluctant to ask questions about personal relationships as they relate to the client's illness or to probe emotionally tinged subjects, such as sexual or occupational adjustment, do their clients a disservice. Clients need to talk about the full particulars of their health issue if they want to make a complete adjustment. Often a client's concerns reflect worry about what will happen next, how he or she will explain their illness, or what the client or family could have done differently to change their situation. Family members may wonder "How will I manage?", "Was it my fault?", "Could I have done more?" The nurse who is astute enough to pick up on the client's or family's stress can prompt discussion of these hidden fears. For example, the nurse might say to the wife of a recent paraplegic, "Seeing your husband like this must be a terrible shock. I would think you might be wondering how you are going to live with John immobilized like this." This type of statement normalizes feeling and allows the client to describe an unexpressed, perhaps personally unacceptable thought and to draw more reasonable conclusions.

It is difficult to answer client questions like "Have I got cancer," "Will this surgery make me impotent," or "Am I going to die?" Usually it is useful to ask the client what prompted the question and to have a good idea of the client's level of knowledge before answering. The answer can be tentative and should reflect the nurse's level of knowledge about the client as well as the condition.

Sometimes the family will ask the physician or nurse not to discuss a terminal diagnosis with a client. This is a tricky situation because the client may intuitively know that their prognosis is grim and yet no one will discuss it with them. Here the nurse can follow the client's questions focused on what the client knows and has concerns about. Communicating this information to the physician or family can be beneficial in helping family members know what is important to the client.

## Theoretical Models of Stress

### Early Models

Cannon (1914) first described stress from the perspective of the body's internal homeostatic processes that undergo change as individuals adapt to change and maintain internal stability in an ever-changing life environment. According to Cannon, when people feel physically well, emotionally centered, and personally secure, they are in a state of *dynamic equilibrium* or **homeostasis.** This internal state is a relatively stable environment that a person does not really have to think about much (Goldberger & Breznitz, 1982).

Stress upsets homeostasis, resulting in disturbances in normal internal physiological processes and emotional arousal in the following way. Internal physiological processes such as blood pressure, respiration, and endocrine functions are regulated by homeostatic regulators that become unbalanced in the face of illness. People respond to prolonged or intense stress with physiological symptoms. Stress affects the immune system and can elevate the response to many physical illnesses (e.g., hypertension, headaches, heart attacks, Graves' disease, ulcers, colitis, human immunodeficiency virus infections, and arthritis) (Ben-Schlomo & Chaturvedi, 1992; Gelent & Hochman, 1992; Niaura & Goldstein, 1992; Perry, Fishman, & Jacobsberg, 1992; Thompson et al., 1992). Severe or untreated prolonged physiological alterations caused by stress can result in death.

Studies (Dantzer, 1997; Roozendaal et al., 1997) suggested that there is more than one physiological pattern associated with stressful events. Different perceptions of stress may produce different physiological consequences. As we develop more effective ways to study brain function and measures of changes in the neuroendocrine system during acute stress, our understanding of the psychophysiological responses to stress and adaptation will become clearer.

### Stress as a Stimulus

In 1967, Holmes and Rahe developed a stress model based on the number of life change events a person experiences and subsequent development of physical illness. Theirs is a cumulative stress model centered around a list of 43 potential life events capable of stimulating a stress reaction. Each life event stressor is given a numerical score. Stressors requiring a significant change in the lifestyle of the individual have a greater impact, as do cumulative stresses that occur within a short period of time (Steptoe, 1991).

Research with the Social Adjustment Rating

Scale suggests that experiencing a significant number of stressors over a short period of time fairly predictably leads to later physical illness. The higher the life events score, the more likely the person is to experience severe distress and perhaps develop a stress-induced physical illness. Although the scale has been criticized for trying to capture a major concept with a single measure, it still remains a widely used measurement of the links between mind and body under stress. Exercise 20–1 is designed as a clinical application of the model.

Although any change in a life situation or relationship can stimulate a stress reaction, the extent to which a transition, change, or crisis alters a person's lifestyle and personal relationships influences the level of stress it creates for that person. A hoped-for event that does not occur in a person's life (e.g., not being promoted or not conceiving a child) can have just as severe an impact on a person's stress level. The stress of missed opportunity can be even more painful because they may not be obvious to anyone else. Most people do not feel as comfortable talking about being passed over for promotion or not being able to conceive a child as they do about sharing a visible illness or job stress.

## Stress as a Physical Response

The concept of stress as a generalized biological response to environmental demands was first described by Hans Selye in 1936. His research found that the body reacts in a predictable manner to any stressor, regardless of its nature. The *stress response* is a term used to describe a nonspecific physiological response to the pressures of daily living.

Not all stress is dangerous. In fact, life would be quite boring with no stress. It is unlikely most people would get out of bed without feeling a certain amount of tension about the day's plans. Selye used the term **eustress** to describe a mild level of stress that acts as a positive stress response with protective and adaptive functions. The increased stress a person feels in completing a project with a deadline is an example of eustress. As a person capitalizes on the additional physiological energy created by the stress of the deadline, the stress can actually improve performance.

---

◆ **Exercise 20–1. Assessing Stress as a Stimulus**

**Purpose:**   To provide practice with understanding stress from a stimulus perspective

**Procedure:**
Analyze the following case example and identify factors using the Holmes and Rahe Life Events Scale, with the case example as the basis for data analysis.

Sally Byrd's father was diagnosed as having Alzheimer's disease a year ago. Her mother, who has been the primary caregiver, recently broke her hip. Her father is ineligible for Medicaid, yet they do not have enough money to pay for the care he needs. Sally's husband fears he will be laid off from his job within the next few months. Her three teenaged sons are normal teenagers who demand her attention and time. As the only child of her aging parents, Sally sees no alternative but to bring her parents to live with her, temporarily and perhaps permanently. If she does assume this responsibility, Sally can expect to experience a significant change in her role, her family routines, and even in her relationships with other family members. The cumulative stressors of her father's chronic disorder, her mother's illness, and her husband's potential job loss create a complex crisis situation for Sally and her family.

**Discussion:**
Using the Holmes and Rahe Life Events Scale (see Box 20–1), how would you rate Sally's level of stress? What individual, family, and environmental factors would you have to consider in planning care? If you were the nurse in this situation, how would you intervene to help Sally and her family reduce the impact of multiple stressors?

## General Adaptation Syndrome

Intense or prolonged stress can produce *distress,* a painful response to a stressor that is capable of creating permanent pathological changes and even death. Selye (1956, 1982) hypothesized that the body tries to respond and compensate for stress through a series of changes referred to as the ***general adaptation syndrome*** (GAS). This biological stress syndrome, diagrammed in Figure 20–1, occurs in three phases. First, the body institutes an initial *alarm phase,* evidenced in changes in the sympathetic nervous system and hormonal secretions of the adrenal glands. To appreciate the physiological effects of the alarm phase, think of the immediate biological response

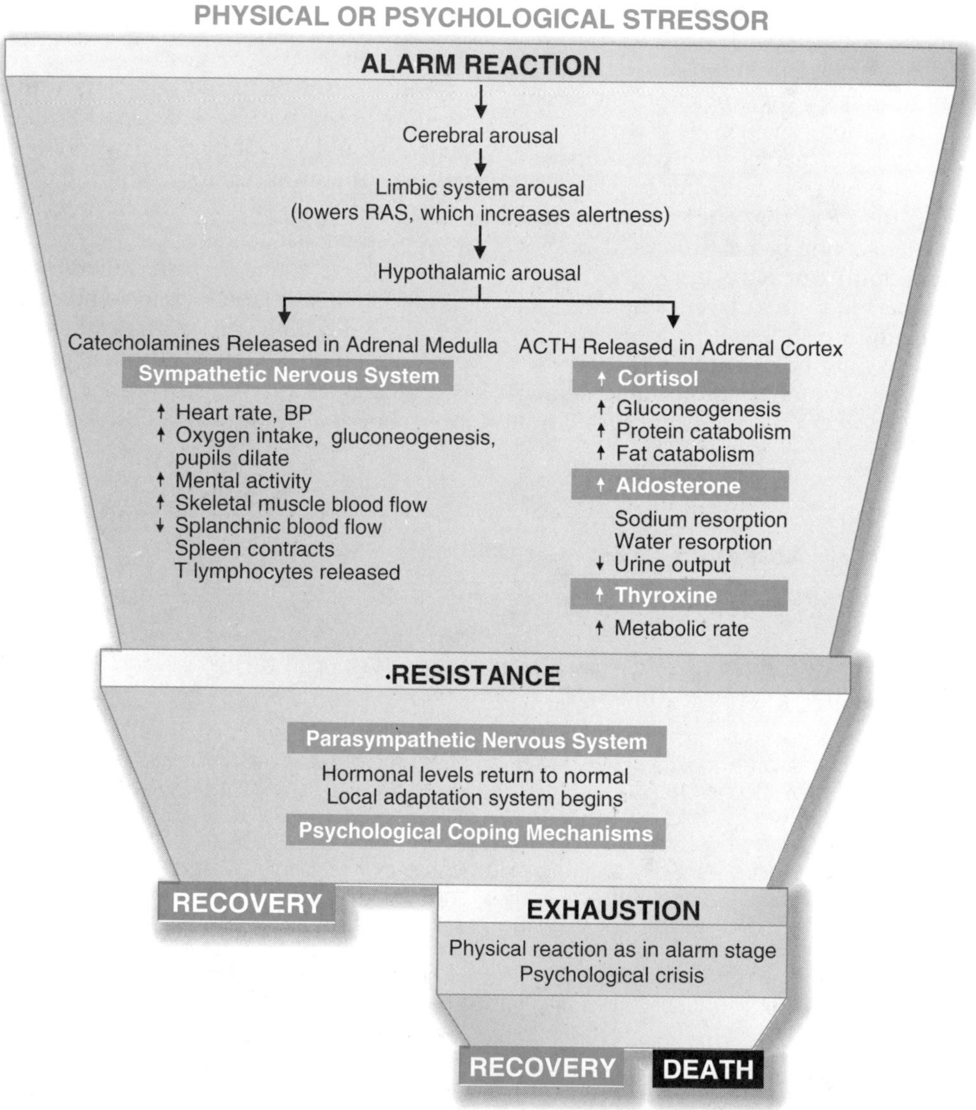

**PHYSICAL OR PSYCHOLOGICAL STRESSOR**

**ALARM REACTION**

Cerebral arousal

Limbic system arousal
(lowers RAS, which increases alertness)

Hypothalamic arousal

Catecholamines Released in Adrenal Medulla

**Sympathetic Nervous System**

- ↑ Heart rate, BP
- ↑ Oxygen intake, gluconeogenesis, pupils dilate
- ↑ Mental activity
- ↑ Skeletal muscle blood flow
- ↓ Splanchnic blood flow
  Spleen contracts
  T lymphocytes released

ACTH Released in Adrenal Cortex

**↑ Cortisol**
- ↑ Gluconeogenesis
- ↑ Protein catabolism
- ↑ Fat catabolism

**↑ Aldosterone**
  Sodium resorption
  Water resorption
- ↓ Urine output

**↑ Thyroxine**
- ↑ Metabolic rate

**·RESISTANCE**

**Parasympathetic Nervous System**

Hormonal levels return to normal
Local adaptation system begins

**Psychological Coping Mechanisms**

**RECOVERY**

**EXHAUSTION**

Physical reaction as in alarm stage
Psychological crisis

**RECOVERY**  **DEATH**

Figure 20–1. Model of the general adaptation syndrome. (From Black JM, Matassarin-Jacobs E. [1993]. Luckman and Sorensen's Medical-Surgical Nursing: A Psychophysiologic Approach [4th ed.]. Philadelphia: W.B. Saunders, p. 46.)

you have when the car in front of you stops unexpectedly and you think you might hit it. You feel a rush of adrenaline, which causes increased breathing, muscle tension, and accelerated heart rate. These sensations subside after you realize you are no longer in danger. You then feel momentarily drained and limp as you realize you are not going to hit the car. Similar sensory experiences occur in individuals experiencing health-related stress, for example, on reacting to an unfavorable diagnosis or responding to a crisis.

The state of alarm cannot exist indefinitely without harming the body. The body tries to adapt to the chronic presence of a stressor, by entering the second phase of the GAS referred to as the *resistance phase*. In the resistance phase, the body produces *endorphins*, naturally occurring internal opiate substances that develop in response to a brain stimulus to restore homeostasis. Their effects are similar to those of morphine in stimulating good feelings in some people (Emrich, 1981).

Knowledge of the role of endorphins in stress management is helpful. Physical exercise, sexual activity, and brief stress increase the production of endorphins, lowering blood pressure and heart rate and acting as a buffer on the unhealthy effects of stress. Consistency and a regular routine enhance the effectiveness of exercise so that a person actually can recover from stress stronger physically and psychologically.

Prolonged or recurrent stress, however, depletes endorphin production. When this occurs, a state of exhaustion develops, in which the body literally gives up the fight. Physical symptoms of stress are wide ranging: sleep disturbances, changes in eating patterns, headaches, stomach and bowel disturbances, heart palpitations, perspiration, muscle tightness, feelings of lightheadedness, back pain, fatigue, and skin eruptions (Fig. 20–2).

The *exhaustion phase* can present as serious physical symptoms, dangerous mental disorganization, physical collapse, and even death. If the stress demands continue to exceed the person's resources, the person may die. Even when the body is able to return to a previous state of resistance and adaptability, residual effects and possible irreversible damage can alter the immune system permanently. Although Selye's theory is faulted because it fails to take into consideration environmental and personal factors influencing the adaptive process, it is a useful model for understanding common physiologic responses to stress.

## Stress as a Transaction

Lazarus and Folkman (1984) used a transactional appraisal model of stress that emphasizes the interaction between person and environment. For stress to occur, there must be a dynamic relationship between a (stressor) situation or circumstance in the environment and the individual experiencing the stressor. This approach emphasizes the personal interpretation of the stressor and the subjective meaning attached to a stressful event as influencing a person's response to it. The cognitive appraisal a person uses evaluates the stressful impact in terms of its impact on self.

### Primary and Secondary Appraisals

Two levels of personal appraisal—primary and secondary—influence the development of a stress response. The first level (primary appraisal) focuses on the event itself. A person determines whether an event is stressful and can draw one of three conclusions: that it is not stressful, that it is a relatively benign stressor, or that it is stressful. Stressors perceived as a major threat to self elicit a stronger stress response than those having less impact on a person's sense of self and significant relationships. Most intense are life events experienced as a personal physical threat to homeostasis, such as a terminal or disfiguring illness, or a psychological threat to self-concept (e.g., job loss) or to significant relationships with family or friends. Primary stress appraisals can include threat of harm or losses that are anticipated but have not yet occurred.

When a primary cognitive appraisal of the stressor determines it to be threat to self, a person automatically switches to a secondary appraisal to determine how to respond (Fig. 20–3). Secondary appraisals are complex internal processes that take into consideration potential coping responses, the likelihood of a response accomplishing its desired effect of reducing a stressor, and the ability of the person to carry it out. Coping resources can include health, energy, problem-solving skills, and amount and availability of social supports and other material resources to cope

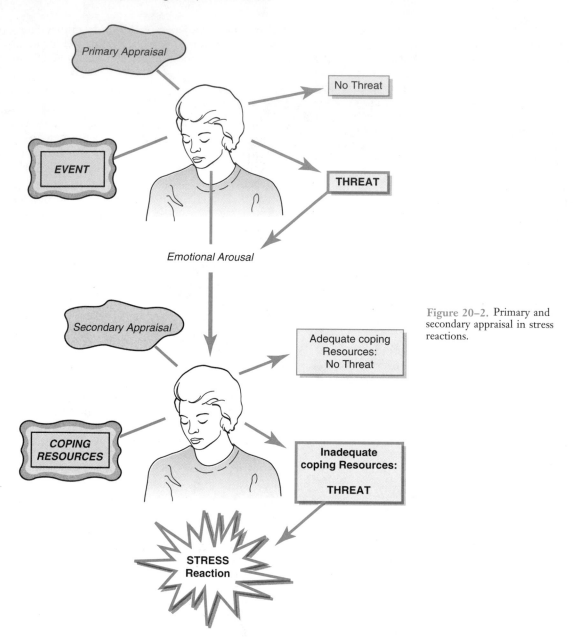

Figure 20–2. Primary and secondary appraisal in stress reactions.

effectively with the stressor (Lazarus & Folkman, 1984). Primary and secondary appraisals do not occur in isolation from one another, but more often occur in close approximation with each other to determine the level of stress an individual experiences.

## Stress as a Subjective Experience

Lazarus and Folkman argued that stress is a subjective experience influenced by a variety of factors, as shown in Box 20–1. Although some stressors are of such magnitude or a person has so many that it would be impossible not to experi-

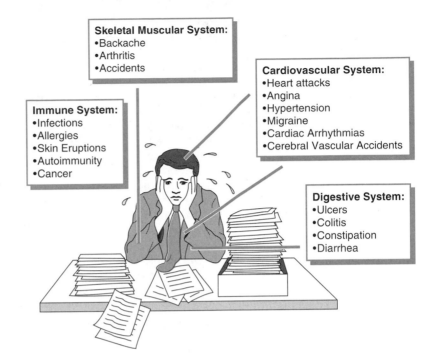

**Skeletal Muscular System:**
•Backache
•Arthritis
•Accidents

**Cardiovascular System:**
•Heart attacks
•Angina
•Hypertension
•Migraine
•Cardiac Arrhythmias
•Cerebral Vascular Accidents

**Immune System:**
•Infections
•Allergies
•Skin Eruptions
•Autoimmunity
•Cancer

**Digestive System:**
•Ulcers
•Colitis
•Constipation
•Diarrhea

Figure 20–3. Physical effects of chronic stress.

ence them as overwhelming, for most life stress, personal responses to the same stressor are highly individual. A set of circumstances can be overwhelmingly stressful for one person, whereas another person can cope with the same circumstances without significant distress (Lazarus & Folkman, 1984). Two college freshmen, for example, may experience their first semester away from home quite differently. For one student, the experience may be a challenging and growth-producing adventure. The other student may feel extremely confused and frightened. How each student personally perceives the meaning of the stressor will influence its impact.

Previous experiences, ability to make friends,

and cognitive maturity can intensify or reduce the impact of the stressor. *Social support,* defined as social environmental factors that contribute to a person's sense of well-being (Edens et al., 1992), can include family, friends, church, work, or school and help people respond to stress productively. Social support can act as a buffer on stress by reducing its intensity (Caplan, 1964). For example, having a supportive roommate and frequent care packages from home can reduce the impact of the stressor for the student who is lonely and unsure during the first semester of college.

## Behavioral Responses to Stress

### Anxiety

The word *anxiety* derives from the Latin root *angere,* "to cause anguish or distress." Anxiety in stressful situations makes the experience more painful than it needs to be. It reduces a person's objectivity and makes it more difficult to envision possibilities, weigh options, make choices, and take action. Acute anxiety causes clients to become hypervigilant of their physical symptoms, particularly pain. Unlike fear, which has a direct,

◆ Box 20–1. Factors Influencing the Impact of Stress

Magnitude of the stressor
Number of stressors
Subjective meaning of the stressor
Developmental level of the client
Availability of social support

identifiable source of discomfort, anxiety is diffuse, and the client may not be able to relate it to an identifiable cause.

People experiencing anxiety as a response to stress have many emotions simultaneously: anger, grief, shame, embarrassment, dread, dismay, all of which may be difficult to sort out as being anxiety. At times, anxiety is expressed directly in nervousness, pacing, inability to concentrate, or insomnia. Other psychological symptoms include inability to recall information, blocked speech, and fear of losing control (Arnold, 1997). In other circumstances, a person does not feel the anxiety directly but experiences this unpleasant emotion as emotional numbness or as images of impending doom, feelings of going crazy, and destructive fantasies. Some people describe their anxious response to a situation as experiencing it as a déjà vu or experiencing it as happening to someone else and not themselves.

Nurses need to help their clients reduce anxiety before providing information and other nonemergency interventions. The consistent, calm presence of the nurse as a source of support is most helpful in helping clients and their families cope with anxiety (Hoff, 1989). People who are anxious need additional information and frequent support delivered in a calm, competent manner (Arnold, 1997). Giving the family progress reports, being available to answer questions, and letting the client and family know who is available to respond to their needs and how to contact the nurse are simple interventions that keep a client and family from becoming more anxious (Hull, 1991; Rushton, 1990). Including a relevant family member in discussions and providing practical information about community resources help reduce client and family anxiety.

## Hostility

Another common reaction to stress is anger. Stressed people say things they do not mean and would not dream of saying in ordinary circumstances. Some clients find it easier to be verbally hostile than to admit feeling totally overwhelmed and powerless. Family members angrily blame each other for an injury, blame the physician for operating—or not operating—on a loved one, and criticize the nurse for not responding quickly enough. If the nurse can recognize the origin of the hostility and see it as a cry for help in coping with escalating stress, it is possible to defuse the stress before it becomes out of control. Verbal hostility can be deflected if the nurse is open to the expression of negative feelings, accepts his or her mistakes, and supports the hostile person without necessarily condoning the behavior.

◆ **Case Example**

**Client:** I don't see any point in talking to you. You can't bring Jenny back, and I don't want what you have to offer me now.

**Nurse** (in a calm, low, slow voice): You're right, Don, I can't bring Jenny back, but what I can offer you is a chance to talk about a very tragic and frightening situation for you. My experience is that talking about it can prove to be healing.

Stress can be transformed into hostility or a demandingness without the person being aware that the underlying emotion is anxiety. In times of stress, the nurse needs to consider two concepts. First, *hostility is a temporary emotional response displaced on you.* It has little to do with you personally other than that you are available; you are the one most involved with the care of the loved one, and you are unlikely to retaliate. Second, *the experience of a serious illness is always an emotional as well as intellectual event for families,* who are emotionally connected to the client (Bluhm, 1987). People can understand intellectually why the nurse is acting in certain ways and what is happening to their loved one, but their emotional understanding may be quite different. When there is a discrepancy between cognitive and emotional understanding, anger is a frequent response. For example, even though Mother is 95 and the family knows intellectually that death is imminent, the emotional remembrance of her is that of someone they do not want to lose just yet. Family members may be angry at the physician or other family members for the decision to let her die without heroic measures. The nurse helps the family accept the fact that there is no way to avoid making very difficult life and death decisions and supports them in their decision making.

Anger projected on the nurse as primary caregiver, even when closely linked with anxiety, can threaten the nurse's energy and commitment. It is hard to be pleasant and caring when someone is attacking you, yet turning frustration, despair, anger, and feelings of being overwhelmed into constructive, meaningful cooperation is highly rewarding and deeply beneficial to the resolution of anger. What a hostile person or family yearns for most despite their behavior is understanding, healing, and human intimacy (Dossey, 1991). What every client and family expects from the nurse is a person who will perceive their pain and confusion and help them to decode the hostile behaviors, feelings, and thoughts that distort reality. For example, the nurse can listen calmly and suggest ways in which the client's concerns can be addressed. Acknowledging the client's right to be angry and simply listening is helpful. If client or family expectations are unrealistic or unable to be met in the current situation, alternative explanations and suggestions reduce anxiety and allow further discussion.

### ◆ Case Example

**Client:** I'm paying a lot of money here and no one is willing to help me. The nursing care is terrible, and I just have to lie here in pain with no one to help me.

**Nurse:** I'm sorry you are feeling so bad. Please tell me a little more specifically what's going on with you, and maybe we can try to do something a little differently to help you.

---

The nurse's first statement acknowledges the feelings of the client. The second statement asks for more information and encourages the client to enter a mutual partnership in correcting the problem. The client feels heard even if the issue cannot be totally resolved as the client wishes. Exercise 20–2 helps the student address the relationship between anger and anxiety. Other strategies for resolving conflict are addressed in Chapter 14.

A major goal in implementing this nursing intervention is to help the client or family replace unrealistic expectations for self, other professionals, and the health care setting with attainable goals. It is usually useless to defend personalities or intentions. A tactful statement acknowledging the client's feeling is helpful: "It sounds as though you are pretty angry with Dr. Moore, and you may have every right to be, but I'd like

to see if there is something we could come up with that might make this situation less frustrating." Such an approach acknowledges feelings, but it also asks the client or family how they might work together with the nurse to make the experience more positive. It takes the focus off nonproductive blaming and helps people refocus on specific productive behaviors. It allows space to contradict false information without making the client lose face.

This strategy is also helpful when the client or family blame themselves for things that are beyond their control. "*If only*'s" are self-defeating because there is nothing anyone can do to change the past. The nurse can help the family reframe their situation as one in which they acted with good intentions on the basis of the knowledge they had at the time. Family members sometimes feel better about circumstances they cannot erase when they can look at a situation this way.

### Grief

Grief is a normal human response to the stress of losing something or someone significant. It derives from a Latin term, "to be robbed." Lindemann (1944) noted that grief as a stress response is accompanied by "sensations of somatic distress occurring in waves lasting from 20 minutes to an hour at a time, a feeling of tightness in the throat, choking with shortness of breath, need for sighing, and an empty feeling in the abdomen, lack of muscular power and an intense subjective distress described as tension or mental pain" (p. 141).

Common psychological characteristics vary. As one person described it, "It felt as though there was a great distance between me and everyone else, as if I was cocooned in cotton wool. Literally numb with shock; no tears, no feelings, just absolute numbness" (Lendrum & Syme, 1992, p. 2425). In health care, denial is a common first response evidenced in statements such as "He's a strong boy . . . I know he is going to make it," even though the child is on a respirator and is not expected to live. This initial disbelief is an emotional buffer protecting one against a powerful assault to the integrity of the self. It does not mean that the client or family is delusional. It simply is an ego defense against a reality that the nurse needs to realize will take time to absorb (Levin, 1998).

---

◆ Exercise 20-2. **Relationship Between Anger and Anxiety**

**Purpose:** To help students appreciate the links between anger and anxiety and how anger is triggered

**Procedure:**

1. Think of a time when you were really angry. It need not be a significant event or one that would necessarily make anyone else angry.
2. Identify your thoughts, feelings, and behavior in separate columns of a table you construct. For example, what were the thoughts that went through your head when you were feeling this anger? What were your physical and emotional responses to this experience? Write down words or phrases to express what you were feeling at the time. How did you respond when you were angry?
3. Identify what was going on with you before experiencing the anger. Sometimes it is not the event itself but your feelings before the incident that make the event the straw that breaks the camel's back.
4. Identify underlying threats to your self-concept in the situation (e.g., you were not treated with respect; your opinion was discounted; you lost status; you were rejected; you feared the unknown).

**Discussion:**

1. In what ways were your answers similar and different from those of your classmates?
2. What role did anxiety and threat to the self-concept play in the development of the anger response? What percentage of your anger related to the actual event and to self-concept?
3. In what ways did you see anger as a multidetermined behavioral response to threats to self-concept?
4. Did this exercise change any of your ideas about how you might handle your feelings and behavior in a similar situation?
5. What are the common threads in the events that made people in your group angry?
6. In what ways could experiential knowledge of the close association between anger and anxiety be helpful in your nursing practice?

---

Grieving behaviors that in ordinary circumstances might be classified as pathological are normal transitory human responses in stressful situations. For example, a client may report seeing or hearing the presence of the lost person or may sense his or her presence through the smell of a flower. Clients who have lost body parts physically feel the sensations or pain in the missed limb. These are not hallucinations brought about by a biological misfiring of neurotransmitters. They are normal temporary responses to extreme stress.

### ◆ Case Example

**Client:** Sometimes when I'm driving home from work, I can actually hear Nancy talking to me. It's eerie, but it feels so real. Am I going crazy?

**Nurse:** Mary, when people have suffered the loss of someone very significant to them, they often do think they hear or see them. It can be very frightening and disorienting, but it really is a very normal response to a powerful loss of someone special.

---

Even though life seems to be back to normal, a chance scene or remarks continue to stir memories. Missing the person can be intense on the anniversary of the death. Clients appreciate the nurse who verbalizes this.

Multiple losses are much more traumatic and take longer to resolve. The most helpful intervention is to focus on one relationship at a time instead of trying to address the losses together. To do the latter can be overwhelming to the client. Reassure the client that responding to multiple loss is more difficult.

### Anticipatory Grief

Anticipatory grief is an emotional response that occurs before the actual loss. It has many of the characteristics of an actual grief reaction with some notable exceptions. With anticipatory grief, there is always the hope that the loss that one anticipates will not occur. The constellation of feelings about the projected loss, the uncertainty, and ambivalence, wishing it would happen soon and simultaneously dreading the finality of the loss, make the grieving process more unstable. Significant others find themselves torn between remaining faithful to the client and needing to start a new life for themselves. There is no way to complete the grieving process.

◆ **Case Example**

Marge's husband Albert was diagnosed with Alzheimer's disease 5 years ago. Albert is in a nursing home. He does not know who Marge is anymore. The doctor told Marge that his disease is progressing rapidly and he most likely will die within the next few years. Marge just turned 60 and has been living with this disorder since she was 55. Although she misses Albert, and feels guilty because she would like a life of her own and has the "other feelings, of wishing he would die so that she can get on with her life, and feeling cheated out of a life she deserves."

## Concepts of Coping

Coping is a conceptual term used to describe the many ways that people respond to the stressors in their life. In their classic work, Pearlin and Schooler (1978) defined *coping* as "any response to external life strains that serves to prevent, avoid, or control emotional distress." They identify three types of coping strategies:

- To change the stressful situation
- To change the meaning of the stressor
- To help the person relax enough to take the stress in stride

The more versatile and flexible a person's coping strategies are, the more likely it is that he or she is able to manage life's challenges. People learn coping strategies from their parents, peers, and the circumstances life presents to them. People with a wide variety of life opportunities and supportive people in their lives have an advantage over those who lack them. Inadequate coping strategies can reflect a life in which a person has not had to respond to danger or lacks the necessary skills to do so.

Coping strategies can be ego enhancing or defensive. *Ego-enhancing strategies* include obtaining more information, seeking practical advice, and taking direct action. Practical advice, emotional support, and a strong belief system provide a wider variety of possible options than a person in the midst of overwhelming stress may have considered. **Ego defense mechanisms** (Box 20–2) are used to buy time or change meanings through misinterpretation. As long-term coping strategies, they are counterproductive. As a temporary strategy, they initially protect clients from painful realities until the initial shock wears off. Exercise 20–3 helps you examine the many dimensions of coping strategies in your own life.

### Defensive Coping Strategies

Knowledge of defensive coping strategies first described by Freud (1940) helps the nurse assess client coping skills. Referred to as ego defense mechanisms, they work unconsciously to protect a person from intolerable anxiety by (1) distorting a threat, (2) substituting another reality, or (3) completely blocking out the threat through denial. As a short-term strategy, they may prove beneficial. People need time to absorb the meaning of a serious stressor.

Over time, ego defense mechanisms can become as a smokescreen to action and prevent a more problem-focused resolution of difficult issues. Carried to an extreme, they lead to ego disintegration (Fig. 20–4). The nurse needs to respect a client's use of defensive coping strategies as needed by the person at that point in time while moving the client toward more adaptive solutions. Providing new information or gently casting doubt can be helpful.

◆ **Case Example**

Lynn was diagnosed as having a high cholesterol count and was advised to go on a low-fat diet. Her friends notice no change in her diet, and Lynn says she sees no reason to modify it. Lynn says she sees no purpose in going on a low-fat diet because "it's all in the genes."

---

◆ Box 20–2. Ego Defense Mechanisms

| Ego Defense Mechanism | Clinical Example |
|---|---|
| Regression: returning to an earlier, more primitive form of behavior in the face of a threat to self-esteem | Julie was completely toilet trained by 2 years. When her younger brother was born, she began wetting her pants and wanting a pacifier at night. |
| Repression: unconscious forgetting of parts or all of an experience | Elizabeth has just lost her job. Her friends would not know from her behavior that she has any anxiety about it. She continues to spend money as if she were still getting a paycheck. |
| Denial: unconscious refusal to allow painful facts, feeling, or perceptions into awareness | Bill Marshall has had a massive heart attack. His physician advises him to exercise with caution. Bill continues to jog 6 miles a day. |
| Rationalization: offering a plausible explanation for unacceptable behavior | Annmarie tells her friends she is not an alcoholic even though she has blackouts, because she drinks only on weekends and when she is not working. |
| Projection: attributing unacceptable feelings, facts, behaviors, or attitudes to others; usually expressed as blame. | Ruby just received a critical performance evaluation from her supervisor. She tells her friends that her supervisor does not like her and feels competitive with her. |
| Displacement: redirecting feelings onto an object or person considered less of a threat than the original object or person | Mrs. Jones took Mary to the doctor for bronchitis. She is not satisfied with the doctor's explanation and feels he was condescending but says nothing. When she gets to the nurse's desk to make the next appointment, she yells at her for not having the prescription ready and taking too much time to make the next appointment. |
| Intellectualization: unconscious focusing on only the intellectual and not the emotional aspects of a situation or circumstance | Johnnie has been badly hurt in a car accident. There is reason to believe he will not survive surgery. His father, waiting for his son to return to the intensive care unit, asks the nurse many questions about the equipment, and philosophizes about the meaning of life and death. |
| Reaction formation: unconscious assuming of traits opposite of undesirable behaviors | John has a strong family history of alcoholism on both sides. He abstains from liquor and is known in the community as an advocate of prohibition. |
| Sublimation: redirecting socially unacceptable unconscious thoughts and feeling into socially approved outlets | Bob has a lot of aggressive tendencies. He decided to become a butcher and thoroughly enjoys his work. |
| Undoing: verbal expression or actions representing one feeling, followed by expression of the direct opposite | Barbara criticizes her subordinate, Carol, before a large group of people. Later, she sees Carol on the street and tells her how important she is to the organization. |

---

Both her parents had high cholesterol, and she claims there is nothing she can do about it, even though the physician has advised her differently.

Lynn's denial is a defense against feeling that she will die like her parents from heart disease. Her defensive coping strategy prevents her from taking action needed to reduce her risk for cardiovascular disease and can result in a heart attack or death. Here the nurse might provide the client with information about the link among diet, exercise, and heart disease and inquire about her parents' lifestyle.

◆ Exercise 20-3. **Coping Exercise**

**Purpose:** To help students experience the wide range of adaptive and maladaptive coping strategies

**Procedure:**
1. Identify all of the ways in which you handle stressful situations.
2. List three personal strategies that you have used successfully in coping with stress.
3. List one personal coping strategy that did not work, and identify your perceptions of the reasons it was inadequate or insufficient to reduce your stress level.
4. List different coping strategies identified by students on a chalkboard or flip chart.

**Discussion:**
1. What common themes did you find in the ways people handle stress?
2. Were you surprised at the number and variety of ways in which people handle stress?
3. What new coping strategy might you use to reduce your stress level?
4. Are there any circumstances that increase or decrease your automatic reactions to stress?

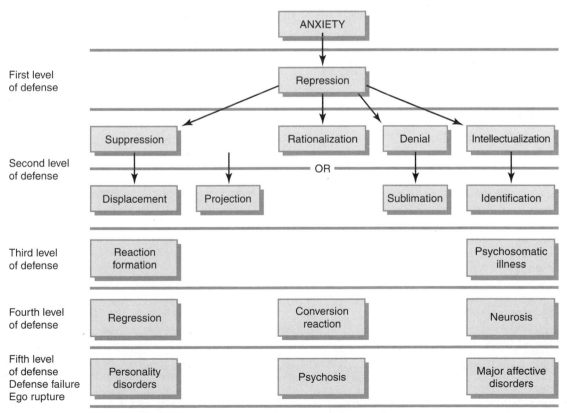

Figure 20-4. Ego defense mechanism: levels of complexity.

## APPLICATIONS
## Nursing Process
### Assessment

Accurate assessment of how an individual is responding to the meaning of the stressor is essential. If the nurse can assess the person's perception of a stressful situation accurately, then the nurse's response can mirror the client's experience. For example, stress perceived as a threat stimulates anxiety, but stress as a loss presents as depression and grief. The strategies the nurse would use to help each of these clients reduce their stress would differ. In the first case, the nurse might suggest stress management techniques. In the second case, the nurse would help the client acknowledge the loss and work through the grieving process.

Understanding stress from the client's perspective is essential in understanding a client's behavior in stressful situations. It is helpful to put yourself in the client or family's position and put into words how you might feel in a similar situation and useful to caution clients not to pass negative judgment on themselves based on one incident. Statements such as "Most people would feel anxious in this situation" or "It would be hard for anyone to have all the answers in a situation like this" remind clients and families to accept the human limitations we all possess.

### Data Analysis

The nurse needs to assess and analyze the factors that influence the impact of stress: suddenness of onset, the magnitude of change the stressor presents, the number and meaning of concurrent stressors in the family, and the biopsychosocial status of the individual and family before the onset of the current situation. In addition, the nurse needs to gather data about the impact of the stress on other family members and to identify likely sources of social support. Listening for relevant themes is important, but so are the communication patterns and what is not being said. A sample assessment tool is presented in Box 20–3.

The nurse would make the following observations as part of a data base:

• Are family members and client communicating with each other?

• What are the family's and client's expectations?
• What does the family or client need from you? From each other?
• Is there a family spokesperson?
• What are the client's cultural, religious, and family values concerning the meaning of the stressor?

The nurse also needs to know what coping strategies the client has used in the past and where the client perceives the greatest difficulty with coping. Assessment of past coping strategies may include questions such as

• What kinds of things increase your stress?
• Are any of your activities limited by your stress level?
• What kinds of leisure activities do you engage in?
• What do you do to relieve your stress?
• What are your usual methods of coping when you do not feel stressed?

The nurse should ask these questions within an informal conversational format and should use the client's reactions as a guide to how much and how quickly the information can be gathered.

### Diagnosis

Nursing diagnoses related to anxiety, grief, and ineffective coping strategies of individuals and families are familiar correlates of stress in health care settings. Lazarus and Folkman (1984) described five coping tasks that clients in health care settings must address:

• Reducing toxic environmental conditions
• Tolerating and adjusting to new and negative realities
• Sustaining a positive self-image
• Maintaining emotional equilibrium
• Maintaining satisfying interpersonal relationships with significant others

### Intervention

Nurses can use several simple measures to help their clients feel less stressed in health care situations, the first of which is to call the client by name and engage the client in a respectful manner (Arnold, Virvan & Kizilay, 1998). This is a simple intervention, but one frequently overlooked in stressful situations when so much else

---

### ◆ Box 20–3. Assessment/Intervention Tool

**Assessment**

A. Perception of stressors
1. Major stress area or health concern
2. Present circumstances related to usual pattern
3. Experienced similar problem: how was it handled?
4. Anticipation of future consequences
5. Expectations of self
6. Expectations of caregivers

B. Intrapersonal factors
1. Physical (mobility, body function)
2. Psychosociocultural (attitudes, values, coping patterns)
3. Developmental (age, factors related to present situation)
4. Spiritual belief system (hope and sustaining factors)

C. Interpersonal factors
1. Resources and relationship of family or significant other(s) as they relate to or influence interpersonal factors

D. Environmental factors
1. Resources and relationships of community as they relate to or influence interpersonal factors

**Prevention as Intervention**

A. Primary
1. Classify stressor.
2. Provide information to maintain or strengthen strengths.
3. Support positive coping mechanisms.
4. Educate client and family.

B. Secondary
1. Mobilize resources.
2. Motivate, educate, involve client in health care goals.
3. Facilitate appropriate interventions; refer to external resources as needed.
4. Provide information on primary prevention or intervention as needed.

C. Tertiary
1. Attain/maintain wellness.
2. Educate or re-educate as needed.
3. Coordinate resources.
4. Provide information about primary and secondary interventions.

Developed by J. Conrad, University of Maryland School of Nursing, 1993.

---

needs to be accomplished quickly. It reinforces the client's identity and respects individuality. Orient the client and family to the unit and provide enough information to familiarize but not overwhelm them as to what they might expect from health care. Take time to explain to the client

- What will happen during tests or surgery
- Who is likely to interview the client
- How the client can best cooperate or assist in his or her treatment process

### Family Involvement

Families suffer significant stress when a family member is critically ill or injured. Coping with the disruptions that such an event produces is difficult and stressful for even the most functional family (Leske, 1998). Family involvement is critical to client stress reduction at all stages of the process for the following reasons: (1) the family is a constant presence in the client's life, whereas health care providers usually have more limited involvement; (2) family members know the client best and can provide valuable data that can affect the type and implementation of treatment; (3) the family will have to be intimately involved with the client's care at home; and (4) providing opportunities for family members to help promote self-confidence and skill development (Whetsell & Larrabee, 1988).

Families feel helpless when all decisions are made by the health care team without consulting them (Abel-Boone et al., 1989). Holding regularly scheduled family conferences helps reduce family stress. If possible, using a team approach, the nurse, physician, social worker, and chaplain can meet with the family to discuss the client's care. These conferences offer the opportunity for two-way communication between the health care team and the client (Ceronsky, 1983). A family conference can be scheduled around any change in the client's condition or the family's ability to cope. Family conferences help families feel they are partners in the care of their loved ones and provide a unique forum for giving information simultaneously to those most involved with the client's well-being.

Less formal interventions act a buffer to stress experienced by families. Provide information about visiting hours and the timing of tests and procedures. This allows family members and clients to plan and, in the process, to gain control over at least some aspects of the hospitalization.

Encourage family and friends to visit, but monitor the client's response. If the client seems bothered or tired by the visit, the client usually appreciates the nurse's intervening. Nurses can act as a sounding board and reality tester related to the family's perception of the stressor and its personalized impact.

The nurse should prepare family members beforehand for their first visit with a client with a visible disfigurement, marked physical or psychological deterioration, or presence of technical apparatus. For example, "Your father will look as though he is sleeping, but he can still hear what you are saying." Another helpful intervention is to furnish the family with an initial verbal statement: "You might want to identify yourself and tell your father you are here with him." Offering such descriptions gives family members permission to ask questions and time to become more comfortable with undesired circumstances surrounding someone they care about deeply.

Offering self as support can be highly reassuring. The presence of the nurse during the initial encounter lessens the shock of a marked change in appearance or function. Sometimes the sight of a family member on a ventilator or with serious injuries overwhelms family members. Accompanying the client's family to the bedside for the first visit strengthens the family member during the initial shock of seeing their family member in such a condition. If the client is intubated, family members should be advised that he or she will not be able to speak.

The nurse may serve as a role model in initiating conversation with a seriously ill or comatose client: "Hello, Mr. James, I have brought your daughter in to see you." By modeling a normal greeting, the nurse indirectly encourages the family to react in their usual manner with the client. Family members also appreciate a suggestion that if they feel uncomfortable, they should feel free to leave the bedside and return when they feel better.

Help family members conserve their strength. This will enable them to be more responsive to the client. Family members in critical care situations often feel that they need be in constant attendance and to become physically and emotionally exhausted in the process. A useful strategy is to suggest that the family members take short breaks. Family members may need "permission" to go to a movie or eat in a restaurant outside the hospital. The family needs assurance that they will be called should there be any change in the client's condition.

Providing simple, practical suggestions helps the family feel more competent. Coaching can relieve stress by helping family members feel like they are "doing something" for the client. In the process, they develop a sense of competency and mastery over at least part of their environment. For example, providing guidelines for families to participate actively in caring for their loved one helps dispel feelings of helplessness. Families can provide simple loving actions, such as moistening the client's lips or stroking the client's hair or hand. The nurse may need to let the family know that it is okay to touch the client and hold his or her hand.

## Stress Reduction Strategies
### Taking Control

Taking control of one's life is perhaps the most important stress reduction strategy. In difficult situations, this coping strategy often becomes lost. Beckingham and Baumann (1990) suggested that it is not simply the identified problem but the accompanying feelings of helplessness and functional immobilization that create a stress state. People use a variety of coping mechanisms—negotiation, specific actions, seeking advice, and rearranging their priorities—to develop different perspectives and modify difficult stressful situations through direct action.

Clients should be encouraged to participate in all aspects of their care planning to whatever extent possible. This simple nursing action conveys the idea that the nurse considers the client a necessary partner in

- Developing a realistic plan to offset stress
- Dealing directly with obstacles as they emerge
- Evaluating action steps
- Making needed modifications in the plan and often lifestyle

The nurse will need to reassure clients and their families that any change will probably provoke feelings of uncertainty and that these feelings will pass as the person develops more familiarity with the changed expectations (Wurzbach, 1992).

### ◆ Case Example

Sam Hamilton received a diagnosis of prostatic cancer on a routine physical exam. His way of coping included obtaining as much information on the disease as possible. He researched the most up-to-date material on treatment options and sought the advice from physician friends as to which surgeons had the most experience with this type of surgery. As he shared his diagnosis with friends and colleagues, he found several men who had successfully survived without a cancer recurrence. Sam used the time between diagnosis and surgery to finish projects and delegate work responsibilities. He attended a support group with his wife and was able to obtain valuable advice on handling his emotional responses to what would happen. When the time came for his surgery, Sam was still apprehensive, but he felt as though he had done everything humanly possible to prepare for it. The actions he took before surgery reduced his stress.

## Ventilating Feelings

In stressful situations, black and white thinking can replace normal thought processes, with little room for negotiation. Clients experiencing stress should be given the opportunity to express their feelings, thoughts, and worries. Crying, anger, and magical thinking are normal reactions to situations that one cannot control.

If there is no immediate jeopardy to treatment, it is best to support the client's right to process a stressful event in his or her own way. Helpful statements can include "This must be very difficult for you to absorb. Can you tell me what you are experiencing right now as you think about . . . ?" This response allows the client to put concerns into words and offers clues about

the role of denial in the current situation. If the client tells the nurse, "I think I'm losing my mind," the nurse might respond, "Many people feel that way. You are not losing your mind. What really is happening is that you are feeling disoriented because of the sudden and unbelievable nature of what is happening here. Can you identify what worries you the most?" By acknowledging the legitimacy of the client's feelings and labeling the nature of it, the nurse reinforces the client's self-integrity and begins to help the client put boundaries on the anxiety by identifying important concerns.

In the process of helping clients ventilate important feelings, the nurse can suggest actions clients can take to increase mastery. Allowing clients to control areas and issues that are not of critical importance to a protocol and helping clients discover the real causes of their frustration can reduce destructive behaviors. Encouraging clients to take one day at a time in their expectations and recovery activities and suggesting referral and concrete resources are helpful strategies the nurse can use to assist clients to take needed action.

## Providing Anticipatory Guidance

Fear of the unknown intensifies the impact of a stressor. When people do not understand what is happening, they frequently try to fill in the gaps, usually with inaccuracies. *Anticipatory guidance* (helping the client foresee and predict potential difficulties) helps the client cope more effectively with the unknown. Exercise 20–4 provides role-playing practice in handling stressful situations.

Anticipatory guidance is particularly useful as a nursing strategy when something new is about to happen: a test, examination, first visitation. Nurses can anticipate the need for information and proactively explain every procedure in detail, using terminology the client understands. For example, the nurse might go through the steps of a procedure, explaining sensations the client can expect to feel at each step. The nurse should take care to repeat important points at intervals. This is particularly important with elderly clients, who have the double stress of adjusting to a change in setting and the stress of an unfamiliar procedure.

---

◆ Exercise 20–4. **Role-Play: Handling Stressful Situations**

**Purpose:** To give students experience in responding to stressful situations

**Procedure:**
Use the following case study as the basis for this exercise.

Dave is a 66-year-old man with colon cancer. In the past, he had a colostomy. Recently, he was readmitted to your unit and had an exploratory laparotomy for small bowel obstruction. Very little can be done for him because the cancer has spread. He is in pain, and he has to have a feeding tube. His family has many questions for the nurse: "Why is he vomiting?", "How come the pain medication isn't working?", "Why isn't he feeling any better than he did before the surgery?" You have just entered the client's room; his family is sitting near him, and they want answers now!

1. Have different members of your group role-play the client, the nurse, the son, the daughter-in-law, and the wife. One person should act as observer.
2. Identify the factors that will need to be clarified in this situation to help the nurse provide the most appropriate intervention.
3. Using the strategies suggested in this chapter, intervene to help the client and the family reduce their anxiety.
4. Role-play the situation for 10 to 15 minutes.

**Discussion:**
1. Have each player identify the interventions that were most helpful.
2. From the nurse's perspective, which parts of the client and family stress were hardest to handle?
3. How could you use what you learned from doing this exercise in your clinical practice?

---

Anticipatory guidance and reassurance can come from other clients as well as from the nurse. Arranging for a client to talk with someone who has survived a similar stressful experience is helpful. Talking with someone who has successfully adjusted and gone on with life can make all the difference for someone who feels life will never be normal again. A word of caution: always check with the other client first. Some people, even with highly successful outcomes, are not ready to talk about their problems.

The nurse can frame the suggestion in the form of a question, leading the client to explore possible alternatives and responding with simple counsel. A starting point is to ask the client what he or she anticipates will be the result of sharing difficult feelings. "What is the worst thing you can imagine happening if you tell your mother (wife, child) about . . . ?" followed by another question about the best way to respond to this concern.

The nurse bears the responsibility to be knowledgeable as well as trustworthy in providing practical suggestions. Do not offer more than what the situation dictates. Encourage the client to expand on the suggestion rather than provide a full plan. The ability of the client to set priorities, to develop a meaningful plan to meet goals, and to establish milestones in the evaluation process stimulates self-confidence and decreases stress.

*Repeating Information*

In stressful situations, most people have difficulty concentrating. Information and directions given in the first 48 hours of an admission should be repeated, maybe more than once, because this is the time of highest stress. Providing written instructions to leave with the client or family after discussing them verbally enhances understanding. Allowing time to answer questions and providing the client's family with a person's name and telephone number to call if other issues arise is helpful.

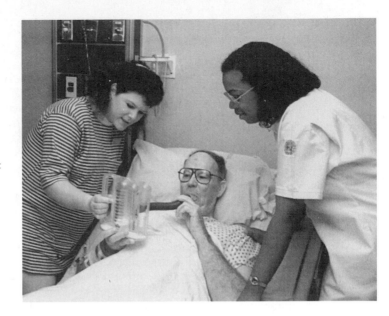

A calm approach and repetition of instructions can help clients in stressful situations relax enough to hear important instructions. (Courtesy University of Maryland School of Nursing)

## Setting Priorities

When people feel stressed, normal problem-solving skills vanish into thin air. Clients need support and encouragement to rework old patterns that compromise the quality of their lives, and they do not always know where to start. The nurse needs to help the client identify the concrete tasks needed to achieve treatment goals, including the people involved, the necessary contacts, the amount of time each task will take, and specific hours or days for each task. Some tasks are more important than others in stressful situations. "Let's see what you need to do right now and what can wait until tomorrow." Tasks that someone else can do and those that not essential to the achievement of goals should be eliminated or ignored. The client should identify a time frame in which to accomplish each short-term goal.

Priority setting also helps reduce hesitation. Putting off tasks and decisions increases stress in health care as well as in personal situations. Most of the time, procrastination occurs when the client or family perceives a task or decision as potentially overwhelming. The nurse can help a client or family think through the elements of a situation and consider which elements are critical and which can be addressed later. Tasks that are appropriate but too overwhelming can be divided into manageable smaller segments. The most important tasks should be scheduled during times when the client or family has the most energy and freedom from interruption.

## Sources of Strength and Hope

In times of stress, people reach out to others for solace and direction. Some people turn to their God, others to family and friends, and still others without these resources turn to community resources. Religion can take on new meaning in times of stress; some people use it to facilitate acceptance of a reality that cannot be changed and others question its validity in the wake of unfavorable news. Some clients experience a spiritual void in times of stress. For many people, belief in a personal God provides an incomparable resource that helps them cope with shattered dreams and incomprehensible life crises. Additionally, religious end-of-life rituals may be extremely helpful in assisting families to experience healing. Carson (1998) noted that "spiritual services staff minister to the emotional, relational and spiritual needs of an individual, recognizing the importance of *healing people*, not diseases" (p. 1077).

Social support is an essential component of

stress management (Lepore et al., 1991). Having contact with other human beings is a resource that most people depend on to help them reduce stress. Social support provides three distinct functions: validation, emotional support, and correction of distorted thinking. Validating the legitimacy of anger, frustration, and helplessness prevents the tunnel vision many clients experience under stress. Emotional support allows a person to feel loved and cared about. Informational support and feedback help a client correct distortions and maintain morale.

Community resources in the form of support groups, social services, and other public health agencies can help clients and families reduce stress. For example, a family caregiver of an Alzheimer's disease victim might find episodic respite care beneficial in reducing the ongoing stress of caring associated with this disorder. The nurse is in a unique position to help clients assess the type of aid they need and the most appropriate community resources (Logsdon & Davis, 1998). Sometimes it is difficult for clients to find community agencies and to obtain access to their services. The more knowledgeable the nurse is about community resources, the better is the client service. Exercise 20–5 is designed to help you become better acquainted with resources in your community.

## Mind–Body Therapies

Mind–body therapies (Pearlin & Schooler, 1978) are coping strategies designed to lessen the intensity of the stressor on a person once the stress response has occurred. The purpose of the mind–body therapies is twofold: to direct a person away from external stressors and to refocus nonproductive physical and psychological energy in a positive health-producing way. In the process of altering physiological reactions such as blood pressure, heart rate, muscle tension, and respiratory rate, most people experience greater calm and peace of mind (Luskin, Newell, Griffith, et al., 1998). Regular practice of these techniques can improve physical and emotional well-being.

## Meditation

Meditation is a stress reduction strategy dating back to early Christian times. Early mystics and holy men used the practice to obtain an altered sense of consciousness that allowed them to experience the presence of God and to transcend the stresses of daily life. In modern times, meditation is used by many people to develop a sense of inner peace and tranquillity. The practice of meditation requires four essential elements: a quiet place, a passive attitude, an object or word symbol to focus on, and a comfortable position

---

◆ **Exercise 20–5. Community Resources for Stress Management**

**Purpose:** To help you become aware of the community resources available in your community for stress management

**Procedure:**
1. Look in the newspaper for ideas, and contact a community agency, social services group, or support group in your community that you believe can help clients cope with a particularly stressful situation.
2. Find out how a person might access the resource, what kinds of cases are treated, what types of treatment are offered, the costs involved, and what you as a nurse can do to help people take advantage of the resource.

**Discussion:**
1. How did you decide which community agency to choose?
2. How difficult or easy was it to access the information about the agency?
3. What information about the community resource did you find out that surprised or perplexed you?
4. In what ways could you use this exercise in planning care for your clients?

(Benson, 1975). A guide to meditation is provided in Box 20–4.

### Biofeedback

**Biofeedback** is a technique that gives a person immediate and continuous information about his or her physiological responses, auditory and visual signals that increase response to external events. Biofeedback provides awareness of minute-by-minute changes in biological activity. This feedback establishes a psychophysiological feedback loop.

Equipment used with biofeedback includes the electroencephalogram, skin temperature devices, blood pressure measures, galvanic skin resistance measurements, and the electromyogram to measure muscle tension. Each device monitors physical information from the client. The data are converted to visual or auditory signals that are reported back to the subject.

Biofeedback has an important role in stress management for clients with chronic stress responses affecting individual body systems such as essential hypertension, migraine headaches, Raynaud's disease, and ulcerative colitis. The major disadvantages of biofeedback are the cost of the equipment, the availability of trained personnel, and the complexity of the stress response in most people.

### Progressive Relaxation

Most people cannot relax on demand. Just wanting to relax and have relief from stress is not enough (Mast et al., 1987a, 1987b). Progressive relaxation is a technique that focuses the client's attention on conscious control of voluntary skeletal muscles. Originally developed by Jacobson (1938), a physiologist physician, the technique consists of alternately tensing and relaxing muscle groups. The client sits in a relaxed position in a chair with arm supports. Feet should be on the ground and legs are placed side by side. To experience the progressive relaxation technique, do Exercise 20–6.

### Guided Imagery

Guided imagery is a technique used frequently with other forms of interventions to help relieve the stress of pain (Papantonio, 1998). Imagery techniques use the client's imagination to stimulate mental pictures in ways that alter consciousness and promote distraction from painful affects or procedures. The guide may use the relaxation techniques described previously to prepare the client for imagery. Positive mental images are associated with improved functioning and reduced pain in clients suffering from intractable pain, cancer, depression, and hypertension. Techniques for using guided imagery are presented in Box 20–5.

## Effects of Stress on the Nurse

Although the primary focus of this chapter is on interventions to reduce stress levels in clients, this portion of the chapter focuses on interventions for the professional nurses who regularly cope with the stress of caregiving in health care. Caring for terminally ill, obnoxious, cognitively impaired, or out-of-control clients places a severe strain on the dedicated caregiver. Yet often nurses do not attend to their own level of stress or that of their coworkers (David, 1991). Nurses sometimes leave the profession because they view this as their only option in managing the unrelenting stress of caring for others. Alternatively,

---

### ◆ Box 20–4. Meditation Techniques

1. Choose a quiet, calm environment with as few distractions as possible.
2. Get in a comfortable position, preferably a sitting position.
3. To shift the mind from logical, externally oriented thought, use a constant stimulus: a sound, word, phrase, or object. The eyes are closed if a repetitive sound or word is used.
4. Pay attention to the rhythm of your breathing.
5. When distracting thoughts occur, they are discarded and attention is redirected to the repetition of the word or gazing at the object. Distracting thoughts will occur and do not mean you are performing the techniques incorrectly. Do not worry about how you are doing. Redirect your focus to the constant stimulus and assume a passive attitude.

Adapted from Benson H. (1975). *The Relaxation Response.* New York, Morrow, pp. 112–113. Used with permission.

◆ Exercise 20-6. **Progressive Relaxation Exercise**

**Purpose:**  To help you experience the beneficial effects of progressive relaxation in reducing tension. This exercise consists of alternately tensing and relaxing voluntary skeletal muscles.

**Procedure:**
1. Sit in a comfortable chair with arm supports. Place the arms on the arm supports, and sit in a comfortable upright position with legs uncrossed and feet flat on the floor.
2. Close your eyes and take 10 deep breaths, concentrating on inhaling and exhaling.
3. Your instructor or a member of the group should give the following instructions, and you should follow them exactly.

I want you to focus on your feet and to tense the muscles in your feet. Feel the tension in your feet. Hold it, and now let go. Feel the tension leaving your feet.

And now I would like you to tense the muscles in your calves. Feel the tension in your calves and hold it. Now let go and feel the tension leaving your calves. Experience how that feels.

Now tense the muscles in your thighs. Most people do this by pressing their thighs against the chair. Feel the tension in your muscles and experience how that feels. Now release the tension and experience how that feels.

Now I would like you to feel the tension in your abdomen. Tense the muscles in your abdomen and hold it. Hold it for a few more seconds. Now release those muscles and experience how that feels.

Now tense the muscles in your chest. The only way you can really do this is to take a very deep breath and hold it. (The guide counts to 10.) Concentrate on feeling how that feels. Now let it go and experience how that feels.

Now I would like you to tense your muscles in your hands. Clench your fist and hold it as hard as you can. Harder, harder. Now release it and concentrate on how that feels.

Now tense the muscles in your arms. You can do this by pressing down as hard as you can on the arm supports. Feel the tension in your arms and continue pressing. Now let go and experience how that feels.

Now I would like you to feel the tension in your shoulders. Tense your shoulders as hard as you can and hold it. Concentrate on how that feels. Now release your shoulder muscles and experience the feeling.

Now feel the tension in your jaw. Clench your jaw and teeth as hard as you can. Feel the tension in your jaw and hold it. Now let it go and feel the tension leave your jaw.

Now that you are in this relaxed state, keep your eyes closed and think of a time when you were really happy. Let the images and sounds surround you. Imagine yourself back in that situation. What were you thinking? What are you feeling?

Now open your eyes. Students who feel comfortable may share the images that emerged in the relaxed state.

**Discussion:**
1. What are your impressions in doing this exercise?
2. Do you feel more relaxed after doing the exercise?
3. If applicable, after doing the exercise, in what ways do you feel differently?
4. Were you surprised at the images that emerged in your relaxed state?
5. In what ways do you think you could use this exercise in your nursing practice?

## ◆ Box 20–5. Using Guided Imagery

Time involved: Reading time, 5 minutes; implementation time, 10 minutes.

Sample situation: Patient is in pain and probably will continue to be for about 30 to 45 minutes while you and/or others are trying to do something more to relieve his pain (e.g., obtain appropriate analgesic orders).

Possible solution: Patient may be willing to try a simple type of imagery or use his own spiritual beliefs.

Expected outcome: Patient will feel his pain is acknowledged and someone cares. He finds that the sensation of pain is relieved by becoming less intense or by changing to a more acceptable sensation. Alternatively, he merely finds the pain more tolerable because this distracts him momentarily. He may note that he feels less anxious.

### Don'ts

1. Do not expect or suggest that imagery will substitute for appropriate pain relief (e.g., adequate analgesic orders).

2. Do not attempt to present imagery for pain relief if you feel unsure or uncomfortable about it. Alternatively, admit these feelings before you proceed, and explain why you think it is worth a try.

3. Do not say there is nothing else anyone can do.

4. Do not tell the patient that he must learn to cope with pain on his own. (He may learn to do this, but not in 10 minutes.)

5. Never tell the patient his pain is not as bad as he thinks.

### Dos

1. Take a deep breath outside his room and relax a little yourself. Plan on spending up to 10 minutes with the patient. You are about to discuss something the patient may find strange; you need to be relaxed and confident.

2. When you enter the room, tell the patient you know he hurts. Be certain that you have assured the patient that you consider his pain real, not imaginary, and that you believe it is just as intense as he says.

3. Tell the patient you are still hoping (searching) for a better alternative, but that meanwhile you would like to offer him the opportunity to try a technique that may ease his pain for just a little while.

4. Explain that you are going to describe a method of using concentration and imagination to help with pain for a brief time. Tell the patient that this may sound strange and he may not want to try it. If so, that is perfectly fine, but you want to offer it just in case it turns out to be something he wants to try and finds helpful.

5. Ask the patient if he daydreams or has a good imagination or if prayer or any kind of faith helps him with pain or illness.

If he gives a negative reply, tell him he may be better at it than he thinks. Ask him whether he remembers a bedroom from his childhood (progress to any bedroom he remembers). Ask him how many windows it had and how many doors. If he can answer with confidence, point out that this is a result of memories that are mental pictures of some sort and not a result of storing numerical information. It is one example of how people who do not even have vivid mental pictures still use their imagination (e.g., images from the past). If he cannot answer these questions, admit that you might be wrong about the appropriateness of this method for him. Ask him whether he wants you to continue. If so, try either of the following.

If he gives a positive reply to daydreaming or a good imagination, use simple symptom substitution, stressing that you are hoping that this will at least reduce unpleasant aspects of the pain for a short time. If the patient cannot concentrate well, try providing another sensation (e.g., cold) to focus on.

If he gives a positive reply to some type of faith, use the ball of healing energy, suggesting that he substitute his personal faith for the healing energy and that this may reduce his pain.

6. Tell the patient you will return to find out if he decided to try this and whether it helped. Tell the patient when you will return, but give yourself leeway. It is better to return early than late.

7. When you return, ask the patient what he decided about the imagery.

*Box continued on following page*

◆ **Box 20-5. Using Guided Imagery** *Continued*

If the patient says he did not try the imagery, tell him you appreciate his considering it.

If it did not work, tell him you admire his willingness to try the technique, reassuring him that it does not always work.

If it did help, tell him you do not expect him to rely on it as his only source of pain relief.

8. In all cases, continue to explore and explain other plans for pain relief.

Adapted from McCaffery M, Beebe A. (1989). Pain: Clinical Manual for Nursing Practice. St. Louis, MO, CV Mosby, p. 213. Reprinted with permission.

they remain in nursing despite low energy and buried resentments, which result in a poorer quality of nursing care (Gray & Diers, 1992; Schaefer & Peterson, 1992).

### Road to Burnout

Physical, emotional, and spiritual exhaustion among caregivers is sometimes called ***burnout.*** Nurses are at high risk for burnout because they care. The road to burnout often begins insidiously (Freudenberger, 1985). It occurs more often in people who have excessive expectations of themselves and who feel they need to do everything right, and nurses are especially prone to this determinant. So strong is the need to be the exemplary nurse, mother, and expert clinician that the compulsion to do the highest quality job takes over at the expense of health and well-being (Freudenberger, 1985).

The need to be perfect does not allow for error or reserve to correct for unexpected events (Porter-Grady, 1998). There is a story about Babe Ruth that applies also to how the professional nurse might approach tasks. Babe was coaching a young, aspiring ball player, and he asked the boy how he was planning to pitch the ball. The boy answered, "I'm going to throw it with all my might and get it right where it needs to go. I'm going to give it 110 percent." Babe Ruth, however, had different advice: "Throw the ball with 80 percent of your might. You will need the reserve to correct for any mistakes." Nurses need the same reserve to correct for the inevitable curve balls of life. Exercise 20–7 can help you assess your own burnout potential.

### Symptoms of Burnout

Physiological, emotional, and spiritual symptoms of burnout are identified in Figure 20–5. Physical

symptoms in the form of increased smoking, drinking or eating, skipping meals, eating compulsively on the run, and sleep disturbances are warning signals of stress. The potential burnout victim begins to feel emotionally drained, constantly tired, "like a robot," or in a constant state of hyperarousal, in which much of life seems irritating.

Conscientiousness becomes confused with the fear of losing control. It becomes increasingly difficult to delegate responsibility because others might not do a task as well. Time begins to slip away, and the nurse finds little time for replenishing the self. Nor is there time for others (e.g., family or friends). Every demand on one's time seems like an intrusion. The person is always tired and preoccupied with work. Emotional pleasures become a thing of the past.

Self needs become buried with rationalizations such as, "As soon as I get the unit staffed . . . ," "As soon as my child finishes college . . . ," "As soon as I get my degree. . . ." Despite working harder and enjoying it less, the nurse feels alone and isolated, misunderstood, and unappreciated. Repressed self-needs find maladaptive expression in overeating, overspending, snapping at family, or avoiding friends. Insomnia during the week, preoccupation with tasks, and utter exhaustion on the weekend or days off suggest a serious imbalance in lifestyle. As one person described the experience

I felt I was looking in at a party—from outside through a window. It was a little dizzying. I knew something was wrong with me but was so resentful that I pushed harder to maintain control of my actions. At work, I'd sit in meetings silently disliking everyone, thinking how bored I was, how stupid everyone sounded, how

◆ Exercise 20–7. **Burnout Assessment**

**Purpose:**  To help students understand the symptoms of burnout

**Procedure:**
Consider your life over the past year. Complete the questionnaire by answering with a 5 if the situation is a constant occurrence, 4 if it occurs most of the time, 3 if it occurs occasionally, 2 if it has occurred once or twice during the last 6 months, and 1 if it is not a problem at all. Scores ranging from 60 to 75 indicate burnout. Scores ranging from 45 to 60 indicate you are stressed and in danger of developing burnout. Scores ranging from 20 to 44 indicate a normal stress level, and scores of less than 20 suggest you are not a candidate for burnout.

1. Do you find yourself taking on other people's problems and responsibilities? _____
2. Do you feel resentful about the amount of claims on your time? _____
3. Do you find you have less time for social activities? _____
4. Have you lost your sense of humor? _____
5. Are you having trouble sleeping? _____
6. Do you find you are more impatient and less tolerant of others? _____
7. Is it difficult for you to say no? _____
8. Are the things that used to be important to you slipping away from you? _____
9. Do you feel a sense of urgency and not enough time to complete tasks? _____
10. Are you forgetting appointments, friends' birthdays? _____
11. Do you feel overwhelmed and unable to pace yourself? _____
12. Have you lost interest in sex? _____
13. Are you overeating, or have you begun to skip meals? _____
14. Is it difficult to feel enthusiastic about your work? _____
15. Do you feel it is difficult to make real contact with others? _____

Tally up your scores and compare your scores with your classmates. Nursing school is a strong breeding ground for the development of burnout (demands exceed resources). To offset the possibility of developing burnout symptoms:

1. Think about the last time you took time for yourself. If you cannot think of a time, you really need to do this exercise.
2. Identify a leisure activity that you can do during the next week to break the cycle of burnout.
3. Describe the steps you will need to take to implement the activity.
4. Identify the time period required for this activity and what other activities will need rearrangement to make it possible.
5. Describe any obstacles to implementing your activity and how you might resolve them.

**Discussion:**
1. Was it difficult for you to come up with an activity? If so, why?
2. Were you able to develop a logical way to implement your activity?
3. Were the activities chosen by others surprising or helpful to you in any way?
4. How might you be able to use this exercise in your future practice?

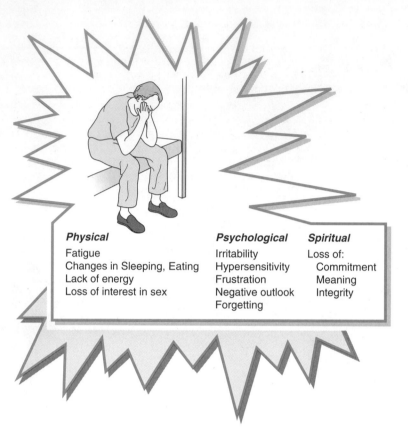

Figure 20–5. Symptoms of burnout.

**Physical**

Fatigue
Changes in Sleeping, Eating
Lack of energy
Loss of interest in sex

**Psychological**

Irritability
Hypersensitivity
Frustration
Negative outlook
Forgetting

**Spiritual**

Loss of:
　Commitment
　Meaning
　Integrity

no one was recognizing how smart I was. I felt like a robot.

(Freudenberger, 1985)

## Burnout Prevention Strategies

Burnout is contagious and can spread quickly in health care settings. Taking the following steps can help prevent burnout (Arnold, 1989).

### Awareness

The first step in burnout prevention is awareness. Deliberately reflecting on the stress in your life immediately puts boundaries on it. If you are in doubt, ask your colleagues to tell you how they experience you. Solutions become possible once the problem is defined appropriately. As you examine your stress behavior, note differences in the way you feel about important people in your life. To what extent have your life, your attitudes, and your thinking become rigid or meaningless?

Emotional awareness requires that you look at the extent to which your ego is involved in the outcome and the extent to which ego involvement is useful. Who are you trying to please, and for what reasons? Often our ego involvement gets in the way. Think about your feelings. Talk to someone who is able to offer you the support and sensitivity you need to become aware of what is going on in your life. Take into consideration what others are telling you about your behavior. A useful exercise is to imagine yourself a year from now and ask yourself how important the conflictive issue would be at that future date.

### Balance

The second step and perhaps the most important is restoring balance in your life.

*A healthy balance* among work, family, leisure, and lifelong learning enhances personal judgments, satisfaction, and productivity. Actively scheduling time for each of these activities is the only way to achieve balance. Anything else falls short of the mark. Good intentions will never cure burnout. Only deliberate actions will provide relief.

## Choice

People experiencing the burnout syndrome usually do not think they have any choice other than to keep doing what they have been doing, but *life is a series of choices and negotiations.* All human beings have choices, and the choices we make create the fabric of their lives. Refusing to delegate work because someone else cannot do it as well and not going out to dinner with friends because you have too much work to do are choices on your part. Making a different choice actually can enhance your productivity, even though this is difficult to appreciate in the throes of a burnout situation. Everyone needs emotional support to nourish the spirit.

## Detachment

The fourth step, detachment, differs from disengagement. With disengagement, there is a withdrawal of emotional energy. *Detachment* allows full emotional involvement in a task or relationship, but not to the degree that it compromises the person's quality of life, values, or needs. It means focusing on a job or project to the best of one's ability and then, at the end of the day or time designated to the project, dropping it completely. Saying to oneself that something is "sufficient for the day" is a stress management strategy that puts boundaries on life tasks.

Emotional detachment means dropping ego involvement when it interferes with balance and integrity. Nothing is so important that friends, coworkers, family, and even oneself should be sacrificed on the altar of achievement. When someone asked Mother Teresa how she was able to remain so energetic and hopeful in the midst of the suffering she encountered in Calcutta, she replied that it was because she did the best she could, realizing that it was important to do her best and not at all important to worry about the outcome. She could not control the outcome but she *could* regulate the quality of her work.

## (Altruistic) Egoism

Potential burnout victims generally put everyone and everything ahead of themselves. Their own needs are ignored or taken for granted. *Altruistic egoism* simply means paying as much attention to your own personal needs as you do to the needs of others. Although this seems obvious, many nurses consider attention to their own needs as being selfish. Nothing is further from the truth. In the long run, a balance between self needs and the needs of others enhances the quality of care one can give to others.

## Focus

People who are focused achieve their goals. Those who are not may reach a goal, but usually it takes longer and it is not as certain. *Focusing full energy* on one thing at a time and finishing one project before starting another have several benefits. First, it is more likely that you will enjoy each activity more. Your full attention will make for a better product. A powerful contributor to the development of burnout is several unfinished projects all demanding similar space in your mind.

## Goals

This seventh step is closely aligned with focus with an emphasis on outcome. *Identifying goals* that are realistic, achievable, and in line with your personal values is an excellent burnout prevention strategy. If you want to go to New York, you do not buy a ticket to California. The same is true of life. Knowing where you want to go and what it takes to get there enhances your chances. It is important to know where you do want to go with your life and to have a realistic sense of what you will find when you get there. Too often people consider only the former and are disappointed when they find it is not where they really want to be!

## Hope

People who feel burned out experience helplessness and hopelessness about ever changing their situation. The despair that accompanies emptiness and futility can be reversed by simply seeking out connections with empathetic others. Their advice and caring support, even in one encounter, can prove a powerful antidote to inner emptiness. It is important, however, to seek support from people who will work with you on developing solutions and not in commiserating with how horrible the situation is. A solution-focused, rather than problem-oriented, approach is essential to the development of hope.

### Integrity

The final step in reversing burnout is to restore your personal integrity. Burnout always leads to some loss of personal integrity in the sense that important values are ignored or devalued. When you begin to forget who you are and to become what everyone else expects of you, you are in trouble. Reclaim yourself! Burnout can be reversed by taking responsibility for yourself and doing what you feel is important. Take the risk to be all that you are as well as all you can be!

Nurses working in high-acuity settings and in chronic care facilities find professional support groups highly effective in providing needed time to reflect on their experience and in finding nurturance from others who understand (Parish et al., 1997).

## SUMMARY

Chapter 20 presents a comprehensive overview of basic concepts related to stress, coping, and crisis. Stress is defined as a physiological and psychological response to the presence of a stressor. A stressor is defined as any demand, situation, internal stimulus, or circumstance threatening a person's personal security and balance. This sense of personal security and balance is referred to as homeostasis, or dynamic equilibrium. Three theoretical models of stress are presented: stress as a stimulus, stress as a physiological response, and stress as a transaction. Factors influencing the development of a stress reaction include the nature of the stressor, the personal interpretation of its meaning, the number of previous and concurrent stressors, previous experiences with similar stressors, and the availability of support systems and personal coping abilities. Hidden stressors can be uncovered if a holistic approach to stress assessment is used.

Coping is defined as any response to external life strains that serves to prevent, avoid, or control emotional distress. People use three types of coping strategies to deal with stressful situations: change the stressful situation, change the mean-

ing of the stressor, and relax enough to take the stress in stride. Accurate assessment allows the nurse flexibility in choosing the most appropriate intervention.

Burnout is a form of stress that frequently occurs in nurses. To reduce the possibilities of burnout, nurses must develop awareness and balance, make appropriate choices, maintain focus, and allow time for self.

## REFERENCES

Abel-Boone H, Dokecki P, Smith M. (1989). Parent and health care provider communication and decision making in the intensive care nursery. Children's Health Care 18(3):133–141.

Aguilera DC. (1990). Crisis Intervention: Theory and Methodology. St. Louis, MO, Mosby Yearbook.

Arnold E. (1989). Burnout as a spiritual issue. In Carson V (ed.), Spiritual Dimensions of Nursing Practice. Philadelphia, WB Saunders.

Arnold E. (1997). The stress connection: Women and coronary heart disease. Critical Care Nursing Clinics of North America 9(4):565–575.

Arnold E, Virvan D, Kizilay P. (1998). Concepts of basic communication. In Leahy J, Kizilay P (eds.), Foundations of Nursing Practice: A Nursing Process Approach. Philadelphia, WB Saunders.

Beckingham A, Baumann A. (1990). The aging family in crisis: Assessment and decision making models. Journal of Advanced Nursing 15:782–787.

Ben-Schlomo Y, Chaturvedi N. (1992). Stress and Graves' disease. Lancet 339:427.

Benson H. (1975). The Relaxation Response. New York, Morrow.

Bluhm J. (1987). Helping families in crisis hold on. Nursing '87 45:44–46.

Cannon WB. (1914). The emergency function of the adrenal medulla in pain and the major emotions. American Journal of Physiology 33:356–372.

Caplan G. (1964). Principles of Preventive Psychiatry. New York, Basic Books.

Carson V. (1998). Spirituality. In Leahy J, Kizilay P (eds.), Foundations of Nursing Practice: A Nursing Process Approach. Philadelphia, WB Saunders.

Ceronsky C. (1983). Family/staff conferences open communication, resolve problems. Hospital Progress 64(8): 58–59.

Dantzer R. (1997). Stress and immunity: What have we learned from psychoimmunology? Acta Physiologica Scandinavica Supplementum 640:43–46.

David J. (1991). How well do nurses care for their own? Journal of Advanced Nursing 16(8):887–888.

Dossey B. (1991). Awakening the inner healer. American Journal of Nursing 91(8):31–34.

Edens J, Larkin K, Abel J. (1992). The effect of social support and physical touch on cardiovascular reactions to mental stress. Journal of Psychosomatic Research 36(4):371–381.

Emmons R. (1991). Personal strivings, daily life events and

psychological and physical well-being. Journal of Personality 59(3):453–472.

Emrich HM. (1981). The role of endorphins in neuropsychiatry. In Ban TA (ed.), Modern Problems of Pharmacopsychiatry. New York, Basal.

Epstein S, Katz L. (1992). Coping ability, stress, productive load and symptoms. Journal of Personality and Social Psychology 62(5):813–825.

Freud S. (1940). An outline of psychoanalysis. In Standard Edition, Vol. 23. London, Hogarth Press.

Freudenberger H. (1985). Women's Burnout. New York, Doubleday.

Gadzella B, Ginther D, Tomcala M, Bryant G. (1991). Differences between men and women on stress producers and coping strategies. Psychological Reports 69(2):561–562.

Gelent MD, Hochman JS. (1992). Acute myocardial infarction triggered by emotional stress. American Journal of Cardiology 69(17):1512–1513.

Goldberger L, Breznitz S. (1982). Handbook of Stress: Theoretical and Clinical Aspects. New York, Free Press.

Gray S, Diers D. (1992). The effect of staff stress on patient behavior. Archives of Psychiatric Nursing 6(1):26–34.

Greene J, Walker L. (1997). Psychosomatic problems and stress in adolescence. Pediatric Clinics of North America 44(6):1557–1572.

Hoff LS. (1989). People in Crisis: Understanding and Helping (2nd ed.). Menlo Park, CA, Addison-Wesley.

Holmes T, Rahe R. (1967). The social readjustment rating scale. Journal of Psychosomatic Research 11:213–218.

Hull MM. (1991). Hospice nurses: Caring support for caregiving families. Cancer Nursing 14(2):63–70.

Jacobson (1938). Progressive Relaxation. Chicago, University of Chicago Press.

Johnson A. (1997). Death in the PICU: Caring for the "other" families. Journal of Pediatric Nursing 12(5):273–277.

LaMontagne L, Pawlak R. (1990). Stress and coping of parents of children in a pediatric intensive care unit. Heart Lung 19(4):416–421.

Lazarus R, Folkman S. (1984). Stress, Appraisal and Coping. New York, Springer.

Leininger M. (1991). Culture Theory: Diversity and Universality (publication no. 152402). New York, National League for Nursing.

Lendrum S, Syme G. (1992). Gift of Tears: A Practical Approach to Loss and Bereavement Counseling. New York, Tavistock/Routledge.

Lepore S, Evans G, Schneider M. (1991). Dynamic role of social support in the link between chronic stress and psychological distress. Journal of Personality and Social Psychology 61(6):899–909.

Leske J. (1998). Treatment for family members in crisis after critical injury. AACN Clinical Issues 9(1):129–139.

Levin B. (1998). Grief counseling. American Journal of Nursing 98(5):69–72.

Lewandowski L. (1996). A parent has cancer: Needs and responses of children. Pediatric Nursing 22(6):518–521.

Lindemann E. (1944). Symptomatology and management of acute grief. American Journal of Psychiatry 101:141–148.

Logsdon M, Davis D. (1998). Guiding mothers of high risk infants in obtaining social support. MCN American Journal of Maternal and Child Nursing 23(4):195–199.

Luskin F, Newell K, Griffith M, et al. (1998). A review of mind-body therapies in the treatment of cardiovascular disease. Alternative Therapies Health Medicine 4(3):46–61.

Mast D, Meyer J, Urbanski A. (1987a). Relaxation techniques: A self-learning module for nurses. Unit I. Cancer Nursing 10:141–147.

Mast D, Meyer J, Urbanski A. (1987b). Relaxation techniques: A self-learning module for nurses. Unit II. Cancer Nursing 10:217–225.

McCaffery M, Beebe A. (1989). Pain: Clinical Manual for Nursing Practice. St. Louis, MO, CV Mosby.

Michalenko C. (1998) The odyssey of Marian the brave: A biopsychosocial fairy tale. Clinical Nurse Specialist 12(1):22–26.

Niaura R, Goldstein MG. (1992). Psychological factors affecting physical condition. Cardiovascular disease literature review. Psychosomatics 33(2):146–155.

Papantonio C. (1998). Alternative medicine and wound healing. Ostomy Wound Management 44(4):44–46, 48, 50.

Parish C, Bradley L, Franks V. (1997). Managing the stress of caring in ITU: A reflective practice group. British Journal of Nursing 6(20):1192–1196.

Pearlin LI, Schooler C. (1978). The structure of coping. Journal of Health and Social Behavior 19:221.

Perry S, Fishman B, Jacobsberg L. (1992). Stress and HIV infection. American Journal of Psychiatry 149(3): 416–417.

Porter-Grady T. (1998). A glimpse over the horizon: Choosing our future. Orthopedic News 17(2 Suppl):53–60.

Roozendaal B, Koolhaas J, Bohus B. (1997). The role of the central amygdala in stress and adaptation. Acta Physiologica Scandinavica Supplementum 640:51–54.

Rushton CH. (1990). Strategies for family centered care in the critical care setting. Pediatric Nursing 16(2):195–199.

Schaefer K, Peterson K. (1992). Effectiveness of coping strategies among critical care nurses. Dimensions of Critical Care Nursing 11(1):28–34.

Selye H. (1956). The Stress of Life. New York, McGraw-Hill.

Selye H. (1982). History and present status of the stress concept. In Goldberger L, Breznitz S (eds.), Handbook of Stress: Theoretical and Clinical Aspects. New York, Free Press.

Stephenson J. (1985). Death, Grief, and Mourning. New York, Free Press.

Steptoe A. (1991). Invited review. The links between stress and illness. Journal of Psychosomatic Research 35(6): 633–644.

Whetsell M, Larrabee M. (1988). Using guilt constructively in the NICU to affirm parental coping. Neonatal Network 6(4):21–27.

Wurzbach ME. (1992). Assessment and intervention for certainty and uncertainty. Nursing Forum 27(2):29–35.

# 21

# Communicating with Clients in Crisis

## Elizabeth Arnold

**OBJECTIVES**

At the end of the chapter, the student will be able to

1. Define crisis and identify its characteristics in health care
2. Identify theoretical frameworks for the study of crisis
3. Identify two types of crises
4. Define crisis intervention
5. Apply the nursing process to the care of the client in crisis
6. Describe crisis intervention applications in selected special situations

*Families come to us—the nurses—scared and seeking, at times not knowing themselves how to sort through what they fear or need most. This is often their first experience of this kind that involves a loved one.*

Kleeman, 1989

◆◆◆ Chapter 21 is designed to provide the nursing student with practical guidelines to use with clients in crisis. Crisis can occur with anyone; it does not respect age, socioeconomic, and sociocultural differences, although those with stronger economic resources and social supports potentially have an advantage in coping with crisis. People experience a crisis as traumatic and personally intrusive. Common crisis situations in health care settings include violence against others or against self, rape, sudden illness, and injury. Family members often experience a crisis state when someone close to them is dying or is critically ill. Parents of infants in the neonatal intensive care unit or of children experiencing acute illness or trauma are particularly vulnerable to experiencing the crisis state. The outcome of a crisis state can be either positive or negative with long-range effects on a person's mental health and consequent behaviors.

## BASIC CONCEPTS

### Definition

A *crisis* is defined as an unexpected and sudden turn of events or set of circumstances that requires an immediate human response (Beckingham & Baumann, 1990). It can be any event that presents a sudden obstacle to important life goals or challenges the self-concept in a critical way. The *crisis state* is characterized as overwhelming internal reaction to stressors that normal coping measures cannot address. This reaction is characterized by an overwhelming sense of extreme emotional imbalance with physical symptoms. It is time limited and pushes for resolution because it is so emotionally uncomfortable.

Webster's dictionary defines crisis as "a turning point." The Chinese word character for crisis is a combination of two symbols: danger and opportunity. Both are suitable descriptors. The danger is that the crisis state will prove so devastating that the client will not be able to function or engage with life again in a full and meaningful way. As an opportunity, a crisis state forces people to reflect on what is truly meaningful to them, and each person's response affects future impact. An adaptive response results in fresh appraisals of life's priorities and offers a second chance to make significant life changes more aligned with personal goals. Working through the crisis strengthens people's coping responses, allowing them to cope with future stressful situations more effectively. With a maladaptive resolution, people may use coping responses such as withdrawal, violence, suicide, or chemical use to ease the emotional pain of the crisis state, none of which helps a person cope better and all of which can be highly self-destructive. Nothing is learned, and future crisis is not likely to be dealt with successfully.

### Characteristics of the Crisis State

Characteristics of the crisis state are identified in Table 21–1. A crisis state is a normal human response to abnormal circumstances and is *not* a mental illness. The client needs to be reassured that a crisis state in not in itself pathological. In a crisis situation, the client experiences the overwhelming emotional pain of an actual or perceived assault on self-concept or the loss of something important that threatens to exceed a person's coping capacities. Crisis states occur when both normal and emergency coping strategies

Table 21-1. **Characteristics of the Crisis State**

| TIME LIMITED | USUALLY LAST 4 TO 6 WEEKS |
| --- | --- |
| Assault to self-concept | Real or perceived loss of something or someone essential to personal well-being. |
| Personalized experience | What creates a crisis for one person does not necessarily do so for another. |
| Inability to cope | There is no frame of reference for coping with the current crisis situation. |
| Change in normal behavior patterns | Functional behaviors appear to self and others as being uncharacteristic. |

fail to reduce internal tension or resolve the crisis. The fact that the crisis state is a personalized response to a crisis situation explains why two people experiencing the same crisis event will respond differently to it.

### Development of a Crisis State

Caplan (1964) described four steps critical to the development of a crisis state (Box 21–1). When the crisis presents itself, there is a rise in tension and a person attempts to use his or her usual problem-solving strategies to resolve it. When these coping strategies fail to reduce the tension, the person experiences escalating psychological discomfort and turns to emergency coping strategies to eliminate the crisis. Here the client may redefine the problem, use avoidance as a coping strategy, or relinquish a goal. If none of the emergency strategies work, tension continues to increase, creating major personality disorganization and a crisis state.

### Clinical Behaviors

Functional behaviors seen in clients experiencing a crisis state appear to self and others as significantly uncharacteristic of regular patterns. This abrupt change in behavior is alarming to the person experiencing a crisis state and often to significant others in the person's life. Clinical manifestations of the crisis state include feelings of extreme fatigue, helplessness, inadequacy, and anxiety (Slaikeu, 1984). Other physical symptoms can involve changes in eating habits, sleep disturbance, and feelings of "leaden paralysis." People describe tunnel vision, and they have trouble seeing beyond the problem or considering options without external feedback in the crisis state. They feel hopeless about returning to normal again.

### Human Response Sequence

Typically, people respond to a crisis state by moving through stages of shock, seen at the time of impact, followed by a period of recoil and inner turmoil as the initial shock subsides and then through an extended period of adjustment. When people are in shock, they display a wide range of behaviors, for example, laughing, crying, anger, hysteria, withdrawal, over-control. Some people describe it as a déjà vu or observer experience almost as if they are watching rather than experiencing the crisis directly. One young woman described feeling almost an out-of-body experience as she went through the funeral of her husband. She said people were amazed that she was able to cope so well but in reality she felt as though she was not really there and this was not happening to her.

During the period of *recoil*, which can last from 2 to 3 weeks, clients' behavior can appear normal, but they describe nightmares, phobic reactions, and flashbacks of the crisis event. Some people describe nonpsychotic hallucinations, and it is important to reassure them that this is a normal response to an overwhelming event.

The recoil stage is followed by a period of *adjustment* that can be either positive or negative. With a positive adjustment, a person begins to take constructive action to rebuild a shattered dream and reestablish identity. For example, Christopher Reeves, after the tragic accident that left him paralyzed, turned his energies to helping other disabled people. Negative adjustments include self-destructive coping strategies such as substance abuse, violence, or avoidance of all men, for example, by a rape victim.

## Theoretical Frameworks

Caplan's (1964) model of preventive psychiatry still forms the basis for much of the current thinking about crisis and crisis intervention (see Table 21–1). According to Caplan, there are many possibilities for personal growth in a crisis situation. The outcome, as either a growth or limiting life experience, depends on the person's interpretation of the crisis within his or her life, perception of coping ability, and the quality of

---

> ◆ **Box 21–1. Developmental Phases in a Crisis Situation**
>
> 1. There is a rise in tension and use of customary problem-solving strategies.
> 2. Coping strategies are insufficient to resolve the crisis; there is an increase in discomfort.
> 3. Emergency coping strategies are used: the problem is redefined and avoided, or goals are relinquished.
> 4. If emergency coping strategies do not work, tension increases, creating major personality disorganization.

human support the person receives to resolve the crisis. Caplan applied concepts of primary, secondary, and tertiary prevention to crisis intervention and viewed the nurse as a key figure in intervention.

Aguilera (1997) and Messick (1978–1990) developed a nursing crisis intervention model that acknowledges the reciprocal nature of environment and person in the development of the crisis state (Fig. 21–1). These theorists believe that a crisis occurs within the larger context of a person's normal life situation either because of a distorted perception of a situation or because the client lacks the resources to cope successfully with it. The client's resources (beliefs or attitudes) and external (environmental) supports, referred to as balancing factors, contribute to the development and resolution of a crisis state. Exercise 21–1 provides practice using Aguilera and Messick's model.

## Types of Crises
### Situational Crises

Most crises in health care situations can be classified as situational. A situational crisis represents an external event or environmental influence perceived as harmful to the organism with a charac-

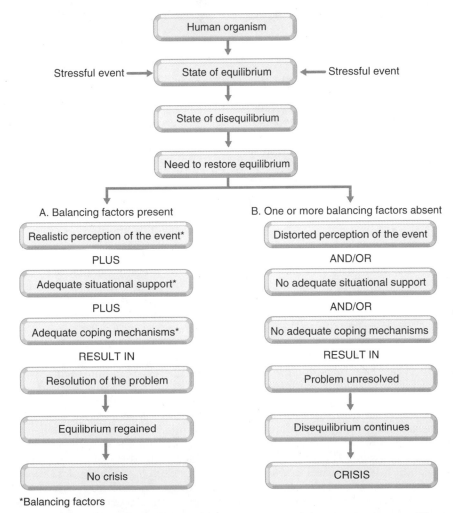

Figure 21–1. Crisis model for intervention. (From Aguilera D [1997]. Crisis Intervention: Theory and Methodology [7th ed.]. St. Louis, Mosby–Year Book, p. 32. Used with permission.)

---

◆ **Exercise 21-1. Understanding the Nature of Crisis**

**Purpose:** To help you understand the elements in the development of a crisis situation. Aguilera's (1997) paradigm of the role of balancing factors is important in assessing and planning communication strategies in crisis situations.

**Procedure:**

1. Describe a crisis you experienced in your life. There are no right or wrong definitions of a crisis, and it does not matter whether the crisis would be considered a crisis in someone else's life.
2. Identify how the crisis changed your roles, routines, relationships, and assumptions about yourself.
3. Apply Aguilera's model to the situation you are describing. Identify balancing factors and other relevant data as they apply to your circumstances.
4. Identify the strategies you used to cope with the crisis.
5. Describe the ways in which your personal crisis strengthened or weakened your self-concept and increased your options and your understanding of life.

---

teristic sudden onset. The event can be physiological, emotional, environmental, or spiritual. Loss of a limb, an automobile accident, rape, diagnosis of cancer, natural disasters, the death of a loved one, loss of a job, and even a job promotion or move to a new area are examples of actual and potential situational crises. In contrast to developmental crises, situational life crises strike randomly and can affect large numbers of people simultaneously.

## Developmental Crises

Developmental crises occur as an internal process that arises in connection with maturational changes. Erikson's (1982) theory of developmental psychosocial crises provides a basis for understanding the role of psychosocial crises at every life stage. A developmental view of crisis takes into consideration interpersonal challenges and stressors that occur at transitional crisis points in the life cycle. Examples of developmental crisis events include conflicts with teachers or parents, unwanted pregnancy, going away to college, marriage, a first job, and caring for aging parents (Slaikeu, 1984). Each of these events calls for interpersonal resources or personal coping strengths a person may not have learned, thus creating a maturational crisis for that person.

A situational crisis may be superimposed on a developmental crisis. For example, a woman

experiencing breast cancer who is about to get married or the loss of a spouse through divorce or death occurring in midlife can be particularly traumatic.

## Crisis Intervention

**Crisis intervention** is defined as "the systematic application of problem-solving techniques, based on crisis theory, designed to help the client move through the crisis process as swiftly and as painlessly as possible and thereby achieve at least the same level of psychological comfort as he or she experienced before the crisis" (Kus, 1985). Although the literature contains a wealth of information on crisis intervention strategies, nursing actions must be adapted to fit each client's individual situation. Differences among clients require the nurse to exercise critical thinking and judgment to make interventions specific to client needs. Crisis intervention treatment strategies compel nurses to examine their personal attitudes and biases toward behaviors common to the crisis state such as denial, hostility, and other forms of acting-out behaviors so that they can understand and respond constructively to clients.

The goal of crisis intervention is to restore individuals to their precrisis state functional level. Treatment strategies are almost exclusively focused on immediate problem solving and strengthening of personal resources of clients and their families for the explicit purpose of reducing the tension associated with the crisis state to a workable level. Nurses are well equipped to help clients and their families identify and treat situations before they escalate into crisis. For example, informal teaching of parenting skills can help prevent child abuse.

## APPLICATIONS
### Safety Issues

The first assessment in any crisis situation is to determine the severity of the crisis and the client's current danger potential. In a state of crisis, people do things they ordinarily would not consider, and the nurse needs to take steps to safeguard these individuals and those around them. Suicide and violence are psychiatric emergencies that present regularly in the emergency departments. If the person in crisis is violent or physically injured, the crisis is treated as a medical emergency first and then as a psychiatric emergency.

The nurse needs to evaluate clients' mental status before attempting crisis intervention. For example, is the client capable at this time of participating in a treatment process? Clients who are psychotic, under the influence of drugs, organically impaired, or temporarily out of control cannot provide a logical, sequential description of their problem, even with the nurse's help. They require immediate triage to stabilize their condition before the nurse conducts an in-depth assessment interview. Table 21–2 provides guidelines for communicating with a client who is unable to cooperate because of an organically related health crisis. In the meantime, a family member or the person accompanying the client can provide assessment data related to the current crisis state (e.g., documenting changes in behavior, ingestion of drugs, medical history).

### Intervention

In the early stages of crisis, *people need to be listened to* rather than to be given much information (Artean & Williams, 1998). It is a period of enormous emotional turmoil, and people can absorb very little compared with their usual capabilities. The nurse acts as advocate, resource, partner, and guide in the crisis intervention, with a strong focus on helping clients mobilize personal resources and use support resources effectively (Hoff, 1991).

**Table 21–2. Guidelines for Choosing Intervention with Different Stages of Aggressive Behavior in the Emergency Department**

| STAGE | CLIENT BEHAVIOR | NURSE ACTIONS |
|---|---|---|
| 1. Environmental trigger | Stress response | Encourage ventilation: avoid challenge, speak calmly, clearly, offer alternative. |
| 2. Escalation period | Movement toward loss of control | Take control: maintain safe distance, acknowledge behavior, medicate if appropriate, remove to quiet area, "show force" if necessary. |
| 3. Crisis period | Emotional/physical discharge | Apply external control: implement emergency protocol, initiate confinement, give focused intensive care. |
| 4. Recovery | Cool down | Reassure: support, no retaliation; encourage to discuss behavior and alternatives; release when in control; assess reaction to release; assist in reentry toward environment; conduct sessions for staff to process all areas of incident. |
| 5. Postcrisis and letdown | Reconciliatory | Demonstrate acceptance while continuing clarification of unit standards and expectations. |

From Steele RL. (1993). Staff attitudes toward seclusion and restraint: Anything new? Perspectives in Psychiatric Care 29(3):28, 1993. Reprinted with the permission of Nursecom, Inc.

People in crisis are very vulnerable. They need to feel that the nurse cares about them and wants to understand their situation. As the nurse, you are their life line for the moment, and they need to see from your body language, eye contact, and the tone of your voice as well as your words that you are fully present to them. It is helpful for the nurse to say, "I think you really did the right thing by coming here" as an opener to demonstrate the partnering in resolving difficult issues. Using a reflective listening response following the client's description of the crisis, such as "it sounds as if you are feeling very sad (angry, lonely) right now," can signal empathy and the human communication link of nurse with client and problem that is so essential in crisis intervention.

Perfetti (1982) proposed a three-step process model of intervention designed to mobilize clients and their families in emergency situations.

## 1. Engaging the Client

The first step in the process of crisis intervention is engaging the client. As with other types of client interviews, the setting should be quiet and conducive to holding a private conversation. Clients in crisis look to the professional to structure the interaction. Here are some guidelines for engaging the client in a crisis state.

- Let clients tell you what they are experiencing. Clients experiencing a crisis need to tell their story in their own words at their own pace. The nurse may use directed questions when needed to keep the client focused on the crisis story but otherwise should not interrupt.
- Respond to clients in brief, concise sentences, and do not explain a lot initially.
- Be specific in asking short questions. Do not interject your opinion, and do not ask irrelevant questions that are nice but not necessary to know.
- Pace the discussion. Follow clients' description; do not let them get ahead of you. Ask for clarification to understand their perspective, but do not anticipate the story. Periodically summarize content so that both parties arrive at the same place simultaneously.
- Present a calm, controlled presence (Kleeman, 1989). Offer realistic support while respecting clients' need to understand the meaning of the crisis in their own way and within their own time frame.
- Reinforce client strengths as you observe them or as clients identify them. Recalling past successes can offer hope to clients that the current crisis also is resolvable.

## 2. Exploring the Problem

The second step in the crisis intervention process involves helping the client explore the crisis problem in more depth. The nurse can help the client focus on the immediate situation by asking directly, "Can you tell me what happened that brought you here?" Letting the client tell his or her story with the nurse directing the conversation by asking (1) for general data, (2) followed by a request for more specific details, and (3) finally for the feelings associated with the immediate crisis can be helpful in defusing client anxiety.

Although telling the story is critical, the nurse needs to help the client stay with the crisis topic and dwell on its meaning. A chronological approach to the story of the crisis provides order and structure to the event in both the client and nurse's mind. Refocus when the client changes the subject, introduces irrelevant material, or seems to be going around in circles. This can be accomplished tactfully by asking the client whether there is a relationship between the new material and the crisis situation, by making an appropriate connection between the content offered and the original stated problem, or by making a comment about the primary problem. Sample statements might include one of the following:

"We need to find out a little more about your immediate situation."

"I think we can help you best if we can understand what led up to this crisis and what its impact is on your life right now."

"How has this crisis (name it) affected your family life, friendships, and physical health?"

The nurse needs to see the crisis through the client's eyes. Because the client's perception of the crisis event is critical to its understanding, inquiry about the crisis event should focus on the client's own words concerning the event, including who was involved, what happened, and when it happened. It is appropriate to inquire how the client is feeling at the present time and to say directly, "This must be devastating for you."

Listen for both facts and feelings, and use reflective listening responses to develop a complete picture of the crisis situation. When either facts or feelings are missing, attempt to bring the missing component into the conversation; for example, "I'm clear that you feel responsible for the baby falling down the stairs, but you say your husband was in the same area. What was he doing when the accident happened?"

Careful inquiry into the feelings of significant others about the meaning of a crisis situation can provide further data. For example, the nurse might ask the client, "How do you see what has happened affecting your present relationships?" "In what ways do you think this will affect your future?" Obviously, the nurse adapts the type of question and how it is asked to each individual situation.

• Inquiring About History

Past coping experiences can be useful data in understanding the current situation. For some clients, living in the crisis mode is a way of life, and the nursing interventions would be different than for someone experiencing a critical life event for the first time. A question the nurse might ask is, "Has anything like this happened in the past?" Previous suicide attempts, drug use, or major psychiatric illness are critical data. Family members can verify known facts and add new information about changes in behavior.

Review of personal family history helps the nurse understand seemingly illogical crisis behavior. For example, Joe was recently divorced. His mother had stomach cancer 2 years ago, and his sister was recently diagnosed with breast cancer. His youngest child will start college in the fall. Although he has handled all of these crises without undue stress, he falls apart when his father is admitted to the coronary unit despite his father having a good prognosis. It is just one stressor too many.

How people have handled stress in the past is important information. People who have demonstrated resiliency and creativity in other aspects of their lives are more likely to weather a crisis satisfactorily, whereas those with few internal resources or social supports have more trouble. The nurse should ask about tension-reducing strategies the client has used in the past (e.g., aerobics, bible study, or calling a friend). Questions the nurse can ask include "What do you usually do when you have a problem?" or "To whom do you turn when you have a difficult problem?" If the client seems immobilized and unable to give an answer about usual coping strategies, the nurse can offer prompts such as, "Some people talk to their friends, bang walls, pray, go to a bar. . . ." Usually with verbal encouragement, a person will identify characteristic coping mechanisms that can be used with the current coping state.

• Assessing Personal Strengths

Crisis intervention is a therapeutic process of helping individuals find adaptive solutions to short-term problems that are causing them significant stress. Often the answers lie within, and coping strategies are already present; they simply need recognition and activation. In a time of crisis, there is a tendency for both nurse and client to focus on what is wrong. It is just as important for the nurse to develop information about what aspects of a person's life are working well as it is to focus on those that are not (Aguilera, 1997). Having a job, financial resources, knowledge, and experience with accessing health care services are important assets in crisis situations (Exercise 21–2). Such strengths can enhance crisis resolution.

• Recognize Concurrent Stressors

Factors in the environment, such as availability of resources and other life responsibilities, legal charges, marital problems, and financial concerns, can intensify a crisis for individuals and their families. Consider the situation of a mother with a 2-year-old recently diagnosed with leukemia. She lives 75 miles from the nearest hospital, and her other four children range in age from 4 to 10 years. Balancing her sick child's needs with those of other family members creates additional stress in the current crisis situation.

• Identify Enabling Factors

Positive social supports and available community resources act as a buffer to the intensity of a crisis state. A healthy, supportive family or a good friend is without peer in the resolution of almost any crisis. Friends and support groups

---

◆ Exercise 21-2. **Personal Support Systems**

**Purpose:** To help you appreciate the breadth and importance of personal support systems in stressful situations

**Procedure:**
All of us have support systems we can use in times of stress, such as church, friends, family, coworkers, clubs, and recreational groups.

1. Identify a support person or system you could or do use in times of stress.
2. What does this personal support person do for you (e.g., listen without judgment; provide honest, objective feedback; challenge you to think; broaden your perspective; give unconditional support; share your perceptions)? List everything you can think of.
3. What factors go into choosing your personal support system (e.g., availability, expertise, perception of support), and which is the most important factor?
4. How did you develop your personal support system?

**Discussion:**

1. What types of support systems were most commonly used by class or group members?
2. What were the most common reasons for selecting a support person or system?
3. After doing this exercise, what strategies would you advise for enlarging a personal support system?
4. What applications do you see in this exercise for your nursing practice?

---

provide practical advice and reaffirm a person's worth during the period of personal questioning that accompanies a crisis. The nurse needs to know what family and social support systems the client has available. Questions the nurse can ask about family and social supports are presented in Box 21-2.

Neighborhood and agency resources can provide the client with needed supports. An important piece of information is whether or not the client is willing to use outside resources, and if so, which ones. For example, it may not be a lack of knowledge that prevents Rose from seeking welfare as a way of stabilizing her financial situation but rather her feelings about welfare. If Rose considers being on welfare as shameful, it is unlikely she will choose it as a viable option.

• Finding the Central Focus

As clients explore their situation in depth with an outside person, they begin to put boundaries on it and to rethink its meaning from a broader perspective. Here the nurse would

*Help the client identify critical elements of the problem.* Breaking down issues of concern into

> ◆ Box 21-2. Questions About Family Support
>
> "Does the client have close family ties?"
>
> "Does the client have close friends?"
>
> "Is the client a member in a social organization (e.g., church, social club)?"
>
> "Who currently is the most important person in the client's life?"
>
> "What is the impact of the crisis event on the client's social relationships (e.g., spouse, children, friends)?"
>
> "Who in the social network can be approached to help the client work through the crisis?"
>
> "Who in the client's network might hinder successful crisis resolution?"
>
> ---
>
> From Slaikeu K. (1984). Crisis Intervention: A Handbook for Practice and Research. Boston, Allyn & Bacon, pp. 130–132. Used with permission.

smaller elements makes the possibility of developing a realistic solution more workable.

*Identify central themes* in the client's story such as powerlessness, shame, and hopelessness to provide a focus for intervention. A useful focusing strategy is to help the client attach feelings to specific events by linking the precipitating event with the observed client response; for example, "Because you think your son is using drugs [precipitating event], you feel helpless and confused [client emotional response], and it seems you don't know what to do next [client behavioral reaction]."

*Provide truth in information.* Being truthful about the circumstances and letting clients know as much as possible about progress, treatment, and consequences of choosing different alternatives allows clients to make informed decisions and reduces the heightened anxiety associated with a crisis situation. Clients appreciate this and often give information they might otherwise not offer.

*Use simple words and repeat them.* The words the nurse uses are important because clients are likely to misinterpret them in a crisis state. Critical elements should be given slowly and repeated at intervals. Including significant others in the discussion helps by giving clients a resource who can confirm or correct what was heard. Sufficient time should be allowed for both processing and asking questions.

*Link crisis content with direct emotional response.* People do not always link the event to specific feelings they are experiencing as emotional responses to a crisis. In the following clinical example, notice the difference when the nurse listens and responds to both the content (experience and thoughts) and the latent feelings in the message. Although all of the responses are appropriate, the last one provides the most complete response.

### ◆ Case Example

**Client:** It's my wife—she's dying. I'm afraid to go in there and see her. I can't act cheerful, and it won't do her any good to see me upset.
**Nurse** (responding to the content of the statement): You don't want your wife to see you're upset because she's dying?
**Nurse** (responding to the speaker's feelings): You're worried that you can't disguise your feelings of sadness?
**Nurse** (responding to the content and feelings expressed by the speaker): You're afraid of getting upset in front of your wife and unsettling her?

*Normalize feelings.* Often clients in crisis feel that their emotional reactions to a situation are abnormal because they feel strange and unwelcome. It is important to point out to the client that a wide array of feelings is quite normal in crisis situations and to suggest common feelings that should be present when they are not. For example, to a person relating a rape incident without expressing any feeling about it, the nurse might say, "You must feel so violated and angry that this happened to you." Should the client respond by saying, "I feel numb," the nurse can assure the client that this "shutdown" of feelings is a common reaction in crisis situations. Even if the client does not respond immediately, linking the crisis event with the feelings about it helps the person in crisis recognize difficult feelings as related to a stressful event. Although it may seem obvious to the nurse, the client may be unaware of the connection. Legitimizing feelings of rage and betrayal helps the victim make meaning of a situation that is perplexing because the thoughts and feelings do not fit together.

*Help the client clarify distortions.* Distinguishing real from unrealistic fears helps clients put a crisis situation in perspective and forces them to look at what can be changed in a situation versus what cannot. For example, the mother of a premature or deformed child often blames herself for a number of reasons: she smoked; she did not really want this baby so God is punishing her; she should not have lifted anything when she was pregnant; and so forth. The nurse can help provide a more objective perspective by gently challenging the validity of her assumptions and providing accurate information about the causes of fetal abnormalities.

### 3. Developing Alternatives

Having options is key to the resolution of a crisis state. Crisis intervention is action oriented and goal directed toward the immediate restoration of an individual to a precrisis functional state. Finding viable solutions helps bring closure to the crisis. Problems not related to the crisis need to handled later. Using the problem-solving strategies described in Chapter 4, the nurse can help the client identify a specific plan of action to cope with the crisis with the following modifications.

- Give the client as much control as possible in developing alternatives. Obviously, the nurse must take control when the client presents a danger to self or others, but when this is not the case, the locus of control should remain with the client to whatever extent possible. Usually clients in crisis feel powerless and need to feel as though they have more control of their lives. Allowing choices encourages clients to take charge of their actions and to take responsibility for the consequences of their choices.

- Examine potential consequences. Helping a client examine the consequences of proposed solutions and breaking tasks to accomplish goals into small, achievable parts empowers clients. Proposed solutions should fit both the problem and the resources of the client. Part of the solution process includes discussing the consequences of one action versus another, for example, "What would happen if you choose this course of action as compared to . . . ?" "What is the worst that could happen if you decided to . . . ?" Using common sense and knowledge of human behavior as a guide for developing solutions, the nurse may provide some alternative actions the client has not yet considered.

- Enlarge perspective. When the facts of a crisis event are overwhelming and cannot be changed, it still is possible to recast their meaning in supportive ways. For example, the loss of an infant at childbirth is undoubtedly one of life's greatest crises. The reality of the child's death cannot be reversed, but the nurse can help the parents integrate the tragic event into their lives in a meaningful way by dressing the child in an infant shirt and diaper, wrapping it in a blanket, and encouraging the family to see the child. Even if the infant is macerated or deformed, the external wrappings can emphasize the normal aspects of the infant, and the nurse through his or her words can emphasize the positive features. Arranging for baptism or religious support acknowledges the existence of the child and is a major source of comfort to many parents.

- Establish follow-up mechanisms. Although the crisis state may have resolved, many clients will need follow-up for problems that cannot be resolved with crisis intervention. The nurse can facilitate the referral process by sharing information and giving the client enough information to follow through. Exercise 21–3 provides an opportunity to practice crisis intervention skills.

## Applications to Specific Situations

### Families in Crisis

A crisis can be a family event experienced as a collective direct hit when disaster strikes or as a more individualized response to the illness or injury of a family member. Bluhm (1987) suggested an image of a family in crisis as "a group of people standing together, with arms interlocked. What happens if one family member becomes seriously ill and can no longer stand? The other family members will attempt to carry their loved one, each person shifting his weight to accommodate the additional burden" (p. 44).

A family's perception of a client's critical illness or injury is a subjective one, colored by the client's role in the family as well as by previous coping, past experience, current support systems, and family traditions (Reeder, 1991). Emotional symptoms of a family in crisis include anxiety, anger, shock, denial, guilt, grief, and hopelessness. These feelings are difficult for most people to put into words for fear of adding to the crisis. For example, how do you tell someone you are angry with him because he is dying? How do you tell your family you are afraid you will never walk again when your family does not want to hear such news? Sample nursing diagnoses are presented in Box 21–3.

The nurse needs to remember that even the most functional family system falters in the face of a critical illness or injury (Leske & Heidrich, 1996). Nurses can help clients voice their concerns within the safety of the nurse–client relationship and can assist family members to develop meaningful ways to communicate effectively with their loved one (Leske, 1998).

Explanations should be kept simple and to the point. Diagrams, simulations, and pictures can sometimes help families understand what is hap-

◆ **Exercise 21–3. Interacting in Crisis Situations**

**Purpose:**  To give you experience in using the three-stage model of crisis intervention

**Directions:**

1. Break up into groups of three. One student should take the role of the client and one the role of the nurse; the third functions as observer.
2. Using the following role-play or others that may represent your current experience, act out your respective parts. The observer uses the counselor rating sheet to provide feedback to the nurse.

**Role-Play:**

Julie is a 23-year-old woman who has been married for 3 years. Her husband, Jack, is 25 and a law student. They were married when she was a senior in college. Although she graduated with a degree in social sciences, she has been unable to find work in her chosen field. As a result, she has been working full time as a secretary. Her husband worked part time as a security guard and attended school full time. During their second year of marriage, Julie unexpectedly became pregnant. Jack had to quit school to support her during her last trimester. He continued to do so 2 months after the baby was born.

Eventually, Jack was able to return to school and Julie to work. Although the baby was a burden, they loved her and were managing. When Julie went back to work, they found a reliable babysitter who lived two doors away. Four days ago she received a call from the hospital to meet with a staff doctor with her husband. When they arrived at the hospital, they were informed by the doctor that their daughter had died at the babysitter's of sudden infant death syndrome.

Both Jack and Julie's parents came to stay with them until the baby's burial. They buried her yesterday morning, and the relatives left in the afternoon. This morning, after Jack left for work and the baby's feeding time came, Julie found herself preparing the baby's formula. She became overcome with feeling and began to cry. She also began feeling angry at her husband and family. She also felt guilty for feeling that way. She says she feels as though she is "going crazy." She can't stop thinking about the baby and has constant vivid images of her whenever she is alone. Julie is flooded with a host of emotions she is unable to identify or control.

To give helpful feedback to the counselor, rate his or her performance with a number from 1 (least effective) to 5 (most effective).

**Rating Scale:**

1. Did the counselor engage the client?    5 4 3 2 1
2. Did the counselor accurately reflect the client's feeling?    5 4 3 2 1
3. Did the client appear to share sensitive emotional information with the counselor?    5 4 3 2 1
4. Did the counselor communicate openness and a nonjudgmental attitude toward the client?    5 4 3 2 1
5. Did the counselor use brief, concise sentences?    5 4 3 2 1
6. Did the counselor use the compound sentence when connecting emotional reactions to stressors?    5 4 3 2 1
7. Did the client and counselor establish a mutually understood definition of the problem?    5 4 3 2 1
8. Did the counselor allow the client to do most of the talking and explaining?    5 4 3 2 1
9. Was the client able to arrive at useful alternatives as a result of the interview?    5 4 3 2 1

*Exercise continued on following page*

◆ Exercise 21–3. **Interacting in Crisis Situations** *Continued*

10. Did the counselor and client plan actions the client could begin using right away?    5 4 3 2 1

**Discussion:**

1. What did you learn from doing this exercise?
2. What would you want to do differently as a result of this exercise when communicating with the client in crisis?
3. What was the effect of using the three-stage model of crisis intervention as a way of organizing your approach to the crisis situation?

Rating scale developed by Perfetti T. (1982). Training Manual for Crisis Counselors. Bethesda, MD, Montgomery County Crisis Center. Used with permission.

pening better than words alone. If the client is capable of understanding, all explanations given to the family should also be given to the client. In a research study of family needs and coping strategies during illness crisis, family members identified the need to know the client's prognosis as being most important. Other needs were for information about the client, being able to stay with the patient, close emotional support, and periodic assurance from the nurse (Twibell, 1998).

Observation of the family's physical state is important. In the face of severe shock, it may not be possible to find out much about the current crisis until the major players have had some rest. Family members may need the nurse's encouragement to take time out and to return for more information. Written information about unit rules may be read at home and used as an

ongoing reference. The family should be given the telephone number of a primary caregiver, because a simple telephone call can relieve hours of potential worry.

### Giving Information

Identifying a primary health care contact is important, because families often feel confused about what they hear, particularly if they receive incomplete or contradictory information. They imagine the worst possible scenario or develop an internal image that has little to do with reality. Similarly, the nurse can advise families to designate one contact person within the family to give information to outsiders and family friends. This intervention helps reinforce the family as the primary unit for information and reduces the possibility of unnecessary or unauthorized calls to the unit. It reduces the chance of misinterpretation because the more people involved in the information loop, the greater is the possibility of misinformation in time of crisis.

Informing the family of a negative change in their loved one's condition should be introduced in incremental stages and in everyday language the client and family can understand. Many decisions the family needs to make—related to surgery, placement of the family member in an alternative treatment center, use or discontinuance of extraordinary measures, and organ donation—have long-term emotional ramifications. It is important for the nurse to support the family's right to make the decision and to offer family members

---

◆ Box 21–3. Sample Nursing Diagnoses for Clients in Crisis

Grieving related to perinatal loss as evidenced by inability to sleep and constant crying

Ineffective coping related to job loss as evidenced by suicide attempt

Anxiety related to rape as evidenced by fear, emotional disorganization, and restlessness

Ineffective family coping related to son's accident, as evidenced by inability to work and expressed desire to dissolve marriage

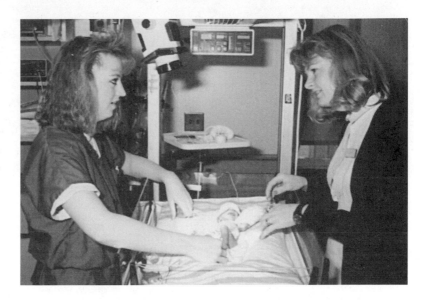

Careful coordination of the information to be shared with family members reduces confusion and allays anxiety in crisis situations. (Courtesy University of Maryland School of Nursing)

honest and compassionate information so that they can make an informed decision. The client's physical and mental condition should be presented in a matter-of-fact, constructive manner with neither a pessimistic or overly optimistic picture. Consequences of using one alternative versus another can be helpful as the nurse gently leads involved family members in developing their own sense of the truth and the best way to proceed. Communication strategies the nurse can use to help families in crisis are presented in Box 21–4.

### Violence

*Violence* is a special form of crisis in that it involves the use of physical force and demands an immediate response for the client's protection as well as that of others in the client's path (Cahill et al., 1991). It is a psychosocial emergency that can be just as critical as a life-threatening medical emergency. Violence is associated with power and control; usually the perpetrator feels powerless or out of control and the behavior is a maladaptive attempt to restore emotional balance.

More often than not, the cause of violent behavior is organic, and the nurse should assume there is an organic component until otherwise indicated. Drugs and alcohol often are implicated. The violent client must be stabilized immediately for the protection of self and others

(Puskar & Obus, 1989). Box 21–5 presents characteristic indicators of increasing tension leading to violence. A recent history of violence, childhood abuse, history of substance abuse, mental retardation, problems with impulse control, and psychosis, particularly when accompanied by command hallucinations, are common contributing factors.

Treatment of violent clients consists of providing a safe, nonstimulating environment. The client should be checked thoroughly for potential weapons and physically disarmed, if necessary. Obviously, prevention of violent behavior is best, and the nurse can use simple strategies such as calling the client by name, using a low, calm tone of voice or a show of force to help the client defuse tension. Encouraging the client to physically walk and to vent emotions verbally can be helpful. Sometimes the environment is overstimulating, and the client calms down if taken to an area that provides less sensory input. Box 21–6 presents some useful guidelines for communicating with a potentially violent client.

### Suicide

Suicide is the ultimate crisis because there can be no return to function. People turn to suicide as an option when they believe there are no other alternatives. It is a myth that people who talk about harming themselves are at less risk. Every

## ◆ Box 21–4. Interventions for Initial Family Responses to Crises

| | |
|---|---|
| Anxiety, shock, fright | Give information that is brief, concise, explicit, and concrete. |
| | Repeat information and frequently reinforce; encourage families to record important facts in writing. |
| | Ascertain comprehension by asking family to repeat back to you what information they have been given. |
| | Provide for and encourage or allow ventilation of feelings, even if they are extreme. |
| | Maintain constant, nonanxious presence in the face of a highly anxious family. |
| | Inform family as to the potential range of behaviors and feelings that are within the "norm" for crisis. |
| | Maximize control within hospital environment, as possible. |
| Denial | Identify what purpose denial is serving for family (e.g., is it buying them "psychological time" for future coping and mobilization of resources?) |
| | Evaluate appropriateness of use of denial in terms of time; denial becomes inappropriate when it inhibits the family from taking necessary actions or when it is impinging on the course of treatment. |
| | Do not actively support denial but neither dash hopes for the future (e.g., "It must be very difficult for you to believe your son is nonresponsive and in a trauma unit"). |
| | If denial is prolonged and dysfunctional, more direct and specific factual representation may be essential. |
| Anger, hostility, distrust | Allow for ventilation of angry feelings, clarifying what thoughts, fears, and beliefs are behind the anger; let them know it's okay to be angry. |
| | Do not personalize family's expressions of these strong emotions. |
| | Institute family control within the hospital environment when possible (e.g., arrange for set times and set person to give them information in reference to the patient and answer their questions). |
| | Remain available to families during their venting of these emotions. |
| | Ask families how they can take the energy in their anger and put it to positive use for themselves, for the patient, for the situation. |
| Remorse and guilt | Do not try to "rationalize away" guilt for families. |
| | Listen, support their expression of feeling and verbalizations (e.g., "I can understand how or why you might feel that way; however, . . ."). |
| | Follow the "howevers" with careful, reality-oriented statements or questions (e.g., "None of us can truly control another's behavior"; "Kids make their own choices despite what parents think and want"; "How successful were you when you tried to control _____'s behavior with that before?"; "So many things have happened for which there are no absolute answers"). |
| Grief and depression | Acknowledge family's grief and depression. |
| | Encourage them to be precise about what it is they are grieving and depressed about; give grief and depression a context. |
| | Allow the family appropriate time for grief. |
| | Recognize that this is an essential step for future adaptation; do not try to rush the grief process. |
| | Remain sensitive to your own unfinished business and, hence, comfort or discomfort with family's grieving and depression. |

---

◆ Box 21-4. Interventions for Initial Family Responses to Crises *Continued*

| Hope | Clarify with families their hopes, individually and with one another. |
|---|---|
| | Clarify with families their worst fears in reference to the situation: are the hopes/fears congruent? Realistic? Unrealistic? |
| | Support realistic hope. |
| | Offer gentle factual information to reframe unrealistic hope (e.g., "With the information you have or the observations you have made, do you think that is still possible?"). |
| | Assist families in reframing unrealistic hope in some other fashion (e.g., "What do you think others will have learned from _____ if he doesn't make it?" "How do you think _____ would like for you to remember him/her?"). |

Adapted from Kleeman K. (1989). Families in crisis due to multiple trauma. *Critical Care Nursing Clinics of North America* 1(1):25. Used with permission.

---

suicidal statement, however indirect, should be taken seriously. Even in clients who have indicated that they are "just kidding," the fact that they have verbalized the threat places them at greater risk. Verbal indicators of potential suicide include statements such as "I don't think I can go on without . . . ," "I sometimes wish I wasn't here," or "People would be better off without me." Less direct indicators are "I don't see anything good in my life." Any of these statements requires further clarification such as "You say you can't go on any longer. Can you tell me more about what you mean?"

Behavioral indicators include giving away possessions, apologizing for previous behavior, writing letters to significant people, more intense sharing of personal data, and frequent accidents. Irrational statements and command hallucinations, abuse of drugs or alcohol, previous suicide gestures, and verbal threats are always matters of concern as is a sudden mood change from vegetative expressions of depression to significantly more energy. The client who verbalizes or behaviorally demonstrates "a weight being lifted off the shoulders" should be watched carefully.

Clients will usually admit to feelings of suicide if they are having them. Having a plan, especially one that could be implemented, no support system, and distorted feelings or thoughts about what the suicide attempt would accomplish increase the risk of suicide (Slaikeu, 1984). The nurse should ask the following questions:

- Are you thinking of hurting yourself?
- Do you have a plan?
- What do you hope to accomplish with the suicide attempt?
- Have you thought about when you might do this?
- What is your support system like? Who are you able to turn to when you are in trouble?

When any combination of these factors is

◆ Box 21-5. Indicators of Potential Violence

| Behavioral Categories | Suggested Indicators |
|---|---|
| Mental status | Confused |
| | Paranoid ideation |
| | Evidence of drug involvement |
| | Organic impairment |
| Motor behavior | Agitated |
| | Pacing |
| Speech patterns | Rapid |
| | Incoherent |
| | Menacing tones |
| | Verbal threats |
| Affect | Belligerent |
| | Labile |

### Box 21–6. Don'ts and Dos in Dealing with the Nonorganically Impaired Violent Client

Don't overlook your feeling that your client is growing hostile and showing inappropriate anger.

Document your observations (even though your client has not behaved in an overtly dangerous way), and share your feelings and suspicions with the staff and the nursing administration.

Request medication as needed (medication prescribed early enough and in adequate doses can help prevent violence).

Review your client's history, searching purposefully for signs of alcoholism, drug addiction, reaction to a change of medication, or a metabolic or emotional disturbance.

Don't undervalue what others (family or staff) tell you about your client's behavior in the belief that he will be different with you or that you can handle it.

Use what the family and other staff members already know about the client. This information is significant, especially information about previous violence, about what is apt to provoke the client, and how the client behaves when provoked.

Don't continue with a treatment or interview if a client is obviously growing more and more agitated. Do not touch or move toward the client. The client may misinterpret your gesture and react with physical aggression.

Ask the client why he or she is angry or agitated and what's making him or her act this way. Also ask the client how he or she handles such feelings ordinarily and what others can do to help him or her. You want the client to know that his or her feelings and point of view are being respected so he or she will feel less powerless, less victimized. Be sure the client understands that violence will not be tolerated.

Don't isolate yourself with a client who has a record of or potential for violence. Don't corner yourself in a setting without a clear exit. (Elevators may prove particularly troublesome because you have no instant exit.)

Put this client in a room near the nurses' station, not at the end of a long, relatively unprotected corridor. Keep the door open when working with this client and face the client (or align yourself literally and figuratively beside him or her), rather than turn your back.

Have a security officer or male aide within immediate call if you suspect violence is imminent.

Study the contents of the client's room carefully, with an eye to what the client could use to harm himself or one of the staff.

Don't disturb this client (with treatments or taking vital signs) any more than is necessary. The client may need his own territory.

Arrange opportunities for physical activities if these seem to help the client siphon off excess energies. Arrange for time out of the room if this seems appropriate and the client agrees to it.

Don't assign a timid, inexperienced nurse to a potentially violent client.

Assign a mature, easy-going, experienced nurse to care for this client. (In this kind of powderkeg situation, it is axiomatic that there should be only one anxious person in the room: the client.)

Don't overlook the significance of gender in the assignment of a nurse to this client.

Therefore, you might want to consider assigning a male staff nurse to a female client who is potentially violent and a female nurse to a male client. Observers have learned that a woman client may be inclined to react negatively to another woman but positively to a male staff member. This gender crossing also works for the male client, who might hesitate to strike or injure a female nurse.

Developed by Joyce Wallskog, PhD, RN, Marquette University, Milwaukee, Wisconsin, 1994. Used with permission.

present, the client should be referred immediately for psychiatric evaluation. Most clients are ambivalent about taking their life and experience relief that the decision has been taken out of their hands. The nurse should explain the reason for the referral with tact and an emphasis on the behaviors that led the nurse to make the referral: "I'm worried that you might harm yourself because of the way you say you are feeling. You have a plan in mind and you have several of the factors that place you at high risk for suicide. I would like you to see Dr. Jones for an evaluation." The nurse should try to address any of the client's reservations while simultaneously reinforcing the idea that the client has little to lose by having the evaluation. If the client declines treatment evaluation, this should be noted with the time and date of refusal written on the chart.

People intent on hurting themselves or others have tunnel vision for the moment and when the nurse has reason to believe that the client is a danger to him- or herself or others, there is a legal and moral responsibility to disclose the information to appropriate parties. Confidentiality is secondary to the goal of saving a human life. It is important, however, to inform the client about the disclosure of information and to whom the information will be given.

"I may need to act on your behalf until your situation is stabilized, and that includes talking with your family and other health professionals involved in your care about what we have just discussed."

The actively suicidal client should never be left alone, and all potential weapons should be confiscated. This includes mirrors, razors, glass frames, and so on. The way this is done can be important to the client's self-esteem. When taking these items, the nurse should explain in a calm, compassionate manner the reason the items should not be in the client's possession and where they will be kept. The client should be assured that the items will be returned when the danger of self-harm resolves. Most people who attempt suicide feel shame and embarrassment about their desire to end their lives. A major part of the intervention is directed toward helping suicidal clients better understand the reasons that led up to the suicide attempt and assisting them to develop alternative strategies. Acceptance of the client is a critical element of rapport. Helping

people to reestablish a reason for living and getting others involved as a support system are critical interventions. Box 21–7 displays the level of supervision warranted by clients demonstrating suicidal behaviors.

If the circumstances are favorable and the client does not have a significant organic impairment, the nurse can establish a no-suicide contract with the client and can help the client develop a prevention plan for responding to difficult life issues. A suicide contract does not wipe out the need for other assessment and intervention strategies, but it provides another safeguard for the client because it forces him to consider the commitment to life. Suicide contracts are contraindicated with clients demonstrating organic involvement, such as overtly psychotic or drug-abusing behaviors.

## Critical Incident Debriefing

Critical incidents in health care are crisis situations that affect the personnel who respond to them. If there is no opportunity to process the meaning of a critical situation, the nurse can become a psychological casualty.

**Debriefing** is a crisis intervention strategy designed to reduce the impact of a crisis event on professional staff and others involved in the crisis situation by processing it as soon as possible after it occurs. A debriefing offers people an opportunity to externalize a traumatic experience through being able to (1) vent feelings, (2) discuss their role in the situation, (3) develop a realistic sense of the big picture, and (3) receive peer support in putting a crisis event in perspective (Curtis, 1995).

Critical incident debriefing also is useful with families witnessing a tragedy with one of their family members (Ragaisis, 1994). The leader uses a group discussion format to provide a safe place in which nurses and those intimately involved with a critical incident can talk about what happened. The debriefing generally is led by a specially trained professional. Only those actively involved in the critical incident attend the debriefing session, and everything said in the session is kept confidential. The leader introduces the purpose of the group and invites each person to identify who they are and what happened from their perspective, including the

494

♦ Box 21-7. Sample of Level of Supervision Warranted by Suicidal Clients

Current checks _____
Any gestures in past 24 hours _____
Number of days of hospitalization _____
Medications available _____

| Off checks | Observation every 30 minutes | Observation every 15 minutes | Close observation every 5–10 minutes | 1:1 Restriction | Restraint or seclusion |
|---|---|---|---|---|---|
| Verbalizes no suicidal ideation. Congruence shown in verbal and behavioral information. 100% compliance with treatment plan. Has perception of support in community. Verbalizes concerns on a feeling level to present nurse. | Verbalizes suicidal ideation. Verbalizes no plan. Verbalizes no intention. Cooperative with treatment plan. Withdrawn, low. Multiple previous attempts. Verbalizes superficially to present nurse. | Verbalizes suicidal ideation with plan and/or intent. No perception of support. Little compliance with treatment plan. Subjective or objective frustration. Anger. Labile affect or mood. Mute or decreased amount of verbalization. Avoidance of staff and others. Withdrawn, high. Intoxicated. Impaired reality testing. Hyperactive. Demonstrates limited problem-solving ability | Sudden change in activity level . . . not chronic anxiety. Unable to agree not to [attempt] suicide. Makes suicidal gesture currently. | Concealing equipment that could be used to harm self with available specific plan. Attempt made while hospitalized to kill self. | Attempt made to kill self in front of staff (i.e., even 1:1 cannot resist impulse to kill self). |

From Bydlow-Brown B, Billman R. (1990). At risk for suicide. In Ismeurt R, Arnold E, Carson V (eds.), Readings in Concepts Fundamental to Nursing. Springhouse, PA, Springhouse Publishing Company, p. 267. Reprinted with permission. Copyright © 1990 Springhouse Corporation. All rights reserved.

role they played in the incident. After the introduction, the leader might ask the participants to recall the first thing they remember thinking or feeling about the incident. As the dialogue expands, the leader asks participants to recall the worst part of the incident and their reaction to it. Participants are asked to discuss any stress symptoms they may have related to the incident. This part of the session is followed by a consideration of psychoeducational strategies to reduce stress. Any lingering questions are answered, and the leader summarizes the high points of the critical incident debriefing for the group (Rubin, 1990).

## SUMMARY

Crisis is defined as an unexpected, sudden turn of events or set of circumstances that requires an immediate human response. Two types of crises were identified: developmental crises, which parallel psychosocial stages of ego development, and situational crises, which occur as unanticipated episodic events unrelated to human development. Crisis must be considered within the social context in which it occurs.

Crisis intervention is a time-limited treatment that focuses only on the immediate problem and its resolution. A three-step model of intervention is proposed, including engaging the client, exploring the problem, and developing alternatives. Guidelines for communication with clients experiencing selected crisis situations, such as violence and suicide, focus on safety and rapid stabilization of the client's behavior. Usually there are signs of impending violence that the nurse can evaluate; having a plan and the necessary tools increases suicide potential.

Critical incident debriefing is a crisis intervention strategy designed to help nurses process critical incidents in health care, thereby reducing the possibility of symptoms.

## REFERENCES

Aguilera D. (1997). Crisis Intervention: Theory and Methodology (7th ed.). St. Louis, Mosby–Year Book.
Artean C, Williams L. (1998). What we learned from the Oklahoma City Bombing. Nursing 98 28(3):52–55.
Beckingham A, Baumann A. (1990). The aging family in crisis: Assessment and decision making models. Journal of Advanced Nursing 15(7):782–787.
Bluhm J. (1987). Helping families in crisis hold on. Nursing '87 17(10):44–46.
Cahill C, Stuart G, Laraia M, Arana G. (1991). Inpatient management of violent behavior: Nursing prevention and intervention. Issues in Mental Health Nursing 12:239–252.
Caplan G. (1964). Principles of Preventive Psychiatry. New York, Basic Books.
Curtis J. (1995). Elements of critical incident debriefing. Psychological Reports 77(1):91–96.
Erikson E. (1982). The Life Cycle Completed. New York, Norton.
Hoff L. (1991). People in Crisis: Understanding and Helping. Menlo Park, CA, Addison-Wesley.
Johnson S, Craft M, Titler M, et al. (1995). Perceived changes in adult family members' roles and responsibilities during critical illness. Image 27(3):238–243.
Kleeman K. (1989). Families in crisis due to multiple trauma. Critical Care Nursing Clinics of North America 1(1):23–31.
Kus R. (1985). Crisis intervention. In Bulechek G, McCloskey J (eds.), Nursing Interventions: Treatments for Nursing Diagnoses. Philadelphia, WB Saunders.
Leske J, Heidrich S. (1996). Interventions for aged families. Critical Care Nursing Clinics of North America 8(1):91–102.
Leske J. (1998). Treatment for family members in crisis after critical injury. AACN Clinical Issues 9(1):129–139.
Perfetti T. (1982). Training Manual for Crisis Counselors. Bethesda, MD, Montgomery County Crisis Center.
Puskar K, Obus N. (1989). Management of the psychiatric emergency. Nurse Practitioner 14(7):9–18, 23, 26.
Reeder J. (1991). Family perception: A key to intervention. AACN Clinical Issues in Critical Care Nursing 2(2):188–194.
Ragaisis K. (1994). Critical incident stress debriefing: A family nursing intervention. Archives of Psychiatric Nursing 8(1):38–43.
Rubin J. (1990). Critical incident stress debriefing: Helping the helpers. Journal of Emergency Nursing 16(4):255–258.
Slaikeu K. (1984). Crisis Intervention: A Handbook for Practice and Research. Boston, Allyn & Bacon.
Twibell R. (1998). Family coping during critical illness. Dimensions of Critical Care Nursing 17(2):100–112.

## PART V

# Professional Issues

# 22

# Communicating with Other Health Professionals

Ann O'Mara

## OBJECTIVES

At the end of the chapter, the student will be able to

1. Identify concepts in professional relationships
2. Describe methods to handle conflict when it occurs through interpersonal negotiation

3. Discuss methods for communicating effectively in organizational settings
4. Apply group communication principles to work groups

*It is not the brains that matter most, but that which guides them—the character, the heart, generous qualities, progressive ideas.*

Fyodor Dostoyevski (1881)

❖❖ Chapter 22 focuses on the development of collegial relationships with other health team members. The principles of communication used in the nurse–client relationship are broadened to include the nature of the communication process in collegial relationships. Specific bridges to communication with other health professionals, such as advocacy, collaboration, coordination, delegation, and networking, are described. Also included in the chapter are strategies to remove barriers to communication with health professionals, such as coping with offensive communication and responding to constructive criticism.

To be effective as a nursing professional, it is not enough to be deeply committed to the client. Ultimately, the work place atmosphere will have an effect on the relationship that takes place between nurse and client even though the connection may not be readily apparent. Professional relationships provide a unique opportunity to approach client care from a holistic perspective by drawing on the expertise of various disciplines such as psychiatry, medicine, dentistry, social work, nutrition, and physical and respiratory therapy. The same thoughtful purpose, authenticity, empathy, active listening, and respect for the dignity of others that underscore successful nurse–client relationships are needed in relations with other health professionals. Caring commitment to developing constructive working relationships with other professionals gives direction, form, and substance to all nursing actions, thereby providing a recognizable pattern of professional nursing practice.

Working with others effectively in health care is a challenge. The nursing profession is in transition; nurses entering the profession need a more complex set of communication skills than was the case a decade ago. Communication with members of other health disciplines, other nurses, allied health personnel, and peers affects how nurses feel about themselves, and this has a

direct, immediate impact on the quality of nursing care given to clients. The human aspect of nursing practice is what causes the nurse to feel the most joy when the inner emotional connections between self and others are truly felt; it causes nurses the most pain as they relive in their minds missed chances and failures to communicate. Communication and human relationships with all those involved in the client's care support the nurse–client relationship as the foundation of nursing practice.

## BASIC CONCEPTS
### Advocacy

Client advocacy is a professional role requiring not only self-awareness but also a broad knowledge base about the client in the health care system. *Advocacy* can be defined as nurses using the skills of teacher, counselor, and leader to protect and support clients' rights (Taylor et al., 1997). The advocacy role is not new to nursing. Nurses have always been involved in promoting the growth and development of the client as a person rather than just treating the diseased or injured part of the body. Nurses have always acted in the interests of clients who cannot act for themselves, such as children and clients who are immobilized, unconscious, or mentally disabled. Furthermore, nurses have been instrumental in giving information to clients about their health problems and in educating clients to care for themselves. More recently, however, client advocacy has received recognition as a formalized component of the professional nursing role.

The client advocate role includes, first, *informing* clients about the nature of their health problems and the choices they have in seeking to resolve or modify their health care needs with nursing intervention. This role is activated whenever the client is unable to assume responsibility for his or her health care needs. Need can arise from a lack of knowledge or skills or from a cognitive, emotional, or financial base. The nurse's role is to help the client gather information and learn the behaviors necessary to execute the chosen option.

Second, the advocacy role is one of **support** when the client has been informed, has made reasoned choices, and must implement them. The client's right to choose health care options is a new phenomenon. It recognizes the client's inherent right to make decisions for self and to take individual responsibility for a chosen decision. The advocacy role requires the nurse to view the client as an equal partner in resolving the client's health care needs. To fulfill this role, the nurse is respectful of client choices, even when the decisions reached are not what the nurse would recommend for the client.

### Types of Advocacy (Box 22–1)

**Anticipatory guidance** is a form of primary prevention. Helping the client foresee and predict potential difficulties decreases the client's stress. For example, respite care is needed at regular intervals in families with severely ill children or elderly family members. Having no relief from caretaking activities fosters strained family relations and potential client abuse. This need should be anticipated for families of clients with sustained handicaps or chronic illness.

For teenage mothers, poverty, inadequate housing, and lack of privacy make it difficult to reach out for needed help as these young women make the transition to motherhood. The adolescent single parent with little financial support usually needs the Women, Infants, Children program for formula and a referral to social services for follow-up. Providing information about ways to obtain public support services can help an adolescent mother meet her child's basic needs.

---

◆ Box 22-1. Types of Advocacy

Anticipatory guidance
Role modeling
Educational support/informing
Professional direction and collaboration
Primary prevention
Mobilization of community resources/referral

---

Children with developmental disabilities benefit if the nurse explains to the parents motor development in infants. Each of these simple nursing actions acts to improve the client or family member's capacity to cope and care.

In the clinical setting, the nurse acts as a **role model** for appropriate behaviors. For example, the nurse can be a role model to a new mother by talking with the infant and smiling and handling the infant in a supportive way. Setting limits in a kind but firm way with toddlers often helps family members focus on minimizing stress and achieving simple, constructive goals in the clinical setting. Asking the child age-appropriate questions in the presence of the parents models an interpersonal approach to clients that the parents may find quite useful. Modeling behaviors combined with anticipatory guidelines for coping with behavioral changes and caretaking strategies help eliminate a sense of confusion and self-doubt.

**Referral** is an important component of client advocacy. Health-related problems are multidimensional and require the services of more than one health discipline. Frequently, the nurse provides educational support as well as specific client data to other health professionals. Support may focus on the client's needs, nursing interventions, or information about the client's family. An interdisciplinary approach to client care in which all members of the health team pool their expertise to develop a workable care plan ensures comprehensive treatment.

### Steps in the Advocacy Process

The nurse, as the client's advocate, uses a four-step informational process, as presented in Box 22–2. The nurse's power base in advocacy is relevant knowledge and information. Basically, the nurse needs to be aware of personal and professional ethics, values, and prejudices. "One needs to have a good knowledge and understanding of personal views on how human beings relate to each other in a framework or philosophy of fairness" (Kohnke, 1982). For example, if the nurse thinks of elderly clients as helpless and equates aging with being taken care of, then the nurse will be likely to "take charge" of all client health activities, even those the client is still capable of performing with little or no assistance. In this ulatory agencies is as important as knowing who is in charge and who is influential in facilitating change. All of these understandings add to the nurse's power base in effecting change on the client's behalf. With this knowledge base, the nurse is in a position to inform and assist the client in making the most of health care choices with the least amount of effort.

Finally, the nurse needs to recognize personal power needs that stem from his or her personal insecurities and to analyze how those needs affect professional relationships with clients. To a greater or lesser extent, everyone has power needs and insecurities. The important thing is to recognize their presence.

### Assessment

Client advocacy is designed to help the client overcome feelings of helplessness and powerlessness in the hospital or health care treatment setting. Questions might center on the following: (1) What does the client believe is the most pressing problem? (2) What aspects of the problem might be a good place to start? (3) What supports—family, minister, rabbi, social services—are in place? (4) What health or social services is the client familiar with or resistant to considering? Powerlessness can be decreased through anticipatory guidance, role-playing, modeling behaviors, education, and mobilization of community resources on the client's behalf.

### Planning

When a problem situation is identified, the nurse acts quickly to mobilize the necessary resources. Consultations are requested. The client or responsible family member is involved in the process of defining the problem and assuming as much responsibility as possible. Sometimes the nurse serves as dual advocate for the client and a family member. In a child abuse situation, for example, the nurse needs to act as an advocate of the child by taking the steps necessary to provide a protective and safe environment for the child, but the nurse must also be an advocate of the parents by referring them to appropriate community resources and helping them develop different methods for coping with situational stressors. As advocate for both client and family, the nurse is a role model for behaviors that foster

situation, personal values have gotten in the way of individualized professional nursing values associated with client advocacy.

Self-awareness is important. Nurses should have a firm understanding of their personal as well as professional goals in nursing situations. Frequently, both goals are unstated and remain a part of the blind self until they are called into conscious awareness by circumstance. For example, the nurse may have an unstated personal goal of wanting to be liked by every client or an unspoken professional goal of never making a mistake in the delivery of clinical nursing care. Each implied goal will have as much effect on the nurse's interpersonal behaviors with clients and coworkers as a stated professional goal of wanting to learn the latest tracheal suctioning technique.

### Understanding the System

To be successful as client advocates, nurses also need to know the environmental, interpersonal, and bureaucratic system within which they work. It is important to understand how the communication flow filters through the different systems. Usually a combination of formal and informal communication with other staff is necessary for complete understanding.

The professional nurse can gain some of this knowledge by observing how communication is passed from person to person and by asking many questions. Knowing how the various units are influenced by outside pressures such as politics, financial constraints, consumer groups, and rega relationship of mutual respect. Once the nurse and client can meet as equal and complementary partners in promoting the interests of the client in health care situations, advocacy becomes an intimate part of the nursing process.

### Implementation

Another component of the advocacy role is to help the client become a self-advocate. More recently, this process has been referred to as empowerment (a model of which is found in Chapter 5). **Empowerment** requires a certain degree of assertiveness on the part of the nurse. Gibson (1991) described the process as assisting individuals in asserting control over the factors affecting their lives. By maximizing clients' independence and minimizing their dependence, nurses are engaging in partnerships with their clients. If a nurse has difficulty being assertive, then the client can hardly be expected to learn assertive interpersonal skills and instead will pick up on the nurse's sense of inferiority and inability to use self in the accomplishment of health promotion goals. Watching the nurse falter and avoid needed confrontations, the client may feel even less powerful and less able to take a stand on important health care issues. Additionally, the nurse should recognize when to speak for the client and when to encourage the client to speak up. In general, encouraging clients to take as much responsibility as possible to speak on their own behalf is more ego enhancing and leads to a higher level of self-esteem.

Finally, as client advocate, the nurse is seen as the client's protector. Client advocacy by nurses is becoming a legitimate role concept, used in the legal system in malpractice and negligence cases. A nurse who does nothing is generally held more liable than one who tries to do something within the scope of nursing practice and fails. The law is particularly interested in client advocacy as it relates to the presence of inadequate or improper medical care of the nurse's client. Therefore, not only must nurses be knowledgeable, they must also be willing and able to assert their knowledge in situations involving poor medical management of a client.

Asserting one's knowledge, however, should not be confused with usurping the client's decision-making power. Advocacy is not paternalism. The elderly have often been viewed as a group reluctant to decide their health care outcomes. Kjervik (1990) warned nurses not to misinterpret this reluctance as the client's decision to confer his or her decision-making power on health care professionals. Instead, the nurse's responsibility in this situation is to work with the client to identify and select an advocate, independent of the health care system, who will preserve the client's autonomy.

Client advocacy acts as a connective link between ethics and the law. Providing appropriate information that allows a client to make an informed choice conforms to client's rights under the law, and supporting the client's right to make a decision that may or may not be compatible with the nurse's recommendation indicates an ethical commitment to ensure the client's self-determination (Kohnke, 1982). Exercise 22–1 provides a clinical situation in which the nurse's advocacy role is in conflict with traditional nursing and medical advice.

### Evaluation

The need for client advocacy can develop in any phase of the nurse–client relationship, but it is a particularly valuable resource when ordinary means of providing information and support fail to meet the client's need. Usually the collective product developed from client advocacy activity expands far beyond the original thoughts and motivations of individual participants in the process.

## Collaboration

Collaboration is an essential component of the professional nursing role in today's social world (Hales, 1998). Never before has the potential for conflict become so visible in the health care system. As society redefines every citizen's right to health, more and sicker clients are demanding higher quality services in spite of declining resources. Society also is struggling to redefine gender role behaviors. Although some of these changes are viewed as necessary and good in that they encourage greater equality, conflicts can emerge. Perhaps the greatest challenge is with physician–nurse relationships because the professional health care alliance has changed from a traditional notion of the nurse as "handmaiden to the physician" to a concept of the nurse as an autonomous professional who collaborates with

◆ Exercise 22-1. **Client Advocate Role Play**

**Purpose:** To understand the nurse advocacy role in difficult and conflictual clinical situations

**Procedure:**

1. Read the following clinical situation and answer the questions in writing.
2. Have one of the students play the role of the client and another play the role of the nurse.
3. After the role-play, examine your written answers. See whether there are any changes you would like to make.
4. Finally, make up a situation and give it to your colleague with the same questions. Role-play the situation with your colleague, this time taking the role of the client.

   A 65-year-old man has been a client on the medical unit for 10 days, and you are assigned to care for him for the next 4 days. Diagnostic workup and tests reveal that he has cancer of the larynx. Surgery is indicated and has been scheduled. The doctor discusses his diagnosis and prognosis with him in your presence.
   During the next 2 days, the client becomes increasingly withdrawn and introspective. Subsequently, he requests to speak with you and the physician. He states that he does not wish to have any surgery performed and no medication given, that he "has lived a good life" and would like you and the health team to accept his decision to die. He asks that no tube feedings be given and no intravenous fluids be given. He asks that you cooperate and support his wishes.

**Discussion:**

1. What would your reaction be in this situation?
2. What does the statement "death with dignity" mean to you?
3. Do you think the client has the right to refuse treatment that may be life sustaining?
4. What nursing care should you provide for this man as he continues to refuse food and fluids (keeping in mind that the client is an equal partner in his care)?
5. What conflicts does this situation pose for you? How would you see yourself dealing with them?
6. How can you as a nurse respect the integrity of a client's decision when it conflicts with promoting maximum client health functions?
7. Does the client's age influence your acceptance of his decision?
8. How will you support the client when faced with other health care professionals who disapprove of the client's decision?
9. What risks will you be taking in supporting the client?

Adapted from Uusral D. (1978). Values clarification in nursing: Application to practice. American Journal of Nursing 78:2058–2063. Used with permission.

the physician to maximize client health goals. It is important to remember that collaboration occurs with a broad spectrum of other health professionals, including occupational, speech, and physical therapists, pharmacists, dietitians, and social workers. However, the most has been written about the manner in which nurses and physicians engage in a collaborative relationship (Stichler, 1995).

### Definition

***Collaboration*** is defined as an interactive process requiring that the involved individuals combine their expertise, skills, and resources to solve a

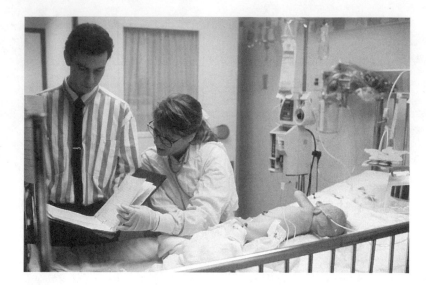

Collaboration is an essential component of the professional nursing role. (Courtesy of the University of Maryland School of Nursing)

problem or achieve a goal (Stichler, 1995). Thus, a broader spectrum of information can be pooled to design a comprehensive care plan for the client (Kalafatich, 1986).

Understanding one another's role needs and responsibilities begins in the educational system. Often health care professionals receive their professional education and training in isolation from one another. Providing interprofessional courses and an informal forum in which nurses and physicians in training can share their role-related expertise would help clarify expectations of one another, lending emphasis to the importance of a collaborative strategy in providing high-quality client care.

The concept of collaboration means working simultaneously at a new relationship with one another and with the client. This new relationship requires that nurses, physicians, other health professionals, and the client communicate effectively with one another and view one another as coming from different perspectives but as having an important joint influence on client care. All members share responsibility to ensure different aspects of holistic, safe, effective, and compassionate care for clients.

Sharing information and ideas with other health care professionals is an important and worthwhile exercise leading to trust and mutual respect. With a nursing perspective, the nurse provides a holistic assessment of health care is-

sues and important information about how likely the client is to accept medical treatment protocols. Because of the nature of their professional responsibilities, nurses are frequently in a better position to help clients explore different options and to plan creatively the most effective approach. A collegial relationship means not only that clients receive better care but that the nurse finds the experience of collaboration personally and professionally affirming (Mauksch, 1981).

## Coordination

*Coordination* is closely related to collaboration, the difference being that with collaboration there may be more joint direct interaction with a client. In coordination, two or more people provide services to a client or program separately and inform each other of their activities. At times, a careful assessment of the nature of the client's adaptive or self-care requirements reveals a need beyond the scope of the nurse's professional practice or level of experience. The nurse needs to identify the health care professional who can best serve the client's need and to contact that person.

To make an appropriate referral, the nurse should have a good sense of personal or professional limitations and an adequate understanding of health, human services, and community resources. Having a knowledge about referral sources allows the nurse to match the client's

---

◆ Box 22-3. Questions to Assess Appropriateness of Resources

1. What are the services like?
2. Does the agency have a sliding fee scale?
3. What are the hours of service?
4. How does the client contact the agency?
5. Does the client need an appointment?
6. How would the client get there?

---

needs and preferences with the best resource. Some referral source factors to be considered include compatibility with the client's expressed need, financial resources, accessibility (time as well as place), and ease of contact. Ease of contact and financial considerations sometimes are forgotten elements in coordination efforts, much to the detriment of the client's welfare. Box 22–3 lists some important questions the nurse should

consider when making a referral for a client. Some of these questions may seem quite basic, and yet for the person in need of health care or human services the answers can be crucial to client compliance efforts. Exercise 22–2 gives practice in exploring community resources.

## Networking

A concept closely related to collaboration and coordination is that of ***networking.*** It is a reciprocal process that validates the nurse's peers as valuable sources of information and reaffirms the individual nurse as a valuable source. As with the previously mentioned roles of collaboration, advocacy, and so on, networking is a relatively new role for the professional nurse. In other professions, networking is an essential component in building professional relationships and ultimately advancing one's status within the profession.

When engaged in networking, nurses are

---

◆ Exercise 22-2. **Community Resources**

**Purpose:** To help you assess different types of health, human services, and community resources

**Procedure:**

1. Contact a health or human services resource of your choosing in the community. The questions cited in the following Discussion section can be used to elicit information.
2. Write down such information as telephone number, address, contact person, and bring it to class.
3. Take turns presenting your findings. You will appreciate having the resource information presented in class; write it down for future reference.

**Discussion:**

1. How did you choose your resource?
2. Where did you find your initial information about it: yellow pages, from a friend, or your own experience?
3. How easy was it to get in touch with someone who could give you relevant information about the resource? Were you treated with courtesy and respect? If not, why? Is there anything you would do differently?
4. What is the fee structure in the agency (e.g., sliding scale)?
5. Are there any restrictions on the allowable number of client visits?
6. Is the service resource accessible by public transportation, or are there any provisions for transportation?
7. Are there any other questions you might have asked based on your experience of contracting the resource?

making contacts with peers from as close as the nursing unit on the floor below to as far as a professional conference 500 miles away. By making contacts, nurses are communicating their expertise and sharing their ideas in a particular area of the profession while they are gathering information from their contacts. This give and take of information is often the bridge in networking with peers. For example, oncology nurses often exchange ideas about the best approach to relieve side effects from chemotherapy and radiation therapy. Extensive networking among oncology nurses was the impetus for the formation of the Oncology Nursing Society. Networking and collaboration will become increasingly important as advanced practice nurses become an active voice in health care reform.

## Professional Rights

All health professionals, including nurses, have rights as well as significant responsibilities in interprofessional relationships with colleagues. Box 22–4 lists Chenevert's (1988) 10 rights of nursing professionals in nursing practice.

Acting responsibly in nursing practice situations requires a willingness to go the extra step

---

> ### ◆ Box 22-4. Chenevert's Rights in Nursing Practice
>
> 1. You have a right to be treated with respect.
> 2. You have a right to a reasonable workload.
> 3. You have the right to an equitable wage.
> 4. You have the right to determine your own reasonable priorities.
> 5. You have the right to ask for what you want, as long it does not interfere with the rights of others.
> 6. You have the right to refuse unreasonable requests without making excuses or feeling guilty.
> 7. You have the right to make mistakes and be responsible for them.
> 8. You have the right to give and receive information as a health professional.
> 9. You have the right to act in the best interest of the client as long as it is not in conflict with agency policy and respects the rights of others involved in the client's care.
> 10. You have the right to be human.

---

in establishing good working relations with professional colleagues, to try different interpersonal communication strategies, and to push on in the face of adversity. Persistence and a good sense of humor are essential characteristics of honest interpersonal relationships with peers, reflecting a dual professional commitment to self and others.

Rights carry with them corresponding responsibilities. Often rightful acceptance of responsibilities fosters the automatic granting of rights by the other person. Think about your professional collegial relationships and your dual professional commitment to self and others. Think about the professional values identified in this book and re-examine the components of professionalism. Each of those components is basically a professional responsibility. Add your ideas for rights next to those responsibilities. Exchange ideas about professional rights and responsibilities with others.

## Delegation

An emerging new aspect to the professional nurse's role and responsibilities is that of delegation. Health care reform and the resulting changes in health care delivery systems have radically altered the manner in which nurses deliver care. Delegation has always been an important component to the nursing role, usually thought of as one professional delegating to another (i.e., peer to peer). This perception no longer holds true in today's health care system. Now nurses are delegating to a variety of unlicensed assistive personnel (UAP), who often possess minimal skills and knowledge. The challenges of maintaining professional integrity and concurrently surviving in today's health care arena are felt by nurses in all settings. Effective and appropriate use of delegation can facilitate the nurse's ability to meet these challenges.

More often than not, novice nurses are inadequately prepared for the demands of delegating much of their nursing tasks to UAPs while retaining responsibility for interpreting patient outcomes. However, the novice nurse is not alone in feeling inadequate; experienced nurses are facing the same dilemmas. Findings from a 1997 study revealed that registered nurses were dissatisfied with UAP's ability to perform delegated nursing tasks, communicate pertinent information, and provide more time for professional nursing activities (Barter et al., 1997).

*Delegation* is defined as "the transfer of responsibility for the performance of an activity from one individual to another while retaining accountability for the outcome." Whether the nurse is delegating to a peer or a UAP, he or she is only transferring the responsibility for the performance of the activity, not the professional accountability for the overall care (American Nurses Association, 1994). In earlier times, delegating and trusting went hand-in-hand, because the nurse was transferring responsibility to a peer and had some assurance of the skills and knowledge of that peer. The present environment poses a much different reality because the nurse is no longer sure of the skills and knowledge of the person to whom she or he is delegating.

Inherent in effective delegation is an adequate understanding of the skills and knowledge of UAPs as well as of the Nurse Practice Act of the state in which the nurse is practicing (Johnson, 1996). Within each state's Nurse Practice Act are specific guidelines describing what nursing actions can and cannot be delegated and to what type of personnel these actions can be delegated. In addition to knowing nurse practice guidelines and the skills and knowledge level of UAPs, the nurse must educate and reinforce the UAP's knowledge base, assess the UAP's readiness for delegation, delegate appropriately, oversee the task, and evaluate and record the outcomes (Adams, 1995; Boucher, 1998). The appropriate implementation of these principles (educating, assessing, overseeing, evaluating) is a costly process both in time and energy. Practice Exercise 22–3 to facilitate your understanding of the principles. The following case example highlights one particular principle.

### ◆ Case Example

After receiving the report on her patient assignments, Monica Lewis, RN, assigns a newly hired UAP to provide routine care (morning care, assistance with meals, vital signs, fingersticks for glucose, and reporting of any changes) to Mrs. Jones, who was recently

---

### ◆ Exercise 22-3. **Applying Principles of Delegation**

**Purpose:** To help you differentiate between delegating nursing tasks and evaluating patient outcomes

**Procedure:**

1. Divide the class into groups: A and B. The following case study is a typical day for a charge nurse in an extended-care facility. After reading the case study, Group A is to describe the nursing tasks they would delegate and instructions they would give the nursing assistants and certified medicine aides (CMAs). Group B is to describe the professional nursing responsibilities related to the delegated tasks. The two groups then share their reports.

Anne Marie Roache is the day shift charge nurse on one of the units at Shadyside Nursing and Rehabilitation Facility. On this particular day, her census is 24, and her staff includes four nursing assistants and two CMAs who are allowed to administer all oral and topical medications. Her nursing assistants are qualified to perform morning care: assist with feedings, obtain and record vital signs, fluid intake and output, and blood glucose fingersticks; turn and position residents; assist with ambulation; and perform decubitus dressing changes. Of the residents, 12 are bedridden, requiring complete bed baths and some degree of assistance with feeding. The remaining 12 require varying degrees of assistance with their morning baths and assistance to the dining rooms for their meals. Nine of the residents are diabetics requiring a.c. blood glucose fingersticks, 7 are recovering from cerebrovascular accidents and display varying degrees of right- or left-sided weakness, 3 require care of their sacral decubiti, and all of the residents are at risk for falling because of varying degrees of confusion, disorientation, or general weakness. The night shift reported that all the residents' conditions were stable and they had slept well. Ms. Roache is ready to assign her staff.

admitted for exacerbation of her type II diabetes. While on routine rounds, during lunch, Monica finds Mrs. Jones unresponsive, with cold, clammy skin, a heart rate of 110, and a fingerstick reading of 60 mg/dL, which the UAP had obtained. Thinking Mrs. Jones was experiencing hypoglycemia, Monica requested the UAP to obtain another blood glucose. While administering high-glucose intravenous solutions to raise Mrs. Jones' blood sugar, Monica observed the UAP violate a number of basic principles in obtaining an accurate blood glucose. Upon further questioning, the UAP admitted never having been taught the proper procedure and thought reading the directions was sufficient. Monica had wrongly assumed all UAPs underwent training on the principles of obtaining blood glucose fingersticks.

## APPLICATIONS
## Conflict Resolution

The relationship between doctor and nurse remains an evolving process, sometimes marked with conflict, mistrust, and disrespect. Although these feelings are changing, it is slow, and some physicians still regard themselves as the only legitimate authority in health care, seeing the professional nurse as an accessory. An attitude that excludes the nurse as a professional partner in health care promotion benefits no one, is increasingly being challenged, and is costly to professionals and patients alike (Forte, 1997). However, the nurse–physician relationship is not the only source of conflict. A number of other sources are listed in Box 22–5.

When the source of conflict is interpersonal, the nurse needs to think through the possible

---

◆ **Box 22–5. Interpersonal Sources of Conflict in the Clinical Area**

Being asked to do something you know would be irresponsible or unsafe

Having your feelings or opinions ridiculed or discounted

Being pressured to give more time or attention than you are able to give

Being asked to give more information than you feel comfortable sharing

Maintaining a sense of self in the face of hostility or sexual harassment

---

◆ **Box 22–6. Steps to Promote Health Goals and Defuse Status Quarrels among Health Care Workers**

Have an objective or a goal clearly in mind.

Set the stage for collaborative communication.

State your position clearly.

Identify the key points.

Be willing to develop alternative solutions in which all parties can meet essential needs.

Depersonalize conflict situations.

Maintain respect for the values and dignity of both parties in the relationship.

---

causes of the conflict as well as his or her own feelings about it and respond appropriately, even if the response is a deliberate choice not to respond verbally. Interpersonal conflicts that are not dealt with leave residual feelings that reappear unexpectedly and affect the nurse's ability to respond realistically and responsibly in future interactions.

Although conflict is inevitable, it is not necessarily detrimental to productivity and job satisfaction. Successful resolution often has a positive effect on both outcomes. Thus, the primary goal in dealing with work place conflict is to find a high-quality, mutually acceptable solution, a win–win strategy. In many instances, a different type of relationship can be developed through the use of conflict management communication techniques. Using purposeful strategies to defuse a negative interaction, the nurse reframes a clinical situation as a cooperative process in which the health goals and not the status relations of the health care providers become the focal object. Steps in the conflict resolution process are presented in Box 22–6.

A clear idea of the outcome one wishes to achieve is a necessary first step in the process. It is important to do your homework by obtaining all relevant information about the specific issues involved and about the client's behavioral responses to a health care issue before engaging in negotiation. Having some idea of what issues might be relevant from the other person's perspective provides important information about the best interpersonal approach to use.

Among the most commonly identified conflict resolution strategies, *confrontation* has been found to be the most effective (Jones et al., 1990). To use confrontation in a productive manner, Jones and colleagues prescribed four essential steps: (1) identify as many concerns as possible from both parties; (2) clarify assumptions; (3) identify the real issue being confronted; and (4) work collaboratively through a problem-solving process to find a solution that satisfies both parties. Exercise 22–4 provides a clinical situation in which the staff's behavior is creating a conflict on the unit.

Knowing your own interpersonal communication strengths and weaknesses as well of those of the other participants is equally important in developing the most appropriate communication strategies. Some people respond better when they have written or oral information before the discussion so they can come prepared. Other people react well to more spontaneous, on-the-spot interactions. The same is true of decision making. Some people need time to absorb the meaning of a situation before coming to a decision, whereas others like to come to decisions at the time of the dialogue. One way of processing and responding to situations is not necessarily better than another, but knowing the characteristics of the other party is an important strength in resolving conflict situations.

Often the professional may not know the communication strengths and weaknesses of the other individual; then it is best to allow some time for the individual to process the information. Few situations are true emergencies that need to be settled immediately. The confronter should allow the recipient to respond later to the issues that are raised. An appropriate way to diffuse the notion of immediacy might be "Let me get back to you when you have had some time to think about what we've talked about today."

If the individual being confronted is forced or coerced into an immediate response, conflict resolution is likely to be less effective.

It is even appropriate to write key points on a 3 × 5-inch card for reference in emotionally tense confrontations. Sometimes this strategy helps the nurse stay focused on the main issue when emotions threaten to preclude direct confrontation or dilute the impact of the issues to

---

◆ **Exercise 22–4. Applying Principles of Confrontation**

**Purpose:** To help you understand the importance of using specific principles of confrontation to resolve a conflict

**Procedure:**

1. Divide the class into two groups: Group A is the day shift (7 A.M.–7 P.M.), and Group B is the night shift (7 P.M.–7 A.M.).

2. The following case study is an example of some problems between the night and day shifts resulting in mistrust and general tension between the two groups. After reading the case study, each group is to use Jones and colleagues' (1990) first three principles, as identified in the text (identify concerns, clarify assumptions, identify real issue). The two groups then share their concerns, assumptions, and what they believe to be the real issue. Finally, both groups are to apply the fourth principle, collaboratively identifying a solution(s) that satisfies both groups.

The night shift's (Group B) responsibilities include completing as many bed baths as possible and the taping report as close to the shift change (7 A.M.) as possible. The day shift (Group A) finds that very few, if any, of the bed baths are completed and that the taped report is usually done at about 5 A.M., reflecting very few of the client changes that occurred between 5 A.M. and 7 A.M.

The day shift is angry with the night shift, feeling they are not assuming their fair share of the workload. The night shift feels the day shift does not understand their responsibilities; they believe they are contributing more than their fair share of work.

be negotiated. Another tactic that stimulates self-confidence is to discuss the issue with a trusted colleague on the unit or with a valued supervisor beforehand to gain a broader perspective. Interpersonal power is increased by an accurate knowledge of the scope of practice boundaries imposed by the institution as well as those of other health providers. Unfortunately, although confrontation frequently is the most effective strategy, it is not the most frequently used.

Setting the stage for goal negotiations is an important part of the process. In the first few minutes, convey the attitude that a major objective of the interaction from your perspective is a better understanding of the issues surrounding the current conflict and a real desire for a relationship. Through words and actions, the nurse needs to demonstrate that the desire is genuine. Discussion should begin with either a statement of the commonalities of purpose or the points of agreement about the issue; for example, "I thoroughly agree Mr. Smith will do much better at home. However, we need to contact social services and make a home care referral before we actually discharge him; otherwise, he will be right back in the hospital again." *Points of disagreement should always follow rather than precede points of agreement.* Empathy and a genuine desire to understand the issues from the other's perspective enhance communication and the likelihood of a successful resolution.

Sometimes there are issues about which the other person feels so strongly that discussion is impossible. Frequently, the person's ego is too intimately involved with the situation or personal goals. Knowing what issues are within one's power to change and what issues cannot be changed helps the nurse to discern the more important and relevant goals and issues for dialogue. Success with a few objectives generally is more productive than attempting to change all of another's deeply held convictions in one or two sessions. Emotional as well as objective data are included in problem analysis because they often represent the most important component of the conflict issue.

During conflict negotiation, it is important to remain flexible, yet not to yield on important, essential dimensions of the issue. Sometimes it is difficult to listen carefully to the other person's position without automatically formulating your next point or response, but it is important to keep an open mind and to examine the issue from a number of perspectives before selecting alternative options. The communication process should not be prematurely concluded. The process of open, flexible communication can be facilitated by using paraphrases and clarifying statements that encourage further disclosure. Sample comments are as follows: "If you did that, what would you see as the outcome?" "So then are you saying that in your opinion, this should . . . ?" "Are you saying, then, that . . . ?" Likewise, reflection phrases are used to gather information about the feelings accompanying the manifest content of the message: "It sounds as if you would be quite disappointed if . . . " "I would imagine it must be quite disconcerting to even think that something like . . . could happen."

It also is appropriate to use open-ended questions and attending behaviors in gathering more data. The more information you have, the more likely it is that the solution will represent the needs of both parties. Finally, no matter how reasoned your personal solution to the problem, unless there is common ground to support ideas, change is unlikely to occur.

Solutions taking into consideration the needs and human dignity of all parties are more likely to be considered as viable alternatives. Backing another health professional into a psychological corner by using intimidation, coercion, or blaming simply is counterproductive. More often than not, solutions developed through such tactics never become implemented. Usually there are a number of reasons for this phenomenon, but the basic issues have to do with how the problem was originally defined and the control issues that were never actually dealt with in the problem-solving discussion.

Essential to the implementation of confrontation strategies are full disclosure and discussion before decisions are made. Both parties must be allowed the opportunity to discuss ideas, concerns, and reasons while searching for proper ways to reach the agreed-on goals (Jones et al., 1990). Whenever people believe that the solution has been predetermined and they have had little input into the outcome, they may feel manipulated and angry. Taking an unrealistic stand with the implicit intent of giving up some of what you truly did not want usually is unworkable over time. It destroys credibility once the manipulative nature of the strategy is uncovered. Furthermore, it stands in the way of a truly creative resolution of the problem. Often the final solution derived through fair negotiation is better than the one arrived at alone by the nurse, the physician, and the client or other health care provider.

## Negotiating with Authority Figures

Negotiating can be even more threatening with a nursing supervisor or an instructor who has direct authority because these people have some control over the future of the staff nurse or student. Usually a poor relationship with a supervisor is tolerated but not shared with peers for fear of damaging the peers' view of oneself or of peers reporting what was said to the supervisor for their own advantage. Not being able to discuss the relationship with colleagues often distorts what is actually happening. Many times, the frustration is played out with the client as the nurse sabotages the supervisor's directives for improved clinical care.

Supervision implies a shared responsibility in the overall professional goal of providing high-quality nursing care to clients. The wise supervisor is able to promote a nonthreatening environment in which all of the aspects of professionalism are allowed to emerge and prosper. In a supervisor–nurse relationship, conflict may arise when expectations for performance are unclear or when the nurse is unable to perform at the desired level. Communication of expectations often occurs after the fact, within the context of an employee performance evaluation. Effective management requires that expectations are known from the beginning and that the nurse is advised of the need for improvement as part of an ongoing, constructive interpersonal relationship. When the supervisor must give constructive criticism, it should be given in a nonthreatening and genuinely caring manner, as presented in Box 22–7.

Receiving criticism is difficult for most people. When a supervisor gives constructive criticism, some type of response is indicated from the person receiving it. Initially, it is crucial that the conflict problem be clearly defined and acknowledged. In addition, Davidhizar (1991) recommended that the nurse:

Defuse personal anxiety.
Listen carefully to the criticism and paraphrase it.
Acknowledge that suggestions for improvement are taken seriously.
Discuss the situation.
Develop a plan for dealing with it.

In studying approaches to authority figures, you are encouraged to analyze your overall personal responses to authority, as in Exercise 22–5.

## Collaborating with Peers

The nurse–client relationship occurs within the larger context of the professional relationship with other health disciplines. How the nurse relates to other members of the health team will affect the level and nature of the interactions that transpire between nurse and client. Interpersonal conflict between health team members periodically is concealed from awareness and projected onto client behaviors.

◆ **Case Example**

On a psychiatric nursing unit, the nursing staff found Mr. Tomkins's behavior highly disruptive. At an inter-

---

◆ Box 22–7. Steps in Giving Constructive Criticism

| Steps | Sample Statement |
| --- | --- |
| 1. Express empathy. | "I understand that things are difficult at home." |
| 2. Describe the behavior. | "But I see that you have been late coming to work three times during this pay period. |
| 3. State expectations. | "It is necessary for you to be here on time from now on." |
| 4. List consequences. | "If you get here on time, we'll all start off the shift better. If you are late again, I will have to report you to the personnel department." |

---

◆ Exercise 22–5. **Feelings about Authority**

**Purpose:** To recognize your feelings about authority

**Procedure:**

1. Lean back in your chair, close your eyes, and think of the work ``authority.''
2. Who is the first person that comes to mind when thinking of that word?
3. Describe how this person signifies authority to you. Next, think of an incident in which this person exerted authority and how you reacted to it.
4. After you have visualized the memory, answer the following questions:

   What were your feelings about the incident after it was over?

   What changes of feelings occurred from the start of the incident until it was over?

   Was there anything about the authority figure that reminded you of yourself?

   Was there anything about the authority figure that reminded you of someone else with whom you once had a strong relationship (if the memory viewed is not mother or father)?

   How could you have handled the incident more assertively?

   Can you see any patterns in yourself that might help you handle interactions with authority figures?

   What about those patterns that are not assertive?

   How could those patterns be improved to be more assertive?

   _____

   Adapted from Levy R. (1972). Self Revelation Through Relationships. Englewood Cliffs, NJ, Prentice Hall. Used with permission.

---

disciplinary conference attended by representatives from all shifts, there was general agreement that Mr. Tomkins would spend 1 hour in the seclusion room—each time his agitated behavior occurred. The order was written into his care plan. The plan was implemented for a week with a noticeable reduction in client symptoms. During the second week, however, Mr. Tomkins would be placed in the seclusion room for the reasons just mentioned, but the evening staff would release him after 5 or 10 minutes if he was quiet and well behaved.

The client's agitated behavior began to escalate again, and another interdisciplinary conference was called. Although the stated focus of the dialogue was on constructive ways to help Mr. Tomkins cope with disruptive anxiety, the underlying issues related to the strong feelings of the day nursing staff that their interventions were being undermined. Equally strong was the conviction of the evening staff that they were acting in the client's best interest by letting him out of the seclusion room as soon as his behavior normalized. Until the underlying behaviors could be resolved satisfactorily at the staff level, the client continued to act out the staff's anxiety as well as his own.

Similar types of issues now and again arise when there is no input from different work shifts in developing a comprehensive nursing care plan. The shift staff may not agree with specific interventions, but instead of talking the discrepancy through in regularly scheduled staff conferences, they may act it out, unconsciously undoing the work of the other shifts. Whenever there is covert conflict among nursing staff or between members of different health disciplines, it is the client who ultimately suffers the repercussions. The level of trust the client may have established in the professional relationship is compromised until the staff conflict can be resolved.

## Responding to Putdowns

At some time in your professional career, you will run into unwarranted putdowns and destructive criticisms. Generally, they are delivered with self-defeating language and have but one intent: to decrease your status and enhance the status of the person delivering the putdown. The putdown or criticism may be handed out because the speaker is feeling inadequate or threatened. Often it has little to do with the actual behavior of the nurse to whom it is delivered. Other times the criticism may be valid, but the time and place of delivery are grossly inappropriate (e.g., in the middle of the nurses' station or in the client's presence). In either case, the automatic response of many nurses is to become defensive and embarrassed and in some way actually to begin to feel inadequate, thus allowing the speaker to project unwarranted feelings onto the nurse.

Recognizing a putdown or unwarranted criticism is the first step toward dealing effectively with it. If a coworker or authority figure's comment generates defensiveness, embarrassment, and doubt about one's professional ability to perform the nursing role, it is likely that the comment represents more than just factual information about performance. If the comment made by the speaker contains legitimate information to help improve one's skill and is delivered in a private and constructive manner, it represents a learning response and cannot be considered a putdown. Learning to differentiate between the two types of communication helps the nurse to separate the "wheat from the chaff."

### ◆ Case Example

A nurse examining a crying child's inner ears notes that the eardrums are red and reports to the head nurse that the child may have an ear infection. The head nurse responds:

When a child is crying, the drums often swell and redden. How about checking again when the child is calm? (Learning response)

Of course they are red when the child is crying. Didn't you learn that in nursing school? I haven't got time to answer such basic questions! (Putdown response)

Whereas the first response allows the nurse to learn useful information to incorporate into practice, the second response serves to antagonize, and it is doubtful much learning takes place. What will happen is that the nurse will be more hesitant about approaching the head nurse again

for clinical information. Again, it is the client who ultimately suffers.

Once a putdown is recognized as such, the nurse needs to respond verbally in an assertive manner as soon as possible after the incident has taken place. Waiting an appreciable length of time is likely to cause resentment in the nurse toward the other person, leaving the staff nurse with feelings of lost self-respect. Furthermore, it may be more difficult later for the other person to remember the details of the incident. At the same time, if the nurse's own anger, not the problem behavior, is likely to dominate the response, it is better to wait for the anger to cool a little and then to present the message in a more dignified and reasoned manner.

The process for responding to putdowns is similar to that described in Chapter 14 for conflict resolution, but the emphasis is a little different. As with all forms of conflict resolution, the nature of the relationship should be considered. Attitudes are important. If you can, look on the incident as an opportunity to learn more about yourself in conflict situations. Respect for the value of each individual as a person should be evidenced throughout the interaction. Try to determine how to respond to this person in a productive way so that you are on speaking terms, but still get your point across. Even if you do not fully succeed in your initial tries, you probably will have learned something valuable in the process. Taking reasoned interpersonal risks is not easy, but generally it is beneficial to the personal and professional growth of the nurse. The process of response follows.

Address the objectionable or disrespectful behaviors first. Briefly state the behavior and its impact on you. It is important to deliver a succinct verbal message without getting lost in detail and without sounding apologetic or defensive. Do not try to give a prolonged explanation of your behavior at this point in the interaction, and do not suggest possible motivations. Instead, emphasize the specifics of the putdown behavior. Once the putdown has been dealt with, you can discuss any criticism of your own behavior on its own merits. Refer only to the behaviors identified, and do not encourage the other person to amplify the putdown.

Because putdowns often catch one by surprise, it is useful to have a standard set of opening replies ready. Examples of openers might include the following:

1. "I think it was out of line for you to criticize me in front of the client."
2. "I found your comments very disturbing and insulting."
3. "I experienced what you said as an attack that wasn't called for by my actions."
4. "I thought that was an intolerable remark."

A reply that is specific to the putdown delivered is essential. The tone of voice needs to be even and firm. In the clinical example given previously, the nurse might have said to the head nurse: "My school is not an issue, and your criticism is unnecessary" or "It seems to me that the assessment of the child's ears, not my school, is the issue, and your superior tone is uncalled for."

An important aspect of putdowns is that they get in the way of the nurse's professional goal of providing high-quality nursing care to clients. The effect of the head nurse's second response is for both nurses to assume the reddened eardrums are from crying and not to reevaluate the child's eardrums. Feeling resentful and less sure of his or her clinical skills, the staff nurse is less likely to risk stirring up such feelings again. If fewer questions are asked, important information goes unshared. In the clinical example just cited, a possible ear infection might not be detected.

## Peer Negotiation

As students, you will encounter situations in which the behavior of a colleague causes a variety of unexpressed differences or disagreement because their interpretation of a situation or meaning of behavior is so different from yours. The conflict behaviors can occur as a result of differences in values, philosophical approaches to life, ways of handling problems, lifestyle, different definitions of a problem, different goals, or alternative strategies to resolve a problem. Nevertheless, they cause friction and turn relationships from collaborative to competitive.

Recognizing the existence of a conflict is the first step toward peer negotiation. Generally, conflict increases anxiety. When interaction with a certain peer or peer group stimulates anxious or angry feelings, the presence of conflict should be considered. Once it is determined that conflict

is present, look for the basis of the conflict and label it as personal or professional. If it is personal in nature, it may not be appropriate to seek peer negotiation. It might be better to go back through the self-awareness exercises presented in previous chapters and locate the nature of the conflict through self-examination.

Sharing feelings about a conflict with others helps to reduce its intensity. It is confusing, for example, when nursing students first enter a nursing program or clinical rotation, but this confusion does not get discussed, and students frequently believe they should not feel confused or uncertain. Because students face several complex interpersonal situations—class and clinical—simultaneously, they may experience loneliness and much self-doubt about their skills compared with those of their peers. These feelings are universal in humans at the beginning of any new experience. By sharing them with one or two peers, one usually finds that others have had parallel experiences. In reviewing Exercise 22–4, think of a conflict or problem that has implications for your practice of nursing, one you would be willing to share with your peers.

Self-awareness is beneficial in assessing the meaning of a professional conflict. For instance, if the nurse's major response to the conflict is emotional, one can be reasonably certain the conflict raises personal feelings from a previous experience. This assumption does not negate the legitimacy of the conflict issue, but it suggests that the personal material needs to be recognized, worked through, and removed from the peer negotiation process. Concrete, observable facts related to the issue should be the focus of discussion; conflictual personal feelings should be discussed elsewhere except as they directly affect the current situation. Now that you have an opportunity to study different types of conflict, work on Exercise 22–6.

## Developing a Support System

Collegial relationships are an important determinant of success as professional men and women enter nursing practice. Although there is no substitute for outcomes that demonstrate professional competence, interpersonal strategies can facilitate the process. Integrity, respect for others, dependability, a good sense of humor, and

## ◆ Exercise 22-6. **Barriers to Interprofessional Communication**

**Purpose:** To help you understand the basic concepts of client advocacy, communication barriers, and peer negotiation in simulated nursing situations

**Procedure:**

1. Following are four examples of situations in which interprofessional communication barriers exist. Refamiliarize yourself with the concepts of professionalism, client advocacy, communication barriers, and peer negotiation.
2. Formulate a response to each example.
3. Compare your responses with those of your classmates, and discuss the implications of common and disparate answers. Sometimes dissimilar answers provide another important dimension of a problem situation.

### Case A

Dr. Tanlow interrupts Ms. Serf as she is preparing pain medication for 68-year-old Mrs. Gould. It is already 15 minutes late. Dr. Tanlow says he needs Ms. Serf immediately in Room 20C to assist with a drainage and dressing change. Knowing that Mrs. Gould, a diabetic, will respond to prolonged pain with vomiting, Ms. Serf replies she will be available to help Dr. Tanlow in 10 minutes (during which time she will have administered Mrs. Gould's pain medication). Dr. Tanlow, already on his way to Room 20C, whirls around, stating loudly, ''When I say I need assistance, I mean now. I am a busy man, in case you hadn't noticed.''

If you were Ms. Serf, what would be an appropriate response?

### Case B

A newly hired nurse is helping a resident draw femoral blood. The nurse states that although she has never assisted with this procedure, she is thoroughly familiar with the procedure through the hospital manual. The nurse requests that, if the resident requires anything different from the manual, he should tell her so. The resident responds, ''You should have practiced this with someone else. I shouldn't be stuck with a neophyte. Ha ha! Get it? Neophyte, instead of needle.''

How should the nurse respond?

### Case C

Mrs. Warfield, the nursing supervisor, remains on Unit C most of the evening with Mr. Whelan, who is working his first evening shift as charge nurse. Toward the end of the evening, Mr. Whelan ask Mrs. Warfield whether there was a special reason she was spending so much time on the unit. Mrs. Warfield replied vaguely that she always does that with first-time charge nurses. Two days later, Mr. Whelan received a written report about his evening as charge nurse that was negative in nature and particularly critical of the fact that the supervisor had to spend so much time on Unit C. A copy of the report went to the head nurse on Unit C and to Mr. Whelan's personnel file.

How would you respond if you were Mr. Whelan?

### Case D

Mrs. Swick had been working the evening shift for 8 months. When she was hired, she was promised in writing that she would be moved to a permanent day shift assignment as soon as a replacement could be found for the evening shift. Recently, two new nurses have been hired and assigned to permanent days.

Writing a note to the supervisor brought no response; Mrs. Swick thus scheduled an appointment to discuss her schedule with her supervisor. After the appointment, her supervisor began scheduling her on days, but her new assignment requires a two-day rotation to nights once a month, a day off (which she used to sleep after her night shift) consistently followed by 5 straight days.

How would you approach this situation if you were Mrs. Swick?

an openness to sharing with others are communication qualities people look for in developing a support system.

Forming a reliable support system to share information, ideas, and strategies with colleagues provides a collective strength to personal efforts and minimizes the possibility of misunderstanding. With problem or conflict situations, getting ideas from trusted colleagues beforehand enhances the probability of accomplishing outcomes more effectively.

### Professional Support Groups

In nursing practice, interpersonal sharing and collaboration are an integral part of effective nursing care. However, there are times the nurse feels overwhelmed with the responsibility and intense feelings associated with work. For example, caring for a young, terminally ill client with a family can raise important existential questions for even the most experienced nurse. Working in critical care settings, nursing homes, and hospices with clients one knows and loves and watching them deteriorate and die despite the best possible nursing care and medical technology leads one to question one's own effectiveness, the meaning of suffering, and even one's own mortality.

It is easy to become hardened to such experiences or to believe that the only recourse is to leave the profession. Frequently, family and friends have a limited understanding of the emotional impact of such experiences or the heartrending toll it takes over time on the individual nurse. A professional support group, composed of individuals with similar work experience, is designed to provide emotional and cognitive support, enabling nurses to work more effectively in high-risk nursing situations.

One of the meanings of the word *comfort* is "to strengthen." In meeting the needs of others in demanding nursing situations, nurses need to take time to strengthen personal resources, and one way to do this is to seek comfort and understanding in a professional support group. Talking it through with others who can support our explorations and commitment, who can both argue and encourage the expression of conflictual feelings from a position of knowledge as well as compassion, is comforting. In professional support groups, members offer themselves as resources and in return fulfill their own needs in the interaction. Giving each other guidance and thoughtful support when we need it is essential to replenish the nurse who is so busy attending to the interpersonal needs of others that there is little time to discover who he or she is as an individual in the situation (Arnold, 1989).

## Understanding the Organizational System

Whenever one works in an organization, either as student or professional, one automatically becomes a part of an organizational system with established political norms of acceptable behavior. Each organizational system defines its own chain of command and rules about social processes in professional communication. Even though your idea may be excellent, failure to understand the chain of command or an unwillingness to form the positive alliances needed to accomplish your objective dilutes the impact. For example, if your instructor has been defined as your first line of contact, then it is not in your best interest to seek out staff personnel or other students without also checking with the instructor.

Although sidestepping the identified chain of command and going to a higher or more tangential resource in the hierarchy may appear less threatening initially, the benefits of such action may not resolve the difficulty. Furthermore, the trust needed for serious discussion becomes limited. Some of the reasons for avoiding positive interactions stem from an internal circular process of faulty thinking. Because communication is viewed as part of a process, the sender and receiver act on the information received, which may or may not represent the reality of the situation. Examples of the circular processes that block the development of cooperative and receptive influencing skills in organizational settings are presented in Box 22–8.

## Guidelines for Communication

Often a person is not directly aware of personal communication blocks in professional relationships. Asking for feedback and engaging in self-reflection give the nurse an honest appraisal of

---

◆ Box 22–8. Examples of Unclear Communication Processes that Block the Development of Cooperative and Receptive Influencing Skills

| Situation | Communication Process |
|---|---|
| Low self-disclosure | No one knows my real thoughts, feelings, and needs.<br>Consequently:<br>I think no one cares about me or recognizes my needs.<br>Others see me as self-sufficient and are unaware that I have a problem.<br>Consequently:<br>Others are unable to respond to my needs. |
| Reluctance to delegate tasks | Other people think I don't believe that they can do the job as well as I can.<br>Consequently:<br>The others work at a minimum level.<br>I don't expect or ask others to be involved.<br>Consequently:<br>Other people don't volunteer to help me.<br>Consequently:<br>I feel resentful, and others feel undervalued and dispensable. |
| Making unnecessary demands | I expect more from others than they think is reasonable.<br>Consequently:<br>I feel the others are lazy and uncommitted, and I must push harder.<br>Other see me as manipulative and dehumanizing.<br>Consequently:<br>Others assume a low profile and don't contribute their ideas.<br>Consequently:<br>Work production is mediocre.<br>Morale is low.<br>Everyone, including me, feels disempowered. |

---

personal communication strategies in professional situations.

## Using a Focused Opening Statement

Most people will respond better when there is an opening statement giving the receiver of the message an overview of the issue to be discussed. This is given in general terms without initially getting into detailed specifics or tangential issues. Such an overview can be accomplished by using an initial focus statement capturing the essence of the communicated message. For example, a nursing student might approach an instructor to discuss problems with the development of a care plan with the focus statement "I'd like to discuss my care plan with you, more specifically, how to individualize my behavioral objectives before I start my next care plan." This type of statement is preferable to an interpersonal approach that shows little forethought (e.g., "I'm not sure what you want from me on this care plan").

## Considering the Ego of the Other Person

The empathy discussed in previous chapters plays an equally important role in reciprocal communications with other professionals. It is useful to find out what the other person's communication style is like before choosing a strategy. For example, some people prefer written communication to verbal discussion, whereas others respond better with more informal interaction. Knowing something about the values and issues of the other person allows the nurse to tailor responses and positions with language and actions clearly recognizing the other person's concerns. It is a more subtle but extremely important element of successful professional communication.

Another aspect of ego consideration in professional dialogue is the potential emotional impact your comments about certain issues may cause in the receiver. Comments requiring a specific interpersonal change in behavior and negative commentaries on behavior can affect the self-esteem of the receiver. Even when the critical statements are valid (e.g., "You do . . ." or "You make me feel . . ."), they should be replaced with "I" statements that define the sender's position. Otherwise, the meaning of the communication will be lost as the individual strives to defend the self against a personally felt attack.

Similarly, statements and attitudes discounting the value of the person can prevent one from achieving professional objectives. For example, verbal expressions using dogmatic language or derogatory adjectives, violating confidences, interrupting a conversation, and asking loaded or offensive questions usually diminish the other person's feelings of personal power and self-esteem. Nonverbal behaviors, such as lateness or withdrawal, serve to disconfirm the importance of the other person.

To be effective, verbal and nonverbal activities should serve a useful purpose in interprofessional dialogue. Otherwise, they can and do stimulate needless hostility on the part of the receiver and, in the end, sabotage the legitimate goals of the communication. Any behavior that makes an individual feel small or less significant is counterproductive.

### Keeping Your Options Open

There is power in keeping your options open in interprofessional dialogue, in not getting so locked into an either/or type of discussion. Having more than one option usually gives both the sender and receiver a greater feeling of flexibility and personal control in responding. It allows the person to respond rather than to react.

The best way to keep your options open is to consider the issue from a variety of perspectives and to listen. Talking situations through with an impartial, trusted colleague or mentor beforehand decreases anxiety and allows the person initiating the dialogue an opportunity to look at the issues from more than one perspective.

The second step, approaching the dialogue with an open mind about which path to take, increases the probability of developing a more satisfactory solution. Approaching a person as a mystery waiting to unfold is useful in that the final answers may be quite different from what either of you might have projected as possibilities. Finally, deliberately choosing words or behaviors that help the other person feel respected as an equal and valuable member of the health team usually strengthens the communication process.

## Professional Work Groups

Throughout a professional nursing career, nurses are involved in peer work-related groups of one kind or another. Multiple group membership is a fact of life in most organizations. Groups found in organizational settings take the form of standing committees, ad hoc task forces, and quality circles to accomplish a wide range of tasks related to the goals of the organization. Nurses traditionally use task and support groups for goal accomplishment in health care settings.

### Work (Task) Groups

Every organization develops permanent and temporary group structures to accomplish its mission. In work groups, just as in therapy groups, there are two main elements: content and process. By contrast with therapy groups, task group content is predetermined by an assignment or charge given to the group. Work groups center their attention on a task to be accomplished or the resolution of difficult interpersonal issues specifically related to the professional work setting.

Emotional issues except as they relate to the accomplishment of group goals are not addressed. Successful groups make this distinction because a work group is not designed to be a personal growth or therapy group. Personal growth may be an important by-product of task accomplishment, but it cannot become the primary concern of the group. Failure to understand the differences between the purposes of a work group and a therapeutic group can be a disruptive side track for the group and a personally devastating experience for individual group members.

## Leadership Style

Flexibility of leadership style is an essential characteristic of successful work groups. Effective leadership develops from leader characteristics, situational features, and member needs in combination with each other. Successful leadership in one group situation does not guarantee similar success in other group situations (Sullivan & Decker, 1997). Different groups require different leadership behaviors. Leadership is contingent on a proper match between a group situation and the leadership style.

The three basic types of leadership styles found in groups are authoritarian, democratic, and laissez faire. Of the three leadership styles, the authoritarian style is the most structured.

Leaders demonstrating an **authoritarian leadership** style take full responsibility for group direction and control group interaction. Dissenting opinions are squelched. The leader makes little attempt to encourage team effort, and decision making is accomplished through authority rule. Authoritarian leadership styles work best when the group needs structure and there is limited time to reach a decision. Most mature groups resist an authoritarian leadership style.

**Democratic leadership** involves members in active discussion and decision making. The leader encourages open expression of feelings and ideas while providing support and encouragement. Democratic leaders are goal directed but allow flexibility in how group objectives and goals are met. In general, a democratic leadership style offers the group structure while preserving individual member autonomy. Member satisfaction is highest in groups with a democratic leadership. A variation of a democratic leadership style is a **participatory leadership** style. Here the group leader maintains final control but actively solicits and uses group member input.

The third leadership style studied is referred to as **laissez faire**. Leaders with a laissez faire style, although physically present, provide little or no structure and essentially abdicate their leadership responsibilities. Group members are free to decide the direction of the group interac-

tion without leader input or structure. Groups with a laissez faire leader are likely to be less productive and satisfying to group members.

## Group Member Responsibilities

Sensitivity to group process and acceptance of personal responsibility as a group member make a person a more effective group participant. Teamwork enhances the probability of goal achievement as well as personal satisfaction with group outcomes and one's own participation (Sheafor, 1991). In a professional work-related group, each group member assumes individual responsibility for the overall functioning of the group and the achievement of group task goals. Effective professional groups need the cooperation of all members. The functional goals in a professional group cannot be dictated by others; they need to emerge from the member roles and responsibilities created in group interaction.

The primary purpose of using a group format to benefit problem resolution is to generate new ideas. A secondary purpose is to involve key individuals directly in clarifying work-related or difficult interpersonal problems and in seeking workable answers to concrete problems. Personal ownership of problem definition and change are essential to successful implementation. Exercise 22–7 is designed to help you focus on your personal involvement as a group member. Building on the assumption that each member is equally responsible for the success or failure of the achievement of the group purposes, the format in Exercise 22–7 can be used as a task or learning contract and re-evaluated at the end of the group task. Using a similar format as you begin membership in a professional group clarifies the nature of the group task and enables you to take personal responsibility for your own actions and learning in a group situation.

## Task Identification in Different Phases

### Pregroup Tasks

Before the group starts, participants should have a clear idea of what the group task commitment will entail in terms of time, effort, and knowledge. Group members should have enough in common to engage in meaningful communica-

◆ Exercise 22-7. **Goals and Objectives in Work Groups**

**Purpose:** To help you identify professional goals in work groups

**Procedure:**

Think of a real or hypothetical work group task related to a clinical or nursing education problem in need of resolution. Answer the following question and be prepared to discuss them in class. Objectives should reflect what you personally hope to achieve as a group participant as well as what you might contribute to the overall group task. Give it some real thought so that you are clear about what you want from the experience and what you have to give to the group.

1. Identify a general goal or goals as they relate to: _____
   Group member _____
   _____

   Group task _____
   _____

   Professional growth _____
   _____

   Supervision (if applicable) _____
   _____

2. Identify short-term objectives, or the steps needed to reach the goals identified previously, as precisely as you can as they relate to the identified group goals and your own professional goals as a member of the group.
   Group member _____
   _____

   Group task _____
   _____

   Professional growth _____
   _____

   Supervision (if applicable) _____
   _____

3. Share your written goals with other members in your group, and include any relevant input from other members.

tion, a willingness to make a contribution to the group solution, and the capability to complete the task. A strong commitment to the group goal is not always a prerequisite because this may develop as part of the group process, but a commitment to engage constructively in the development of a viable solution is essential. Participants with conplementary views rather than the same views on task group issues ensure a more lively discussion and a potentially stronger outcome.

## Forming

Clear goal identification is important because the objectives and specific nature of the group problem will determine the number of members required to accomplish the task. The leader responsible for convening the group explains the group purpose and structural components—time, place, commitment—in detail. Group members take personal responsibility for clarifying and modifying group goals. A task group with vague or poorly understood goals can breed boredom or frustration, leading to power struggles and inadequate task resolution.

### Norming

Member responsibilities are outlined clearly and understood by all members. In general, all data developed within the group context should be kept confidential until officially ready for publication. Otherwise, the grapevine is likely to distort information and sabotage the efforts of the group.

Members need to be held accountable for regular attendance. If administrative staff are part of the group membership, it is essential that they attend every meeting. Few circumstances are more threatening to a work-related group than having a supervisor enter and exit the task group at will.

### Performing

Once norms are in place, attention turns directly to the designated work of the group. Leader interventions should be consistent and well defined. The process the group would use to develop an understanding of the problem is listed next.

1. Description of relevant background and historical data
2. Definition of problem, goal, and task objectives
3. Feedback and refining of problem statement and goals
4. Identification of potential resources and obstacles to goal achievement

Exercise 22–8 provides work group practice. After identification of basic data relevant to the work of the group, the group members begin to analyze possible solutions. Brainstorming is a strategy used to generate ideas quickly. In addition to creating innovative ideas, brainstorming usually is a stimulating and pleasant experience for group members. The following are some guidelines for brainstorming:

1. All ideas are entertained without censure.
2. More promising ideas are tested for legitimacy.
3. For each idea chosen, possible consequences are explored.
4. Personnel and resources are identified (need for and availability).
5. A final group solution is developed.

---

### ◆ Exercise 22–8. **Problem Diagnosis Exercise**

Unless you can define a problem accurately, it cannot be solved. This exercise should be done individually and without consultation with other members. Think of a work-related problem in need of resolution. Define the problem in such a way that the group can work on it successfully with its current resources (i.e., current membership). Complete each question before going on to the next one.

1. Identify the problem you wish to work on. Describe the problem as you see it now.
2. Most problem statements can be rephrased so that they describe two things: the situation as it is now and the situation as you would like it to be (the ideal). Restate your problem situation in both these terms.
3. Define the changes you think you might have to make, as a member of the group, to make your ideal situation become reality.
4. Define the changes you think others in the group might have to be willing to make to make your ideal situation become reality.
5. Describe how you would envision your functioning vis-à-vis other group members to bring about an ideal situation from your perspective so that this group would be most meaningful.

---

Group members are partners in the brainstorming process. The process of pulling diverse ideas together in a group means that each member has a clear understanding of the problem and personal satisfaction of contributing to the group goals. Exercise 22–9 provides practice in the use of brainstorming.

Group formats are particularly useful for facilitating changes in organizational life. Sufficient time and administrative support for proposals are essential components of successful group work. Most of the failed efforts to implement change occur because of a lack of understanding of the processes needed to effect change, insufficient

---

◆ Exercise 22–9. **Brainstorming: A Family Dilemma**

**Purpose:** To increase self-awareness and provide practical experience with the use of brainstorming as a group activity

**Procedure:**

1. Using the format on brainstorming identified in this chapter, consider the following clinical problem:

◆ Mrs. Joan Smith is an 80-year-old woman living in Florida. Her husband recently suffered a stroke, which has affected his speech. All he is able to say to his wife is that he loves her, although he seems to understand her words to him. He is paralyzed on one side. When he tried to get out of bed, he fell and broke his hip, so he is confined to a wheelchair. No longer able to care for him, Mrs. Smith moved to Virginia to be close to her daughter, and Mr. Smith is being cared for in a nearby nursing home. She is living temporarily in her daughter's home, sleeping on the couch because her daughter has a 15-year-old boy and a 3-year-old girl occupying the bedrooms.

   Mrs. Smith visits her husband every day and entertains the idea that he will get well enough that they will be able to return to Florida. She tries to be there at mealtime because she thinks no one will feed him if she doesn't, and he can't eat by himself. Now that the evenings are getting darker, her daughter fears her driving after dark. She hesitates to bring up the idea of selling the house in Florida for fear it will distress her mother. Mrs. Smith is not sleeping at night and seems driven to be with her husband. Her daughter worries that her mother will collapse if she keeps up her current pace. Meanwhile, the house in Florida remains empty, her mother has taken no steps to secure legal advice, and the current living situation is becoming more permanent by default.

2. Divide the group into smaller groups of three to six students depending on class size.
3. Each group should identify a spokesperson to the larger group. Use a flip chart or board to record ideas.
4. Follow the steps described in the format to generate ideas for a practical solution to the Smith family's problem. Allow 15 minutes for the first part of the exercise and 20 minutes for the brainstorming section.
5. Describe your group's solution and give the rationale for your selection.

**Discussion**

1. In the larger group, each spokesperson presents the smaller group's solution to the Smith family's problem.
2. How did your group's answers compare with those of other groups?
3. What did you learn about the brainstorming process as a problem-solving format?
4. What was the most difficult part of the process for your group?
5. As you listen to how other groups implemented the process, what ideas came to mind?
6. How might you use this format in your nursing practice?

administrative support, unclear expectations, and poor communication with those who are affected by the change. Although it is beyond the scope of this text to describe all dimensions of the organizational change process, Box 22–9 summarizes guidelines that nurses can use in groups responsible for developing changes in organizational settings.

**Termination Phase**

Termination in professional groups can be a group experience that all members share when the group task is accomplished and there is no further need for the group, or it can take place for one individual leaving the group. For the single individual leaving an intact group, it is important for that person to know that he or she was valued as a group member. The remaining group members need an opportunity to express their feelings of loss to and about the departing member. If the termination is unplanned and affects the work of the group, the group may need to discuss the matter further after the loss of the member.

Usually it is better to overestimate rather than underestimate the extent of relationship in groups. Although most people will not deny that an important work-related group is ending, they frequently ignore or minimize their feelings about it. It seems harder to acknowledge that important interactions with our peers are ending than it is to admit this with our clients. As a

---

◆ **Box 22-9. Guidelines for Use by Groups Planning Organizational Changes**

1. Clarifying plans
   Make one person responsible for implementation plans.
   Formulate clear, simple, time-bound goals.
   Make specific plans with milestones and outcomes.
   Make plans public.
   Give and solicit frequent face-to-face feedback.

2. Integrating new practices
   Limit the amount of change introduced at any one time.
   Slow the change process.
   Introduce the change to receptive users first.
   Ensure that the rationale and procedure for change are well known.

3. Providing education
   Involve the end users and incorporate their experience.
   Provide "hands-on" training whenever possible.
   Design training from end users' perspectives.
   Train motivated or key end users first.
   Evaluate the effects of training or work practices and end users' attitudes.

4. Fostering ownership
   Ensure that the change improves end users' ability to accomplish work.
   Provide incentives for end users applying the change.
   Specify milestones for obtaining end user feedback.
   Incorporate end user suggestions in the implementation plans.
   Publicize end user suggestions.

5. Giving feedback
   Document and communicate the expected outcomes of the change.
   Ensure frequent face-to-face feedback.
   Identify clear milestones.
   Make sure feedback includes the large organization.
   Acknowledge key successes.

From Schoonover S, Dalziel M. (1988). Developing leadership for change. In Cathcart R, Samovar L (eds.), Small Group Communication: A Reader (5th ed.). Dubuque, IA, William C. Brown, p. 397. Used with permission.

result, it is not unusual for group members to allow one of their peers to leave without saying a genuine good-by.

## SUMMARY

In Chapter 22, the same principles of communication used in the nurse–client relationship are broadened to examine staff conflicts and the nature of communication among health professionals. Similar elements of thoughtful purpose, authenticity, empathy, active listening, and respect for the dignity of others that underscore successful nurse–client relationships are needed in relations with other health professionals. Building bridges to professional communication with colleagues involves concepts of collaboration, coordination, and networking. Modification of barriers to professional communication includes negotiation and conflict resolution. Self-concept changes and evolves with increasing knowledge, life stage crises, and experiences. Self-awareness as a nursing student will be different from that of the beginning nurse. The interpersonal competencies of the new nurse will be different from those experienced by the nurse 10 years later: "for the entirety of our lives we must continually assess and reassess where our responsibilities lie in the everchanging course of events" (Peck, 1978).

Work groups are an important part of organizational life. Although the focus is different from client-centered groups, work groups follow a similar pattern of growth and development.

One needs to recognize self-changes and be able to assess how those changes influence one's professional self in collegial relationship with physicians, nursing supervisors, and peers. This chapter can be reviewed and used throughout one's nursing career because it provides self-assessment exercises and applies self-awareness strategies to enhance the quality of professional relationships. In turn, successful collegial relations strengthen the nurse–client relationship.

## REFERENCES

Adams D. (1995). Teaching the process of delegation. Seminars for Nurse Managers 3(4):171–174.

American Nurses Association. (1994). Registered Professional Nurses and Unlicensed Assistive Personnel. Washington, DC, American Nurses Association.

Arnold E. (1989). Burnout as a spiritual issue. In Carson V (ed.), Spiritual Dimensions of Nursing Practice. Philadelphia, WB Saunders.

Baggs JG, Ryan SA. (1990). ICU nurse-physician collaboration and nursing satisfaction. Nursing Economics 8:386.

Barter M, McLaughlin FE, Thomas SA. (1997). Registered nurse role changes and satisfaction with unlicensed assistive personnel. Journal Nursing Administration 27(1):29–38.

Boucher MA. (1998). Delegation alert! American Journal of Nursing 98(2):26–33.

Brammer L, MacDonald G. (1996). The Helping Relationship: Process and Skills (6th ed.) Boston: Allyn & Bacon.

Chenevert M. (1988). Stat: Special Techniques in Assertiveness Training for Women in the Health Professions (3rd ed.). St. Louis, MO, CV Mosby.

Davidhizar R. (1991). Impressing the boss who criticizes you. Advances in Clinical Care 6(2):39–41.

Davidhizar R, Bowen M. (1988). Confrontation: An underused nursing management technique. Health Care Supervisor 8:1, 29–34.

Dostoyevski F. (1881). In Steele S (ed.), Creativity in Nursing. Thorofare, NJ, Charles B. Slack.

Forte PS. (1997). The high cost of conflict. Nursing Economics 15(3):119–123.

Gibson CH. (1991). A concept analysis of empowerment. Journal of Advances in Nursing 16:354.

Hales A, Karshmer J, Montes-Sandoval L, Fiszbein A. (1998). Preparing for prescriptive privileges: CNS-physician collaborative model. Clinical Nurse Specialist 12(2):73–82.

Johnson SH. (1996). Teaching nursing delegation: Analyzing nurse practice acts. Journal Continuing Education in Nursing 27(2):52–58.

Jones MA, Bushardt SC, Cadenhead G. (1990). A paradigm for effective resolution of interpersonal conflict. Nursing Management 21:64B.

Kalafatich A. (1986). Nursing interfacing with nursing. In England D (ed.), Collaboration in Nursing. Rockville, MD, Aspen Publications.

Keenan GM, Cooke R, Hillis SL. (1998). Norms and nurse management of conflicts: Keys to understanding nurse-physician collaboration. Research in Nursing and Health 21(1):59–72.

Kjervik DK. (1990). Empowerment of the elderly. Journal of Professional Nursing 6:74.

Knaus W, Draper E, Wagner D, Zimmerman J. (1986). An evaluation of outcome from intensive care in major medical centers. Annals of Internal Medicine 104:410.

Kohnke M. (1982). Advocacy: Risk and Reality. St. Louis, MO, CV Mosby.

Mauksch I. (1981). Nurse-physician collaboration. A changing relationship. Journal of Nursing Administration 6:35.

Nobel KA, Rancourt R. (1991). Administration and interdisciplinary conflict within nursing. Nursing Administration Quarterly 15(4):36–42.

Peck MS. (1978). The Road Less Traveled. New York, Simon & Schuster.

Schoonover S, Dalziel M. (1988). Developing leadership for change. In Cathcart R, Samovar L (eds.), Small Group

Communication: A Reader (5th ed.). Dubuque, IL, William C. Brown.

Sheafor M. (1991). Productive work groups in complex hospital units: Proposed contributions of the nurse executive. Journal of Nursing Administration 21(5):25–30.

Stichler JF. (1995). Professional interdependence: The art of collaboration. Advanced Practice Nursing Quarterly 1(1):53–61.

Sullivan E, Decker P. (1997). Effective management in Nursing (4th ed.). Redwood City, CA, Addison-Wesley.

Taylor C, Lillis C, LeMone P. (1997). Fundamentals of Nursing: The Art and Science of Nursing (3rd ed.). Philadelphia, Lippincott-Raven.

Uusral D. (1978). Values clarification in nursing: Application to practice. American Journal of Nursing 78: 2058–2063.

# 23

# Documentation in the Age of Computers

Kathleen Underman Boggs

**OBJECTIVES**

At the end of the chapter, the student will be able to

1. Define computer information systems
2. Describe and document the essential components of a nursing assessment of an individual client
3. Discuss the advantages and disadvantages of various charting formats

4. Describe four charting formats
5. Identify legal aspects of charting
6. Discuss application of basic rules for writing professional forms of documentation
7. Describe and analyze interactions between nurse and client in a written process recording

*Documentation is the key element of communication between the provider of . . . services and the third party payer.*

A. M. Baeten (1997)

❖❖ The process of obtaining, organizing, and conveying information to others in a print format is referred to as *documentation.* Documentation serves four purposes: it provides a record of care received, shows pertinent information about the client's condition and response to treatment interventions, substantiates the quality of care by showing adherence to care standards, and provides evidence for reimbursement. This chapter focuses on emerging computer applications for documentation of nursing care. It discusses some legal implications of documentation and also describes the use of interpersonal process records.

## BASIC CONCEPTS
## Documenting Client Information for Records

Written documentation of client care must be complete and accurate. Standards of documentation must meet the specifications of government, health care agency, professional practice regulators, third-party payers, and the courts (Gryfinski & Lampe, 1990; Lampe, 1985). Every health care agency has its own version of forms to be filled out. For most, written documentation includes a client history (often this data base also includes a summary list of health problems and needs), a client-centered nursing care plan (NCP), daily records of client progress, and evaluation of outcomes. These daily records often run to multiple pages and may include flow sheets, nursing notes, and intake and output forms (which may not become part of the permanent record), and medication records (Table 23–1).

### Computer Information Systems

Computer information systems (CISs) promote entry and storage of all information about each client. CISs allow ease of access, portability of records between in-patient and out-patient agencies, easy retrieval of information, uniform categories of data for quality assurance (utilization review), and aggregation for research purposes. CISs include client data bases, knowledge bases, health care information, and expert systems. The discussion in this chapter focuses on the client data base. In the early 1990s, the U.S. govern-

Table 23–1. **Nine Reasons Nurses Document**

1. To communicate to others what you know about a client to facilitate care planning and delivery
2. To identify individual patterns or norms so that deviation from these is noted as soon as possible
3. To communicate to other caregivers what still needs to be done
4. To show how the planned care interventions have been tailored to the individual so that care outcome can be evaluated
5. To protect yourself and your employer from threats of malpractice
6. To provide a record on which to base the billed cost to the client
7. To provide evidence of acuity to make decisions about staffing
8. To build a client data base to improve care
9. To adhere to standards of care (of JCAHO and other regulatory bodies).

From Iowa Intervention Project 1997. Proposal to bring nursing into the information age. Image 29(3):275.

ment moved toward fostering development of computerized information for storage of client health-related data, including nursing care. Several grants have supported development of methods to classify types and intensity of nursing care interventions.

### The OASIS System

In 1998 and 1999, home care agencies phased in a new taxonomy developed by the Health Care Financing Administration (HCFA). The taxonomy called **OASIS** (**O**utcome and **As**sessment **I**nformation **S**et) was the result of a partnership between Medicare and the home care industry. It requires home health care agencies to monitor and improve outcomes of care. The components of OASIS are essential items for documenting a comprehensive assessment for adult home care patients and measuring patient outcome for agency outcome-based quality improvement.

OASIS data items include the sociodemographic, environmental, support system, health status, and functional status attributes of nonmaternity adult patients and the attributes of health service utilization. OASIS was not developed as a comprehensive assessment tool, and home care agencies need to supplement the assessment items. The items of OASIS have evolved over a 10-year period and are the result of a national research program funded by HCFA and co-funded by the Robert Wood Johnson Foundation.

When this new taxonomy is fully implemented, home health agencies will be required to electronically transmit OASIS data to a designated state site. The state agency will then have the responsibility of collecting OASIS data that can be retrieved from a central repository. These data will provide a national picture of health status, outcome, and cost of Medicare enrollees who require home health care. To learn more, visit HCFA's Medicare web site at *www.hcfa.gov/medicare/hsqb/oasis/hhoview.htm.*

*Contributed by David R. Langford, RN, DNSc.*

## Advantages

Computerized systems reduce redundancy, increase time efficiency, reduce cost, decrease data errors, and force compliance with standards and policies (Hohnloser et al., 1996; Poirrier et al., 1996). An automated system can be more than an electronic patient record. In addition to management of records, it can be used for client education, can send reminders of appointments, can assist the providers of health care with decision-making prompts, monitor medications, and use Internet connections to interface with information resources (Hofdijk, 1996; Safran et al., 1996).

## Disadvantages

At this early developmental stage, there are tremendous problems because multiple types of CISs have been developed using software programs that do not interface, so data cannot be exchanged or pooled (Dolin, 1997). There also is a lack of a commonly accepted, universal language. A system needs to be able to meet the needs of all the staff in different kinds of agencies. Another problem is access to information about clients who obtain care from multiple providers such as the hospital, the home health agency, the primary physician, and the specialists to whom the client has been referred. What agency keeps the computerized record? Do all other agencies have access to it? One potential solution is to develop a Worldwide Web–based format in which client records are stored using "html," so that all providers can have access through the Internet (Giuse & Mickish, 1996; Rind et al., 1997). Another possibility being attempted is use of a "memory card" or a "smart chip health card," which is portable and has a large storage capacity (Engelbrecht, 1996).

## Electronic Patient Record

The use of computers is now the norm in most agencies, if only for billing and appointment purposes. Under managed care's focus on cost containment, agencies are moving away from use of paper documents to streamline data for easy recording and retrieval. Eventually, the adoption of comprehensive computer information systems may simplify routine functions by changing the way information flows through the health care delivery system. For example, after the client's admission to an acute care hospital, the physician's orders entered into the computer are transmitted simultaneously and directly to the pharmacy, the laboratory, and the nursing unit. This hastens communication by making the results of laboratory tests available to care providers as soon as the lab technician makes an entry. Computerized records also permit easy data retrieval for billing and reimbursement. Use of computers for client record keeping is referred to in the medical literature as the electronic clinical record, electronic patient record, or electronic health record. Using computers for charting is discussed later in this chapter.

## Universal Language

As computerized client record systems proliferate, the challenge is to move toward a universally accepted language and classification system that can be modified quickly to accommodate changing care and still meet the multiple needs of the many disciplines involved in delivering health care. An initial step has to be developing adequate common vocabulary so communication can occur. The language has to be comprehensive and applicable across all health care settings. The National Library of Medicine maintains a metathesaurus for a unified medical language. The Joint Commission on Accreditation of Health

Care Organizations (JCAHO), which accredits health care organizations, has developed standards for uniform data for agencies it accredits. The American Nurses Association (ANA) has accepted several different taxonomies to establish common vocabularies for nursing care, which are potentially codable. The National League for Nursing has developed teaching tools to upgrade skills of nurses by familiarizing them with standardized classification systems.

## Coding Systems

For computerization, information needs to be categorized by number. To do this, several *coding systems* have been developed in medicine and in nursing that lend themselves to computer records. Assigning a code to client diagnosis or treatment can aid in direct client care, statistical reporting, automated computer-assisted decision making, scheduling of return visits, and so on. Coded data also assist in conducting research and provide information to standardize length of stay, type of care, and so on. Historically, providers of health care have each had to develop their own applications, because traditional coding systems only synopsize information from the client record and do not provide information about all the client's care. Classification and medical coding systems are described next. This chapter describes systems like International Classification of Diseases-9 (ICD-9), Current Procedural Terminology (CPT), and drug-related groups (DRGs), which are already in wide use. A major drawback for nursing is that they do not measure nursing contributions to client health care. Ongoing modifications are being made by agencies to provide enough detail to meet many specific needs. Figure 23–1 shows how coding allows a

Coding Nursing Practice Provides Information:

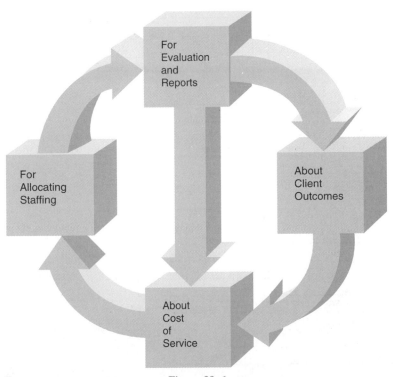

Figure 23–1

client's data to be easily aggregated with other cases to produce a larger picture describing health care delivered by the agency (Cimino, 1996).

**ICD-9 CM Codes.** One of the most common coding systems is the ICD-9 codes or ICPC for primary care. It gives numerical values to record diagnosis and care interventions. ICD-9 codes have been modified by the U.S. Center for Health Statistics to provide more detailed information (ICD-9 CM codes). Generally, diseases are classified according to body system. For example, circulatory diseases all have numbers ranging from 390 to 459. An additional fourth and fifth digit may be added to describe the diagnosis more specifically. For example, hypertensive heart disease is coded 402 but by adding a fourth digit (e.g., 402.1) we further define it as benign, by adding a fifth digit (e.g., 402.11) we know it is benign hypertensive heart disease with congestive failure. Many insurance corporations will not reimburse unless the information is coded to its highest level of specificity.

**CPT.** The American Medical Society developed CPT codes to provide further coding for diagnostic procedures. Figure 23–2 shows an ab-

| PREVENTIVE MEDICINE — ESTABLISHED PATIENT | | | |
|---|---|---|---|
| 9939100 | Under 1 year | 99391 | |
| 9939200 | Early Childhood (1 – 4) | 99392 | |
| 9939300 | Late Childhood (5 –11) | 99393 | |
| 9939400 | Adolescent (12 – 17) | 99394 | |
| 9939500 | 18 – 39 yrs. | 99395 | |
| | | | |
| SURGERY | | | |
| 1012000 | Foreign Body, Removal | 10120 | |
| 1006000 | I & D Abscess | 10060 | |
| 1008000 | I & D Pilonidal Cyst | 10080 | |
| | | | |
| PROCEDURES | | | |
| 9466400 | Aerosol or Vapor Inhalation | 94664 | |
| 9300000 | Electrocardiogram, Complete | 93000 | |
| 9255100 | Hearing Test, Pure Tone | 92551 | |
| | | | |
| IMMUNIZATIONS | | | |
| 9070200 | DT | 90702 | |
| 9070100 | DTP | 90701 | |
| 9074400 | Hepatitis B (NB to 11 yrs.) | 90744 | |
| 9074600 | Hepatitis B (adult) | 90746 | |
| 9072400 | Influenza | 90724 | |
| | | | |
| LABORATORY | | | |
| 8052400 | CBC | 85024 | |
| 8001900 | Chem 24 | 80019 | |
| 8016620 | Digoxin Level | 80162 | |
| 8294700 | Glucose Serum | 82947 | |

Figure 23–2. Sample CPT codes; partial example of coding sheet. I&D, incision and drainage; DT, diphtheria, tetanus; DTP, diphtheria, tetanus, pertussis; CBC, complete blood count.

breviated example. The reimbursement process for billing third-party payers such as private insurance companies and government Medicaid-Medicare programs relies on these codes to quantify the type of care. The chart must provide sufficient information about a diagnosis so that the insurance company computer accepts the diagnostic test as relevant and necessary for reaching a correct diagnosis. For example, if a digoxin level was ordered by a provider (CPT code 8016620), this would be appropriate related to a diagnosis with a ICD-9 CM code of 402.11 for hypertension with congestive failure, but would not be appropriate or reimbursable for a diagnosis code 345.9, which is the code for epilepsy.

**DRGs.** These were orginally developed for use in prospective payment for the Medicare program. DRG coding provides a small number of codes for classifying client hospitalizations based on diagnosis and severity of illness (Cimino, 1996).

**Nursing Codes.** Like others in health care, nursing must be able to demonstrate the value and effectiveness of care. In the past, nursing has been unable to establish a cost for its contributions to client care. Nowhere on a client's hospital bill does the cost of nursing care appear. It traditionally has been part of the "room charge."

The diagnostic and billing codes just described were derived from the medical community and do not contain number codes for many nursing activities, such as variations of patient teaching or case management. Society demands that costs be better controlled and that health care resources be better managed and controlled. The nursing profession has been very active in developing coding systems for classification of nursing care. If nursing cannot classify care, it will not be recognized and reimbursed. The ANA reported on data bases to support nursing clinical practice as early as 1994. Use of computers allows for entering data and retrieving needed information. To do this successfully, nurses must universally develop and use a common vocabulary of standard terms.

**Nursing Minimum Data Sets.** To develop a unified nursing language, several projects in the United States and internationally have developed nursing minimum data sets (NMDS). NMDS includes three categories: service items like client demographics, nursing care, and services pro-vided. Nursing care elements includes nursing diagnoses, nursing interventions, outcomes, and level of intensity of care (a measure of the time required for the nursing care) (Blewitt & Jones, 1996).

### Advantages

Potential advantages of implementation of NMDS would be improved access to care, better documentation of nursing care, development of a method to establish the cost of nursing care, and improved quality assurance (McLeay, 1998). By linking all categories to representative numbers, nursing activities could be computerized. Computerized charting by its nature is more difficult to chart improperly (Gravely & Brick, 1997).

### Disadvantages

Some nurses have expressed concern that we will lose the richness of individualized care if nurses are forced to conform to preset, codable activities. Confidentiality is another important issue. Cautions about the need to guard client confidentiality and privacy are expressed by many (Graveley & Brick, 1997; Thadkurdas et al., 1996). Whenever there are multiple users, there are risks that they or others may access confidential information. This is particularly true for computerized data but also is a concern with any data transmitted by telephone line, such as information sent by FAX. For computers with a central server, security safeguards include requirements for passwords, preset log-on time limitations, and internal computer system safeguards to prevent tampering with data.

### Nursing Care Plan

Historically, nursing care plans were designed to promote continuity of care and improve nurse-to-nurse communication about client treatment. They were used as short summaries of client care to assist nurses in communicating about nursing interventions for the client. Once client health problems were identified in the form of diagnoses, problem lists, and so on, goals for desired client outcomes were developed. These were recorded in the plan of client care. These care plans were generally discarded after discharge rather than being filed as a part of a permanent record.

In recent times, the plan of care is often incorporated into a comprehensive documentation system such as that described in the sections on the OASIS or the Omaha systems or the section on Critical Pathways.

## Assessment and Care Data Base

As with nursing care plans, the trend is to incorporate the client assessment into comprehensive types of client data bases that organize information into codable categories. Logical organization of assessment information is essential to specifying the types of interventions that can be made effectively. Use of an assessment guideline derived from a holistic model leads the nurse to collect complete data before implementing the other steps of the nursing process.

The term *nursing assessment* implies that the nurse conducts a systematic inquiry into the client's past and present health status. The five assessment activities include collecting data, validating data, organizing data, identifying patterns, and communicating this assessment. If the entire agency uses the same format, paperwork is simplified. Basing this assessment on a sound framework, such as one developed by a nurse theorist, ensures that the information-gathering phase will be comprehensive and will proceed in an organized manner. The final result will be the compilation of a data base containing enough information to identify problems, make appropriate diagnoses, plan interventions, and evaluate client outcomes.

Documentation of assessment data facilitates care by sharing client information with all those giving care to the client. JCAHO, the organization that accredits many agencies, in the past required that nurses repeat information recorded by the physician. Now documentation may consist merely of completing and updating an intake history form supplied by the agency.

Communication skills are the essential tools nurses need to compile a client data base, which can be understood by nurses and others. A nursing data base begins with a client assessment but is usually far more comprehensive than the type of information collected by physicians using a body systems format. It often includes psychosocial information, coping strategies, family function information, and so on. Explaining the purpose of the data base, the information that is needed, and the manner in which the information will be used helps the client respond in a more meaningful way to the short-answer questions on a data base form. Box 23–1 lists information commonly included in a nursing data base.

## Nursing Diagnoses and Problem Lists

One early effort to promote a standard common vocabulary for nurses to communicate was the use of a nomenclature system for identifying client diagnoses. Nursing diagnoses label actual or potential client conditions (response to health or illness) that professional nurses are able and legally responsible to treat. Thus, diagnoses describe a clinical judgment and define the nurse's

---

◆ **Box 23–1. Elements of Comprehensive Client Assessment Data Base**

1. Demographic information identifying the client's name, age, sex, marital status, and family constellation; primary language, occupation, social support relationships with significant others, cultural or religious preferences that might impact on care

2. Information about prior health status (medical history)

3. Information about current problems, concerns, stressors, or alterations in current health status, as perceived by the client or client's family (e.g., current comfort status; other information about coping patterns, developmental needs, health maintenance behaviors; problem-solving methods also included

4. Objective observations by the nurse about the client's current physiological and psychosocial status, including activity level, ability to perform self-care, health needs and goals, and level of understanding of health status; data base usually, but not always, includes information obtained from the nurse's physical examination

5. A written list of client health problems, nursing diagnoses, or other summary of the nurse's analysis of the assessment data

practice. Potentially, they also provide data for reimbursement purposes. The nursing process provides a basis for nursing practice. As a part of nursing process, nursing diagnosis gives direction for activities of therapeutic nursing intervention (Duespohl, 1986). Within nursing, there several systems of classification are used. It remains to be seen which one will be universally adopted.

**North American Nursing Diagnosis Association.** The North American Nursing Diagnosis Association (NANDA) has developed more than 100 standardized terms to describe information about the client as a nursing diagnosis. Initially, this system was primarily designed to classify the problems of hospitalized ill clients, but later work expanded nursing diagnoses to include community. In fact, some efforts are being made toward developing diagnoses for individual, family, and community (Janken, 1998). A nursing diagnosis is not another name for a medical diagnosis. Rather, it delineates areas of independent nursing functions. When the primary intervention must be initiated by a physician, the nursing actions are collaborative, secondary interventions, including monitoring and managing physician-

prescribed interventions (Carpenito, 1992). A sample of some of the 100 NANDA diagnoses is provided in Table 23–2 with the intent of generating enough material for application in the accompanying learning exercises. The reader should refer to books on nursing diagnoses, some of which are listed at the end of this chapter, for complete information on the use of nursing diagnoses. Writing nursing diagnoses takes practice. Exercises 23–1 and 23–2 are designed to provide experience in writing diagnoses that are relevant to client relationships.

### Advantages

Nursing diagnoses can save time by improving communication among staff members. They ensure consistent care in the writing of nursing care plans, charting nursing notes, retrieving client data, conferring with health team members or giving oral reports, and communicating with community health care agencies for follow-up services (Tartaglia, 1985).

### Disadvantages

Lack of completeness has been a continuing problem. A number of nurses have expressed

**Table 23-2. Sample Nursing Diagnoses**

Nursing diagnosis problem statement relevant to interpersonal relationships

Directions: when writing a diagnostic statement for an actual nursing diagnosis (which describes a human response the nurse can treat), the nurse should use the PES formula: Stating the *Problem*, the *Etiology*, and the *Symptoms* or signs of risk factors that validate the diagnosis. Take any of the case studies in this book and practice writing a diagnosis.

Example: impaired verbal communication related to inability to speak English as manifested by inability to follow instructions in English and verbalizing requests in Spanish (Alfaro, 1990).

**SAMPLE DIAGNOSES**

Re: interpersonal relationships
  Altered parenting associated with . . .
  Social isolation related to . . .
  Altered role performance related to . . .
Re: cognitive functioning—sensory-perceptual alterations
  Visual sensory alteration associated with . . .

Re: coping patterns
  Ineffective individual coping related to . . .
  Ineffective family coping: compromised . . . (specify)

sexual dysfunction
altered family processes related to . . .
parental role conflict associated with . . .

Altered thought processes associated with . . .

From NANDA. 1996. Nursing Diagnoses: Definitions and Classifications. Philadelphia, North American Nursing Diagnosis Association. Used with permission.

◆ Exercise 23-1. **Charting Nursing Diagnoses**

**Purpose:** To clarify diagnoses

**Procedure:** Discuss in small groups which of the following examples help provide a direction for independent nursing interventions.

*Example 1*
Incorrect: inability to communicate related to deafness
Correct: social isolation related to limitations in communication secondary to deafness, as evidenced by refusal to interact with other clients

**Discussion:**

1. What additional information is provided in the correct diagnosis?
2. Why would the first statement be incorrect? Are all people who are deaf unable to communicate?

*Example 2*
Incorrect: acute lymphocytic leukemia
Correct: pain during ambulation related to leukemic process as evidenced by limping, grimacing, and increased pulse

**Discussion:**
Could a nurse make any independent intervention based on the information provided by the diagnosis ``acute lymphocytic leukemia''?

◆ Exercise 23-2. **Developing Nursing Diagnoses**

**Purpose:** To increase familiarity with phychosocial nursing diagnoses

**Procedure:**

1. Take each of the standard diagnoses listed in Table 23-2 and write a second component to tailor it to a specific client with whom you have worked. Some examples are:

   a. Impaired verbal communication . . . (associated with Japanese spoken as a first language)
   b. Moderate anxiety . . . (associated with separation from kin)
   c. Chronic low self-esteem . . . (related to profound sensory impairment

2. In a group or dyad discussion, compare your statements with those of other students.

**Discussion:**
What can the listener tell you about the client just from reading a diagnosis written by another nurse? What is the most difficult aspect of writing diagnoses? What problems were identified that were not easily found among the listing of accepted diagnoses?

VISITING NURSE ASSOCIATION OF THE MIDLANDS SKILLED VISIT REPORT

H.H.# 59241   Client Name Earl, Esther   Date 11/17/99   Time 2:00 a.m. (p.m.)   Unscheduled ( ) Explain

Homebound Due to dyspnea w/amb, on $O_2$ cont.   Compromised cv status

INTERVENTION SCHEME CATEGORIES

I. Health Teaching, Guidance, and Counseling
II. Treatments and Procedures
III. Case Management
IV. Surveillance

TARGETS

01. Anatomy/physiology
02. Behavior modification
03. Bladder care
04. Bonding
05. Bowel care
06. Bronchial hygiene
07. Cardiac care
08. Caretaking/parenting skills
09. Cast care
10. Communication
11. Coping skills
12. Daycare/respite
13. Discipline
14. Dressing change/wound care
15. Durable medical equipment
16. Education
17. Employment
18. Environment
19. Exercises
20. Family planning
21. Feeding procedures
22. Finances
23. Food
24. Gait training
25. Growth/development
26. Homemaking
27. Housing
28. Interaction
29. Lab findings
30. Legal system
31. Medical/dental care
32. Medication action/side effects
33. Medication administration
34. Medication set-up
35. Mobility/transfers
36. Nursing care, supplementary
37. Nutrition
38. Nutritionist
39. Ostomy care
40. Other community resource
41. Personal care
42. Positioning
43. Rehabilitation
44. Relaxation/breathing techniques
45. Rest/sleep
46. Safety
47. Screening
48. Sickness, injury care
49. Signs/symptoms-mental/emotional
50. Signs/symptoms-physical
51. Skin care
52. Social work/counseling
53. Specimen collection
54. Spiritual care
55. Stimulation/nurturance
56. Stress management
57. Substance use
58. Supplies
59. Support group
60. Support system
61. Transportation
62. Wellness
63. Other (specify)

| CLIENT PROBLEMS (Circle #) | SUBJECTIVE/OBJECTIVE | CAT | TARG | RX | INTERVENTIONS/COMMENTS |
|---|---|---|---|---|---|
| ENVIRONMENTAL: (12) Emotional stability | Bland affect. Talked about rel. w/ mother — deceased 1 yr ago. (upset that 20 yr. son planning marriage — thinks he's too young. | I | 49 | | Allowed to vent feelings, active listening. |
| PHYSIOLOGICAL: 21. Speech and language: | | | | | |
| 24. Pain: | | | | | |
| 26. Integument: Lesion Depth Diameter Drainage | | | | | |
| 27. Neuro-musculo-skeletal function: | | | | | |
| 28. Respiration: $O_2$ @2ℓ per nc cont. Rate 22 Resting clear Activity Lung sounds clear | SOB w/walking. Doesn't like to use wc. See data base | | | | |
| (29) Circulation: Pulse 78 Apical Radial R 168/70 Pedal Lying Sitting Standing | ↑edema in ankles. ↑ascites 12# wt.↑. States has ↓ activity which has caused ↑ in s/s & wt. | IV III | 50 31 | | Will report s/s to MD for fu |
| Edema 2 + ankles Weight 243# Temp. | | | | | |
| 30. Digestion-hydration: | | | | | |
| 31. Bowel function: | | | | | |
| 32. Genito-urinary function: Incontinent ( ) (Other) | | | | | |
| HEALTH RELATED BEHAVIORS: (35) Nutrition Intake | c/o ↓ appetite  Diff w/fluid restriction | I | 37 | | Reviewed food diary. Disc ↓ Na+ foods |
| 38. Personal hygiene: HHA SUPERVISORY VISIT POC ( ) Appropriate ( ) Inappropriate | | | | | |
| 41. Health care supervision MD Visit Date | See data base | I | 32 33 | | |
| (42) Prescribed med(s): Know  Comply Lasix (Yes) No  Yes (No) Lanoxin (Yes) No  (Yes) No | | | | | |
| 43. Technical procedure | | | | | |

Assessment ↑ s/s requiring medical fu. Interested in learning about diet, meds. s/s depression evident

Plan: Frequency and Reason RV 1 wk to cont. surv & teaching. Report to MD & set up appt.

Signature Susan Stevens, CSN4   RN   LPN   RPT   OTR   SP   MSS   Employee #

Figure 23-3. Example of the Omaha System.

CLIENT FAMILY NAME  Earl, Esther

HOUSEHOLD NUMBER  59241

### INTERIM NOTES

| DATE | |
|------|---|
| 11/17/99 | TC to Dr. Brian Allen. Reported ↑ edema, ascites & wt. Made app't |
| | to see her in his office  11/19/99 at 10:30 am.  Susan Stevens CSN4 |
| 11/17/99 | Tc to pt. to inform of MD app't.  Says she will be able to go – will |
| | have friend Ann take her.                    Susan Stevens CSN4 |

**Figure 23–3** *Continued.*

frustration with categorizing client problems that did not seem to fit easily into a standard diagnosis. NANDA did accept "wellness diagnoses" that reflect the client's positive adaptation to a situation. However, the greatest problem has been that nursing diagnoses were never incorporated into clinical records and data bases maintained by health care agencies. Further work has been done to develop a comprehensive and validated taxonomy of nursing diagnoses (McLeay, 1988).

**The Omaha System of Client Problems.** In the late 1970s and 1980s, the Omaha classification system was developed to meet the needs of community health nurses. It is a comprehensive client record amenable to computer record keeping because it uses codes and standard names. There are four levels of problem classification. Level 1 defines the area or domain of concern: environmental, psychosocial, physiological, or health related. Level 2 identifies and classifies the problem by number. Level 3 modifies or further defines the problem by describing who owns it and what risk factors exist. Level 4 lists symptoms and category of intervention and describes extent of client outcome (ranging from 0, continual problems, to 5, sustained successful intervention). For further information, consult appropriate references, in particular *The Omaha System* (Martin & Scheet, 1992) for sample charting forms. Refer to Figure 23–3 for an example of this format.

### ◆ Case Example

Jody S., age 24 years:

Level 1, domain: physiological

Level 2, problem 24: pain 1 day postoperative

Level 3, modifier: individual, actual

Level 4, signs/symptoms: 01, expressed complaint incisional pain; 03, guarding; 05, facial grimaces

Category and target for intervention scheme: category II, treatment (2 Tylenol #3) & IV surveillance (reassess in 1 hour).

Outcome status: 05, no signs/symptoms pain; 06, re-evaluate in 4 hours.

## Clinical Pathways

**Clinical pathways** are a more comprehensive documentation system using standardized plans of care. Each specific disease or procedure has a standard path developed by an interdisciplinary team. The path describes expected care for each day and also permits the nurse to record care given. They are discussed in greater detail later in the chapter when charting is discussed.

## Nursing Interventions Classification and Nursing Outcomes Classification

The trend has been to evaluate outcomes of health care. To reduce cost, unnecessary care must be reduced. This requires that outcomes of different types of care are identified. Once client data are coded and computerized, comparisons of outcomes can be made. In the 1990s, it became apparent that nursing care needed to be a part of these large data sets (Maas et al., 1996).

**Nursing interventions classification** (NIC) was developed as a standardized language describing direct and indirect care that nurses perform in all settings relevant to illness prevention, illness treatment, or health promotion. NIC can be used in conjunction with a standardized list of diagnoses (NANDA) or problems (Omaha). NIC has three levels of classification: 6 client domains, 27 classes, and more than 400 nursing interventions, as shown in the following case example (Henry, 1997). These interventions also can be used in conjunction with nursing outcomes classification (NOC).

### ◆ Case Example (Adapted from Henry, 1997)

Joe, 1 day postoperation for heart valve replacement

Domain: physiological

Class:

Intervention:

    Label: airway management

    Definition: facilitation of patency

    Activities: instruct how to cough effectively; monitor respiration q4h; assess oxygenation q4h.

Findings from a study by Henry and associates (1997) suggest that NIC is superior to CPT for categorizing nursing activities because it describes nursing activities more fully.

NOC was developed in an effort to identify and measure how nursing care affects client outcomes. Client states that are more affected by nursing care are called "nursing sensitive outcome indicators."

### Advantages

NIC-NOC measures nursing care so that it becomes visible and defines professional practice. It helps develop realistic standards of care. Potentially you could set the desired level of achievement for your client based on your initial assessment and then measure his or her actual level of achievement. Your agency could use this classification system to bill for your nursing care. This system is more universally adaptable to both inpatient and out-patient settings than some other systems (Iowa Intervention Project, 1997).

### Disadvantages

NIC-NOC needs to gain acceptance by the business interests who manage health care. Use requires advanced, expensive technology not yet in place in many agencies. Another difficulty is that client outcomes for a nursing intervention may not occur immediately. For example, teaching about a health promotion activity, like changing to a low cholesterol diet, may not result in client outcome for many months.

## Charting Formats for Documenting Nursing Care

Charting is one of the most common forms of written nurse-to-other communication. This documentation is also the key element of communication between care provider and third-party payer (Baeten, 1997). All agency contact with clients is documented in some written or electronic format, including the individual's office file, hospital chart, or clinic record. Quality care depends on finding a complete, accurate, and easily used charting system. Charting practices that worked in the 1980s and 1990s will not be useful in the new century. Health care, perhaps driven by managed care concepts, is moving to paperless charting. Although the electronic patient record is becoming the norm, current systems are flawed. The perfect charting system has yet to be developed.

According to Smith and Duell (1989), there are three purposes for charting: (1) communication with the health team; (2) provision of a permanent client record for future reference (a possible legal document should litigation occur); (3) provision of a record of employee performance, which assists supervisory personnel to evaluate day-by-day staff performance. Next to direct care, charting is one of the nurse's most important functions.

JCAHO has revised standards for nursing care delivery. These revised standards were designed to provide agencies with guidelines that would help ensure higher quality, more cost-effective care. These standards affect broad areas of nursing practice, including documentation, by establishing criteria for charting client care. In the past, nurses spent up to 40 percent of their time collecting and documenting client information (McHugh, 1986). Recent literature is filled with articles advocating more streamlined forms of charting. According to JCAHO, written nursing notes no longer need to restate information listed elsewhere in the client's chart.

### Traditional Narrative Charting

Narrative charting is defined as a chronological record of events happening to the client. Traditional charts of the past typically contained separate sections for each source from which information was obtained. For example, data from the laboratory would be found in a section of the chart marked "Lab." Likewise, information about nursing care would be in a section called "Nursing Notes." Generally, nurses using the narrative format wrote chronological notes each shift, as depicted in the following example.

---

◆ **Case Example**

0700   Morning care given. Appetite good. K. Boggs, RN

1100   To x-ray for chest film. Tom Mark, LPN

1400   Reviewed medication information in anticipation of discharge tomorrow. Visitors in; no complaints. K. Boggs, RN

---

Because the narrative format was inefficient and time consuming and did not focus on the client's health problem, it is no longer routinely used. Instead, the narrative nurse's note is used to describe only a specific deviation in assessment or care.

### Problem-Oriented Record

**Problem-Oriented Record Using the SOAP Format.** In the 1970s, problem-oriented charting format was developed by Dr. Weed, a physician. The problem-oriented record (POR) focused on the client's identified list of health problems. A problem list was intended to be developed by the health team, but typically the identified problems are medical diagnoses (Griffiths, 1989). In POR, nurses refer to the problem list and chart their observations by referring to the listed problem by number or name or both. Information about the client's progress in each problem area was documented only when some measurable change occurred.

A specific format (called SOAP) is used to record data relevant to each problem. The first part of the four-step suggested method of documentation lists all the client's subjective comments (*S*) relevant to the identified problem. The second section lists all the current objective information (*O*) noted by the nurse. Then comes the nurse's analysis or problem assessment (*A*) of the client's current progress. Finally, there is a list of the nurse's intended future interventions or plans for care (*P*).

### ◆ Case Example

Problem 4: Alteration in skin integrity: decubitus related to immobility as evidenced by excoriation and drainage.

S:  I think my leg looks better today. It doesn't hurt anymore.

O:  4 cm × 2 cm excoriation on outer aspect of left thigh. App. 2 cm of serous drainage noted on old dressing. Sensitive to touch. Unable to note skin color due to purple staining from gentian violet treatments. Peripheral area red and puffy.

A:  Less drainage than yesterday, less peripheral inflammation noted; healing decubitus.

P:  Continue applications of 1/2-strength $H_2O_2$ and NS every 4 hr. Apply gentian violet every 8 hr; cover with DSD, monitor for signs of infection. 1400: K. Boggs, RN

### Advantages

SOAP notes focus on the status of the client's progress in terms of identified problems.

### Disadvantages

There is a tendency to focus on medical diagnoses and there is difficulty in maintaining interdisciplinary contributions, although psychosocial problems may be documented in the same manner (Lampe, 1985). Exercise 23–3 gives practice in using the POR format.

**Problem-Oriented Record Using PIE Format.** An expanded variation of the SOAP format containing additional information about implementation interventions and evaluation of outcome is known as SOAPIE, or PIE for short. In this version, charting information is as follows: (P) = the plan (goals), (I) = the interventions, and (E) = an evaluation of outcome.

### ◆ Case Example (Iyer, 1991)

| 1/15/94 | 1000 | S: "I have abdominal pain." |
| | | O: grimacing, rubbing abdomen. |
| | | A: abdominal pain. |
| | | P: medicate for pain. |
| | | I: Demerol 75 mg, IM, RD. |
| | | K. Boggs, RN |
| | 1045 | E: verbalized relief of pain. |
| | | K. Boggs, RN |

### Focus Charting

*Focus charting* is readily understood by nurses and is adaptable to many settings (Iyer, 1991). It is similar to the POR except that the "focus" does not have to be limited to a clinical problem—it also lists strengths. A focus may be a sign or symptom, a nursing diagnosis, a behavior, a condition, a significant event, or an acute change

---

### ◆ Exercise 23–3. **Utilization of Nursing Diagnosis in POR Charting Formats**

**Purpose:**  To provide practice developing a relevant nursing assessment using a POR charting format

**Procedure:**  Take the sample nurse's notes provided in the section on ''Traditional Narrative Charting'' and convert the information to a problem-oriented format.

**Discussion:**
Discuss the advantages and disadvantages of each approach. Which documentation provides the greatest clarity? Identify the nursing diagnosis in each example. Discuss whether the nursing diagnosis should be assessed in the *A* section of SOAP.

in condition. This charting method, by listing a focus, is designed to provide a quick description of the client's current status. This is a brief statement about what is happening to the client. The SOAP is replaced by DAR: *D*ata, *A*ction, and *Re*sponse.

The nurse charts information in columns. The left-hand column, "Data," lists all subjective and objective assessment information, patient behaviors, patient status, and nursing observations to substantiate the problem or strength (the focus). In the next columns, "Action" includes the nursing plan and interventions and the nursing orders for the identified focus, and "Response" includes all evaluations and information indicative of the client's response to the interventions (Driedger & Dick, 1988; Lampe, 1985, 1990; Lucatonto et al., 1991). A nursing care plan would be in a similar format, listing the focus and then the expected client outcomes. This method is supplemented by a client data base, flow sheets, graphs for vital signs, and check lists because only relevant data are selected for documentation. The focused charting method streamlines documentation in some cases and has the advantage of capturing the critical thinking and decision-making process of the professional nuse (Driedger & Dick, 1988; Lampe, 1985, 1990).

---

### ◆ Case Example (Iyer, 1991)

| | |
|---|---|
| 1/15/94 | Pain |
| | D: grimacing, c/o burning-abdomen |
| | A: Demerol 75 mg, IM, Rt.D. |
| | R: verbalized relief of pain. |
| | S. Solomon, RN |

---

### Advantages

In one study, the use of focus charting saved 90 minutes of registered nurse time in a 24-hour period, a 36 percent reduction (Lucatonto et al., 1991), whereas another study found a 73-minute (per 8-hour shift) time savings (Griffiths, 1989).

### Disadvantages

This technique is not used by medical staff. There are legal questions regarding the lack of comprehensiveness.

## Charting by Exception

***Charting by exception*** began in Milwaukee in 1983. It is based on a system of predetermined standards of care protocols. It requires that staff have a clear understanding of standards of care. Although this method evolved from the POR, it is well suited to use with clinical pathways or other standards of practice protocols. Charting by exception uses flow sheets with predefined assessment and client progress parameters, based on written standards (Charles, 1997). The nurse then charts by initialing the flow sheet for normal findings. "Rather than charting all of the individual steps of your nursing care, you initial the necessary protocols, and your initials indicate that you performed all of the required interventions in the required way" (Stearly, 1997, p. 61). Only abnormal or significant deviations, called exceptions, are charted in a long-hand descriptive format.

**Flow Sheets.** Flow sheets are graphs with preprinted categories of information. For example, in assessing lung sounds, the nurse needs to merely check or circle "clear" if that information is normal. Deviations from norm must be charted either in narrative notes or some space on the form designated for this information. In some agencies, flow sheets containing assessment information are kept at the client's bedside, including the vital signs and intake graphic record, nursing-physician order sheet, and patient teaching records (Murphy et al., 1988). These flow sheets include a column for recording narrative notes in the event of an abnormal finding.

### Advantages

This technique can be efficient and time saving.

### Disadvantages

Charting by exception does not allow for qualitative information or for variation. If you fail to perform even one step of the protocol, you are guilty of falsifying the client's record. Legal decisions in the early 1990's found that nurses using the charting by exception method to be negligent by virtue of items not charted (Stearley, 1997).

**Clinical Pathways–Critical Pathways.** The trend toward more streamlined, meaningful charting is exemplified in clinical paths. This is a comprehensive tool, whose goals are to provide a structured tool for planning the highest quality of care; encourage interdisciplinary communication; decrease the time spent charting, because you are charting by exception; focus care on expected client outcomes; and facilitate quality assurance evaluations (Aronson & Maljanian, 1996). Most agencies give the client a copy of the pathway at the time of admission, so he or she understands what is expected each day (Fig. 23–4). For example, Short (1997) described a six-day pathway for postoperative recovery and discharge for clients in her institution, which is given to the client admitted for total hip replacement. Thus, the pathway becomes a teaching tool for client education and to measure quality. Unlike POR, the pathway is truly an interdisciplinary tool. It allows the entire health team to monitor the client's progress compared with a standard time frame for progress. A variance or exception occurs when a client does not progress as anticipated or an expected outcome does not occur. A variance is a red flag, alerting staff of a need for further action to assist the client. Computer software packages are available that transform pathway data into a codable format for reimbursement, quality assurance, and aggregation for research about client outcomes.

### Advantage

By providing a concise method for documenting routine care, nurses direct attention to abnormal or significant findings rather than spending time detailing normal findings. Murphy, and associates (1988) reported a 44 percent decrease in registered nurse documenting time and a 53 percent drop for the licensed practical nurse. Short (1997) found that charting by exception integrated with clinical pathways took on average 0.82 hours per shift in charting time compared with other forms, which required up to 2.5 hours. Fewer pages are needed for each record. Data are easily retrievable. In another study, use of pathways reduced hospital stay for total hip arthroplasty by nearly 3 days, reduced delays in testing and rehabilitation, and reduced cost by 8.5 percent (American Academy of Orthopedic Surgeons, 1997).

### Disadvantages

This technique is labor intensive to develop; it requires "buy-in" by physicians and nursing staff, because in the current malpractice climate nurses tend to repeat flow sheet information in the "Nursing Notes" section.

## Computer-Assisted Charting

Computer-assisted charting facilitates the recording of nursing notes. At a video monitor located in the nurse's station or in client care areas, each nurse enters his or her own identification number and then enters data into the client's computer file. Most systems use a mouse or light pen and standard groupings or categories of client care information. When the operator points the pen at the correct phrase displayed on the video terminal, data are entered into an individual's computer "chart." The nurse displays entries and makes corrections before storing data in the client's permanent computer record. Because the computer has preset pathways, the nurse needs to learn the correct sequence for entering data. However, once skill is developed in using the system, computer charting considerably reduces the nurse's volume of written work (McHugh, 1986).

### Advantages

Computer-assisted charting results in reduced workload; uniformity of charting, because the computer will only allow one to chart in the way in which it has been programmed; and clarity and legibility because all entries are typed. Paper print-outs can be made anytime the nurse desires. Up-to-the minute care plans and medication orders are available to each nurse at the beginning of and during his or her shift. Each person, including the student nurse caring for a client, can print out his or her own copy of the current orders, plan of care, and so on. In addition to saving time, with computer-assisted charting, specific categories of client care are listed and may be selected. These categories act as a prompt to the nurse to ensure that the nursing notes are complete.

### Disadvantages

A delay may occur between administering medication and recording it on the computer. There are also risks to confidentiality. Power system failures can make client records inaccessible for the period of time that the computer is "down."

Patient Name _____

DRG# _____

Date _____

Expected LOS _____ <23 hours

| | Preprocedure | Preoperative | Intraoperative | Postoperative Phase I PACU | Postoperative PHASE II PACU | Discharge | Postoperative PHASE II PACU |
|---|---|---|---|---|---|---|---|
| Medication | Review medical history | Start IV | Administer meperidine | Administer naloxone, flumazenil pm | Pain med prm | Start on Rx omeprazole | Continue medications |
| Diagnostic tests | H & P chest x-ray, ECG, blood work | Review tests | Endoscopy procedure | None, unless complications | None | None | None |
| Diet | Regular | NPO | NPO | NPO | Clear liquids & progress | Regular | Regular |
| Activity | Not restricted | Ambulate | None | Turn, cough, and deep breathe | Increase activity to ambulation | Normal ambulation | Not restricted |
| Nursing action | Assessment | Vital signs | Vital signs, O₂ saturation | Vital signs, level of consciousness, O₂ saturation | Monitor as before | Prepare for discharge | Follow-up evaluation via phone |
| Teaching/ Discharge planning | Phone call | Patient education about procedure | Transport to PACU | Discharge when Aldrete criteria I met | Discharge when Aldrete criteria II met | Instructions reviewed | Phone call for follow-up |

Figure 23–4. Clinical pathway for endoscopy. DRG, diagnosis-related group; LOS, length of stay; PACU, postanesthesia care unit; IV, intravenous; prn, as needed; H&P, history and physical; ECG, electrocardiogram; NPO, nothing by mouth; O₂, oxygen. (From Monahan FD, Neighbors M. [1998]. Medical-Surgical Nursing: Foundations of Clinical Practice, 2nd ed. Philadelphia, WB Saunders, p. 116.)

## Other Electronic Devices

**Portable Computers.** Some home health agencies are using laptop or notebook computers for recording clinical data.

**Tracker System** (Contributed by Anne Hakenewerth, MS, Director of Health Informatics, University of North Carolina Charlotte). The Nightingale Tracker System is one of several systems being developed that help document client information electronically. This system gives nurses in the community the ability to collect client data electronically while in the client's home. The nurse carries a small, user-friendly handheld computer. This device has a touch sensitive screen, so the nurse can enter information using a finger or penlight. The device contains a custom-designed client data base that is based on the Omaha system of clinical vocabulary. Before seeing clients for the day, the nurse copies to the device any already existing information about the client from a central server via a standard telephone line. During a home visit, new nursing notes are charted into this device. At the end of the day, the nurse plugs the device into a telephone line and copies the data back to the central server. All client records are thus archived in a central, secure location. In addition to documenting client records, this device can receive electronic mail, FAX, or voice mail; send reports to physician offices; and download drug or health care information from the Internet.

**Mobile Telephones and Pagers.** Mobile call telephones provide easy access back to the agency, to the client's primary physician, and so on. Some community nurses prefer pagers, which notify them of telephone messages so they can return calls. Other electronic devices used for communication about client status include modems, which allow a home health nurse to transmit client data directly over a telephone to the computer system of the primary provider, similarly to a FAX. For example, some devices directly transmit the client's uterine contractions to the primary provider via modem and telephone line. In another example, a device has been developed that allows the client with asthma to transmit respiratory function information (peak flow readings) across a telephone line directly to the physician's office.

**Automated Decision Support.** With the advent of computerized client information systems, another potential asset is the development of computerized "clues" or prompts to assist in clinical decision making. One example is the computer program for medication dispensing used by pharmacists. All the medications prescribed for a specific client are stored in the data base. When a new drug is entered, the program not only alerts the provider about whether the prescribed dose exceeds maximum standard safety margins but the program also cross-compares the new medicine with those the client is already taking to check for potential drug interactions (Forsstrom, 1996).

## Documentation: JCAHO Standards

Any of several charting systems is acceptable to regulators at JCAHO, but the agency must demonstrate consistency across similar units. All charting, regardless of method, must address the client's current status according to a prioritized needs list. Beginning in 1995, JCAHO shifted emphasis in documentation to focus on client outcomes of care. For example, in a rehabilitation facility "medical records must provide evidence of ongoing reassessment of patient's response to treatment, change of condition, degree of goal attainment and patient status relative to discharge planning" (Dunovan, 1997). Documentation must show that assessment was used to identify need for care, response to care, and response to medication (Chase, 1997).

## Legal Aspects of Charting

Management literature emphasizes the need for less repetitive, less time-consuming methods of documentation, which reflects the nursing process. At the same time, all documentation must be legally sound. The legal assumption is that the care was not given unless it is documented in the client's record (Fiesta, 1991a; NSO Risk Advisory, 1997; Stearley, 1997). Malpractice settlements have approached the multimillion-dollar mark for individuals whose charts failed to document safe, effective care. Aside from issues of legal liability, third-party reimbursement depends on accurate recording of care given. Major insurance companies audit charts and contest any charges that are not documented in the written record.

**If It Is Not Charted, It Was Not Done.** This statement stems from a legal case (Kolesar v. Jeffries) heard before Canada's Supreme Court, in which a nurse failed to document the care of a client on a Stryker frame before he died. Because the purpose of the medical record is to list care given and client outcomes, any information that is clinically significant must be included. Legally all care must be documented. As Cone (1996) stated, "Since documenting is fundamental to continuity and quality of care, care delivered but not documented is, from a legal perspective, care not done." Gravely and Brick (1997) noted that juries are skeptical when nurses claim to remember what happened but was not charted 4 to 8 years ago, which is the average time it takes for a case to go to trial.

Any method of charting that provides comprehensive, factual information is legally acceptable. This includes graphs, check lists, and all of the types of charting discussed earlier in this chapter. "Long, narrative paragraphs should be a necessary part of charting only infrequently and in exceptional circumstances" (Fiesta, 1991a, p. 17). However, by initialing a protocol, the nurse is documenting that every step was carried out. If a protocol exists in a health care agency, you are legally responsible for carrying it out (Stearley, 1997).

**Errors.** Corrections to the medical record should be made in such a way that the incorrect information is still legible and never obliterated. In the preferred method of correction, the nurse draws a line through the incorrect entry and adds his or her initials and the date. Additions to existing charting, even if added shortly afterward, are not a problem in the courtroom. Additions that occur after the defendant has been notified that the client is contemplating legal action are difficult to defend in court.

Table 23–3 lists some recommended rules for charting to keep you legally safe. For further information, Fiesta (1991b) provided an excellent overview of the legal process involved in malpractice claims. Alternatively, contact your national professional agency such as the American Nurses Association's Marketing Division for a copy of *Liability Prevention and You—What Nurses and Employers Need to Know.* Table 23–4 lists common charting mistakes to avoid

**Table 23–3. Charting Rules**

**CONTENT**

Chart promptly but never ahead of time.
Document complete care.
Document noncompliant behavior and the teaching-information you gave the client, and the reason.
When care or medicine is omitted, document action and rationale: who was notified and what was said.

**FORMAT**

Use black or blue ink or appropriate computerized entry system.
Use military time.
Use correct spelling and grammar.
Do not leave blank spaces.

Compiled from Bergerson SR. (1988). More about charting with a jury in mind. Nursing '88 18:51–56; Iyer P. (1991). Thirteen charting rules. Nursing '91 21(1):40–44; Iyer P. (1991). Six more charting rules. Nursing '91 21(2):48

(The NSO Risk Advisor, http://www.nso.com/common.html).

**Written Orders.** Nurses are required to question orders that they do not understand or those that seem to them to be unsafe. Failure to do so puts the nurse at legal risk. "Just following orders" is not an acceptable excuse.

Persons licensed or certified by appropriate government agencies to conduct medical treatment acts include physicians, advanced nurse practitioners (nurse practitioners), and physician assistants. These providers have their own prescribing number and must abide by government rules and restrictions. One of the restrictions has been a requirement that the responsible physician must cosign within a given period of time. Another restriction example is that nurse practitioners in most places cannot prescribe controlled substances unless they obtain a Drug Enforcement Agency number. Consult your agency policy regarding who is allowed to write client orders for you to carry out.

**FAXing Orders.** The physician or practitioner may choose to send you a FAXed order. Because this is a form of written order, it has been shown to decrease the number of errors that occur when translating verbal or telephone orders. However, FAXing can pose a threat to client confidentiality. To safeguard this, some

Table 23-4. **Charting Mistakes to Avoid**

1. Failing to record complete, pertinent health information
2. Making subjective conclusions rather than recording objective data. (Do not describe the client in derogatory terms. Clients have a legal right to read their record if their lawyer obtains it, and angry clients are more likely to sue.)
3. Not charting in a legible manner, or erasing or using White-Out to obliterate comments
4. Using incorrect or obscure abbreviations
5. Making "untimely" entries (i.e., charting after the fact, later than past the end of your day)
6. Failure to record drug information and administration
7. Not recording all nursing actions
8. Recording on the wrong chart
9. Failing to document a discontinued medication
10. Failing to record outcome of an intervention such as a medicine
11. Not documenting a change in the client's condition
12. Advertising incident reports in the Nurses' Notes. (Do not attach a copy to the chart.)

Data from NSO Risk Advisor. (1997). http://www.nso.com/common.html; Bergerson SR. (1998). More about charting with a jury in mind. Nursing '88 18:51–56.

recommendations include keeping the FAX machine in a private area, having one designated person to monitor incoming transmissions, sealing the orders in an envelope before delivering them, obtaining a legal release before sending out any client records.

**Verbal Orders.** Many times a change in client condition requires the nurse to telephone the primary physician or hospital staff resident to obtain new orders. The nurse transcribes these verbal orders onto the order sheet, adding a notation that these are verbal orders (v.o.). Legal requirements specify a time frame by which the physician, nurse practitioner, or physician assistant must personally sign these. Most primary providers work in group practices, so it is necessary to determine who is "on call" or who is covering your client when the primary provider is unavailable. It may be necessary to call for new orders if there is a significant change in the client's physical or mental condition as noted by vital signs, lab value reports, treatment or medication reactions, or response failure. Before calling for verbal orders, obtain the chart, familiarize yourself with current vital signs, medications, infusions, and other relevant data.

With the growth of unlicensed personnel, there is greater likelihood that a verbal order will be relayed through someone with this status. The legality is vague, but basically if harm comes

to the client through miscommunication of a verbal order, the licensed nurse will be held accountable.

◆ **Case Example**

Tracy, the secretary on your unit, answers the telephone. Dr. U. gives her an order for a medication for a patient. Tracy asks him to repeat the order as soon as she gets a registered nurse to take the call. If you cannot answer the telephone immediately, have her tell him you will call back in 5 minutes to verify the order.

**Charting for Others.** It is not a wise practice to chart for others, although sometimes you may be required to cosign an entry.

◆ **Case Example**

Juanita worked day shift. At 6 P.M. she calls you, says she forgot to chart Mr. Reft's preoperative enema and asks you to chart the procedure and his response to it. Can you just add it to your notes? In court this would be portrayed as an inaccuracy. The correct solution is to chart "1800: Nurse Diaz called and reported. . . ."

## Written Communication with Other Professionals

Just as primary physicians, consultants or specialists, dietitians, social workers, and others use the *progress notes* in the client's chart to communicate with each other, nurses have developed a number of methods of communicating about client status in addition to the chart and the nursing care plan.

A professional nurse is called on daily to communicate with other professionals in some type of written format. Written communication has several advantages over other forms of communication. Written text provides a potentially permanent record of information and may diminish miscommunication. The natural tendency to distort verbal messages or forget components over time is alleviated when there are written records to refer to, particularly when the topic being discussed is complex or when the communication is directed at larger groups of people.

A number of types of written documentation may be used to improve communication with nurse colleagues within the agency or to supplement verbal communication mechanisms (i.e., shift reports and staff meeting reports). Some examples are memos, communication books, minutes from staff meetings, and professional newsletters.

In dealing with colleagues in an organization, Claus and Bailey (1977) advised nursing leaders to improve their chances of being understood by combining spoken words with other forms of communication, including memos, letters, and other written messages. They identify prerequisites for effective formal communication. First, the sender of the message must have credibility by having demonstrated trustworthiness, positive regard for others, and consistency. Second, the message must be composed in such a way as to be understandable to the recipients. Finally, the sender needs feedback to verify that the message was correctly interpreted.

Rules for written communication vary with the type of situation. The three principles of written communication are (1) be accurate, (2) be brief, (3) be complete. As with the acquisition of psychomotor skills or problem-solving skills, development of competent writing skills requires extensive practice. Most school curricula offer many opportunities to develop and improve basic writing skills. However, many of us require additional practice with professional writing before we feel comfortable as well as proficient. Box 23–2 lists some tips for written communication.

---

◆ **Box 23–2. Guidelines for Written Communication**

1. Use the format appropriate to the situation, one familiar to the individuals with whom you are communicating.
2. Use vocabulary or terminology at a level the intended recipients understand.
3. Avoid unnecessary jargon and abbreviations.
4. Be clear; use exact dates and times.
5. Use correct grammar and spelling.
6. Try to organize your message logically (introduction, rationale, content, conclusion).

---

# APPLICATIONS
## Computer Literacy

To practice nursing in coming years, it is clear that all nurses will need to become proficient in use of computers for data entry, word processing, obtaining information from the Internet, and perhaps even using spread sheets.

## Professional Publications

Nurses, like members of other professions, are obligated to contribute to the body of the discipline's knowledge. In part, this contribution is made through publication in professional journals.

## Documenting Client Information for Learning: Interpersonal Process Records

Frequently in a relationship interactions occur that either help or hinder the progression of the relationship. Often, however, we remain unaware of exactly what helped move us along or what disrupted communication. The written ***interpersonal process record*** is a tool to help analyze interpersonal communication.

A process record helps you synthesize communication theory by applying concepts to clinical situations. Over a period of time, this activity leads to an increased sensitivity to one's own communication strengths and weaknesses. It may also promote an increased acceptance of one's own thoughts and feelings. It involves active participation of the learner, closely followed by an opportunity to interpret the effectiveness of the process.

There are three essential parts to the process record. First, a written anecdotal record is made of both the client's words and the nurse's words along with notes about their nonverbal behavior. Second, a written analysis of the interaction process is done, identifying specific communication skills and interventions used. This analysis is an evaluation of the effectiveness of the nurse's communication skills in fostering the goals of the interaction. The goal of analyzing a process record is to promote use of more effective nursing interventions, so the third component of the process is to add written suggestions for making more effective comments. The writer suggests alternative communication responses that might enhance the therapeutic interaction. Focus is placed on better strategies to help the client solve problems. At the very least, analyzing a conversation can help the nurse determine which communication techniques work and which are ineffective, perhaps finding clues to psychosocial factors that influence the interaction. These may help identify any recurring communication patterns and enable the nurse to discover why certain intervention strategies do not work.

Educators often recommend sharing the written process record with a more experienced professional. An objective reader is often able to discern patterns the learner does not see. The reader may also be able to help the learner by critiquing the written record's analysis and suggesting more effective communication strategies.

Use of the written process record is an effective but time-consuming process. To obtain maximum benefit from this learning tool, the nurse needs to record a series of nurse–client interactions, conduct a self-analysis, and obtain feedback for each interaction from a reader. Confidentiality must be maintained at all times to protect the client and the therapeutic nature of the nurse–client relationship. Anonymity can be ensured on the process record by using only client initials rather than full names and by omitting identifying demographic information.

## Instructions for Using Process Records for Learning

To be able to review an interaction objectively, it is necessary first to record the content of the conversation. Figure 23–5, which illustrates one standard format for listing this information, may be photocopied for use. The written process record is designed to be used after the nurse has finished interacting with a client. Some experts suggest that notes be taken during the conversation. Writing while talking, however, may be extremely disruptive to the conversation as well as to the overall nurse–client relationship.

A better approach is to find a quiet, private spot as soon after the interaction as possible and to write down the content of the interaction. An example of this content is provided in columns 1 and 2 of Figure 23–6. Because this form is a tool for learning, space is provided for self-analysis of the therapeutic components of the interaction. Any interaction between a nurse and a client can be recorded and analyzed to learn better communication skills. As Travelbee (1971) noted, "No nurse is without some degree of skill in being able to purposefully use the communication process; neither is any nurse a communication expert in the sense that she cannot develop further skill."

A form similar to that shown in Figure 23–5 can be used to list interpersonal interactions. The process record should contain some information about the client and location, such as the client's initials and the data of the interaction. The immediate preceding event should be listed, such as medication for pain with a strong narcotic, which might affect the way the client responds.

A complete listing should be made of all comments. Notes about tone of voice may also be made. This record should be as accurate as possible. The nurse should resist the natural inclination to edit or "improve" the comments made to the client. The list should record the conversation in the order in which it occurred. Although the nurse may forget some of the words used, he or she should strive to make as accurate a recording as possible. Because it is often difficult to recall extensive information, limit the actual interaction to be described on the process recording to 10 to 15 minutes.

Because nonverbal behaviors can significantly affect the nature of a communication, all relevant

INTERPERSONAL PROCESS RECORD

Student's Name ——————————————  Client's Initials ——————————————
Process Record # —————————————  Background Information ——————————
Date & Time of Interaction ——————  ————————————————————————
Setting ————————————————————  ————————————————————————

| Client | Nurse | Analysis |
| --- | --- | --- |
|  |  |  |

Figure 23–5. Interpersonal process record.

nonverbal behaviors exhibited by either the nurse or the client are also listed along with verbal responses. Of particular interest are comments about the nurse's thoughts and feelings during the interaction. The nurse should describe his or her "gut-level" responses during the course of the interaction—whether he or she felt comfortable, uncomfortable, helpless, or knowledgeable—by making comments in parentheses (see column 2 of Figure 23–5).

The last column in Figure 23–5 is for analysis of the content and meaning of the interaction. After careful reflection, the nurse should write an interpretation of each of the statements made by the client and the nurse's response. Each specific communication skill should be identified along with the rationale for using it and a critique of its effectiveness. Commentary about transitions in the conversation, such as the rationale for changing the subject, should be entered. A brief analysis of identified predominant emotions should be recorded in the third column as well as any conscious and perhaps unconscious feelings held by the client or nurse during the interaction. Note the effects of client or nurse values, such as age difference or reli-

gious orientation, on the course of the conversation.

The nurse then makes an overall summary, evaluating the process of interaction and the effectiveness of the nurse's interventions. Possible alternative interventions should be listed that, in retrospect, might have more effectively accomplished client or nurse goals for the interaction. This brief summary may also contain information about any factors or client needs that might affect the future course of the client–nurse relationship. For example, a consistent behavior pattern of lateness may indicate the need to focus on underlying feelings about the relationship.

Some of the most effective learning may occur as a result of analysis of less-than-perfect responses. Column 2 of Figure 23–6 clearly reveals errors made by the nurse during the course of the interaction. Many individuals have commented that some of their best learning has occurred when they "bomb." It is potentially threatening to write up comments that may not reveal ourselves in a favorable light. This is particularly true for students when an instructor reads the process record and makes comments on it or

Date: 1/18/94–9:23 A.M. Intake Interview in Clinic, private exam room. Mrs. S's second visit for weight reduction.

| Client | Nurse | Analysis |
|---|---|---|
| Hello, Ms. Foy. | Hi, Mrs. S.<br>I brought you those booklets on dieting I promised you. | |
| Thank you. | I'd like to spend time today talking about them with you. | Establishing trust |
| I've been on every diet published in every magazine. I gain on them all. | You have tried dieting several times before? | Tried to clarify |
| Yes, I've had a weight problem for five years. Diets don't help.<br>(loud voice, sad face) I get disgusted with them after two or three weeks. | You've had trouble actually losing weight on these diets? | Paraphrased to verify |
| Yes, I'd like to be slimmer. For years I pictured myself as a lump in a bathing suit but every time I resolve to diet, I end up stuffing myself. I always reward myself with a treat when I've had a hard day at work like I'm a big nothing . . . just a weak-willed slob. (started crying) | You find dieting discouraging. (attentive posture)<br><br>(I began to feel uncomfortable when she got off into these negatives) | Reflection<br>Silence |
| | Well, I see it upsets you. Let's review these booklets now. I have a lot to cover today. | Acknowledgment of nonbehavioral feelings but changed subject. My own anxiety led me to focus on my own needs. |
| No comments. (avoided eye contact, slumped in chair) | Mrs. S., you look like this conversation is getting you down. Maybe we should talk about how you're feeling and discuss the exchanges later. You've mentioned that being overweight makes you feel bad about yourself. What is it about the weight that bothers you most? | Attempt to salvage discussion by refocusing on client's problem<br><br>Open-ended question to facilitate communication. |
| I find it most depressing to fail on a diet because of the way it makes me feel, but I also can't accept not fitting into a size less than 16. | Okay, Mrs. S., I think I have a better idea of how you feel. You feel equally bad being overweight and failing to successfully lose weight on a diet.<br>To help me better understand your usual eating patterns, I'd like you to fill out this daily record of food intake. With each meal entry, also list a rating of 1 to 10, bad to good, of how you feel.<br>Next week when you come for your appointment, we'll go over this notebook together and look for clues to help you succeed in losing weight. | Summarization |
| Thanks, I'll be glad to try something constructive. Good-by. | (I felt great!) | Summary<br>Figured I'd really turned around a bad situation. Her mood change let me know I might be on the right track. (1) She needs to develop insight into her eating patterns. (2) Participating in the process of selecting her diet may be a more effective plan than teaching exchange groups. |

**Figure 23–6.** A sample process recording. This example illustrates beginning-level student analysis appropriate for a communications course. A more in-depth analysis would be expected of an advanced student practicing in a psychiatric clinical setting.

◆ Exercise 23-4. **A Process Record**

**Purpose:** To provide the student with practice in writing process records

**Directions:**

1. Conduct a 10-minute interaction with a client.
2. Photocopy the format in Figure 23-5 to write the actual interaction as soon as possible after your contact with the client. Fill in any needed data about the client, time, or place of the interaction. Identify your goal for the interaction: what you intended to accomplish. Then fill out only the first two columns, listing raw data (i.e., all the comments made by both the client (column 1) and the nurse (column 2) in the order in which they occurred). Some inaccuracies will naturally occur, but try to write as faithful a record as you can recollect. In parentheses, note nonverbal behaviors obvserved in the client or any feeling you recall that accompanied your conversation with the client.
3. After recording all the raw data, begin your analysis (column 3). Read through each exchange between you and the client (usually, initially, an exchange constitutes only one or two sentences from each of you). The analysis should be guided by the purpose for doing the process recording. Essential components usually are development of communication skills and identification of client problems requiring nursing assessment and intervention.

   a. Identify each communication skill used.
   b. Describe your rationale for using each skill in your responses. Suggest alternative skills for areas in which the listed skill did not achieve the desired results.
   c. Describe relevant feelings not previously identified in Column 2, particularly if they are related to your choice of the next intervention.
   d. Make comments about what you think went on in the process of the conversation. List any opinions, tentative interpretations, or hypotheses you can make about the recorded behavior. In particular, highlight your interpretation of the client's behavior. Apply principles from communication theory to help identify the underlying process/ that occurred during the interaction.
   e. Conclude with a statement summarizing those aspects in the process that seem relevant for your future interactions with the client. For example, certain inferences made from this record may need to be checked or validated with the client in your next interaction.

grades it. However, a reader's critique is based not on right or wrong answers but on the writer's ability to analyze the interactive process correctly and insightfully to apply concepts from communications theory. The amount of learning will depend on the nurse's willingness to be vulnerable, especially in regard to the ability to perceive accurately deficits in his or her communication skills. Exercises 23–4 and 23–5 are provided to give practice in writing process records and to help you further your understanding of process records.

## SUMMARY

Chapter 23 focuses on the use of written communication in the nurse–client relationship. Documentation refers to the process of obtaining, organizing, and conveying information to others in a written format. Three areas of content are discussed: written tools used in developing communication skills, transcribed documentation of the nursing process, and the reporting of client information in professional records. Learning to write process records, to chart accurately, and to

◆ **Exercise 23-5. The Interpersonal Process: Related Concepts**

**Purpose:** To help you analyze interpersonal responses in process records. The process recording is an effective tool for developing increased awareness of process problems and use of communications skills. Alternatively, audio or video recordings may accomplish the same purpose. The following exercise may be used to supplement process records or may be used alternately with process records.

**Directions:** Answer the following questions after completing a nurse–client interaction.

1. Were your goals or objectives for the interaction achieved?
2. To what extent were they not achieved?
3. Cite evidence to document that your objective was achieved. (This is usually in the form of a behavioral change noted in the client.)
4. Identify why some goals were not achieved.

    a. Were your goals realistic?
    b. Were they mutual goals or just your goals as a nurse?

5. Were any client goals achieved or needs fulfilled?
6. What were your preconceptions or feelings before this interaction? To what extent did they affect the outcome of the interaction?
7. What did you learn about the client that you were not aware of before?
8. What particular communication skills were you uncomfortable using? Which were ineffective?
9. What new nursing diagnoses or client problems did you identify after this interaction?

provide clear written communication to other health professionals is an essential component of successful nurse–client relationships.

## REFERENCES

Alfaro R. (1990). Applying Nursing Diagnosis and Nursing Process: A Step-by-Step Guide (2nd ed.). Philadelphia, JB Lippincott.

American Academy of Orthopedic Surgeons. (1997). News release: Clinical pathways cut costs for total hip arthroplasty. Available at http://www.aaos.org.

Aronson B, Maljanian R. (1996). Critical path education: Necessary components and effective strategies. Journal of Continuing Education in Nursing 27(5):215–219.

Baeten AM. (1997). Documentation: The reviewer perspective. Topics in Geriatric Rehabilitation 13(1):14–22.

Bergerson SR. (1998). More about charting with a jury in mind. Nursing '88 18:51–56.

Blewitt DK, Jones KR. (1996). Using elements of the nursing minimum data set for determining outcomes. Journal of Nursing Administration 26(6):48–56.

Carpenito LJ. (1992). Handbook of Nursing Diagnosis. Philadelphia, WB Saunders.

Charles EJ. (1997). Charting by exception: A solution to the challenge of the 1996 JCAHO's nutrition care standards. Journal of the American Dietetic Association 97(Suppl 2):S131–S138.

Chase SK. (1997). Charting critical thinking: nursing judgments and patient outcome. Dimensions of Critical Care Nursing 16(2):102–111.

Cimino JJ. (1996). Review paper: Coding systems in health care. Methods of Information in Medicine 35:273–284.

Claus KE, Bailey JT. (1977). Power and Influence in Health Care. St. Louis, MO, CV Mosby.

Cone KJ, Anderson MA, Johnson J. (1996). Documentation of assessment in the emergency department. Chart 93(1):9.

DeMilliano M. (1997). Eight Common Charting Mistakes to Avoid. Available at *http://www.nso.com/common/html*.

Dolin RH. (1997). Outcome analysis. MD Computing 14(1):50–56.

Driedger LS, Dick J. (1988). Patient focused charting. Canadian Journal of Nursing Administration 1(2):20–22.

Duespohl TA. (1986). Nursing Diagnosis Manual for the Well and Ill Client. Philadelphia, WB Saunders.

Dunovan KA. (1997). Review of Documentation Requirements to Meet Joint Commision Standards. Topics in Geriatric Rehabilitation 13(1):61–71.

Dykes PC, Wheeler K. (1997). Planning, Implementing and Evaluating Critical Pathways. New York, Springer.

Engelbrecht R, Hildebrand C, Brugues E. et al. (1996). DIABCARD—an application of a portable medical record for persons with diabetes. Medical Informatics 21(4):273–282.

Fiesta J. (1991a). If it wasn't charted, it wasn't done. Nursing Management 22(8):17.

Fiesta J. (1991b). Legal procedure. Nursing Management 22(7):12–13.

Forsstrom JJ. (1996). Linking patient medication data with laboratory information system. International Journal of Bio-Medical Computing 42(1–2):111–116.

Graveley EA, Brick J. (1997). Security and legal issues associated with the computerized patient record. Seminars in Perioperative Nursing 6(2):87–93.

Griffiths A. (1989). Focus charting in rehabilitation. Rehabilitation Nursing 14(3):142–148.

Gryfinski JJ, Lampe SS. (1990). Implementing focus charting, process and critique. Clinical Nurse Specialist 4(4): 201–205.

Guise DA, Mickish A. (1996). Increasing the availability of the computerized patient record. In Proceedings of the AMIA Annual Fall Symposium, pp. 633–637.

Henry SB, Holzemer WL, Randell CR, Hsieh S, Miller TJ. (1997). Comparison of nursing interventions classification and current procedural terminology codes for categorizing nursing activities. Image 29(2):133–138.

Hofdijk J. (1996). The proactive medical record. International Journal of Bio-medical Computing 42(1–2):51–58.

Hohnloser JH, Purner F, Kadlec P. (1996). Coding medical concepts: A controlled experiment with a computerized coding tool. Medical Informatics 21(3):199–206.

Iowa Intervention Project. (1997). Proposal to bring nursing into the information age. Image 29(3):275.

Iyer PW. (1991). New trends in charting. Nursing '91 21(1):48–50.

Janken J. (1998). Personal communication.

Joint Commission on Accreditation of Health Care Organizations. (1991). The New Standards for Nursing Care. Oakbrook Terrace, IL. Author.

Lampe SS. (1985). Focus charting: Streamlining documentation. Nursing Management 16(7):43–46.

Lampe SS. (1990). Focus charting assists the nurse manager. Primary Nursing 9(5):1–2.

Lucatonto M, Petras D, Drew I, Zbuckvich I. (1991). Documentation: A focus for cost savings. Journal of Nursing Administration 21(3):32–36.

Maas ML, Johnson M, Moorehead SO. (1996). Classifying nursing-sensitive patient outcomes. Image 28(4):295–302.

Martin KS, Scheet NJ. (1992). The Omaha System: Applications for Community Health Nursing. Philadelphia, WB Saunders.

McHugh ML. (1986). Increasing productivity through computer communications. Dimensions of Critical Care Nursing 5(5):294–303.

McLeay JE. (1998). Nursing minimum data sets: Are you ready? Available on Internet at http://www.unc.edu/courses/nurs117/evaluation/jmfinal.html.

Murphy J, Belinger J, Johnson B. (1988). Charting by exception: Meeting the challenge of cost containment. Nursing Management 19(2):56–72.

North American Nursing Diagnosis Association. (1996). Nursing Diagnoses: Definitions and Classifications. Philadelphia, author.

Poirrier GP, Wills EM, Broussard PC, Payne RL. (1996). Nursing Information Systems Applications in Nursing Curricula. Nurse Educator 21(1):18–22.

Rind DM, Kohane IS, Szolovits P, et al. (1997). Maintaining the confidentiality of medical records shared over the Internet and the World Wide Web. Annals of Internal Medicine 127(2):138–141.

Safran C, Rind DM, Sands DZ, et al. (1996). Development of a knowledge-based electronic patient record. M.D. Computing 13(1):46–51.

Short MS. (1997). Charting by exception on a clinical pathway. Nursing Management 28(8):45–46.

Smith S, Duell D. (1989). Clinical Nursing Skills (2nd ed.). Los Altos, CA, National Nursing Review.

Stearley H. (1997). Nursing and the Law: An Update on Charting by Exception. Revolution—The Journal of Nurse Empowerment Fall:60–61.

Tartaglia MJ. (1985). Nursing diagnosis: Keystone of your care plan. Nursing '85 15(34).

Thakurdas P, Coster G, Gurr E, Arroll B. (1996). New Zealand general practice computerisation, attitudes and reported behavior. New Zealand Medical Journal 109(1033):419–422.

Travelbee J. (1971). Interpersonal Aspects of Nursing (2nd ed.). Philadelphia, FA Davis.

## Electronic References

http://www.unc.edu/courses/nurs117/evaluation/jmfinal.html. (a formal paper on nursing minimum data sets)

http://www.nursing.uiowa.edu/nic/overview.htm. (information on nursing intervention classification)

http://www.hcn.net.au/clinical. (an education package about clinical pathways; cost $150.00)

http://www.nso.com/common.html. (The NSO Risk Advisor)

http://www.aaos.orq. (information on clinical pathways)

http://www.hcfa.gov/medicine/hsqb/oasis/hhoview.htm. (information on Medicaid charting system, OASIS)

## Suggested Reading

Chase SK. (1997). Charting Critical Thinking: Nursing Judgements and Patient Outcomes. Dimensions of Critical Care Nursing 16(2):102–111.

Comstock LG, Moff T. (1991). Cash effective, time effective, time efficient charting. Nursing Management 22(7):44–48.

France FHR. (1996). Control and Use of Health Information: A Doctor's Perspective. Ireland, Elsevier Science Ltd.

Hartman D, Knudson J. (1991). A nursing data base for initial patient assessment. Oncology Nursing Forum 18(1):125–130.

# Glossary

*(The number at the end of the entry indicates the chapter(s) in which the term is defined.)*

**Accommodation:** A desire to smooth over a conflict through cooperative but nonassertive responses. **(14)**

**Accountability:** Assuming full responsibility for one's actions: for the care given, and for maintaining the necessary knowledge, skills, and competencies to render safe, effective nursing care. **(6)**

**Acculturation:** The natural learning of cultural roles and behaviors, as with little children learning from their elders; the process by which a person learns and accepts the values of a new culture. **(6, 11)**

**Active listening:** A dynamic interpersonal process whereby a person hears a message, decodes its meaning, and conveys an understanding about the meaning to the sender. **(10)**

**Advocacy:** Interceding or acting on behalf of the client to provide the highest quality of care obtainable. **(22)**

**Affective learning:** Emotional learning; changes in attitude that inform and direct behaviors. **(15)**

**Aggressive response:** A response in which the individual acts to defend the self, to deflect the emotional impact of the perceived threat to the self through personal attack, blaming, or an extreme reaction to a tangential issue. **(14)**

**Androgogy:** The art and science of helping adults to learn. **(15)**

**Anticipatory guidance** Helping the client foresee and predict potential difficulties. **(20)**

**Anxiety:** A vague, persistent sense of impending doom. **(5, 20)**

**Aphasia:** A neurologic linguistic deficit; a speech-language pathology that is most frequently associated with neurologic trauma to the brain. **(17)**

**Apraxia:** The loss of ability or the inability to take purposeful action even when the muscles, senses, and vocabulary seem intact. **(19)**

**Assertive behavior:** Setting goals, acting on these goals in a clear and consistent manner, and taking responsibility for the consequences of one's actions. **(14)**

**Authoritarian leadership:** The style in which the leader takes full responsibility for group direction and controls group interaction. **(22)**

**Autonomy:** Decision-making power; the nurse supports autonomy by leaving decision making to the client whenever possible and by supporting the client's decisions unless there is a chance of harm to the client or others. **(4)**

**Avoidance:** Withdrawal from conflict. **(14)**

**Bias:** Generalizations representing expectations and prejudgments about people and behaviors. **(5)**

**Biofeedback:** Immediate and continuous information about a person's physiological responses; auditory and visual signals that increase one's response to external events. **(20)**

**Body image:** The physical dimension of self-concept; thoughts and feelings about one's physical appearance, body parts, movements, and body functions. **(3)**

**Body language:** A system of communication that includes facial expression, eye movements, body movements, posture, gestures, and proxemics. **(9)**

**Burnout:** A state in which a person's physical, psychosocial, and spiritual resources are exhausted. **(20)**

**Caring:** An intentional human action, characterized by commitment and a sufficient level of knowledge and skill, that allows the nurse to support the basic integrity of the person being cared for. **(5)**

**Catastrophic reactions:** Outbursts of a dementia victim that represent an angry, disorganized set of responses in reaction to real or perceived frustration. Warning signs may be restlessness, refusals, or general uncooperativeness. **(19)**

**Charting by exception:** A type of charting in which normal data are charted using check marks on flow sheets, with only abnormal/significant findings, called exceptions, being charted in a long-hand descriptive format. **(23)**

**Circular questions:** Questions that focus on the interpersonal context in which an illness occurs. In contrast, *linear questions* focus on a description of the physical situation. **(10)**

**Clinical pathways:** Documentation systems using standardized plans of care; each specific disease or procedure has a "path" that describes expected care for each day. **(2, 23)**

**Closed questions:** Questions that can be answered with a yes, no, or one-word answer. **(10)**

**Coding systems:** Numerical systems (such as ICD-9, CPT, and DRGs) for recording client diagnosis or treatment. **(23)**

**Cognitive dissonance:** The holding of two or more conflicting values at the same time. **(7)**

**Cognitive learning:** Knowledge obtained from information a person did not have before. **(15)**

**Cohesiveness:** The degree of positive attachment and investment that members have for the group. **(12)**

**Collaboration:** Two or more people working together to solve a common problem and sharing responsibility for the process and outcome. **(22)**

**Communication:** An interpersonal activity involving the transmission of messages by a source to a receiver for the purpose of influencing the receiver's behavior; a complex composite of verbal and nonverbal behaviors integrated for the purpose of sharing information. **(1, 9)**

**Competition:** A response style characterized by domination; a contradictory style in which one party exercises power to gain personal goals regardless of the needs of others. **(14)**

**Complementary relationships:** Relationships that involve unequal distribution of power. **(13)**

**Computer-assisted charting:** Entry of client data into a computer file, most often by selecting from standard groupings or categories of client care information. These "electronic files" are stored in the computer and can be updated and printed out as needed. **(23)**

**Concepts:** Broad comprehensive ideas that serve as building blocks to present key ideas that make up models in a logical and focused manner. *Assumptions* are belief statements that form the basis for developing concepts. *Propositions* describe the relationship between concepts. **(1)**

**Conceptual models:** Mental images or abstract representations of nursing that operate as a frame of reference to describe person, environment, health, and nursing. **(1)**

**Concrete operations period:** Piaget's developmental stage in which a child can play cooperatively and employ complex rules. **(18)**

**Confidentiality:** Respect for another's privacy that involves holding and not divulging information given in confidence, except in cases of suspected abuse, commission of a crime, or threat of harm to self or others. **(2, 4, 5)**

**Confirming responses:** Validation of the client as a person and of the client's thoughts and feelings in the context of the situation. **(10)**

**Conflict:** A mental struggle resulting from incompatible or opposing needs, drives, wishes, or internal demands; a hostile encounter. It may be *overt* (observable) or *covert* (hidden or buried). **(14)**

**Connotation:** The personalized meaning of a word or phrase. **(9)**

**Context:** A person's environment, defined as all of the intrapersonal and interpersonal circumstances influencing client behaviors. **(3)**

**Coordination:** Two or more people providing services to a client or program separately and keeping one another informed of their activities. **(22)**

**Coping:** Any response to external life strains that serves to prevent, avoid, or control emotional distress. **(20)**

**Countertransference:** Personal feelings or attitudes the helping person may feel toward a client that emerge as a reaction to the client's behavior or from the nurse's past life experiences. **(1)**

**Crisis:** A sudden, unanticipated, or unplanned event that necessitates immediate action to resolve the problem. A crisis may be *situational* (an external event or environmental influence) or *developmental* (an internal process that arises in connection with maturational changes). **(21)**

**Crisis intervention:** The systematic application of problem-solving techniques, based on crisis theory, designed to help the client move through the crisis process as swiftly and painlessly as possible and thereby achieve at least the same level of psychological comfort the client experienced before the crisis. **(21)**

**Critical thinking:** A framework for problem solving by which a person can identify and analyze the assumptions underlying the actions, decisions, values, and judgments of themselves and others. **(16)**

**Cultural diversity:** Differences between cultural groups. **(11)**

**Cultural relativism:** The belief that cultures are neither inferior nor superior to one another and that there is no single scale for measuring the value of a culture. **(11)**

**Culture:** Collective beliefs, values, and shared understandings and patterns of behavior of a designated group of people. **(11)**

**Debriefing:** A crisis-intervention strategy designed to help nurses and others process critical incidents in health care, thereby reducing the possibility of symptoms. **(21)**

**Delegation:** The transfer of responsibility for the performance of an activity from one individual to another while retaining accountability for the outcome. **(22)**

**Democratic leadership:** The style in which the leader involves members in active discussion and decision making, encouraging open expression of feelings and ideas. **(22)**

**Denial:** Unconscious refusal to allow painful facts, feelings, and perceptions into conscious awareness. **(8)**

**Denotation:** The generalized meaning assigned to a word. **(9)**

**Dependent nursing interventions:** Nursing actions that require an oral or written order from a physician. **(2)**

**Discrimination:** Situations and actions in which a person is denied legitimate opportunity offered to others because of bias or prejudice. **(5)**

**Distress:** A stress response capable of creating permanent pathological changes and even death. **(20)**

**Documentation:** The process of obtaining,

organizing, and conveying information to others in a written format. **(23)**

**Double-bind communication:** A communication that sends two conflicting messages at once. **(13)**

**Dysfunctional communication:** A communication style in which messages are defensive or distorted and do not inform or enhance communication between people. It usually develops in families suffering from chronic low self-esteem. **(13)**

**Dysfunctional conflict:** Conflict in which information is withheld, feelings are expressed too strongly, the problem is obscured by a double message, or feelings are denied or projected onto others. **(14)**

**Dysfunctional receiving:** Communication in which a receiver fails to listen, disqualifies what is said, responds with negativity, or fails to validate the message. **(13)**

**Dysfunctional sending:** Communication that occurs when part or all of a message fails to express the truth or is expressed in such a way that the receiver experiences the message as a personal attack. **(13)**

**Ecomap:** Diagram of a family member's relationship with people, agencies, and institutions outside the family. **(13)**

**Ego defense mechanisms:** Conscious and unconscious coping methods used by people to change the meaning of a situation in their minds. **(20)**

**Empathy:** The capacity to understand another's world and to communicate that understanding. The ability of one person to perceive and understand another person's emotions accurately and to communicate the meaning of feelings to the other through verbal and nonverbal behaviors. **(1, 5)**

**Empowerment:** Helping a person become a self-advocate; an interpersonal process of providing the appropriate tools, resources, and environment to build, develop, and increase the ability of others to set and reach goals. **(4, 5, 22)**

**Environment:** All the cultural, developmental, physical, and psychosocial conditions external to an individual that influence a person's perception and involvement. **(1)**

**Ethical dilemma:** (*also* moral dilemma) Conflict of two or more moral issues; a situation in which there are two or more conflicting ways of looking at a situation. **(7)**

**Ethnic group:** A social grouping of people who share a common racial, geographic, religious, or historical culture. **(11)**

**Ethnocentrism:** The belief that one's own culture is superior to others. **(11)**

**Eustress:** A moderate level of stress that acts as a positive stress response with protective and adaptive functions. **(20)**

**Family:** A self-identified group of two or more individuals whose association is characterized by special terms, who may or may not be related by bloodlines or law, but who function in such a way that they consider themselves to be a family. **(13)**

**Feedback:** The response given by the receiver to the sender about the message. **(1)**

**Focus charting:** A charting format using a focus (a sign or symptom, a nursing diagnosis, a behavior, a condition, a significant event, or an acute change in condition) and three steps: Data, Action, and Response (DAR). **(23)**

**Formal operations period:** Piaget's developmental stage in which abstract reality and logical thought processes emerge; independent decisions can be made. **(18)**

**Functional communication:** Communication in which the content and relational aspects of the message are clearly and directly sent and received; it is based on valid assumptions, trust, and a firm sense of self. **(13)**

**General adaptation syndrome (GAS):** A series of changes caused by the body's response to and compensation for stress: (1) *alarm phase*, the immediate biological response, including increased breathing, muscle tension, and accelerated heart rate; (2) *resistance phase*, in which the body produces endorphins and the brain attempts to restore homeostasis; (3) *exhaustion phase*, the result of unremitting stress, the stage during which serious physical symptoms, dangerous mental disorganization, physical collapse, and even death may occur. **(20)**

**Genogram:** Family diagram that records information about family members and their relationships for at least three generations. **(13)**

**Grief:** Mourning, bereavement, the journey toward healing and recovering from the pain of a significant loss. **(8)**

**Group:** A gathering of two or more individuals who share a common purpose and meet over a period of time in face-to-face interaction to achieve an identifiable goal. **(12)**

**Group dynamics:** All of the communication processes and behaviors that take place within a group. **(12)**

**Group process:** The identifiable structural development of the group that is needed for a group to mature. **(12)**

**Group think:** Fear of expressing conflicting ideas and opinions because loyalty to the group and approval by other group members have become so important. **(12)**

**Health:** A broad concept that is used to describe an individual's state of well-being and level of functioning. **(1)**

**Health teaching:** A flexible, person-oriented process in which the helping person provides information and support to clients with a variety of health-related learning needs. **(16)**

**Holistic construct:** The unified whole of a person, with each functional aspect of self-concept fitting together, and each single element affecting all other parts. **(3)**

**Homeostasis:** (*also* dynamic equilibrium) A person's sense of personal security and balance. **(20)**

**I–thou relationship:** A relationship in which each individual responds to the other from his or her own uniqueness and is valued for that uniqueness in a direct, mutually respected, reciprocal alliance. **(1)**

**Independent nursing interventions:** Nursing interventions that nurses can provide without a physician's order or direction from another health professional. **(2)**

**Informed consent:** Assurance that the client fully understands what is happening or is about to happen in his or her health care and knowingly consents to care. **(2, 16)**

**Intercultural communication:** Communication in which the sender of a message is a member of one culture and the receiver is from a different culture. **(11)**

**Interpersonal competence:** The ability to interpret the content of a message from the point of view of each of the participants and the ability to use language and nonverbal behaviors strategically to achieve the goals of the interaction. **(9)**

**Interpersonal process record:** A three-part record of the nurse–client interaction: (1) a written anecdotal record of the client's and the nurse's words as well as their nonverbal behavior; (2) a written analysis of the interaction, identifying communication skills and interventions; and (3) written suggestions for making more effective comments. **(23)**

**Knowing, patterns of:** (1) *Empirical*, knowledge based on scientific principles; (2) *personal*, intuitive understanding of and response to another human; (3) *aesthetic*, use of literature, art, and music to connect with a person; (4) *ethical*, knowledge of what is right and wrong, making choices in the best interest of the client, attention to standards and codes. **(1)**

**Leadership:** Interpersonal influence, exercised in situations and directed through the communication process, toward the attainment of a specified goal or goals. **(12)**

**Leveling:** Communication that is healthy and direct. **(13)**

**Maintenance functions:** Group role functions that foster the emotional life of the group. **(12)**

**Message:** A verbal or nonverbal expression of thoughts or feelings intended to convey information to the receiver and requiring interpretation by that person. **(1)**

**Message competency:** The ability to use language and nonverbal behaviors strategically to achieve the goals of the interaction. **(9)**

**Metacommunication:** All of the factors that influence how a message is received. **(9)**

**Modeling:** The transmission of values by presenting oneself in an attractive manner and living by a certain set of values, hoping that others will follow one's lead; teaching by performing a behavior that another observes. **(7, 16)**

**Moral distress:** A feeling that occurs when one knows what is "right" but is bound to do otherwise because of legal or institutional constraints. **(7)**

**Moral uncertainty:** Difficulty deciding which moral rules (values, beliefs, etc.) apply to a given situation. **(7)**

**Motivation:** The forces that activate behavior and direct it toward one goal instead of another. **(15)**

**Multiculturalism:** A term used to describe a heterogeneous society in which diverse cultural world views can coexist with some general characteristics shared by all cultural groups and some perspectives that are unique to each group. **(11)**

**Mutuality:** Agreement on problems and the means for resolving them; a commitment by both parties to enhance well-being. **(5)**

**Narrative charting:** A chronological record of events happening to the client. **(23)**

**Networking:** A form of peer collaboration whereby individuals take advantage of making and using contacts. **(22)**

**Nurse Practice Acts:** Legal documents developed at the state level that define professional nursing's scope of practice and outline the nurse's rights, responsibilities, and licensing requirements in providing care to individuals, families, and communities. **(2)**

**Nursing:** Involved interaction with persons in a caring mode. **(1)**

**Nursing interventions classifications (NIC):** A standardized language describing direct and indirect care that nurses perform. NIC and nursing outcomes classification (NOC)—the measure of how nursing care affects client outcomes—attempt to quantify nursing care so that it becomes visible and defines professional practice. **(23)**

**Objective data:** Data that are directly observable or verifiable through physical examination or tests. **(2)**

**Open-ended question:** A question that is open to interpretation and that cannot be answered by yes, no, or a one-word response. **(10)**

**Optacon:** A reading device that converts printed letters into a vibration, which can be felt by the deaf-blind person. **(17)**

**Orientation phase:** Period in the nurse–client relationship when the nurse and client first meet and set the tone for the rest of their relationship, assessing the client's situation and setting goals. **(4)**

**Paradigm:** A world view reflecting the knowledge developed about a phenomenon of interest within a scientific discipline. **(1)**

**Paralanguage:** The oral delivery of a verbal message expressed through tone of voice and inflection, sighing, or crying. **(9)**

**Paraphrasing:** Transforming the client's words into the nurse's words, keeping the meaning intact. **(10)**

**Participatory leadership:** The style in which the leader maintains final control but actively solicits and uses the input of group members. **(22)**

**Perception:** A personal identity construct by which a person transforms external sensory data into personalized images of reality. **(3)**

**Person:** A unitary concept that includes physiological, psychological, spiritual, and social elements. **(1)**

**Personal space:** An invisible and changing boundary around an individual that provides a sense of comfort and protection to a person and that is defined by past experiences and culture. **(5)**

**Position:** An external context that formalizes roles and makes them understandable to others in the community or group; relates to the status one holds in the community. **(6)**

**Preoperational period:** Piaget's developmental stage in which learning by the toddler is developed through concrete experiences and devices and the child is markedly egocentric. **(18)**

**Prevention:** A way of thinking and being that actively promotes responsible behavior and the adoption of lifestyles that are maximally conducive to good health. **(15)**

**Primary group:** Spontaneous group formation characterized by an informal structure and social process; it can be automatic, like a family, or based on a common interest; it has no defined time limit. **(12)**

**Problem-oriented record (POR):** A chart containing four basic sections: a data base, a list of the client's identified problems, a treatment plan, and progress notes. **(23)**

**Profession:** A calling requiring specialized knowledge and often long and intensive academic preparation. **(6)**

**Professional boundaries:** Invisible structures imposed by legal, moral, or professional standards of nursing that respect nurse and patient rights. **(4)**

**Proxemics:** The study of an individual's use of space. **(5)**

**Psychomotor learning:** Learning a skill by taking knowledge and applying it with "hands on." **(15)**

**Receiver:** The recipient of a message, the person who decodes or translates the message into word symbols that make sense to the receiver. **(1)**

**Reflection:** A communication strategy linking the client's apparent emotion with the content of the client's message; it is used to clarify what the client is feeling and to affirm that the client's feelings are acceptable. **(10)**

**Reframing:** A strategy in which the nurse helps the client look at a situation in a new way. **(10)**

**Reinforcement:** (*also* conditioning): The consequences of performing identified behaviors; positive reinforcement increases the probability of a response, and negative reinforcement decreases the probability of a response. **(16)**

**Role:** A set of expected standards of behavior established by the society or community group to which a person belongs; role represents the social aspects of self-concept. **(6)**

**Role ambiguity:** A situation in which roles are not clearly defined. **(6)**

**Role conflict:** An incompatibility between one or more role expectations. **(6)**

**Role performance:** A person's capacity to function as expected in social roles, in sexual relations with a partner, in family, and in a job. **(6)**

**Role pressures:** The external or internal circumstances, which are capable of change, that interfere with role performance. **(6)**

**Role stress:** A subjective experience of mental, physical, and social fatigue often accompanied by a loss of meaning in what was previously important and exciting. **(6)**

**Scope of practice:** The legal boundaries of practice for professional nurses established by each state and defined in written state statutes. **(2)**

**Secondary groups:** Groups that are formally established to achieve certain agreed-on goals; they have a prescribed structure and a designated leader, and they last for a specified length of time. **(12)**

**Self-actualization:** The level of development in which a person balances interdependence with individual self-awareness. **(1)**

**Self-awareness:** The means by which a person gains knowledge and understanding of all aspects of self-concept. **(3, 6)**

**Self-concept** (*also* self, self-system): An abstract structural construct that is used to describe the different images that make up the self in each person's mind. All of the psychological beliefs and attitudes people have about themselves: perceptual, cognitive, emotional, and spiritual. **(3)**

**Self-differentiation:** The capacity to stay involved in one's family or group without losing one's identity. **(13)**

**Self-esteem:** The value and significance people place on their self-concepts; an emotional process of self-judgment; an orientation to the self, ranging on a continuum from feelings of self-efficacy and respect to feelings that one is fatally flawed as a person. **(3)**

**Self-talk:** A cognitive process that produces a thought or thoughts, which then lead to a feeling about a situation. **(3)**

**Sender:** The source or initiator of a message. **(1)**

**Sensorimotor period:** Piaget's developmental stage in which the infant explores its own body as a source of information about the world. **(18)**

**Shaping:** Changing a person's behavior through a behavioral learning process. **(16)**

**SOAP format:** A four-step method of documentation that lists all of the client's subjective (*S*) comments, all of the current objective (*O*) information noted by the nurse, the nurse's analysis or assessment (*A*), and future interventions or plans (*P*) for care. **(23)**

**Social cognitive competency:** The ability to interpret message content within interactions from the point of view of each participant. **(9)**

**Social support:** All of the social and environmental factors that contribute to a person's sense of well-being. **(20)**

**Stereotyping** (*also* bias): Attributing characteristics or behavior, generalized opinions, attitudes, and beliefs to a group of people as if all persons in the group possessed them. **(5)**

**Stress:** A physiological and psychological response to the presence of a stressor. **(20)**

**Stressor:** Any demand, situation, internal stimulus, or circumstance that threatens a person's personal security and balance. **(20)**

**Subculture:** An ethnic, regional, or economic group of people who are joined together by distinguishing characteristics that differentiate the group from the predominant culture or society. **(11)**

**Subjective data:** The client's perception of the data and what the client says about the data. **(2)**

**Summarization:** Reworking a lengthy interaction or discussion into a few succinct sentences. **(10)**

**Symmetrical relationship:** Relationship in which each person has equal power and the exchanges mirror each other. **(13)**

**Task functions:** Group role functions that facilitate goal achievement. **(12)**

**Tellatouch:** A portable machine into which the nurse can type a message that emerges in Braille. **(17)**

**Termination:** The deliberate separation of two or more persons from an intimate and meaningful relationship. **(8)**

**Termination phase** (*also* resolution): The period in the nurse–client relationship when the nurse and client examine and evaluate their relationship and its goals and results; the time when they deal with the emotional content (if any) involved in saying good-by. **(4)**

**Theory:** An organized, conceptual representation or explanation of a phenomenon. **(1)**

**Therapeutic communication:** A goal-directed, focused dialogue between nurse and client that is fitted to the needs of the client. **(10)**

**Transference:** Behaviors in which the client projects irrational attitudes and feelings from the past onto people in the present. **(1)**

**Triangle:** A three-person emotional system in which there is tension between two members and a third person steps in to stabilize the relationship. **(13)**

**Trust:** Reliance on the consistency, sameness, and continuity of experiences that are provided by an organized combination of familiar and predictable things and people. **(5)**

**Validation:** A form of feedback involving verbal and nonverbal confirmation that both participants have the same basic understanding of the message. **(1)**

**Values:**  A set of personal beliefs and attitudes about truth, beauty, and the worth of any thought, object, or behavior. Attitudes, beliefs, feelings, worries, or convictions that have not been clearly established are called *values indicators.* **(7)**

**Values acquisition:**  The conscious assumption of a new value. **(7)**

**Values clarification:**  A process that encourages one to clarify one's own values by sorting them through, analyzing them, and setting priorities. **(7)**

**Violence:**  Physical force used by one person against another. **(21)**

**Working phase:**  The period in the nurse–client relationship when the focus is on communication strategies, interventions for problem resolution, and enhancement of self-concept. **(4)**

# Index

Note: Page numbers in *italics* indicate boxed material and illustrations; those followed by t indicate tabular material.

— **H** —